Mechanical Testing of Bone *and the* Bone–Implant Interface

Mechanical Testing of Bone *and the* Bone–Implant Interface

edited by

Yuehuei H. An, M.D.
Robert A. Draughn, D.Sc.

CRC Press
Boca Raton London New York Washington, D.C.

Library of Congress Cataloging-in-Publication Data

Mechanical testing of bone and the bone-implant interface / edited by
    Yuehuei H. An and Robert A. Draughn.
        p.   cm.
    Includes bibliographical references and index.
    ISBN 0-8493-0266-8 (alk. paper)
    1. Bones—Mechanical properties. 2. Orthopedic implants.
    3. Bones—Effect of implants on. 4. Biomechanics. I. An, Yuehuei H.
    II. Draughn, Robert A.
        [DNLM: 1. Bone and Bones—physiology. 2. Biocompatible Materials.
    3. Biomechanics. 4. Materials Testing—methods. 5. Prostheses and
    Implants. 6. Stress, Mechanical. 7. Surface Properties.
    8. Tensile Strength.   WE 200 M4856 1999]
    QP88.2.M424 1999
    617.4'71—dc21
    DNLM/DLC
    for Library of Congress   99-36531
                                                                      CIP

No claim to original U.S. Government works
International Standard Book Number 0-8493-0266-8
Library of Congress Card Number 99-36531
Printed in the United States of America 1 2 3 4 5 6 7 8 9 0
Printed on acid-free paper

Foreword

The skeletal system gives the body its form, facilitates movement, and protects internal organs from traumatic forces. Any disease, drug, or biological process that influences bone directly influences the fundamental mechanical function of the skeleton. Skeletal imaging data and quantitative assessments of bone composition and histomorphology are often important only because they reflect something about mechanical competence. To truly assess the mechanical competence of the skeleton, however, it is imperative that we assess the mechanical characteristics of the bone and bone–implant constructs.

Early investigations of the mechanical properties of bone in the last half of the twentieth century by Evans, Yamada, Katz, Ascenzi, Currey, Burstein, Bonfield and Lanyon helped form the modern foundation for how bones should be tested and viewed from a mechanical and material perspective. From these initial pioneers, new investigators began to build a research literature and a series of laboratory approaches for the mechanical testing of bone and bone–implant systems. The mechanical testing of bone and the bone–implant interface has progressively become an important aspect of a wide variety of research projects on bone growth, adaptation, regeneration, and aging. This work has resulted in a better understanding of the material mechanical properties of bone and greater standardization of testing protocols.

This collection by editors Yuehuei H. An and Robert A. Draughn marks a transition in the role of mechanical testing of bone and bone–implant systems. It addresses the field of bone mechanics not so much as an arena of basic science but rather as a compendium of practical research tools and mechanical assay techniques. It is a wonderful addition to the literature in that it summarizes much of the data generated in recent years. The greatest value of the book, however, is that it provides a synopsis of laboratory approaches that a broad range of investigators have used and continue to use in their research.

The treatise begins at a very basic level and can therefore serve as an effective introduction to those without significant previous experience in bone mechanics. The 39 chapters of the book are separated into three sections that progress from concise descriptions of techniques used to characterize and test bone to more specialized laboratory studies. The perspectives of the many contributors to the book who work in many different laboratories contribute to the richness and breadth of the book. The coherence of the book is maintained under the clear direction of the editors. The emphasis is on teaching the reader "how to do it." This theme is maintained throughout and is surely enhanced by the involvement of the editors as coauthors in many chapters.

This book serves as a comprehensive primer for the mechanical testing of bone. For new investigators in this area, it is an invaluable tool. For the more experience investigators, it serves as a touchstone for evaluating new testing protocols and data. This text has a great deal to offer all of us.

Dennis R. Carter, Ph.D.
Director, Palo Alto VA Rehabilitation R&D Center
Professor, Biomechanical Engineering Division
Mechanical Engineering Department
Stanford University

Preface

Biomechanics is an integral part of the study of bone as an organ or tissue. Mechanical testing of bone specimens is a basic method in bone-related research. The mechanical properties of whole bones or bone tissues and bone–implant interfaces are equally important as their morphological or structural aspects. The former is evaluated by mechanical testing and the latter is mostly studied using histological techniques.

This book is an outgrowth of the editors' own quest for information on mechanical testing of bone and, more importantly, a response to significant needs in the orthopaedic research community. Most researchers are not well trained in biomechanics and assistance from an expert is not always readily available. What many researchers really need to know are basic mechanical principles in bone-related research and most importantly how to conduct mechanical testing of bone specimens. This book is designed to be an experimental guide for orthopaedic or dental residents, bioengineering graduate students, orthopaedic or dental researchers, biomaterials scientists, laboratory technicians, and anyone not well trained in biomechanics who plans to conduct mechanical testing of bone specimens. Most readers belong to societies in the fields of orthopaedic or dental research, biomechanics, or biomaterials, such as the Orthopaedic Research Society, American Society of Biomechanics, American Society of Mechanical Engineers, American Society for Bone and Mineral Research, Society for Biomaterials, or Materials Research Society. This text is intended to be a "beginner's" guide, and no prior training in biomechanics is required to understand the contents. It should also serve as a useful handbook for biomechanical and bioengineering researchers and students at all levels.

This is the first inclusive and organized reference book on how to perform mechanical testing of bone. The topic has not been adequately covered by any existing textbook on bone biomechanics. The 39 chapters of this book are divided into three major parts: Section I — mechanical properties of bone and general considerations and basic facilities for mechanical testing; Section II — specific mechanical testing procedures on bone tissues; and Section III — mechanical testing procedures on the bone–implant interface.

The book is designed to be concise as well as inclusive and more practical than theoretical. The text is simple and straightforward. Numerous diagrams (~150), tables (~150), line drawings (~150), and photographs (~150) are included to help readers better understand the main principles. Full bibliographies at the end of each chapter guide readers to more detailed information. A book of this length cannot discuss every method in biomechanical testing of bone that has been conducted over the years, but it is hoped that major methods and their applications have been included.

Yuehuei H. An, M.D.
Charleston, South Carolina

The Editors

Yuehuei H. (Huey) An, M.D., graduated from the Harbin Medical University, Harbin, Northeast China in 1983. He completed residency training in orthopaedic surgery at Ji Shui Tan Hospital in Beijing, China and went on to a fellowship in hand surgery at Sydney Hospital in Sydney, Australia. In 1991, Dr. An joined Dr. Richard J. Friedman in the Department of Orthopaedic Surgery at the Medical University of South Carolina to establish the MUSC Orthopaedic Research Laboratory, which is now a multifunctional orthopaedic research center.

Soon after beginning his career in orthopaedic research, Dr. An developed an interest in bone mechanics and he learned much about practical mechanical testing by "trial and error." His understanding of the importance of biomechanical principles and mechanical testing techniques to researchers in bone-related fields of work led to his desire to organize this effort.

Dr. An has published more than 70 scientific papers and book chapters and more than 60 research abstracts. He has edited three reference books. His first book, *Animal Models in Orthopaedic Research*, a major contribution to orthopaedic research, was published by CRC Press in 1998. His third book, *Handbook of Bacterial Adhesion — Principles, Methods, and Applications*, will be published by Humana Press in late 1999. He created many of the line drawings used in his books and papers. He is an active member of eight academic societies including the American Society of Biomechanics, Orthopaedic Research Society, Society for Biomaterials, and the Tissue Engineering Society. Dr. An's current research interests include bone and cartilage repair using tissue engineering techniques, bone or soft tissue ingrowth to implant surfaces, bone structure and biomechanics, bacterial adhesion and prosthetic infection, and animal models in orthopaedic research.

Robert A. Draughn, D.Sc., is Professor and Chairman of the Department of Materials Science at the Medical University of South Carolina, Charleston, South Carolina. He is also an Adjunct Associate Professor of Bioengineering at Clemson University, Clemson, South Carolina. Dr. Draughn earned his Doctor of Science degree in Materials Science from the University of Virginia in 1968. He has been on the faculty of the College of Dental Medicine at the Medical University of South Carolina since 1973. His principal research interests have been in the general area of biomedical applications of composite materials. The emphasis of much of his work has been the mechanical properties of particle-reinforced polymers and hard tissues as well as studies of adhesive bonding processes.

Dr. Draughn has over 70 publications and over 90 research presentations and published abstracts. He is active in several professional organizations. His activities have included Chairperson of the Biomaterials Section of the American Association of Dental Schools, Chairperson of the Gordon Research Conference on the Science of Adhesion, and membership on the executive committee of the Adhesion Society.

Contributors

C. Mauli Agrawal, Ph.D.
Associate Professor
Department of Orthopaedics
University of Texas Health Science Center
  at San Antonio
San Antonio, Texas

Yuehuei H. An, M.D., M.Sc.
Associate Professor and Director
Orthopaedic Research Laboratory
Department of Orthopaedic Surgery
Medical University of South Carolina
Charleston, South Carolina
and
Adjunct Assistant Professor
Department of Bioengineering
Clemson University
Clemson, South Carolina

Antonio Ascenzi, Ph.D.
Professor Emeritus
Department of Experimental Medicine
  and Pathology
University of Rome La Sapienza
Rome, Italy

Maria-Grazia Ascenzi, Ph.D.
Mathematical Researcher
Department of Sciences
University of California Extension
Los Angeles, California

Kyriacos Athanasiou, Ph.D., P.E.
Associate Professor of Orthopaedics
  and Engineering
Director of Musculoskeletal
  Bioengineering Center
Director of Orthopaedic Biomechanics
The University of Texas Health Science Center
  at San Antonio
San Antonio, Texas

William R. Barfield, Ph.D.
Assistant Professor
Orthopaedic Research Laboratory
Department of Orthopaedic Surgery
Medical University of South Carolina
Charleston, South Carolina

Christopher V. Bensen, M.D.
Orthopaedic Surgery Resident
Department of Orthopaedic Surgery
Medical University of South Carolina
Charleston, South Carolina

Alessandro Benvenuti, Ph.D.
Research Associate
Department of Experimental Medicine
  and Pathology
University of Rome La Sapienza
Rome, Italy

Aivars Berzins, M.D.
Assistant Professor
Department of Orthopaedic Surgery
Rush Medical College
Rush-Presbyterian-St. Luke's Medical Center
Chicago, Illinois

Ermanno Bonucci, Ph.D.
Professor and Chairman
Department of Experimental Medicine
  and Pathology
University of Rome La Sapienza
Rome, Italy

Matthew S. Crum, B.Sc.
Undergraduate Student
Department of Mechanical Engineering
Clemson University
Clemson, South Carolina

John M. Cuckler, M.D.
Professor and Chairman
Department of Orthopaedic Surgery
University of Alabama
Birmingham, Alabama

A. U. (Dan) Daniels, Ph.D.
George Thomas Wilhelm Endowed Professor
Department of Orthopaedic Surgery
University of Tennessee
Memphis, Tennessee

James R. Davis, B.Sc., FRCS
Research Fellow
Department of Orthopaedic Surgery
University of Maryland
Baltimore, Maryland

Wouter J. A. Dhert, M.D., Ph.D.
Professor
Department of Orthopaedics
Utrecht University Hospital
Utrecht, the Netherlands

Robert A. Draughn, D.Sc.
Professor of Materials Science
Department of Materials Science
College of Dental Medicine
Medical University of South Carolina
Charleston, South Carolina
and
Adjunct Associate Professor of Bioengineering
Department of Bioengineering
Clemson University
Clemson, South Carolina

Lisa A. Ferrara, M.Sc.
Director
Spine Research Laboratory
Department of Neurosurgery
Cleveland Clinic Foundation
Cleveland, Ohio

José Luis Ferretti, M.D., Ph.D.
Director
Centro de Estudios de Metabolismo
  Fosfocalcico (CEMFoC)
Hospital del Centenario
National University of Rosario
and
Instituto/Fundacion de Investigaciones
  Metabolicas (IDIM)
Buenos Aires, Argentina

Richard J. Friedman, M.D., FRCSC
Professor
Department of Orthopaedic Surgery
Medical University of South Carolina
Charleston, South Carolina
and
Adjunct Professor of Bioengineering
Department of Bioengineering
Clemson University
Clemson, South Carolina

Benjamin R. Furman, M.S.
Research Associate
Division of Biomaterials
Department of Restorative Dentistry
University of Texas Health Science Center at
  San Antonio
San Antonio, Texas

Vasanti M. Gharpuray, Ph.D.
Associate Professor
Department of Bioengineering
Clemson University
Clemson, South Carolina

Steven A. Goldstein, Ph.D.
Henry Ruppenthal Family Professor of
  Orthopaedic Surgery and Bioengineering
Professor of Mechanical Engineering and
  Applied Mechanics
Director of Orthopaedic Research
Interim Associate Dean for Research and
  Graduate Studies
University of Michigan
Ann Arbor, Michigan

C. Edward Hoffler, M.S.
M.D./Ph.D. Candidate
Orthopaedic Research Laboratories
The University of Michigan
Ann Arbor, Michigan

Sarandeep S. Huja, Ph.D., B.D.S.,
M.D.S., M.Sc.
Graduate Dental Student
Section of Orthodontics
Indiana University School of Dentistry
Indianapolis, Indiana

Ivan Hvid, M.D., D.M.Sc.
Professor
Department of Orthopaedics
Aarhus University Hospital
Aarhus, Denmark

Kenneth S. James, Ph.D.
Associate Director of Orthopaedic Programs
Tissue Engineering, Inc.
Boston, Massachusetts

John A. Jansen, D.D.S., Ph.D.
Professor and Head
Department of Biomaterials
University of Nijmegen Dental School
Nijmegen, the Netherlands

Riyaz H. Jinnah, M.D., FRCS
Professor of Orthopaedic Surgery
The University of Maryland School of
  Medicine
Baltimore, Maryland

Qian Kang, M.D.
Associate Chief Surgeon
Department of Orthopaedic Surgery
Beijing Ji Shui Tan Hospital
Beijing, China
Former Research Fellow (1995–1997)
Orthopaedic Research Laboratory
Department of Orthopaedic Surgery
Medical University of South Carolina
Charleston, South Carolina

Thomas R. Katona, Ph.D., DM.D.
Associate Professor of Orthodontics
Indiana University School of Dentistry
Associate Professor of Mechanical Engineering
Purdue University School of Engineering
  and Technology
IUPUI Biomechanics and Biomaterials
  Research Center
Indianapolis, Indiana

J. Lawrence Katz, Ph.D.
Professor, Department of Biomedical
  Engineering
Case Western Reserve University
Cleveland, Ohio

Tony S. Keller, Ph.D.
Associate Professor
Department of Mechanical Engineering
University of Vermont
Burlington, Vermont

Fadi M. Khoury, M.Sc.
School of Engineering and Applied Science
University of Pennsylvania
Philadelphia, Pennsylvania

Ivars Knets, Ph.D.
Professor of Biomechanics
Department of Mechanical Engineering
Riga Technical University
Riga, Latvia

David H. Kohn, Ph.D.
Associate Professor
Department of Biologic and Materials Sciences
School of Dentistry
University of Michigan
Ann Arbor, Michigan

Michael A. K. Liebschner, Ph.D.
Orthopaedic Research Laboratory
University of California at Berkeley
Berkeley, California

Frank Linde, M.D., DM.Sc.
Consultant Orthopaedic Surgeon
Department of Orthopaedics
Aarhus University Hospital
Aarhus, Denmark

Robert A. Lofthouse, M.A., FRCS
Research Fellow
Department of Orthopaedic Surgery
University of Maryland School of Medicine
Baltimore, Maryland

Mandi J. Lopez, D.V.M., M.S.
Postdoctoral Fellow
Comparative Orthopaedic Research Laboratory
School of Veterinary Medicine
University of Wisconsin-Madison
Madison, Wisconsin

Mark D. Markel, D.V.M.
Professor
Comparative Orthopaedic Research Laboratory
School of Veterinary Medicine
University of Wisconsin-Madison
Madison, Wisconsin

Barbara R. McCreadie, M.S.
Ph.D. Candidate
Orthopaedic Research Laboratories
University of Michigan
Ann Arbor, Michigan

Brodie E. McKoy, M.D.
Orthopaedic Surgery Resident
Department of Orthopaedic Surgery
Medical University of South Carolina
Charleston, South Carolina

Peter L. Mente, Ph.D.
Assistant Professor
Department of Biological and Agricultural
  Engineering
North Carolina State University
Raleigh, North Carolina

Sanjiv H. Naidu, M.D., Ph.D.
Assistant Professor
Department of Orthopaedic Surgery
Pennsylvania State University
Hershey, Pennsylvania

Takashi Nakamura, M.D., Ph.D.
Professor
Department of Orthopaedic Surgery
Kyoto University
Kyoto, Japan

Shigeru Nishiguchi, M.D.
Research Assistant
Department of Orthopaedic Surgery
Graduate School of Medicine
Kyoto University
Kyoto, Japan

George M. Pharr, Ph.D.
Professor
Department of Mechanical Engineering and
  Materials Science
Rice University
Houston, Texas

William S. Pietrzak, Ph.D.
Director
Resorbable Technology
Biomet Co.
Warsaw, Indiana

Jae-Young Rho, Ph.D.
Assistant Professor
Department of Biomedical Engineering
University of Memphis
Memphis, Tennessee

W. Eugene Roberts, D.D.S., Ph.D.
Professor of Orthodontics
Indiana University School of Dentistry
Professor of Physiology and Biophysics
Indiana University School of Medicine
and
Professor of Mechanical Engineering
Purdue University School of Engineering
  and Technology
Indianapolis, Indiana

Timothy C. Ryken, M.D.
Assistant Professor
Division of Neurosurgery
University of Iowa School of Medicine
Iowa City, Iowa

Subrata Saha, Ph.D.
Professor
Department of Bioengineering
Clemson University
and
Director
Bioengineering Alliance of South Carolina
Clemson, South Carolina

David R. Sarver, B.Sc.
Product Development Engineer
Biomet Co.
Warsaw, Indiana

Naoki Sasaki, D.Sc.
Associate Professor
Division of Biological Sciences
Graduate School of Science
Hokkaido University
Sapporo, Japan

Rakesh Saxena, Ph.D.
Department of Mechanical Engineering
The University of Vermont
Burlington, Vermont

Chris W. Smith, Ph.D.
Research Fellow
Department of Engineering
University of Exeter
Exeter, United Kingdom

Erica A. Smith, M.S.
Ph.D. Candidate
Orthopaedic Research Laboratories
University of Michigan
Ann Arbor, Michigan

Dale R. Sumner, Ph.D.
Professor and Chairman
Department of Anatomy
and
Professor
Department of Orthopaedic Surgery
Rush Medical College
Rush-Presbyterian-St. Luke's Medical Center
Chicago, Illinois

John A. Szivek, Ph.D.
Professor
Orthopaedic Research Laboratory
Department of Surgery
University of Arizona School of Medicine
Tucson, Arizona

Charles H. Turner, Ph.D.
Associate Professor and Director of
  Orthopaedic Research
Department of Orthopaedic Surgery and
  Biomechanics and Biomaterials
  Research Center
Indiana University Medical Center
Indianapolis, Indiana

Rong-Ming Wang, Ph.D.
Associate Professor
Head of Metal Physics and
  Failure Analysis Laboratory
Beijing Institute of Aeronautical Materials
Beijing, China

Xiaodu Wang, Ph.D.
Assistant Professor
Department of Orthopaedics
University of Texas Health Science Center
  at San Antonio
San Antonio, Texas

Keith R. Williams, B.Sc., Ph.D.
Reader
Department of Basic Dental Science
Dental School
University of Wales College of Medicine
Cardiff, Wales, United Kingdom

Franklin A. Young, Jr., D.Sc.
Professor
Department of Materials Science
College of Dental Medicine
Medical University of South Carolina
Charleston, South Carolina

Peter Zioupos, Ph.D., MIPEM
Lecturer
Department of Materials and Medical Sciences
Cranfield University
Shrivenham, United Kingdom

Acknowledgments

The editors would like to acknowledge Kylie Martin for her tireless assistance in communication with contributors, manuscript review, and editorial assistance. We would also like to thank Drs. Christopher Bensen and Brodie McKoy for revising manuscripts and preparing figures. We are also grateful to Drs. Richard Friedman and Angus McBryde, Jr. and all members of the Departments of Orthopaedic Surgery and Materials Science of the Medical University of South Carolina for their continuous administrative support of our work. Finally, we wish to thank Liz Covello, Acquiring Editor at CRC Press, for her help on this and the previous text, *Animal Models in Orthopaedic Research*.

To Kay Q. Kang, M.D.
Without her love, inspiration, and support,
this book would not have been possible

Yuehuei H. An, M.D.

To Donna, Sally, and Margaret

Robert A. Draughn, D.Sc.

Contents

Section II — Methods of Mechanical Testing of Bone

Section I

General Considerations

1 Basic Composition and Structure of Bone

Ermanno Bonucci

CONTENTS

I. INTRODUCTION

Bone is a specialized tissue which, although apparently immobilized in a petrified state, has fundamental physiological functions. First, together with the intestine and kidney, it contributes to the regulation of calcemia. This can, in fact, be decreased by the diversion of calcium ions from the serum into the bone matrix during its mineralization, or be increased by the passage of calcium ions from osteoclasts into the bloodstream during bone resorption. Besides this fundamental metabolic activity, which requires the participation of bone cells and systemic and/or local factors,[1] bone is devoted to vital mechanical functions.[2] Its hardness, moderate elasticity, and very limited plasticity and brittleness make it an ideal tissue for standing and moving, i.e., for the insertion of muscles, the formation of levers able to make muscles respond, and the protection of soft tissues and organs, including bone marrow. Moreover, the arrangement of its microstructures and the presence of cavities in its interior give bone an optimum mass-to-strength ratio. These well-known properties seem to be common to all skeletal segments, as the structure and composition of bone appear at first glance to be the same in all cases. On closer examination, bone turns out to be a highly heterogeneous tissue; its composition and structure both vary in a way that depends on skeletal site, physiological function, the age and sex of subjects, and the type of vertebrate species. In contrast with this heterogeneity, the basic components of the tissue are remarkably consistent.

II. BASIC COMPONENTS OF BONE MATRIX

Calcified bone matrix contains two components: the organic matrix and the mineral substance.

A. ORGANIC MATRIX

The organic matrix of bone mainly consists of type I collagen fibrils, which account for over 90% of the whole matrix, with the remaining 10% corresponding to noncollagenous proteins, proteoglycans, and phospholipids.[3]

1. Collagen Fibrils

Several surveys[4-6] deal with the structure and composition of collagen fibrils, which are only summarized here. Collagen fibrils are formed by the assemblage of filamentous molecules which are themselves made up of three polypeptide chains arranged in a helical configuration. These chains may include a variety of amino acid sequences, so that the molecules may show diversity. Type I collagen consists of relatively thick fibrils (mean diameter 78 nm) resulting from the assemblage of molecules consisting of two $\alpha_1(I)$ chains and one $\alpha_1(II)$ chain. The molecules are assembled in such a way as to give the fibrils a characteristic periodic banding (repetitive axial period of about 66.8 nm) when examined under the electron microscope (Figures 1.1A,B). According to the classical bidimensional model of Hodge and Petruska,[7] parallel collagen molecules overlap in such a way that they are staggered by approximately a quarter of their length; the aligned chemical groups give rise to periodic bands, and the quarter staggering to gaps or "holes" (Figure 1.1A). The molecules are stabilized by intra- and intermolecular cross-links, which are essential for the tensile strength of the fibrils and their mineralization.[8] The three-dimensional assemblage of collagen molecules in the fibril is not known precisely; the subject has been discussed in several surveys.[4,6,9]

2. Noncollagenous Components

The noncollagenous components of bone include noncollagenous proteins, proteoglycans, phospholipids, glycoproteins, and phosphoproteins. Detailed information can be found in several surveys.[10-12] Moreover, the calcified matrix contains growth factors[13] and enzymes such as alkaline phosphatase[14,15] and metalloproteinases.[16,17] The distribution and amounts of noncollagenous proteins (osteopontin, osteonectin, bone sialoprotein) are variable according to types of bone[18,19] and zones of bone matrix where they are located: substantial amounts of bone sialoprotein and osteopontin are present in the cement lines and in discrete interfibrillary patches;[20-23] osteocalcin is found in lamellar bone[19]; woven bone is unique in containing the bone acidic glycoprotein-75.[19] The function of noncollagenous proteins seems to vary, too.[10,11,24-27] The degree of calcification may be a contributing factor in this connection,[28] while calcification may itself be influenced by noncollagenous proteins.[29,30] Proteoglycans may have a regulatory effect, although their role as inhibitors or promoters of the calcification process is still under discussion.[11,31] Phospholipids, which are present in the calcifying matrix,[32] are also considered to have a significant role in calcification.[33]

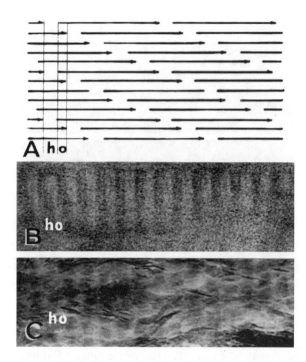

FIGURE 1.1 (A) Diagram showing the arrangement of the collagen molecules according to the model of Hodge and Petruska; note that the shifting of molecules gives rise to zones of holes (*h*) and zones of overlapping (*o*). (B) Under the electron microscope, decalcified ultrathin sections show that the period of collagen fibrils is due to the repetition of two main bands, which correspond to the *h* and *o* zones. Uranyl acetate and lead citrate, ×100,000. (C) During early calcification, the mineral substance forms "bands" corresponding to the *h* zones of the collagen fibrils. Note the presence of needlelike crystals. Unstained, ×100,000.

Several growth factors are involved in bone cell differentiation and recruitment. One substance of special interest is bone morphogenetic protein, which has osteoinductive properties and is found in the calcified bone matrix.[34]

B. MINERAL SUBSTANCE

The mineral substance of bone is a calcium phosphate hydroxyapatite.[35] The problems arising from its molecular structure, mechanism of formation, and deposition in bone matrix have been discussed in several surveys.[3,35-37] Morphologically, the inorganic substance of bone, which appears homogeneous under the light microscope, can be resolved into characteristic crystallites under the electron microscope (Figure 1.1C). Surprisingly, there is no complete agreement about their shape and dimensions, or about their relationship with the organic components.[38] The results of electron microscope and X-ray diffraction studies have led to their being described as tablets,[39] or as tablet-, rod-, and needlelike crystals.[40] Needles and tablets may occur simultaneously (Figure 1.1C), the former apparently deriving from the latter.[41]

Investigation of the problem of the crystal shape and location in bone may contribute much to an understanding of the biophysical properties of the tissue. The ultrastructural evidence that the mineral substance forms "bands" corresponding to the collagen period[3,40] (Figures 1.1C and 1.2A) and, more exactly, to the "holes" zones,[3] suggests that the crystals fit exactly into the holes. This would allow the crystals to be located inside the fibrils without disrupting their structure. However, this possibility is called into question by the observation that with the progression of the calcification

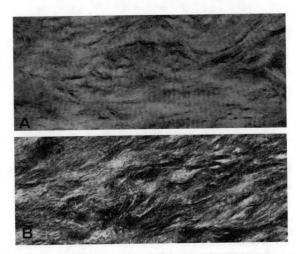

FIGURE 1.2   Electron microscope pictures of a low calcified (A) and fully calcified (B) bone matrix: at low degree of calcification, the mineral substance gives rise to "bands" corresponding to the period of collagen fibrils; as calcification increases, the periodic pattern is masked by filament- and needlelike crystals. Unstained, (A) ×36,000; (B) ×80,000.

process the mineral periodic "bands" are obscured by needlelike and filament-like crystals (Figure 1.2B) whose length may be greater than that of the holes:[40,42] if located inside the collagen fibrils, they would have to perforate the walls of the holes and the fibril molecular organization to attain such a length.[43,44] As a result, although collagen solubility should increase with the degree of calcification, bone collagen from fully calcified chick metatarsals has been found to be insoluble in reagents which solubilize the collagen from soft tissues.[45] This discrepancy has been explained by assuming that (1) the intrafibrillary space is increased by the connection of holes with pores;[3] (2) crystal elongation can occur not only through crystal growth but also through the multiplication of mineral particles which fill all the available space;[3] (3) only short, platelike crystals are located in the fibril holes, whereas the long needle-like crystals are located in the interfibrillar spaces.[38] In reality, the organic–inorganic relationships in bone are still incompletely known. On the other hand, they may vary according to the type of bone,[19] and may change during the calcification process.[46] This lack of information is not without consequences, because the strength, elasticity, and other biophysical characteristics of bone largely depend on the amount of inorganic substance, the relative loss of water and organic material during calcification, the integrity of collagen fibrils, and above all the relationship between collagen fibrils and crystals. In any case, all the biophysical properties of bone may be altered by treatments (dehydration, fixation, embalming) which modify the organic components of the bone matrix[47] or lead to the removal of the inorganic substance (decalcification).[48]

III. WHOLE BONE

The variable assemblage of the basic components reported above leads to the formation of bone as a tissue. Whole bone, i.e., bone as an organ, consists not only of calcified bone matrix and bone cells, but also of nonosseous cells, blood vessels, nerve fibres, and bone marrow, whose relative proportions change with the type and age of the bone. Obviously, the physiological properties of bone are closely dependent on the variable presence of these soft structures. However, they can be neglected if bone is considered strictly as a calcified tissue.

Depending on the skeletal sites, bones may appear as long, tubular segments (long bones), bilaminar plates (flat bones), or short, irregularly prismatic structures (short bones). In long bones three different regions can be distinguished (Figure 1.3): the diaphysis, that is, the central shaft

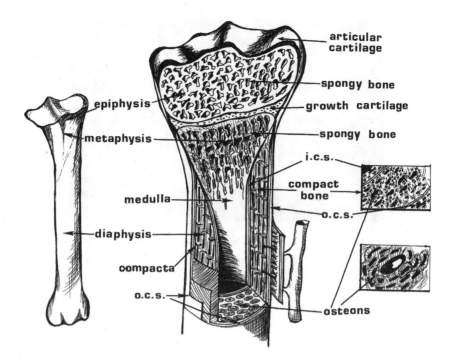

FIGURE 1.3 Schematic representation of the upper third of the tibia, an example of long bone; i.c.s. = inner circumferential system; o.c.s. = outer circumferential system.

which represents the longest part; the epiphyses, which are present at the two extremities; and the metaphyses, which lie between. A cartilaginous layer, the so-called growth cartilage, separates the metaphysis from the epiphysis in the growing skeleton, but tends to disappear as the skeleton matures. The long bones are present in the peripheral or appendicular skeleton, i.e., the limbs, and in ribs and clavicles; the flat bones are typically found in the skull, scapula, and pelvis; and the short bones in the axial skeleton (vertebrae, sternum), carpus, and tarsus. With the exclusion of the membranous bones (skull, clavicle, part of the mandible and of the facial skeleton) which develop on the basis of a fibrous anlage, all other bones are formed by the ossification of a cartilaginous model (endochondral ossification). Articular cartilage covers the part of the external epiphyseal surface that has an articular function; the periosteum covers the outer bone surface.

Independently of their macroscopic anatomy, all skeletal segments consist of an outer layer of compact bone (also called the compacta, or cortical bone) and an inner zone (the medulla), which contains bone marrow (see Figure 1.3). The relative proportion between the compacta and the medulla varies with the skeletal segments and their function (Figures 1.3, 1.4, 1.5), but the maximum strength-to-weight ratio retains its validity. The diaphysis of long bones shows a thick compacta, in which about 90% of the volume is calcified, and a medulla, which corresponds to an axial, more or less eccentric cylinder containing red, hemopoietic bone marrow in youth, and yellow, fat-repleted, nonhemopoietic marrow in adults (see Figure 1.3). The thickness of the compacta diminishes as the flared metaphyseal zone is approached (see Figure 1.5). The flat and short bones (see Figure 1.4), as well as the epiphysis and metaphysis of the long bones (see Figure 1.5), have a thin outer compacta. The medulla is prevalent and consists of a frame of interlacing laminar or rodlike osseous trabeculae (see Figures 1.4, 1.5) which delimit irregular, intercommunicating spaces containing bone marrow, blood vessels, nerve fibres, and other soft structures. For this reason, the area covered by the medulla is much greater than that covered by the compacta, although the calcified matrix covers only 20 to 25% of the total volume in the former, but as much as 95% in the latter.

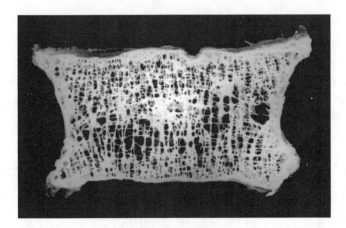

FIGURE 1.4   Section of the body of a lumbar vertebra, showing the thin outer compacta (left and right side of the vertebral section), and the vertical and horizontal trabeculae which form the spongy bone of the medulla. The upper and lower surfaces correspond to articular cartilage, which is in continuity with the intervertebral disk.

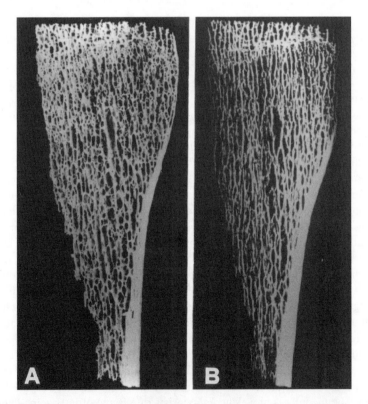

FIGURE 1.5   (A) Section of one half of the upper third of the tibia and (B) its microradiograph. The spongy bone of the metaphysis consists of comparatively thick vertical trabeculae connected by thin transverse trabeculae; the thickness of the compacta decreases from the diaphysis to the metaphysis. The degree of calcification is rather uniform.

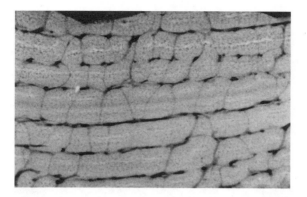

FIGURE 1.6 Microradiography of primary bone in the shaft of an embryonal long bone. Note the parallel trabeculae, and the interposed vascular canals, of the inner circumferential system (bone marrow canal partly visible above), ×15.

IV. TYPES OF BONE

The outer compacta of the skeletal segments consists of compact bone (see Figures 1.3 through 1.5); the inner medulla corresponds to the bone marrow cylinder in long bones, to interlacing osseous trabeculae in short and flat bones, and in long bone epiphyses (see Figures 1.4 and 1.5). The osseous trabeculae form the spongy, cancellous, or trabecular bone. These denominations do not refer to a basic difference in the aggregation state of the bone tissue. Although the true density of fully calcified cancellous bone is a little lower (3%), and its proteoglycan content a little greater, than those of the fully calcified compact bone and in spite of other minor differences, the two types of bone (compact and trabecular) have a very similar basic composition and degree of aggregation (however, see below for the differences between lamellar and woven bone). The real difference between compact and spongy bone depends on its porosity: that of compact bone, mainly due to the voids provided by osteon canals, Volkmann's canals, osteocytes and their canaliculi, and resorption lacunae (see below), varies from 5 to 30% (apparent density about 1.8 g/cm^3); the porosity of cancellous bone, chiefly due to the wide vascular and bone marrow intertrabecular spaces, ranges from 30 to more than 90% (apparent density 0.1 to 0.9 g/cm^3).[49]

A. COMPACT BONE

Starting as soon as a few months after birth (for bone structure and osteogenic activity during embryonic and fetal life see the survey by Gardner[50]), a cross section cut through the middiaphysis of a long bone shows that the cortical, compact bone is structured in three main concentric systems: an outer circumferential system, an intermediate osteonic area, and an inner circumferential system (see Figure 1.3). The names of these systems are due to their microscopic configuration. Both circumferential systems consist of concentric layers of bone trabeculae running parallel to the periosteal (outer system) or endosteal (inner system) surface (Figure 1.6). Both the inner and outer systems are conspicuous at birth (see primary bone) and are then partly substituted by osteonic, or secondary, bone (Figure 1.7), so that their width progressively decreases; in particular, the inner system may become inconspicuous in the elderly.[49] The intermediate area, which enlarges with age at the expense of the circumferential systems, contains Haversian systems or osteons (see below, and Figure 1.8). The thin compacta of the flat and short bones shows both trabeculae and osteons, but the typical three-system arrangement of the long bones is not apparent.

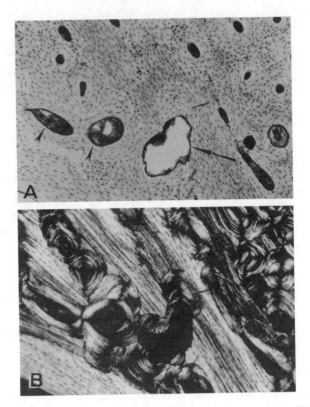

FIGURE 1.7   Cross section of the diaphysis of neonatal long bone as seen under the light (A) and polarization (B) microscope: the primary, parallel-fibered bone (which crosses the picture obliquely) is partly substituted by secondary osteonic bone. The arrow points to still unrepaired resorption lacuna; arrowheads point to two osteons, which are still under construction as shown by their wide vascular canals. Unstained section prepared by grinding, ×35.

B. CANCELLOUS BONE

Cancellous, or spongy, or trabecular bone is present in the medulla of flat and, above all, short bones, and in the epiphysis and metaphysis of long bones. It is almost absent in the central part of the diaphysis, whereas increasing numbers of trabeculae protrude from the inner, endosteal surface into the marrow cavity as the metaphyses are approached. The name of this type of bone derives from its architecture; it consists of trabeculae, that is, osseous structures having a sheetlike, tubular, or barlike configuration, which interlace and anastomose to form a cancellous (lattice-like) or spongy structure (see Figures 1.4 and 1.5). As shown by the variability of the apparent density (see above), the dimensions of the holes in this lattice are extremely variable, the variation increasing with age.[51]

C. WOVEN AND PARALLEL-FIBERED BONE

According to the arrangements of the collagen fibrils, both compact and spongy bones can be of woven or parallel-fibered type.[52]

1. Woven Bone

Woven bone, also called coarse-fiber bone, is characterized by the presence in the matrix of coarse, irregularly oriented collagen fibrils which, under the polarization microscope, appear as uneven anisotropic structures. They encircle osteocyte lacunae of globular shape which are irregularly distributed in the matrix (osteocyte morphology and function have been reviewed elsewhere[1,53-55]). Moreover, they surround relatively large canal-like structures which are penetrated by capillary vessels. When these canals are small, they correspond to primary osteons (see below) and the appearance of bone is compact; when they are conspicuous, their appearance is that of spongy bone and the intertrabecular spaces contain bone marrow elements. The matrix of woven bone is characterized by the presence of wide interfibrillary spaces which contain abundant interfibrillar noncollagenous material[18] and relatively abundant proteoglycans, as shown by its metachromasia after toluidine blue staining.[56] Moreover, woven bone is unique in containing BAG-75 (bone acidic glycoprotein-75).[19] Woven bone is the bone formed first during skeletal embryogenesis. After birth, it is gradually removed by the process of bone remodeling, and is substituted by lamellar bone.[57] It can, however, be formed again in pathological conditions, such as callus formation, bone tumors, and ectopic ossification. This is in line with the suggestion that woven and lamellar bone are the result of a rapid and a slow osteogenic process, respectively.[58]

2. Parallel-Fibered Bone

Parallel-fibered bone consists of relatively thin, parallel-oriented collagen fibrils. In reality, their orientation is only prevalently parallel, because many of them interlace during their course[59]; moreover, they may be regularly organized into unit layers called lamellae (see below). Because collagen fibrils in parallel-fibered bone are rather uniformly oriented, they appear anisotropic when their axis is perpendicular to the optical axis of the polarization microscope (see Figures 1.7B). In this type of bone, as well as in lamellar bone, osteocytes have an elongated, ovoidal shape; however, they do not show the regular distribution they have in lamellar bone.[55]

D. PRIMARY AND SECONDARY BONE

Because of its appearance early in life, woven bone is often called primary, or immature, bone. However, primary and woven bone are not synonymous, because the former may consist of collagen fibrils that run parallel to each other, with an orderly arrangement (see parallel-fibered bone, and Figures 1.6 and 1.7). On the other hand, lamellar bone is also called secondary or mature bone, because it replaces bone of woven or primary type as it is resorbed after birth, and because it is formed at the end of the life span of the basic multicellular units during the process of bone remodeling.[60,61] As already mentioned, lamellar bone can be found in primary bone. Both primary and secondary bone may be structured as osteons or trabeculae.

V. OSTEONS AND TRABECULAE

A. OSTEONS

As mentioned, osteons, or Haversian systems, can be found both in primary and secondary bone. Primary osteons are formed as the primitive vascular spaces are filled up by growing bone. As a result, they merge into the surrounding bone matrix without any precise delimitation, and repeat its structural characteristics. Secondary osteons are formed during, and because of, bone remodeling. They are new entities which substitute previously formed structures removed by osteoclastic resorption. For this reason, they are separated from the surrounding matrix by a reversal, or cement line (see below, osteon remodeling).

Osteons (see Figure 1.8) are more or less regular cylindrical structures, whose length, although hardly measurable and varying according to animal species and age, ranges from 3 to 6 mm, and can reach 12 mm in branched osteons.[62] Their mean cross-sectional area varies too, and changes with the animal species and bone site;[63] it has been reported to be $5.16 \pm 5.12 \cdot 10^{-4} cm^2$ in human tibial cortical bone,[64] or $17.45 \ \mu m^2$ in males and $17.62 \ \mu m^2$ in females.[65] In horse metacarpal bone

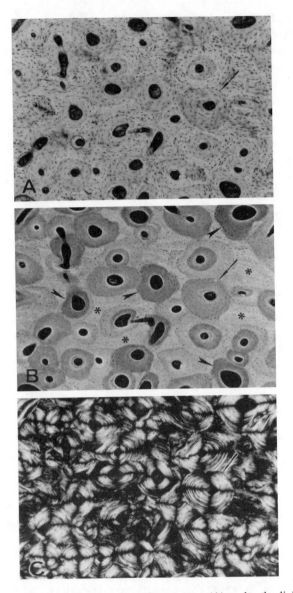

FIGURE 1.8 Cross-sectioned osteons of compact bone as seen (A) under the light microscope; (B) in a microradiograph; and (C) under the polarization microscope (arrows point to the same osteon). Note in (B) that osteons have different degrees of microradiographic density, i.e., of calcification, that the less calcified ones have the largest Haversian canals (arrowheads), that the highest degree of calcification is that of the interstitial bone (asterisks), and that the border of the Haversian canals is apparently hypermineralized. Note in (C) that most of the osteons are of "intermediate" type. Unstained section prepared by grinding, ×35.

the osteon diameter shows a range comprising 156 μm in the dorsal region, 179 μm in the medial region, and 182 μm in the lateral region.[63] The osteons are oriented parallel to the axis of bone,[66] but with an inclination varying from 5 to 15°,[66] so that they have a spiral diaphyseal distribution.[68-70] Their major axis consists of a vascular canal (or Haversian canal). Because osteons are built in a centripetal way, at the beginning of their formation the canal is wide (see Figures 1.7 and 1.8), with the inner wall lined by a layer of plump, active osteoblasts (for osteoblast morphology and function see Marks and Popoff,[1] Scherft and Groot,[71] and Marks[72]); subsequently, the canal gradually narrows, and the osteoblasts become flat,[73] so that at the end of the process the canal is bordered by so-called lining cells.[74] Adjacent osteons may anastomose; moreover, they can be connected by other vascular canals (Volkmann's canals) which arise from the periosteum or the endosteum and run obliquely or transversally through the bone.

1. Microradiography of Osteons

The discovery of microradiography[75] cast new light on the physiology of bone, by allowing the demonstration that osteon calcification is variable: it is at a maximum in primary osteons, whose calcification is rapid and occurs soon after their formation (the same is true of woven bone), while it can range from a minimum to a maximum in secondary osteons, where a sudden but partial initial calcification of the organic matrix is followed by slow mineral deposition which lasts until completeness is reached[75] (see Figure 1.8B). Due to the process of bone remodeling, osteons are renewed continuously. As a result, osteons at different degrees of calcification are always present in adult compact bone: those at the initial stage of formation are less calcified and more transparent to X rays than those at the final stage of formation, which are fully calcified; intermediate patterns are easily recognizable (see Figure 1.8B). Because of their different degrees of calcification, osteons and other bone structures can be distinguished on the basis of their different microhardness,[76] and can be separated by means of density gradient fractionation.[28,77,78]

The degree of microradiographic density may not be uniform in single osteons. The borders of their vascular canals often appear to be hypermineralized (see Figure 1.8B), a condition that has been thought to be an early sign of bone matrix destruction or "delitescence."[79] Moreover, adjacent lamellae may display different degrees of X-ray density.[80,81] Both these microradiographic patterns may depend on X-ray scattering rather than on differences in mineral content.[82]

2. Osteon Remodeling

Although secondary osteons are already present in bone during the last period of intrauterine life, most of them develop after birth.[57] This means that they replace the already present primary bone, while they in their turn will be replaced by other secondary osteons during the continuous process of bone remodeling. Because resorption is usually partial and asymmetric, osteon remains persist between the newly formed ones (see Figures 1.8A,B). These remains appear as irregularly polygonal fragments of fully calcified lamellar matrix, which connect osteons at various degrees of calcification. They represent the so-called interstitial bone. The new osteons are surrounded, with separation from the interstitial bone, by a continuous, laminar structure, called the cement or reversal line. This provides proof that the osteon formation has been preceded by bone resorption, because the matrix of the cement line is the first to be laid down on the wall of the Howship's lacunae at the end of osteoclast activity (the structure, morphology, and function of osteoclasts have recently been reviewed[1,83-87]). Cement lines are reported to be highly mineralized;[88] however, they seem to contain significantly less Ca and P and more S, and to have a lower Ca/P ratio, than the surrounding bone matrix.[89] Moreover, they contain substantial amounts of bone sialoprotein[23] and osteopontin.[21] This may act as an interfacial adhesion promoter and may help to maintain the integrity of the tissue and regulate cell dynamics.[20,90]

3. Lamellae

The arrangement and orientation of collagen fibrils in secondary bone may give rise to lamellae. For this reason, it is often called lamellar bone, although lamellae may be found in primary bone (see above). Lamellae can be seen under the light microscope if thin sections are examined (Figure 1.9A), and are best recognized under the polarization (Figures 1.8C and 1.9B) and electron microscopes (Figure 1.9C). However, the organization of collagen fibrils in them, and above all in osteons, is still controversial. When examined under a polarization microscope, lamellar and osteonic bone may show an alternation of isotropic and anisotropic lamellae which implies a

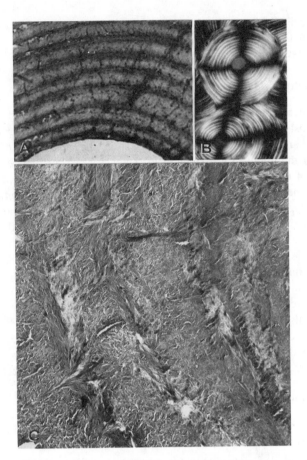

FIGURE 1.9   (A) Cross-section of part of an "intermediate" osteon (vascular canal below), showing the lamellar arrangement of its matrix. Thin section (about 1 μm thick) stained with Azure II–Methylene blue, ×450. (B) Cross section of "intermediate" osteons, which show alternating bright and dark lamellae under the polarization microscope, ×120. (C) Electron microscope picture of an "intermediate" osteon, showing alternating thin and thick lamellae. Unstained, ×6000.

different orientation of the collagen fibrils in successive lamellae (Figures 1.8C and 1.9B). This optical pattern was explained by Gebhardt[91] by assuming that the collagen fibrils have a helical course around the osteon axis, and that the fibrils which have the same spiral orientation form a lamella; the fibril course in one lamella is opposite and more or less perpendicular to the course in the adjacent lamellae. On the basis of this classic model, and of the findings obtained by polarization microscopy, three types of osteons have been described in cross sections of diaphyseal bone: bright, i.e., anisotropic; dark, i.e., isotropic; and intermediate, i.e., with alternate bright and dark lamellae.[92] These optical patterns have been considered to depend on the arrangement of collagen fibrils in successive lamellae, corresponding to a transversal spiral course in all lamellae (bright osteons), a longitudinal spiral course in all lamellae (dark osteons), and a transversal spiral course in one lamella and a longitudinal spiral course in the next (alternate osteons).[92] Obviously, these types constitute paradigms of the different lamellar arrangements the osteon can have and refer to extreme, sharply differentiated models, without consideration of the intermediate arrangements the lamellae may have. If these are examined in depth, other osteon models can be described on the basis of their birefringence.[63,93] On the other hand, even the early studies (reviewed by Frank et al.[94] and Smith[95]) slightly modified Gebhardt's model. By considering both staining and optical properties, Smith[95] described three types of lamellar arrangement in osteons: type I, characterized by alternate lamellae of similar density with longitudinal or transversal fibrils; type II, the same as type I, but with different lamellar density; type III, without any evident lamellar arrangement. On the basis of transmission electron microscope findings, two lamellar arrangements were considered possible, one consisting of dense lamellae alternating with arched lamellae, another showing a herringbone pattern.[94] A goniometric control of the ultrastructural findings has prompted the suggestion that the various lamellar patterns partly depend on the direction of the section plane, and that the lamellae derive from the arrangement of the fibrils according to either a "cylindrical twisted plywood" or a "cylindrical orthogonal plywood," which may coexist in the same osteon.[96] The twisted plywood pattern could account for the "alternate" appearance the osteons can have under the polarization microscope. Five arrays of parallel collagen fibrils, each offset by 30°, have been proposed as components of individual lamellae in a plywoodlike structure.[97] On the basis of scanning electron microscope studies, several models have been proposed: the classic alternate osteon pattern and the twisted plywood pattern;[98] alternation of fibril orientation in adjacent lamellae, with domains of differently oriented fibrils in the same lamella, and with fibrils connecting adjacent lamellae;[99] thin and thick lamellae with a structure like "rotated plywood";[100] variable fibrillar architectures in the same osteon;[101] interlamellar transitional zones, in which both the fibrils and the crystals have an intermediate orientation.[102] Again, on the basis of SEM results, lamellar bone has been considered to consist of two types of lamellae, one "dense," or collagen rich, another "loose," or collagen poor, the former thinner and less calcified than the latter, the only one containing osteocyte lacunae, both showing a highly interwoven arrangement of collagen fibrils.[59,103-105]

Whatever the ultrastructural pattern of the lamellae may be, the polarization microscope permits the selection of differently structured osteons whose mechanical properties are closely related to their optical characteristics and lamellar conformation. In agreement with theoretically predictable results, dark, isotropic osteons best resist tensile forces,[106] whereas bright, anisotropic osteons best resist compressive ones.[92] Other mechanical properties of lamellar bone are consistent with this structure–function relationship.[107] Also the distribution of different osteon types within the skeleton reflects the forces which predominate in a specific skeletal segment.[70,107,108]

B. Trabeculae

Trabeculae are the unit components of the cancellous bone. Usually, they are described as rod- or sheetlike structures. In the calcaneus, both types of trabeculae are present; however, many (up to 83%) of those of rodlike conformation are tubular, due to the vascular canal running through them, so that they are similar to Haversian systems.[109] Microradiography shows different levels of calcification in these trabeculae; the polarization microscope shows that in their outer portion the collagen fibrils mostly run parallel to the long axis, whereas in the inner, osteonic portion they run perpendicular. This basic structure is probably common to the tubular trabeculae of all spongy bones, because it has been found in the cancellous bone of the mastoid, and the epiphysis of the femur and tibia.[110]

The microarchitecture of spongy bone appears random; however, the connections and orientation of the trabeculae are found to have precise patterns which are believed to be related to the specific mechanical properies. The structure of spongy bone in the head and neck of the femur is classically put forward as an example of the correlation between the orientation of the trabeculae and the linear distribution of the principal forces during load bearing — so-called stress trajectoral theory.[111] The possibility that the distribution of trabeculae depends on the prevailing direction of the mechanical forces has been viewed by some authors[112] as being in line with the mathematical calculations, but it has been evaluated cautiously by others, especially because of the complicated effects the traction of muscles may have on the overall load.[113] In any case, there is a close relationship between the numbers and arrangement of trabeculae and the strength of spongy bone.[114,115] This is confirmed by the fractures which can follow the age-induced loss of trabeculae, whose total volume can fall, at least in the iliac crest, from about 25% in youth to about 12% in the elderly.[116-121] The loss is rather selective, as is shown by the falling frequency of transverse trabeculae and the persistence of vertical ones in the central zone of the osteoporotic vertebral bodies,[122] and by the total disappearance of individual trabeculae in elderly women, and the generalized, sharp fall in their numbers in elderly men.[51,123] This selective effect may be very dangerous because it causes not only a fall in bone volume, but also a breakdown in bone's "connectivity,"[114] that is, the trabecular frame which greatly contributes to the strength of spongy bone.[124,125]

The possibility that trabeculae may be lost in a selective way introduces an important concept, which is that spongy bone contains some bundles of trabeculae whose main function is that of resisting mechanical forces, while others have chiefly metabolic functions. These last must not be confused with those of the spongy bone which is classically considered "metabolic," on account of its being completely devoid of mechanical function, for example, the medullary bone of egg-laying birds. This bone is formed under estrogen stimulation, represents a reserve of calcium for eggshell formation, and is characterized by high amounts of acid proteoglycans and glycoproteins in its matrix.[126] The possibility that the trabeculae of the metaphyseal spongy bone may be pre-ponderantly "metabolic" or "mechanic" is in line with their behavior under different stimulations. Thus, in growing animals the osteogenic activity is higher in the peripheral (or "tubular") than in the central (or "lamellar") spongiosa, whereas in adult animals, in which osteogenesis mainly depends on bone metabolism, the results are just the opposite.[127] The already mentioned loss of transverse trabeculae in the central zone of aged vertebral bodies[122] points in the same direction. The same is true of the osteoporosis which follows ovariectomy in rats: the fall in the concentration of estrogens stimulates bone resorption in the central metaphyseal trabeculae, whereas the peripheral trabeculae are to a large extent preserved.[128-130] Thus, not only is spongy bone more active meta-bolically, and more susceptible to variations in mechanical conditions, than compact bone,[19] but inside it single trabecular zones may have metabolic rather than mechanical functions.

VI. CONCLUSIONS

Bone is a heterogeneous tissue because its basic components are assembled in different ways, the main structural determinants being the type of bone, age, loads, and metabolic activity. The type of bone essentially depends on the density of its structures, which ranges from a very compact state in cortical bone to a spongelike appearance in cancellous bone, and from a compact aggregation of collagen fibrils in lamellar bone to their comparatively loose state in woven bone. Age chiefly induces a transformation of woven bone into lamellar bone soon after birth, and a late, almost physiological loss in bone volume with alterations to connectivity.[131] The mechanical functions are responsible for the maintenance of the architecture of bone,[132,133] and the metabolic ones for its renewal[1]; both are mediated by the various aspects of bone remodeling, which induces the erosion and reconstruction of trabecular segments in spongy bone,[131] and of osteons and other lamellar structures in compact bone.[134] The heterogeneity of the tissue fully justifies the study of single components dissected and isolated from the bone context, such as osteons, trabeculae, and lamel-lae.[135] Clearly, structural heterogeneity by itself greatly contributes to osseous properties such as stiffness, elasticity, hardness, and strength, which are necessarily those of bone as a whole. The study of a tissue as complex as bone calls for careful analysis of all its variables.

ACKNOWLEDGMENTS

The preparation of this chapter and the personal research mentioned supported by grants from the Italian Ministry of University and Scientific and Technological Research (MURST), the Italian National Research Council (CNR), and the University of Rome La Sapienza. The author is grateful to Paola Ballanti, Silvia Berni, Carlo Della Rocca, and, above all, Giuliana Silvestrini for their suggestions, discussions, and technical assistance.

REFERENCES

1. Marks, S.C. and Popoff, S.N., Bone cell biology: the regulation of development, structure, and function in the skeleton, *Am. J. Anat.*, 183, 1, 1988.

2. Keaveny, T.M. and Hayes, W.C., Mechanical properties of cortical and trabecular bone, in *Bone,* Hall, B.K., Ed., CRC Press, Boca Raton, FL, 1993, 285.

3. Glimcher, M.J., Composition, structure, and organization of bone and other mineralized tissues and the mechanism of calcification, in *Handbook of Physiology: Endocrinology,* Greep, R.O. and Astwood, E.B., Eds., American Physiological Society, Washington, D.C., 1976, 25.

4. Chapman, J.A. and Hulmes, D.J., Electron microscopy of the collagen fibril, in *Ultrastructure of the Connective Tissue Matrix*, Ruggeri, A. and Motta, P.M., Eds., Martinus Nijhoff Publishers, Boston, 1984, 1.

5. van der Rest, M., The collagens of bone, in *Bone,* Vol. 3: *Bone Matrix and Bone Specific Products*, Hall, B.K., Ed., CRC Press, Boca Raton, FL, 1991, 187.

6. Veis, A. and Sabsay, B., The collagen of mineralized matrices, in *Bone and Mineral Research,* Vol. 5, Peck, W.A., Ed., Elsevier Science Publishers, Amsterdam, 1987, 1.

7. Hodge, A.J. and Petruska, J.A., Recent studies with the electron microscope on ordered aggregates of the tropocollagen molecules, in *Aspects of Protein Structure*, Ramachandran, G.N., Ed., Academic Press, London, 1963, 289.

8. Yamauchi, M., Chandler, G.S., and Katz, E.P., Collagen cross-linking and mineralization, in *Chemistry and Biology of Mineralized Tissues*, Slavkin, H. and Price, P., Eds., Elsevier Science Publishers, Amsterdam, 1992, 39.

9. Chapman, J.A., Molecular organization in the collagen fibril, in *Connective Tissue Matrix*, Hukins, D.W.C., Ed., Macmillan, London, 1984, 89.

10. Boskey, A.L., Noncollagenous matrix proteins and their role in mineralization, *Bone Miner.*, 6, 111, 1989.

11. Butler, W.T., Matrix macromolecules of bone and dentin, *Collagen Relat. Res.*, 4, 297, 1984.

12. Seyedin, S.M. and Rosen, D.M., Matrix proteins of the skeleton, *Curr. Opinion Cell Biol.*, 2, 914, 1990.

13. Seyedin, S.M. and Rosen, D.M., Unique bone-derived cytokines, in *Cytokines and Bone Metabolism*, Gowen, M., Ed., CRC Press, Boca Raton, FL, 1992, 109.

14. Bonucci, E., Silvestrini, G., and Bianco, P., Extracellular alkaline phosphatase activity in mineralizing matrices of cartilage and bone: ultrastructural localization using a cerium-based method, *Histochemistry*, 97, 323, 1992.

15. de Bernard, B., Bianco, P., Bonucci, E., et al., Biochemical and immunohistochemical evidence that in cartilage an alkaline phosphatase is a Ca^{2+}-binding glycoprotein, *J. Cell Biol.*, 103, 1615, 1986.

16. Eeckhout, Y. and Delaisse, J.M., The role of collagenase in bone resorption. An overview, *Pathol. Biol.*, 36, 1139, 1988.

17. Jilka, R.L., Procollagenase associated with the noncalcified matrix of bone and its regulation by parathyroid hormone, *Bone*, 10, 353, 1989.

18. Bonucci, E. and Silvestrini, G., Ultrastructure of the organic matrix of embryonic avian bone after en bloc reaction with various electron-dense "stains," *Acta Anat.*, 156, 22, 1996.

19. Gorski, J.P., Is all bone the same? Distinctive distributions and properties of non-collagenous matrix proteins in lamellar vs. woven bone imply the existence of different underlying osteogenic mechanisms, *Crit. Rev. Oral Biol. Med.*, 9, 201, 1998.

20. McKee, M.D., Farach-Carson, M.C., Butler, W.T., et al., Ultrastructural immunolocalization of non-collagenous (osteopontin and osteocalcin) and plasma (albumin and $_{\alpha 2}$HS-glycoprotein) proteins in rat bone, *J. Bone Miner. Res.,* 8, 485, 1993.

21. McKee, M.D., Glimcher, M.J., and Nanci, A., High-resolution immunolocalization of osteopontin and osteocalcin in bone and cartilage during endochondral ossification in the chicken tibia, *Anat. Rec.*, 234, 479, 1992.

22. McKee, M.D. and Nanci, A., Postembedding colloidal-gold immunocytochemistry of noncollagenous extracellular proteins in mineralized tissues, *Micros. Res. Tech.*, 31, 44, 1995.

23. Riminucci, M., Silvestrini, G., Bonucci, E., et al., The anatomy of bone sialoprotein immunoreactive sites in bone as revealed by combined ultrastructural histochemistry and immunohistochemistry, *Calcif. Tissue Int.*, 57, 277, 1995.

24. Bianco, P., Ultrastructural immunohistochemistry of noncollagenous proteins in calcified tissues, in *Ultrastructure of Skeletal Tissues,* Bonucci, E. and Motta, P.M., Eds., Kluwer Academic Publishers, Boston, 1990, 63.

25. Ingram, R.T., Clarke, B.L., Fisher, L.W., and Fitzpatrick, L.A., Distribution of noncollagenous proteins in the matrix of adult human bone: evidence of anatomic and functional heterogeneity, *J. Bone Miner. Res.,* 8, 1019, 1993.

26. Silbermann, M., Von der Mark, H., and Heinegard, D., An immunohistochemical study of the distribution of matrical proteins in the mandibular condyle of neonatal mice. II. Non-collagenous proteins, *J. Anat.,* 170, 23, 1990.

27. Sommer, B., Bickel, M., Hofstetter, W., and Wetterwald, A., Expression of matrix proteins during the development of mineralized tissues, *Bone,* 19, 371, 1996.

28. Mbuyi-Muamba, J.M., Dequeker, J., and Gevers, G., Collagen and non-collagenous proteins in different mineralization stages of human femur, *Acta Anat.,* 134, 265, 1989.

29. Cowles, E.A., DeRome, M.E., Pastizzo, G., et al., Mineralization and the expression of matrix proteins during *in vivo* bone development, *Calcif. Tissue Int.,* 62, 74, 1998.

30. Fisher, L.W. and Termine, J.D., Noncollagenous proteins influencing the local mechanisms of calcification, *Clin. Orthop.,* 200, 362, 1985.

31. Buckwalter, J.A., Proteoglycan structure in calcifying cartilage, *Clin. Orthop.,* 172, 207, 1983.

32. Silvestrini, G., Zini, N., Sabatelli, P., et al., Combined use of malachite green fixation and PLA_2-gold complex technique to localize phospholipids in areas of early calcification of rat epiphyseal cartilage and bone, *Bone,* 18, 559, 1996.

33. Boyan, B.D., Schwartz, Z., Swain, L.D., and Khare, A., Role of lipids in calcification of cartilage, *Anat. Rec.,* 224, 211, 1989.

34. Sakou, T., Bone morphogenetic proteins: from basic studies to clinical approaches, *Bone,* 22, 591, 1998.

35. Posner, A.S., Bone mineral and the mineralization process, in *Bone and Mineral Research,* Vol. 5, Peck, W.A., Ed., Elsevier Science Publishers, Amsterdam, 1987, 65.

36. Eanes, E.D., Dynamics of calcium phosphate precipitation, in *Calcification in Biological Systems,* Bonucci, E., Ed., CRC Press, Boca Raton, FL, 1992, 1.

37. Glimcher, M.J., Mechanism of calcification: role of collagen fibrils and collagen–phosphoprotein complexes *in vitro* and *in vivo, Anat. Rec.,* 224, 139, 1989.

38. Bonucci, E., Role of collagen fibrils in calcification, in *Calcification in Biological Systems,* Bonucci, E., Ed., CRC Press, Boca Raton, FL, 1992, 19.

39. Robinson, R.A., An electron-microscopic study of the crystalline inorganic component of bone and its relationship to the organic matrix, *J. Bone Joint Surg.,* 34-A, 389, 1952.

40. Ascenzi, A., Bonucci, E., and Steve Bocciarelli, D., An electron microscope study of osteon calcification, *J. Ultrastruct. Res.,* 12, 287, 1965.

41. Höhling, H.J., Kreilos, R., Neubauer, G., and Boyde, A., Electron microscopy and electron microscopical measurements of collagen mineralization in hard tissues, *Z. Zellforsch.,* 122, 36, 1971.

42. Ascenzi, A., Bonucci, E., Ripamonti, A., and Roveri, N., X-ray diffraction and electron microscope study of osteons during calcification, *Calcif. Tissue Res.,* 25, 133, 1978.

43. Bonucci, E., The locus of initial calcification in cartilage and bone, *Clin. Orthop.,* 78, 108, 1971.

44. Bonucci, E., The structural basis of calcification, in *Ultrastructure of the Connective Tissue Matrix,* Ruggeri, A. and Motta, P.M., Eds., Martinus Nijhoff, Boston, 1984, 165.

45. Glimcher, M.J. and Katz, E.P., The organization of collagen in bone: the role of noncovalent bonds in the relative insolubility of bone collagen, *J. Ultrastruct. Res.,* 12, 705, 1965.

46. Pugliarello, M.C., Vittur, F., de Bernard, B., et al., Chemical modifications in osteones during calcification, *Calcif. Tissue Res.,* 5, 108, 1970.

47. Evans, F.G., Factors affecting the mechanical properties of bone, *Bull. N.Y. Acad. Med.,* 49, 751, 1973.

48. Bonucci, E. and Reurink, J., The fine structure of decalcified cartilage and bone: a comparison between decalcification procedures performed before and after embedding, *Calcif. Tissue Res.,* 25, 179, 1978.

49. Carter, D.R. and Spengler, D.M., Mechanical properties and composition of cortical bone, *Clin. Orthop.,* 135, 192, 1978.

50. Gardner, E., Osteogenesis in human embryo and fetus, in *The Biochemistry and Physiology of Bone,* Bourne, G.H., Ed., Academic Press, New York, 1971, 77.

51. Aaron, J.E., Makins, N.B., and Sagreiya, K., The microanatomy of trabecular bone loss in normal aging men and women, *Clin. Orthop.*, 215, 260, 1987.

52. Smith, J.W., Collagen fiber patterns in mammalian bone, *J. Anat.*, 94, 329, 1960.

53. Aarden, E.M., Burger, E.H., and Nijweide, P.J., Function of osteocytes in bone, *J. Cell. Biochem.*, 55, 287, 1994.

54. Bonucci, E., The ultrastructure of the osteocyte, in *Ultrastructure of Skeletal Tissues*, Bonucci, E. and Motta, P.M., Eds., Kluwer Academic, Boston, 1990, 223.

55. Marotti, G., Canè, V., Palazzini, S., and Palumbo, C., Structure–function relationships in the osteocyte, *Ital. J. Miner. Electrol. Metab.*, 4, 93, 1990.

56. Hancox, N.M., *Biology of Bone*, Cambridge University Press, Cambridge, U.K., 1972, Chapter 3.

57. Amprino, R., and Bairati, A., Processi di ricostruzione e di riassorbimento nella sostanza compatta delle ossa dell'uomo. Ricerche su cento soggetti dalla nascita sino a tarda età, *Z. Zellforsch.*, 24, 439, 1936.

58. Amprino, R. La structure du tissu osseux envisagée comme expression de différences dans la vitesse de l'accroissement, *Arch. Biol.*, 58, 315, 1947.

59. Marotti, G., The structure of bone tissues and the cellular control of their deposition, *Ital. J. Anat. Embryol.*, 101, 25, 1996.

60. Bonucci, E., The basic multicellular unit of bone, *Ital. J. Miner. Electrol. Metab.*, 4, 115, 1990.

61. Parfitt, A.M., Bone remodeling: relationship to the amount and structure of bone, and the pathogenesis and prevention of fractures, in *Osteoporosis: Etiology, Diagnosis, and Management*, Riggs, B.L. and Melton, L.J.I., Eds., Raven Press, New York, 1988, 45.

62. Filogamo, G., La forme et la taille des ostéones chez quelques mammifères, *Arch. Biol.*, 57, 137, 1946.

63. Martin, R.B., Gibson, V.A., Stover, S.M., et al., Osteonal structure in the equine third metacarpus, *Bone*, 19, 165, 1996.

64. Black, J., Mattson, R., and Korostoff, E., Haversian osteons: size, distribution, internal structure, and orientation, *J. Biomed. Mater. Res.*, 8, 299, 1974.

65. Broulik, P., Kragstrup, J., Mosekilde, L., and Melsen, F., Osteon cross-sectional size in the iliac crest, *Acta Pathol. Microbiol. Immunol. Scand. Sect. A*, 90, 339, 1982.

66. Benninghoff, H., Spaltlinien am Knochen, eine Methode zur Ermittlung der Architektur platter Knochen, *Verh. Anat. Ges.*, 34, 189, 1925.

67. Hert, J., Fiala, P., and Petrtyl, M., Osteon orientation of the diaphysis of the long bones in man, *Bone*, 15, 269, 1994.

68. Cohen, J. and Harris, W.H., The three-dimensional anatomy of Haversian systems, *J. Bone Joint Surg.*, 40-A, 419, 1958.

69. Petrtyl, M., Hert, J., and Fiala, P., Spatial organization of the Haversian bone in man, *J. Biomech.*, 29, 161, 1996.

70. Portigliatti Barbos, M., Bianco, P., Ascenzi, A., and Boyde, A., Collagen orientation in compact bone: II. Distribution of lamellae in the whole of the human femoral shaft with reference to its mechanical properties, *Metab. Bone Dis. Relat. Res.*, 5, 309, 1984.

71. Scherft, J.P. and Groot, C.G., The electron microscopic structure of the osteoblast, in *Ultrastructure of Skeletal Tissues*, Bonucci, E. and Motta, P.M., Eds., Kluwer Academic, Boston, 1990, 209.

72. Marks, S.C.J., The structural basis for bone cell biology. A review, *Acta Med. Dent. Helv.*, 2, 141, 1997.

73. Marotti, G., Decrement of volume of osteoblasts during osteon formation and its effect on the size of the corresponding osteocytes, in *Bone Histomorphometry*, Meunier, P.J., Ed., Armour Montagu, Paris, 1976, 385.

74. Miller, S.C., de Saint-Georges, L., Bowman, B.M., and Jee, W.S.S., Bone lining cells: structure and function, *Scanning Microsc.*, 3, 953, 1989.

75. Amprino, R. and Engström, A., Studies on X-ray absorption and diffraction of bone tissue, *Acta Anat.*, 15, 1, 1952.

76. Marotti, G., Favia, A., and Zambonin Zallone, A., Quantitative analysis of the rate of secondary bone mineralization, *Calcif. Tissue Res.*, 10, 67, 1972.

77. Engfeldt, B. and Hjerpe, A., Density gradient fractionation of dentine and bone powder, *Calcif. Tissue Res.*, 16, 261, 1974.

78. Engfeldt, B. and Hjerpe, A., Glycosaminoglycans and proteoglycans of human bone tissue at different stages of mineralization, *Acta Pathol. Microbiol. Scand. Sect. A*, 84, 95, 1976.

79. Dhem, A., Etude histologique et microradiographique des manifestations biologiques propres au tissu osseux compact, *Bull. Acad. Med. Bel.*, 135, 368, 1980.

80. Engström, A. and Engfeldt, B., Lamellar structure of osteons demonstrated by microradiography, *Experientia*, 15, 19, 1953.

81. Vincent, J., Microradiographie des lamelles de l'os haversien, *Arch. Biol.*, 69, 561, 1958.

82. Bohatirchuk, F.P., Campbell, J.S., and Jeletzky, T.F., Bone lamellae, *Acta Anat.*, 83, 321, 1972.

83. Baron, R., Molecular mechanisms of bone resorption. An update, *Acta Orthop. Scand.*, 66, 66, 1995.

84. Göthlin, G. and Ericsson, J.L.E., The osteoclast. Review of ultrastructure, origin, and structure-function relationship, *Clin. Orthop.*, 120, 201, 1976.

85. Hall, T.J. and Chambers, T.J., Molecular aspects of osteoclast function, *Inflamm. Res.*, 45, 1, 1996.

86. Sasaki, T., Recent advances in the ultrastructural assessment of osteoclastic resorptive functions, *Microsc. Res. Tech.*, 33, 182, 1996.

87. Suda, T., Nakamura, I., Jimi, E., and Takahashi, N., Regulation of osteoclast function, *J. Bone Miner. Res.*, 12, 869, 1997.

88. Philipson, B., Composition of cement lines in bone, *J. Histochem. Cytochem.*, 13, 270, 1965.

89. Schaffler, M.B., Burr, D.B., and Frederickson, R.G., Morphology of the osteonal cement line in human bone, *Anat. Rec.*, 217, 223, 1987.

90. McKee, M.D. and Nanci, A., Osteopontin at mineralized tissue interfaces in bone, teeth, and osseointegrated implants: ultrastructural distribution, and implications for mineralized tissue formation, turnover, and repair, *Microsc. Res. Tech.*, 33, 141, 1996.

91. Gebhardt, W., Ueber funktionell wichtige Anordnungsweisen der grösseren und feineren Bauelemente der Wilbertierknochens. II. Spezieller Teil. Der Bau der Haversschen Lamellensysteme und seine funktionelle Bedeutung, *Arch. Entwicklungsmech. Org.*, 20, 187, 1906.

92. Ascenzi, A. and Bonucci, E., The compressive properties of single osteons, *Anat. Rec.*, 161, 377, 1968.

93. Vincentelli, R., Relation between collagen fiber orientation and age of osteon formation in human tibial compact bone, *Acta Anat.*, 100, 120, 1978.

94. Frank, R., Frank, P., Klein, M., and Fontaine, R., L'os compact humain normal au microscope électronique, *Arch. Anat. Microsc. Morphol. Exp.*, 44, 191, 1955.

95. Smith, J.W., The arrangement of collagen fibres in human secondary osteones, *J. Bone Joint Surg.*, 42-B, 588, 1960.

96. Giraud-Guille, M.-M., Twisted plywood architecture of collagen fibrils in human compact bone osteons, *Calcif. Tissue Int.*, 42, 167, 1988.

97. Weiner, S., Arad, T., Sabanay, I., and Traub, W., Rotated plywood structure of primary lamellar bone in the rat: orientations of the collagen fibril arrays, *Bone*, 20, 509, 1997.

98. Raspanti, M., Guizzardi, S., Strocchi, R., and Ruggeri, A., Collagen fibril patterns in compact bone: preliminary ultrastructural observations, *Acta Anat.*, 155, 249, 1996.

99. Pannarale, L., Braidotti, P., d'Alba, L., and Gaudio, E., Scanning electron microscopy of collagen fiber orientation in the bone lamellar system in non-decalcified human samples, *Acta Anat.*, 151, 36, 1994.

100. Weiner, S., Arad, T., and Traub, W., Crystal organization in rat bone lamellae, *Fed. Eur. Biochem. Soc.*, 285, 49, 1991.

101. Raspanti, M., Guizzardi, S., Strocchi, R., and Ruggeri, A., Different fibrillar architectures coexisting in Haversian bone, *Ital. J. Anat. Embryol.*, 100, 103, 1995.

102. Ziv, V., Sabanay, I., Arad, T., et al., Transitional structures in lamellar bone, *Microsc. Res. Tech.*, 33, 203, 1996.

103. Marotti, G., The original contribution of the scanning electron microscope to the knowledge of bone structure, in *Ultrastructure of Skeletal Tissues*, Bonucci, E. and Motta, P.M., Eds., Kluwer Academic, Boston, 1990, 19.

104. Marotti, G., A new theory of bone lamellation, *Calcif. Tissue Int.*, 53, S47, 1993.

105. Marotti, G. and Muglia, M.A., A scanning electron microscope study of human bony lamellae. Proposal for a new model of collagen lamellar organization, *Arch. Ital. Anat. Embriol.*, 93, 163, 1988.

106. Ascenzi, A. and Bonucci, E., The ultimate tensile strength of single osteons, *Acta Anat.*, 58, 160, 1964.

107. Ascenzi, A., The micromechanics vs. the macromechanics of cortical bone — A comprehensive presentation, *J. Biomech. Eng.*, 110, 357, 1988.

108. Carando, S., Portigliatti Barbos, M., Ascenzi, A., and Boyde, A., Orientation of collagen in human tibial and fibular shaft and possible correlation with mechanical properties, *Bone*, 10, 139, 1989.

109. Lozupone, E., The structure of the trabeculae of cancellous bone 1. The calcaneus, *Anat. Anz.*, 159, 211, 1985.

110. Lozupone, E. and Favia, A., The structure of the trabeculae of cancellous bone. 2. Long bones and mastoid, *Calcif. Tissue Int.*, 46, 367, 1990.

111. Bell, G.H., Bone as a mechanical engineering problem, in *The Biochemistry and Physiology of Bone*, Bourne, G.H., Ed., Academic Press, New York, 1956, 27.

112. Koch, J.C., The laws of bone architecture, *Am. J. Anat.*, 21, 177, 1917.

113. Rybicki, E.F., Simonen, F.A., and Weis, E.B., Jr., On the mathematical analysis of stress in the human femur, *J. Biomech.*, 5, 203, 1972.

114. Kleerekoper, M., Villanueva, A.R., Stanciu, J., et al., The role of three-dimensional trabecular micro-structure in the pathogenesis of vertebral compression fractures, *Calcif. Tissue Int.*, 37, 594, 1985.

115. Parfitt, A.M., Trabecular bone architecture in the pathogenesis and prevention of fracture, *Am. J. Med.*, 82, 68, 1987.

116. Ballanti, P., Bonucci, E., Della Rocca, C., et al., Bone histomorphometric reference values in 88 normal Italian subjects, *Bone Miner.*, 11, 187, 1990.

117. Birkenhäger-Frenkel, D.H., Courpron, P., Hüpscher, E.A., et al., Age-related changes in cancellous bone structure. A two-dimensional study in the transiliac and iliac crest biopsy sites, *Bone Miner.*, 4, 197, 1988.

118. Hoikka, V. and Arnala, I., Histomorphometric normal values of the iliac crest cancellous bone in a Finnish autopsy series, *Ann. Clin. Res.*, 13, 383, 1981.

119. Malluche, H.H., Sherman, D., Meyer, W., and Massry, S.G., Quantitative bone histology in 84 normal American subjects, *Calcif. Tissue Int.*, 34, 449, 1982.

120. Melsen, F., Melsen, B., Mosekilde, L., and Bergmann, S., Histomorphometric analysis of normal bone from the iliac crest, *Acta Pathol. Microbiol. Scand. Sect. A*, 86, 70, 1978.

121. Schnitzler, C.M., Pettifor, J.M., Mesquita, J.M., et al., Histomorphometry of iliac crest bone in 346 normal black and white South African adults, *Bone Miner.*, 10, 183, 1990.

122. Atkinson, P.J., Variation in trabecular structure of vertebrae with age, *Calcif. Tissue Res.*, 1, 24, 1967.

123. Compston, J.E., Mellish, R.W.E., and Garrahan, N.J., Age-related changes in iliac crest trabecular microanatomic bone structure in man, *Bone*, 8, 289, 1987.

124. Goldstein, S.A., Goulet, R., and McCubbrey, D., Measurement and significance of three-dimensional architecture to the mechanical integrity of trabecular bone, *Calcif. Tissue Int.*, 53, S127, 1993.

125. Parfitt, A.M., Mathews, C.H.E., Villanueva, A.R., et al., Relationship between surface, volume, and thickness of iliac trabecular bone in aging and in osteoporosis, *J. Clin. Invest.*, 72, 1396, 1983.

126. Bonucci, E. and Gherardi, G., Histochemical and electron microscope investigations on medullary bone, *Cell Tissue Res.*, 163, 81, 1975.

127. Lozupone, E., A quantitative analysis of bone tissue formation in different regions of the spongiosa in the dog skeleton, *Anat. Anz.*, 145, 425, 1979.

128. Ballanti, P., Martelli, A., Mereto, E., and Bonucci, E., Ovariectomized rats as experimental model of postmenopausal osteoporosis: critical considerations, *Ital. J. Miner. Electrol. Metab.*, 7, 243, 1993.

129. Miller, S.C., Bowman, B.M., Miller, M.A., and Bagi, C.M., Calcium absorption and osseous organ-, tissue-, and envelope-specific changes following ovariectomy in rats, *Bone*, 12, 439, 1991.

130. Yoshida, S., Yamamuro, T., Okumura, H., and Takahashi, H., Microstructural changes of osteopenic trabeculae in the rat, *Bone*, 12, 185, 1991.

131. Parfitt, A.M., Age-related structural changes in trabecular and cortical bone: cellular mechanisms and biomechanical consequences, *Calcif. Tissue Int.*, 36, S123, 1984.

132. Frost, H.M., Changing concepts in skeletal physiology: Wolff's law, the mechanostat, and the "Utah Paradigm," *Am. J. Hum. Biol.*, 10, 599, 1998.

133. Frost, H.M., Ferretti, J.L., and Jee, W.S.S., Perspectives: some role of mechanical usage, muscle strength, and the mechanostat in skeletal physiology, disease, and research, *Calcif. Tissue Int.*, 62, 1, 1998.

134. Parfitt, A.M., Osteonal and hemi-osteonal remodeling: the spatial and temporal framework for signal traffic in adult human bone, *J. Cell. Biochem.*, 55, 273, 1994.

135. Ascenzi, A., Microscopic dissection and isolation of bone constituents, in *Skeletal Research: An Experimental Approach*, Kunin, A.S. and Simmons, D.J., Eds., Academic Press, New York, 1983, 185.

2 Basic Concepts of Mechanical Property Measurement and Bone Biomechanics

Yuehuei H. An, William R. Barfield, and Robert A. Draughn

CONTENTS

I. INTRODUCTION

Mechanics is a physical science that assesses the effects of force on objects. Mechanical properties of bone are basic parameters which reflect the structure and function of bone and can be measured by testing whole anatomical units or specimens prepared to isolate particular structural components. Within this context the fracture of bone can represent failure of whole bone at the structural level and bone tissue at the material level. The mechanical behavior of bone in normal physiological situations is similar to that of an elastic material with no visible change in external appearance. Bone, however, can be degraded and still retain its morphological features for an indefinite period of time. Unlike inorganic materials, bone has adaptive mechanisms which give the tissue the ability to repair itself, altering its mechanical properties and morphology in response to increased or decreased function. This chapter covers common mechanical concepts and terminology used in the field of bone biomechanics and mechanical property measurement.

TABLE 2.1
Common Symbols Used in the Field of Bone Biomechanics

Symbol	Meaning	Common SI Units Used
A	Surface area	m^2
E	Elastic modulus or Young's modulus	Pa (N/m^2), MPa, GPa
F	Force	N
I	Area moment of inertia of cross section	m^4
J (joule)	SI unit of energy (work)	N·m
J	Polar moment of inertia	m^4
L	Length or span	m
M	Mass	kg
P	Load	N
r	Radius	m
S	Strength	Pa (N/m^2), MPa, GPa
S_b	Bending strength	Pa (N/m^2), MPa, GPa
S_c	Compressive strength	Pa (N/m^2), MPa, GPa
S_t	Tensile strength	Pa (N/m^2), MPa, GPa
S_s	Shear strength	Pa (N/m^2), MPa, GPa
T	Torque or torsional moment	N·m
W	Weight	N
ε	Strain	mm/mm, %
ε_y	Yield strain	mm/mm, %
ε_{ult}	Ultimate strain	mm/mm, %
η	Viscosity	Pa·sec
ν	Poisson's ratio	length/length
ρ_a	Apparent density	kg/m^3, g/cm^3, mg/mm^3
ρ_{ash}	Ash density	kg/m^3, g/cm^3, mg/mm^3
σ	Stress	Pa (N/m^2), MPa, GPa
σ_y	Yield stress	Pa (N/m^2), MPa, GPa
σ_{ult}	Ultimate stress	Pa (N/m^2), MPa, GPa
τ	Shear stress	Pa (N/m^2), MPa, GPa

Source: Low, J. and Reed, A., *Basic Biomechanics Explained,* Butterworth Heinemann, London, 1996. With permission.

II. CONCEPTS RELEVANT TO MECHANICAL TESTING

There are two main unit systems for measurements, the British system and the SI system. The British system uses pound, foot, and second as its basic units and the SI system uses kilogram, meter, newton, second, and Celsius (°C). Most journals or publishers prefer the SI system due to its simplicity. Measurement involves two groups of parameters, scalars and vectors. A scalar is a quantity, such as temperature, length, or mass, which provides information regarding magnitude only. Vector quantities possess both magnitude and direction. Measures such as force, moment, and torque are typical examples. Symbols commonly used in the field of bone biomechanics are listed in Table 2.1.

A. STATICS AND DYNAMICS

Mechanics deals with the effects of forces on the form or motion of bodies or subjects, and can be divided into two categories, statics and dynamics. Statics studies bodies at rest or when there is equilibrium of forces. The state of equilibrium means that the sum of the forces and the sum of

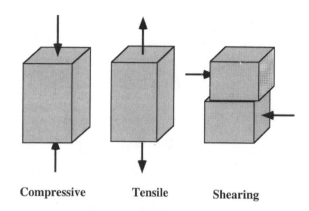

Compressive   **Tensile**   **Shearing**

FIGURE 2.1 Three types of pure forces.

the moments is equal to zero. There must be no overlapping resultants. Dynamics studies moving bodies and is subdivided into kinematics and kinetics. Kinematics describes the relations among displacements, velocities, and accelerations in all kinds of motion without regard to the forces involved and has been described as geometry of motion. Kinetics deals with the forces causing movement. Most of the concepts, studies, methods of evaluation, and findings presented in this book fall into the category of statics.

B. Force and Displacement

Force (**F**) or load, the primary physical entity in mechanics, is a measurable vector, which has a magnitude, direction, and point of application. Forces act on a body and tend to change the velocity of the body (external effect) or shape of the body (internal effect). Changes in shape are determined by changes of the relative positions of the structural elements within a body. The changes in shape, structure, or morphology of bodies or objects (such as bone) result from the effects of the forces. For instance, movements of an implant relative to the bone in which it resides is likely the result of external forces, although micromovement that occurs at the bone–implant interface is also impacted by concentric and eccentric muscle forces. Force is a vector quantity, meaning that it has both intensity and direction. There are basically three types of fo2525rces: tensile, compressive, and shear force, which are determined by the direction and effect of the force(s) acting on the body (Figure 2.1).

The magnitude of a force is expressed in the SI system of units as newtons. A newton is the force required to give 1 kilogram mass an acceleration of 1 meter per second per second (m/sec^2). Small forces can be expressed in units of dynes. A dyne is the force that gives 1 gram mass an acceleration of 1 centimeter per second per second (cm/sec^2).

In most measurements of mechanical properties the applied force is measured by a load cell and changes in specimen dimensions are indicated by the motion of the load application system. In a mechanically actuated test machine (a "screw" machine) the motion of the crosshead defines the total displacement of the specimen and the test fixture. In a hydraulically actuated test system, the movement of the actuator piston proscribes the displacement. While a test object is being loaded, a load–displacement curve is recorded by a chart recorder or computer (Figure 2.2). The load–displacement (P–D) curve defines the total deformation of the specimen in the direction of force application. Actually, the displacement includes the deformation of the specimen and the deformation of the testing system, such as in the case of an unstable or soft interface between the specimen and the machine. P–D curves are particularly useful for measuring the strength and stiffness of whole structures; however, to compare behavior of different materials, stress–strain curves are needed for standardization. When transforming the load–displacement curve to a stress–strain curve, force and deformation are normalized as stress and strain by the dimensions of the sample.

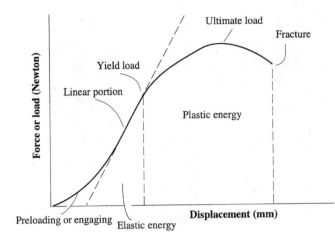

FIGURE 2.2   A typical load–displacement curve.

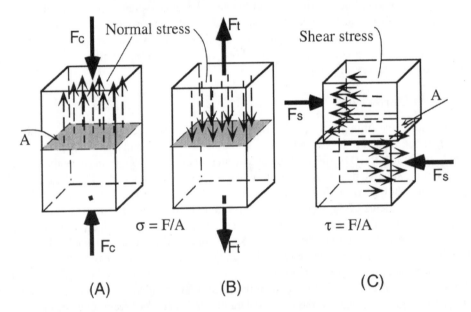

FIGURE 2.3   Illustration of (A, B) normal stress (σ) and shear (C) stress (τ).

C. STRESS AND STRAIN

Stress is the internal resistance of a material body to a force acting upon it (Figure 2.3). In bone, stress (σ) arises from the forces or bonds between molecules, between collagen fibers, and the bonding between collagen and hydroxyapatite crystals. In solid mechanics, stress is a normalized force. It is a ratio (i.e., force per unit area) which is calculated by the magnitude of the force (**F**) divided by the surface area (A) over which the force acts:

$$\sigma = \mathbf{F}/A \tag{2.1}$$

Axial or normal stresses are categorized as either compressive or tensile stresses. Pressure is a normal stress acting on the surface of an object. Shear stress (τ) exists when the force is applied parallel to the surface of a material body. For example, when long bones are subjected to a torsional load, shear stresses are developed in the bone.

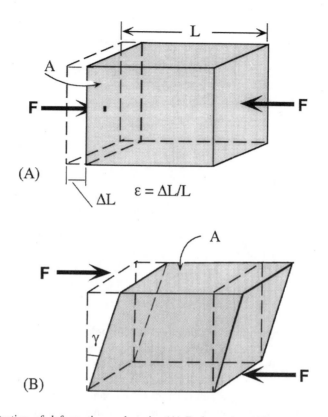

FIGURE 2.4 Illustration of deformation and strain. (A) Deformation (ΔL) and normal strain (ε) under a compressive load (F). (B) shows that a shearing force (F) acting parallel to the surface (A) of the cube produces shear strain (γ).

The standard unit of stress (SI system) is the pascal (Pa), which is 1 N force distributed over one square meter (1 N/m^2). The pascal is a small unit and typically stress is expressed as multiples of pascals including kilopascal (kPa or 10^3 N/m^2), megapascal (MPa or 10^6 N/m^2), and gigapascal (GPa or 10^9 N/m^2). The physiological stress levels for bone are generally below the megapascal range. The unit of stress in English units is pounds/in.^{2} (psi).

Stress concentration is the increase in stress around a defect in a material, such as a screw hole or a defect in bone, and is discussed in detail in other chapters in this text.

Strain represents the dimensional changes of a subject or body under the action of a force or several forces. When force is applied, the object changes its dimensions (Figure 2.4). This change in dimension is termed deformation (ΔL). Deformation per unit length (L) is strain (ε):

$$\varepsilon = \Delta L/L \qquad (2.2)$$

Strain is a dimensionless measure since it is the ratio of two quantities, both in units of length. Strain is defined as the geometric change in a material in response to force application and is also known as a normalized displacement. The types of strains in a body are the same as the types of force producing them: normal strain (compressive or tensile) and shear strain. The latter is defined as the angular deformation of the material measured in radians.

Normal and shearing strains are concepts analogous to normal and shear stress. Normal strain is a measure of the change in length per unit length and shear strain is half the change of an original 90° angle and usually is measured in radians.[1] Shear strain can also be defined as the angle between original and deflected locations on the edge of a material (γ) (Figure 2.4).[2] Ultimate strain (ε_{ult}) is the strain that

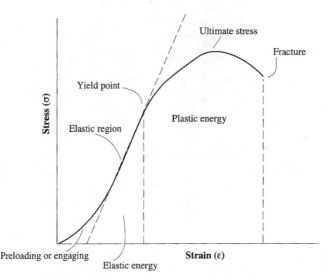

FIGURE 2.5   A typical stress–strain curve.

occurs at fracture. Strain can be measured directly and is recorded as length per unit length (such as cm/cm or mm/mm) or can also be reported as a percentage. Positive strain occurs when material is subjected to tensile stress in the direction of the applied load, reflected as an increase on the length of the material. If the material is compressed, the length is decreased and the strain is negative. Strain rate is the deformation per unit time, which is an important parameter for viscoelastic materials such as bone. Strain rate is discussed in more detail in the section on viscoelasticity.

Strain can be measured by bonding strain gauges directly to bone or with extensometers, brittle lacquer coatings, or birefringent plastic coatings.[3] Uniaxial gauges allow for single directional measures, while triaxial gauges or rosettes permit direction and magnitude of principal strains to be determined. Several technical manuscripts offer detailed information with regard to how these procedures are carried out. [4]

A stress–strain curve (Figure 2.5) displays the relationships between applied stress and resulting strain in a mechanical property measurement test. The curves are generated by conversion of applied force data into units of stress or plotting against directly measured values of strain. Modern computer-based data acquisition systems significantly facilitate the generation of stress–strain curves. From the stress–strain curve, the following properties can be determined:

1. The beginning of the elastic portion, which represents the engagement of the machine specimen;
2. The proportional limit or the limit to which stress and strain are proportional (PL);
3. The elastic limit or the limit at which the greatest stress can be applied without leaving permanent deformation upon removal of the load;
4. The elastic range, that part of the curve where strain is directly proportional to stress;
5. The yield point, or point at which permanent deformation occurs;
6. The range of plastic deformation, the part of the curve from the yield point to the failure point;
7. The breaking point or ultimate stress or ultimate strength; and
8. The amount of energy absorbed by the specimen prior to failure.

The stress–strain plot also allows calculation of the elastic modulus of the material by measuring the slope of the curve in the elastic region.

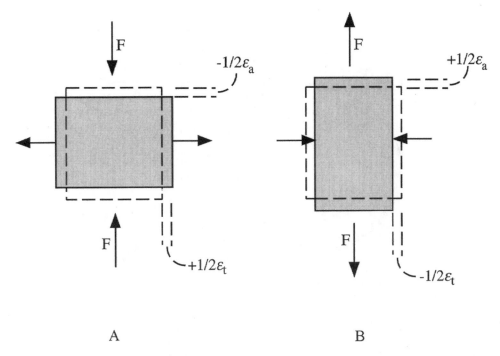

FIGURE 2.6 Illustration of Poisson's effect: (A) axial direction; (B) transverse direction.

D. CONCEPTS RELATED TO MATERIAL DIMENSIONS

When a material specimen is subjected to a compressive uniaxial force, its dimension decreases in the axial (loading) direction and increases in the transverse direction (Figure 2.6). The relationship between these two strains is given by Poisson's ratio (ν):

$$\nu = \varepsilon_t/\varepsilon_a \tag{2.3}$$

where ε_t is transverse strain and ε_a is axial strain. Poisson's effect applies as well in the opposite sense, tensile loading. In general, Poisson's ratio is less than 0.5 which means the volume of the material under simple tensile load cannot diminish and that compression cannot increase a volume of the material. The Poisson's ratio of human cancellous bone is 0.2 to 0.3.[5,6] The clinical implications of Poisson's ratio may be minor, although there may be technical implications with regard to the accuracy of mechanical testing, especially in trabecular bone.[7]

A moment is the tendency to produce rotation, and is the product of force magnitude and perpendicular moment arm length. Like forces, moments have both internal and external effects upon their objects. The external effect of a moment is to change, or attempt to change, the angular or rotational velocity of the body. The internal effects of a moment is to cause a state of strain.

Inertia, a fundamental characteristic of all matter, is the property that causes a body to remain at rest or in uniform motion in one direction unless acted upon by an external force that changes the body with respect to the state of rest, velocity, or direction (Newton's first law). Areal moment of inertia (I) is the structural feature governing stiffness in bending. If a bone is considered to be a hollow cylinder, the areal moment of inertia is calculated by

$$I = \pi \, (a^3b - a'^3b')/64 \tag{2.4}$$

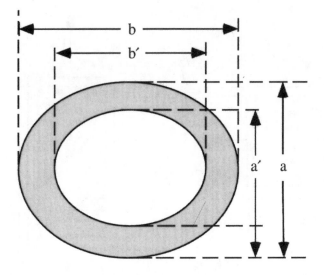

FIGURE 2.7 Illustration of the external and internal anteroposteral and side-to-side diameters for the cross sections at the loading points of the bone.

where a, a', b, and b' are the mean external and internal anteroposteral and side-to-side diameters for the cross sections at the loading points of the bone (Figure 2.7). The external diameters (a and b) are measured before testing by use of a digital caliper. After testing, the pieces are glued together and cut transversely at the break point. The dimensions of the medullary canal (a' and b') are then measured. I, as a geometric parameter, expresses the characteristics of the cross-sectional distribution relative to the transverse axis. Simply put, this explains the large differences in bending resistance of a meterstick held flat compared with when it is held on the edge and bent.[8] Polar moment of inertia is a structural feature governing stiffness in torsion and is a function of the distance the individual masses of the object are located from the axis of rotation. Basically, the further the individual masses of bone are from the axis of rotation, the greater will be the moment and the more resistant the material will be to deformation.[9]

E. LOADING MODES

Depending upon the direction of application, a force applied to an object or body can be axial (compressive and tensile), bending, torsional, or multiaxial and can be static or cyclic (repeated).

1. Compressive or Tensile Loading

In compressive or tensile loading, the force is applied perpendicular to the surface of the body or object. Typical examples are the *in vitro* compressive and tensile tests. Compressive and tensile loading can be thought of as numerous small loads directed toward or away from the surface of the structure, with maximal compressive or tensile stress occurring in a plane perpendicular to the applied load. Compressive loading *in vivo* creates a shortening and widening of the bone and is commonly seen in human vertebra. Clinically, fractures that result from tensile loading are commonly seen in cancellous bone, as in the calcaneus fracture when a strong contraction from the triceps surae occurs. Another similar condition is the avulsion fracture of the medial epicondyle of the humerus.

2. Bending

Although bones are not beams, frequently they are modeled as such, especially bones of the appendicular skeleton. Due to the general curvature of long bones, they are subjected to axial and

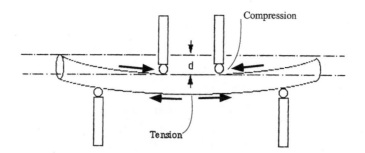

FIGURE 2.8   Illustration of bending of diaphyseal bone.

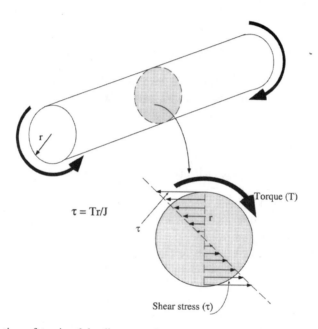

FIGURE 2.9   Illustration of torsional loading. τ = shear stress, T = torque, J = polar moment of inertia, R = the distance from the center of the cylinder to any point.

bending forces *in vivo*. Bending loads on bone may occur with three-point bending such as that seen in the tibia during a boot-top fracture which occurs when skiers fall forward over their skis. Bending causes tensile forces and lengthening on the convex side of the bone and compressive forces and shortening on the concave side. In bending, stress and strains are maximal at the surfaces of the beam and are zero at the neutral axis (Figure 2.8). Frequently, bending forces are coupled with axial and transverse loading. Because bone is best able to resist compressive loads, muscle contraction of the triceps surae, in the ski-boot-top fracture, may work to attenuate the tensile forces seen on the posterior (convex) side of the tibia, thereby reducing the chance of fracture.[3,8]

3. Torsional Loading

In torsional loading a cylinder of long bone is twisted under a torsional test, and shear stress develops (Figure 2.9). Shear stress due to torsion is expressed as:[2]

$$\tau = Tr/J \tag{2.5}$$

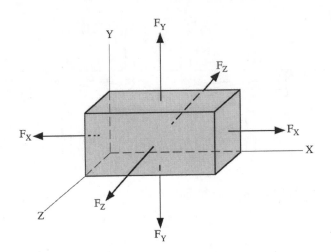

FIGURE 2.10 Multiaxial loading with applied forces in the *x, y,* and *z* directions.

where T is the torque or torsional moment of the applied force, r is the radial distance from the neutral axis to the point in the cross section at which the shear stress acts, and J is the polar moment of inertia.

4. Multiaxial Loading

While considerable progress has been made in the study of uniaxial compressive and tensile properties of bone tissue in the last several decades, multiaxial loading of bone to measure material mechanics has lagged due to the complexity and difficulty of the processes of loading and recording. Living bone is seldom loaded in one direction, but is mostly multidirectional and therefore multiaxial. For this reason, the study of multidimensional loading and the effect on bone is essential. Basically, multiaxial loading uses the same concepts as in uniaxial loading, but extends the concepts to two- and three-dimensional space. Consideration in multiaxial loading must be given for normal stresses and strains as well as shear stresses and strains. Three-dimensional analysis generally provides a more realistic assessment of the material loading complexity and may involve as many as nine material property characteristics to describe the anisotropic sample completely. Analysis of the mechanical properties of the material can be simplified by assuming symmetry and/or isotropy in two or more of the principal planes.[2] In Figure 2.10, biaxial and three-dimensional tensile loading is shown. The concepts are equally applicable to compressive loading when the force vectors would be reversed.[10]

In vivo loading of bone is difficult to assess because of the irregular geometric properties of bone and the fact that bone is commonly exposed to multiple indeterminate loads. Recent *in vivo* measures have been calculated for walking and jogging and these convincingly demonstrate the complexity of multiaxial loading. As might be expected, compression occurs at heel strike and toe-off and are tensile during the stance phase. Shear forces normally occur during the late phases of gait, and torsional forces are seen during external rotation of the tibia, as part of the screw home mechanism, as stance approaches. Running, as might be anticipated, creates a totally different loading pattern.[11]

5. Static or Cyclic

In seeking the answers to tolerable levels of force that a bone can withstand prior to fracture, the static ultimate properties of bone are of interest; however, repetitive, submaximal trauma is frequently the more significant area of concern.[12]

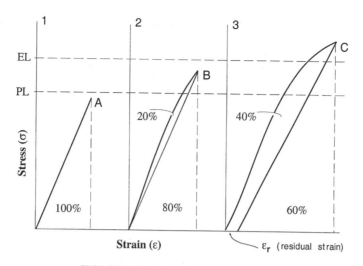

FIGURE 2.11   A typical hysteresis loop.

Loading a bone specimen cyclically with progressively higher forces produces a highly nonlinear stress–strain curve. For example, in Figure 2.11, the bone specimen is loaded up to point *A*. When the force is removed, the specimen exhibits reversible behavior and returns to its original unloaded length. The load that causes the stress–strain curve up to point *B* also permits the material to return to its original length, although the time required to return to normal is longer. Stress–strain up to point *C* produces a permanent change in the original length of the material and is not reversible. The loading and unloading curves do not overlap, but rather create a closed loop, known as a hysteresis loop, which is indicative of the inefficiency of storing and releasing of strain energy. The area under the unloading curve represents strain energy release during unloading. The area enclosed by the hysteresis loop represents energy dissipated within the material through mechanical damage and internal friction.[12]

Test-type influences the mechanical properties that bone will exhibit. Cyclic loading produces microdamage that accumulates with each cycle and the damage increases as the intensity of testing increases. Intensity can be varied through change in the load magnitude and through the number of cycles to which the specimen is exposed. Lessons learned from cyclic loading include that, once a crack occurs, the number and cyclical load required for propagation of the fracture decreases rapidly and that there is a strong negative correlation between load intensity and number of cycles needed for failure.[12]

F. Strength

Strength can be defined as the internal resistance of a material to deformation and ultimately failure or fracture. Proportional limit is the point on the load–displacement curve where the load is no longer proportional to the deformation. At this point there begins a brief region of relatively large strain for little increase in stress. It indicates that a portion of the bone structure starts to fail or crack and the structure becomes plastic. Yield strength (σ_y) is defined as the stress corresponding to a specific amount of permanent deformation. Ultimate strength defines the stress required to fracture the bone or the bone–implant interface. It is called the strength, or ultimate stress. The magnitude of strength is calculated from a mechanical test, based on the load, deformation, and the dimensions of the specimen.

G. Elasticity (Stiffness and Elastic Modulus) and Compliance

Elasticity is the ability of a material to return to its original shape when an applied stress is removed. Elasticity is quantified by a simple stiffness value or elastic modulus. Stiffness is the ability of a

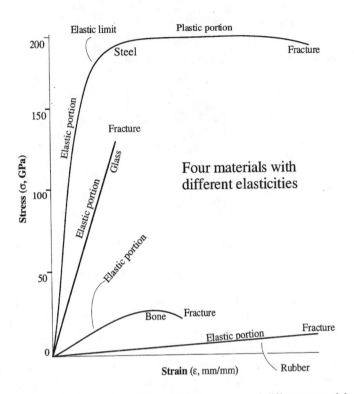

FIGURE 2.12 Illustration of the elasticities of several different materials.

material to resist being deformed when a force is applied to it. A simple stiffness value is any force divided by its corresponding deformation within the elastic range of the load–displacement curve.

$$S = F/d \qquad (2.6)$$

Elastic modulus is a standardized stiffness value and is the ratio between stress (σ) and strain (ε) or any $\Delta\sigma/\Delta\varepsilon$ within the linear portion of the stress–strain curve (Equation 2.7). The elastic modulus determined in a tensile test is also called Young's modulus.[13] The modulus of elasticity is computed in terms of force per unit area from the slope of the elastic region of the stress–strain curve. The slope is usually obtained by drawing a line tangent to the stress–strain curve. The ratio of stress to strain is not a function of the size and shape of the material being tested, but rather is a measure of the ability of the material to maintain shape under application of external loads and is therefore material dependent (Figure 2.12). The property of elasticity is time independent and completely reversible.

$$E = \sigma/\varepsilon = \Delta\sigma/\Delta\varepsilon \qquad (2.7)$$

Linearly elastic materials obey Hooke's law, which proposes that the stress and strain are linearly related and mathematically expressed as

$$\sigma = E\varepsilon \qquad (2.8)$$

The mechanical properties of biological tissues, such as bone, typically are not linear throughout their physiological range due to the nonlinear characteristics of their fluid component.

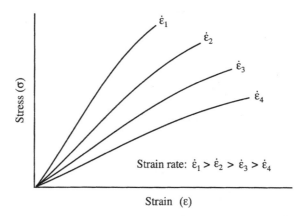

FIGURE 2.13   Effect of strain rate on elastic properties of a viscoelastic material.

Compliance is the inverse of stiffness or modulus and is defined as the ratio of deformation to load or strain to stress.[14]

$$\text{Compliance} = \varepsilon/\sigma \qquad (2.9)$$

Relative to other biological materials, bone has relatively high E values (high slope of stress–strain curve) and low compliance values. Compliant materials, such as cartilage or skin, have low E values and high compliance values. Mechanical testing machines are constructed of high-modulus materials (E of steels $\approx$ 200 GPa), so their compliance is considered as zero when testing softer materials such as cortical bone (E = 5 to 21 GPa) or cancellous bone (E < 1 GPa). If several fixture parts are used in the testing assembly, a significant machine compliance can exist. A routine testing for machine compliance is recommended by testing the fixture column without the specimen in place.

H. Fracture Energy and Toughness

The area under the stress–strain curve represents the energy absorbed when the object is loaded. This energy is stored as elastic strain energy and can be dissipated as heat. Work of fracture (toughness) is the energy required per unit volume of a material to produce fracture. The unit for work and toughness is the joule (N·m).

I. Viscoelasticity

Viscoelasticity describes the time-dependent mechanical characteristics of materials. Bone is a viscoelastic material, which means that the stress developed within bone is dependent on the rate at which the bone specimen is strained (strain rate). With increasing strain rates, the material appears stiffer and stronger, with smaller deformations (Figure 2.13). Most biological materials exhibit some degree of viscoelasticity. Two behaviors of viscoelastic materials which are important in quantifying the mechanical properties of bone are (1) stress relaxation and (2) creep. Stress relaxation is the decay of stress within a material subjected to a constant strain (Figure 2.14). Stress relaxation rate is the slope of the stress–time curve determined under a constant strain.[13] Creep is the gradual increase in strain of a material subjected to a constant load (or deformation under constant load). A creep curve displays strain vs. time under a constant force or stress (Figure 2.15). In a linearly viscoelastic material energy is dissipated by plastic or viscous flow within the material. So, the loading and unloading curves do not overlap, instead forming a closed hysteresis loop.

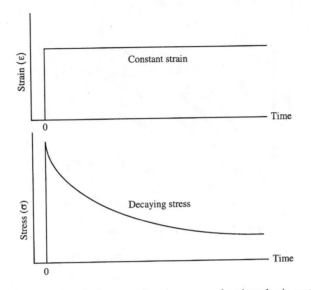

FIGURE 2.14   A typical stress relaxation curve of a viscoelastic material.

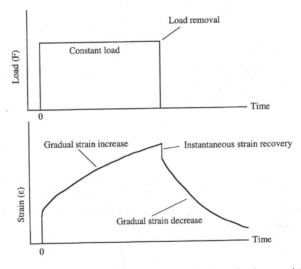

FIGURE 2.15   A typical creep curve of a viscoelastic material.

J. FAILURE, FRACTURE, FATIGUE, FATIGUE FRACTURE, BUCKLING, AND CRACKING

Failure is the degradation of a material property beyond a set limit,[13] or loss of material continuity. Fatigue is the damage due to repetitive stresses below the ultimate stress. Fatigue is a slow progressive process, as opposed to an acute, catastrophic event which results when the ultimate strength of a material is surpassed. Typically, repetitive cyclical loading (smaller than the ultimate strength) causes a crack through a material with subsequent separation of the object into pieces. Fatigue fracture in whole bone is a common finding that frequently results from the stresses imposed on the skeletal system by the muscular system during locomotion. The failure is referred to as stress fracture and is more common in females than males. The mechanism of the injury commonly occurs when there are acute bouts of strenuous exercise over an extended period of time which

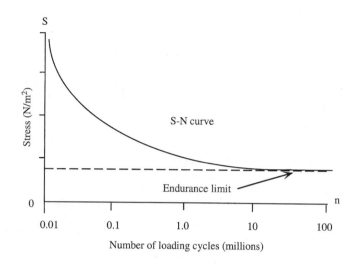

FIGURE 2.16   A typical S–N curve shows the fatigue characteristics of materials.

was immediately preceded by a relatively sedentary period. Typically, there are no prodromal signs.[15] Fatigue fractures *in vivo* result when the remodeling process is outpaced by the microdamage which accumulates with repetitive loading.[9,11] From a biomechanical point of view stress fracture is most likely to occur when the bone is repeatedly loaded at the elastic limit region.[16]

Endurance (fatigue) limit is the maximum stress that a material can sustain repeatedly without failure. Some materials, especially steels, have an endurance limit below which the material will withstand an infinite number of cycles without failure. An S–N curve is the stress–number curve representing the relationship between stress and minimum number of loadings at the stress required to produce fracture (Figure 2.16). The S–N curve is illustrated with stress plotted on the ordinate and the logarithm of the corresponding number of cycles to cause failure plotted on the abscissa. The fatigue life of a material can be affected microscopically and macroscopically by stress concentration, specimen surface geometry, and the surrounding environment.[17,18] Two distinct features of the S–N curve are (1) the lower the stress magnitude the greater the number of cycles prior to failure, and (2) the material will either demonstrate an endurance limit at or below where the material can be stressed an infinite number of times without fracture or the S–N curve will curve monotonically downward and the specimen eventually fracture no matter how low the applied load.[15]

According to a report by Choi and Goldstein,[19] trabecular specimens had significantly lower moduli and lower fatigue strength than cortical specimens, despite their higher mineral density values. Fracture surface and microdamage analyses illustrated different fracture and damage patterns between trabecular and cortical bone tissue, depending upon their microstructural characteristics.[9] When long, slender columns are considered, similar to long bones in the body, collapse of the wall of the tube laterally can produce local buckling failure, which leads to subsequent complete buckling and material failure.[2]

Cracking is incomplete loss of material continuity with near absence of unrecoverable strain, dependent somewhat on the ductility of the specimen material.[13] When stress is applied through plastic deformation, the material will ultimately break with complete molecular separation. Brittle bone cracks more readily than bone that is healthier.[20] The crack may be initiated as a stress riser, such as an indentation, scratch, or hole. Stresses near these areas can be concentrated, thereby creating local material failure with ultimate propagation of the crack.[18] Cracks will spread when energy release from the material as the crack spreads exceeds energy necessary to extend the crack and/or when stress at the crack tip reaches a value that exceeds the cohesive strength of the atoms just ahead of the crack. The latter parameter is known as the critical stress intensity factor.[15]

III. MECHANICAL MODELING AND SIMULATION

Finite-element analysis (FEA), originally developed in the 1950s, is the most popular methodology for modeling bone structure and its mechanical properties. FEA has had a profound impact on the field of orthopaedics and the modeling of bone by assisting researchers and physicians in the quantitative analysis of bone and other complex biological structures. FEA is especially useful for the modeling of irregularly shaped bones, such as vertebra and for identification of high-stress areas on bone.[21]

Basically, FEA makes use of simple shapes, known as elements (building blocks), which are assembled to form complex geometric structures which are used to solve complex problems, most of which can be represented with one or more partial differential equations.[22] The elements are connected at points known as nodes. In a model, a finite number of elements (or shapes) are connected at nodes to form a mathematical representation of a structure such as bone. The process of dividing the structure into elements of interest to create the finite-element mesh is known as discretization. The governing equations are only approximately satisfied at nodal points; therefore the finite-element technique involves replacement of partial differential equations having an infinite number of degrees of freedom with a more discrete system with a finite, albeit sometimes large, number of degrees of freedom.[22] As forces are applied to the model or as the model is deformed, elaborate equations predict the stress and strain responses of the structure to loading. The complexity of a finite-element model is determined by the imagination of its creator, the level of mathematical sophistication, and computing power.

The finite-element method (FEM) originated as a tool to assist engineers in the design of structures. The FEM approach often requires lengthy and complex calculations and therefore became tractable only with the advances in computer technology. Originally, its use was restricted to experts specializing in FEM who used large, mainframe computers to solve problems. As computer technology advanced, FEM became more accessible to nonspecialists via commercially available FE program packages. In recent years biomechanists have found finite-element modeling to be a valuable tool for investigating a wide range of biological problems, such as designing better artificial hip joints.

The three basic phases of FEM are (1) creation of the model; (2) solution; and (3) validation and interpretation of the results.

The goal of modeling is the creation of a mathematical finite description of nodes, elements, material properties, boundary and interface conditions, and load application. This is the most labor-intensive phase of FEA and can takes weeks or months, although computer technology has hastened the modeling phase. One of the initial steps is determining whether the model will be one, two, or three dimensional. Because bone is a three-dimensional structure, the model will include linear (two nodes per side) and quadratic elements (three nodes per side). Common three-dimensional elements include the linear eight-node brick and the quadratic 20-node brick, although tetrahedral and linear wedge models are also available. The costs for a three-dimensional FEM are higher than for a two-dimensional model, although limitations in the two-dimensional model frequently dictate three-dimensional use. There are two primary questions that influence whether a two-dimensional or a three-dimensional model is used: What mechanical characteristic does the third element provide? Is it necessary to solve the problem at hand?[22]

The material property specifications for FEA can be difficult when modeling bone due to the inhomogeneity and anisotropic behavior of the material. In the biomechanics literature, bone is mostly modeled as linear elastic material in a nonimpact loaded state.

Load specifications and boundary and interface conditions are the final tasks in modeling. Loads include joint reaction forces, musculotendinous forces, and ligament forces such as exist during gait, rising from a chair, or stairclimbing. Many of these loads (bending and torsion) have been identified in the recent past *in vivo* as being out-of-plane for traditional two-dimensional FEA. Symmetrical and asymmetrical boundary conditions consist of displacement constraints which are required to prevent rigid-body motion. For structures that are constructed of different materials the interface can affect the system response and needs to be accounted for. For example, in a prosthetic joint, cartilage, metal, cement, bone, and polyethylene regions need to be accounted for in the FEM.[22]

The solution requires an FEA computer program that is based on the input data from the model. Computer time, which is usually through a batch process, rather than interactive, is a function of the model nodes and numbers of degrees of freedom per node. The solution phase is completed when nodal displacements and derived quantities (stresses, strains) have been calculated and stored in digital form.

FEA validation is assessed with two distinct issues, validity and model accuracy. That is, does the model represent the true system of interest based on the modeling phase? Convergence can be used to measure the accuracy of the model. Convergence testing involves repeated refinement of the finite-element mesh and subsequent reanalysis to determine how the changes affect the predictions of the model. If possible, the validation should include comparisons of strain gauge data, *in vivo* load-sensing implants, and other analytical solution techniques.

Interpretation of results involves interactive graphics based on a postprocessing program. Contour plots and color fringe plots are common methods of stress and strain display. A common pitfall, especially in orthopaedics, is overemphasis on stress and strain variables, because despite the most accurate models the values are idealized at some level. The results of FEA need to be interpreted based on meaningful measures: Will the bone fracture? Is the prosthesis appropriate for the bone stock available? Will the prosthesis loosen as a result of activity?

Due to the variability and uncertainties with use of FEA one should view FEA as more of a qualitative tool than as a quantitative measurement device, although when the FEA of today is compared with the same technique from 20 years ago it is clear that the technique is becoming more relevant, accessible, and valuable.[22]

IV. SUMMARY

Bone is a nonlinear, viscoelastic, anisotropic, and heterogeneous material and therefore can be complex to analyze mechanically. The fact that bone has the inherent ability to adapt continually to metabolic and environmental changes *in vivo* provides even more complexity, further limiting our understanding of specific bony mechanisms. Many of the basic mechanical concepts presented in this chapter are currently in use and will continue to be utilized to explore the mechanical behavior of bone and other biological tissues. Despite the fact that the major points in this chapter were divided into sections, it is important to note that all of the concepts are interrelated in challenging and fascinating ways. Analytical models, including FEA, which account for bone geometry and its heterogeneous properties, depend on appropriate material and mechanical estimates. While sophisticated, complex testing is demanded in some circumstances to answer relevant questions, it is wise to begin testing with simple ideas and hypotheses. The long-term objective for a majority of bone studies is to characterize and better understand the relationship between the structure and mechanical behavior of bone. The central issue, however, for all researchers in bioengineering is to identify the most appropriate variables for their area of interest and then to blend them into understandable and useful contexts.

REFERENCES

1. Cowin, S.C., Mechanics of materials, in *Bone Mechanics*, Cowin, S.C., Ed., CRC Press, Boca Raton, FL, 1989, 16.
2. Biewener, A.A., Overview of structural mechanics, in *Biomechanics, Structures and System. A Practical Approach*, Biewener, A.A., Ed., IRL Press, Oxford, 1992.
3. Frankel, V.H. and Burstein, A.H., *Orthopaedic Biomechanics*, Lea & Febiger, Philadelphia, 1970.

4. Ashman, R.B., Experimental techniques, in *Bone Mechanics*, Cowin, S.C., Ed., CRC Press, Boca Raton, FL, 1989, 91.
5. Vasu, R., Carter, D.R., and Harris, W.H., Stress distributions in the acetabular region — I. Before and after total joint replacement, *J. Biomech.*, 15, 155, 1982.
6. Brodt, M.D., Swan, C.C., and Brown, T.D., Mechanical behavior of human morselized cancellous bone in triaxial compression testing, *J. Orthop. Res.*, 16, 43, 1998.
7. Keaveny, T.M. and Hayes, W.C., A 20-year perspective on the mechanical properties of trabecular bone, *J. Biomech. Eng.*, 115, 534, 1993.
8. Hayes, W.C. and Bouxsein, M.L., Biomechanics of cortical and trabecular bone: implications for assessment of fracture risk, in *Basic Orthopaedic Biomechanics*, Mow, V.C. and Hayes, W.C., Eds., Lippincott-Raven, Philadelphia, 1997, Chapter 3.
9. Einhorn, T.A., Biomechanics of bone, in *Principles of Bone Biology*, Bilezikian, J.P., Raisz, L.G., and Rodan, G.A., Eds., Academic Press, San Diego, CA, 1996, 25.
10. Whiting, W.C. and Zernicke, R.F., Biomechanical concepts, in *Biomechanics of Musculoskeletal Injury*, Whiting, W.C. and Zernicke, R.F., Eds., Human Kinetics, Champaign, IL, 1998, 41.
11. Nordin, M. and Frankel, V.H., Biomechanics of whole bones and bone tissue, in *Basic Biomechanics of Skeletal System*, Frankel, V.H. and Nordin, M., Eds., Lea & Febiger, Philadelphia, 1980, 15.
12. Burstein, A.H. and Wright, T.M., *Fundamentals of Orthopaedic Biomechanics*, Williams & Wilkins, Baltimore, MD, 1994.
13. Black, J., *Orthopaedic Biomaterials in Research and Practice*, Churchill Livingstone, New York, 1988.
14. An, Y.H., Kang, Q., and Friedman, R.J., Mechanical symmetry of rabbit bones studied by bending and indentation testing, *Am. J. Vet. Res.*, 57, 1786, 1996.
15. Currey, J., *The Mechanical Adaptations of Bones*, Princeton University Press, Princeton, NJ, 1984.
16. Chamay, A., Mechanical and morphological aspects of experimental overload and fatigue in bone, *J. Biomech.*, 3, 263, 1970.
17. Caputo, A.A. and Standlee, J.P., Eds., *Biomechanics in Clinical Dentistry*, Quintessence Publishing, Chicago, 1987.
18. Tencer, A.F. and Johnson, K.D., *Biomechanics in Orthopedic Trauma. Bone Fracture and Fixation*, M. Dunitz, London, 1994.
19. Choi, K. and Goldstein, S.A., A comparison of the fatigue behavior of human trabecular and cortical bone tissue, *J. Biomech.*, 25, 1371, 1992.
20. Low, J. and Reed, A., *Basic Biomechanics Explained*, Butterworth Heinemann, London, 1996.
21. Ranu, H.S., The role of finite-element modeling in biomechanics, in *Material Properties and Stress Analysis in Biomechanics*, Yettram, A.L., Ed., Manchester University Press, Manchester, 1989, 164.
22. Beaupré, G.S. and Carter, D.R., Finite element analysis in biomechanics, in *Biomechanics — Structure and Systems*, Biewener, A.A., Ed., Oxford University Press, Oxford, 1992, 150.

3 Mechanical Properties of Bone

Yuehuei H. An

CONTENTS

I. INTRODUCTION

Before and during the process of testing bone mechanical properties, the researcher has to learn the basic structural and mechanical properties of bone. These properties include cortical and cancellous bone at the level of whole bones, bone tissues, osteons or trabeculae, bone lamellae, and ideally the nano- or ultrastructure such as collagen fibers, fibrils, molecules, and mineral components.[1,2] These basic structural and mechanical data are searchable in the journal literature and also have been written about in numerous textbooks.

Bone has a hierarchical structure and coherent mechanical properties as proposed initially by Katz[3] in 1970s and further developed recently by Rho et al.[4] and Hoffler et al. (see Chapter 8). In general, this hierarchical structure and the related mechanical properties can be investigated and considered at the five levels shown in Table 3.1.

The author believes that one of the reasons to separate whole bone and bone tissue blocks is that the mechanical determinants of these two levels of structures are different. For example, the bending mechanical properties of a long bone are determined by its tubular shape and bone densities, while that of a cortical cut beam are by bone densities and osteonal direction (see Section IIB). As pointed out by Katz[3] nearly 20 years ago, it is essential to understand the "form–function" (structure–mechanics) relationship of the bone specimen to be tested. The bone hierarchical composite modeling is based on both the structural evaluations and mechanical measurements at different levels.

TABLE 3.1
The Hierarchical Levels of Bone

Level	Elements (Specimens)	Main Factors Determining Bone Strength
Macrostructure (whole bone)	Femur, humerus, vertebrae, frontal bone, phalangeal bones, calcaneous, etc.	Macrostructure such as tubular shape, cross-sectional area, and porosity of long bone, cortical bone-covered vertebrae, or the irregular pelvic bone
Architecture (tissue level)	Compact bone or cancellous bone blocks, cylinders, cubes, or beams	Densities, porosity, the orientations of osteon, collagen fibers, or trabeculae
Microstructure (osteonal or trabecular level)	Osteons, trabeculae	Loading direction, with maximum strength along their long axis
Submicrostructure (lamellar level)	Lamella, large collagen fibers	Collagen-HA fibrils are formed into large collagen fibers or lamellar sheets with preferred directions. The orientations of the fibrils define directions of maximum and minimum strengths for a primary loading direction
Ultrastructure (nanostructure)	Collagen fibril and molecule, mineral components	HA crystals are embedded between the ends of adjoining collagen molecules; this composite of rigid HA and flexible collagen provides a material that is superior in mechanical properties to either of them alone, more ductile than hydroxyapatite, allowing the absorption of more energy, and more rigid than collagen, permitting greater load bearing

Adapted from the work by Rho et al.[4] and Hoffler et al. in Chapter 8.

However, due to the scope of this text, this chapter covers only the basic mechanical properties of cortical and cancellous bone at whole bone, bone tissue, and microstructural levels (osteon and trabeculae), the effects of porosity and densities on mechanical properties, the anisotropic and heterogeneous characteristics of bone mechanical properties, and some basic considerations of the validity of the continuum assumption commonly used in mechanical testing.

For more detailed descriptions of basic and theoretical mechanics of bone, one can refer to several books, including *Strength of Biological Materials* by Yamada (1970),[5] *Mechanical Properties of Bone* by Evans (1973),[6] *The Mechanical Adaptations of Bones* by Currey (1984),[7] *Bone Mechanics,* edited by Cowin (1999),[8] and *Skeletal Tissue Mechanics* by Martin et al.,[9] and several book chapters or journal articles by Nordin and Frankel (1980),[10] Albright (1987),[11] Einhorn (1996),[12] Hayes and Bouxsein (1997),[13] Whiting and Zernicke (1998),[14] and Rho et al.[4]

II. MECHANICAL PROPERTIES OF CORTICAL BONE

A. GENERAL MECHANICAL PROPERTIES

For mechanical testing, cortical bones are often used as a whole bone or tailored into beams or rods. A whole diaphyseal bone is commonly tested using bending and torsional tests. A beam is a bar or rod with constant cross-sectional shape and area, which can be spherical, square, or rectangular. A variable beam is a beam with inconsistent cross-sectional shape and area, such as long bones. A cantilever beam is a beam that is fixed at one end and usually used for cantilever bending tests. A dumbbell sample is a dumbbell-shaped bone specimen made specifically for mechanical testing, such as tensile or torsional tests. The dense nature of cortical bone determines its strong and stiff mechanical properties compared with cancellous bone. For comparison, Figure 3.1 gives the elastic modulus and strength of bone (cortical bone) and several other common tissues and biomaterials.

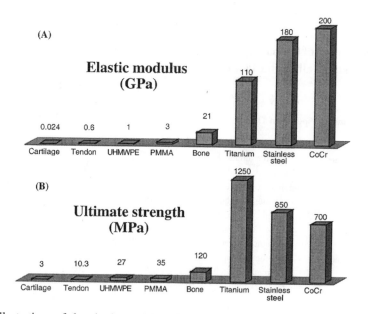

FIGURE 3.1 Illustrations of the elastic modulus (A) and strength (B) of bone (cortical bone) and other common tissues and biomaterials.

The mechanical properties of cortical bone depend on the type of mechanical testing. According to the data collected in Table 3.2, the strength and elastic modulus by compression tests range from 133 to 295 MPa (200 ± 36 MPa) and from 14.7 to 34.3 GPa (average 23 ± 4.8 GPa), respectively. The strength and elastic modulus by tensile tests range from 92 to 188 MPa (average 141 ± 28 MPa) and from 7.1 to 28.2 GPa (average 19.6 ± 6.2 GPa), respectively. The strength and elastic modulus by torsional tests range from 53 to 76 MPa (average 65 ± 9 MPa) and from 3.1 to 3.7 GPa, respectively. The tensile strength is about $2/3$ that of compression strength. The torsional (shear) strength is approximately $1/3$ to $1/2$ of the values of the longitudinal strength (tested by bending, tensile, or compressive tests) (Table 3.3). And the torsional (shear) modulus is only about $1/6$ to $1/5$ of the longitudinal modulus. Although the tensile test is the standard method for testing mechanical properties of cortical bone, bending tests are used the most often.

The bending strength and elastic modulus of cortical bone ranges from 35 to 283 MPa and from 5 to 23 GPa, respectively (excluding the questionable values marked with [c], Tables 3.3 and 3.4). Note the significant differences between the two levels.

As mentioned earlier, the bending mechanical properties of a long bone are determined by its tubular shape and bone densities, while that of cortical cut beams are by bone densities and osteonal direction. Table 3.5 contains the average values of the individual reports listed in Tables 3.3 and 3.4. It clearly shows that the values of strength and elastic modulus of the two levels of bone tissue are different. Both the strength and elastic modulus of whole bone are about 60% of that of cortical bone beams. One should be aware of the fact that besides the true difference between the two levels of structures, there are several other factors possibly playing important roles, such as the equations used for calculations, the specimen aspect ratio (larger for beams), or the size of the specimens tested. These speculations have already been partially addressed by Sedlin and Hirsch.[25] Further studies are still needed to determine the relevance of each of these factors.

B. BONE DENSITY

The material density of cortical bone is the wet weight divided by the specimen volume. It is a function of both the porosity and mineralization of the bone materials. Cortical bone has an average

TABLE 3.2
Mechanical Properties of Human and Bovine Cortical Bones Tested by Compression, Tensile, and Torsional Testing (all at the tissue level)

Species	Bone	Specimen Dimensions	Strength (MPa)	Elastic Modulus (GPa)	Reference
Compression Test					
Human	Femur	2 × 2 × 6 mm dumbbell	167–215[a]	14.7–19.7[a]	Reilly 1974[15]
		2 × 2 × 6 mm dumbbell	179–209[a]	15.4–18.6[a]	Burstein 1976[16]
		3 mm diam. cylindrical dumbbell	205–206[a]	—	Cezayirlioglu 1985[17]
	Tibia	2 × 2 × 6 mm dumbbell	183–213[a]	24.5–34.3[a]	Burstein 1976[16]
		3 mm diam. cylindrical dumbbell	192–213[a]	—	Cezayirlioglu 1985[17]
Bovine	Femur	3.8 × 2.3 × 76 mm dumbbell	133	24.1–27.6[a]	McElhaney 1964[18]
		2 × 2 × 6 mm dumbbell	240–295[a]	21.9–31.4[a]	Reilly 1974[15]
	Tibia	4 × 5 mm rectangular	165	23.8 ± 2.2	Simkin 1973[19]
		2 × 2 × 6 mm dumbbell	228 ± 31	20.9 ± 3.26	Reilly 1974[15]
		3 mm diam. cylindrical dumbbell	217 ± 27	—	Cezayirlioglu 1985[17]
Means ± SD (n^b)			200 ± 36 (10)	23.0 ± 4.8 (7)	
Tensile Test					
Human	Femur	3.8 × 2.3 × 76 mm dumbbell	66–107[a]	10.9–20.6[a]	Evans 1951[20]
		2 × 2 × 6 mm dumbbell	107–140[a]	11.4–19.7[a]	Reilly 1974[15]
		2 × 2 × 6 mm dumbbell	120–140[a]	15.6–17.7[a]	Burstein 1976[16]
		3 mm diam. cylindrical dumbbell	133–136[a]	—	Cezayirlioglu 1985[17]
	Tibia	2 × 2 × 6 mm dumbbell	145–170[a]	18.9–29.2[a]	Burstein 1976[16]
		1.7 × 1.8 × 25 mm beam	162 ± 15	19.7 ± 2.4	Vincetelli 1985[21]
		3 mm diam. cylindrical dumbbell	154–158[a]	—	Cezayirlioglu 1985[17]
Bovine	Femur	3.8 × 2.3 × 76 mm dumbbell	92	20.5	McElhaney 1964[18]
		2 × 2 × 6 mm dumbbell	129–182[a]	23.1–30.4[a]	Reilly 1974[15]
		3 mm diam. cylindrical dumbbell	162 ± 14[a]	—	Cezayirlioglu 1985[17]
	Tibia	4 × 5 × 30 mm dumbbell	136	7.1 ± 1.1	Simkin 1973[19]
		2 × 2 × 6 mm dumbbell	152 ± 17	21.6 ± 5.3	Reilly 1974[15]
		2 × 2 × 6 mm dumbbell	188 ± 9	28.2 ± 6.4	Burstein 1975[22]
Means ± SD (n^b)			141 ± 28 (13)	19.6 ± 6.2 (10)	
Torsional Test					
Human	Femur	?	53	—	Hazama 1964[23]
		?	54 ± 0.6	3.2	Yamada 1970[5]
		2 × 2 × 6 mm dumbbell	—	3.1–3.7[a]	Reilly 1974[15]
		3 × 3 × 6 mm dumbbell	65–71[a]	—	Reilly 1975[24]
		3 mm diam. cylindrical dumbbell	68–71[a]	—	Cezayirlioglu 1985[17]
	Tibia	3 mm diam. cylindrical dumbbell	66–71[a]	—	Cezayirlioglu 1985[17]
Bovine	Femur	3 × 3 × 6 mm dumbbell	62–67[a]	—	Reilly 1975[24]
		3 mm diam. cylindrical dumbbell	76 ± 6	—	Cezayirlioglu 1985[17]
Means ± SD (n^b)		65 ± 9 (7)	3.3 ± 0.1 (2)		

[a] Range of average values from different subjects.
[b] Number of data sets from the literature.

apparent density of approximately 1.9 g/cm^3.[1,2] For cortical bone, apparent density and material density are basically the same, as there is no marrow space in compact bone. Therefore, "cortical bone density" is commonly used to describe the density of cortical bone. There is a positive correlation between apparent density of cortical bone and its mechanical properties.[45] The true meaning of bone mineral density (BMD) is bone mineral mass per unit bone volume, or "ash

TABLE 3.3
Bending Properties of Cortical Bones at the Bone Tissue Level

Species	Bone	Specimen	Strength (MPa)	Elastic Modulus (GPa)	Reference
Human	Femur	2 × 5 × 50 mm beam	181	15.5	Sedlin 1966[25]
		3 × 3 × 30 mm beam	103–238[a]	9.82–15.7[a]	Keller 1990[26]
		0.4 × 5 × 7 mm beam	225 ± 28	12.5 ± 2.1	Lotz 1991[27]
		2.0 × 3.4 × 40 mm	142–170[a]	9.1–14.4[a]	Curry 1997[28]
Cattle	Femur	2 × 3.5 × 30 mm beam	—	18.5 ± 2.8	Curry 1988[29]
		2 × 4 × 35 mm beam	228 ± 5	19.4 ± 0.7	Curry 1988[30]
		2 × 30.4 mm beam	209 ± 13	18.1 ± 0.5	Curry 1995[31]
	Tibia	4 × 4 × 35 mm beam	—	14.1	Simkin 1973[19]
		4 × 10 × 80 mm beam	230 ± 18	21.0 ± 1.9	Martin 1993[32]
Horse	Femur	2 × 2 × 40 mm beam	204–247[a]	17.1–19.9[a]	Schryver 1978[33]
		2 × 3.5 × 30 mm beam	—	21.2 ± 1.9	Curry 1988[29]
	Radius	2 × 2 × 40 mm beam	217–249[a]	16.2–20.2[a]	Schryver 1979[33]
	Metacarpus	2 × 2 × 40 mm beam	226–240[a]	17.0–18.4[a]	Schryver 1978[33]
	3MT, 3MC[b]	1.8 × 4.5 × 70 mm	195–226[a]	14–16[a]	Bigot 1996[34]
Sheep	Metatarsus	2 × 3.5 × 30 mm beam	—	18.9 ± 2.2	Curry 1988[29]
Donkey	Radius	2 × 3.5 × 30 mm beam	—	17.6 ± 2.0	Curry 1988[29]
Goose	Femur	0.75 × 0.75 × 25 mm beam	232–283[a]	16.9–20.7[a]	McAlister 1983[35]

[a] Range of average values.

[b] Third metatarsus and third metacarpus.

density" if an ashing (or burning) method is used.[26,46] Similarly, the true meaning of bone mineral content (BMC) describes the ratio of unit weight of the mineral portion to dry bone unit weight and is frequently reported as a percentage.

BMD and BMC are positively correlated with the strength and stiffness of various bones, such as human ulna,[47] human femur and tibia,[45,48] bovine femur and tibia,[32,46] feline femur,[49] and a wide variety of animal bones.[50] Using tension testing of wet bovine Haversian cortical bone, Burstein et al.[22] demonstrated the role of mineral content on mechanical strength. Progressive surface decalcification of this bone with dilute hydrochloric acid resulted in progressive decreases in the tension yield point and the ultimate stress with no change in the yield strain or ultimate strain unless decalcification was complete. Their findings are consistent with an elastic-plastic model for the mineral phase of bone tissue in which the mineral contributes the major portion of the tension yield strength. Currey[51,52] and Schaffler and Burr[46] found that small changes in the amount or mineral density of cortical bone exert a more pronounced influence on its elastic property than would similar changes in trabecular bone. Currey studied the relationship between the bending and tensile elastic modulus of cortical bone from 17 vertebrate species to porosity and mineralization. He found that these two factors together accounted for 84% of the stiffness variation.[30] Recently, the influence of wet and dry apparent density, percentage of mineral on the tension and shear fracture toughness of tubular bone have been studied by Yeni et al.[45] They found that compositional parameters altogether can explain 35 to 59% of the variation in fracture toughness of the cortical bone.

Many reports have shown linear or exponential increases in bone stiffness with increasing mineralization, such as the one proposed by Schaffler and Burr:[46]

$$E = 89.1M3.91$$ (3.1)

where E is compressive elastic modulus and M is mineralization of bovine cortical bone.

TABLE 3.4
Bending Properties of Cortical Bones at the Whole Bone Level

Species	Bone	Specimen	Strength (MPa)	Elastic Modulus (GPa)	Reference
Monkey	Tibia	Whole bone	—	9.0 ± 1.3	Kasra 1994[36]
Dog	Humerus	Whole bone	193 ± 35	2.7 ± 0.6[c]	Kaneps 1997[37]
Pig	Femur	Whole bone	39.9	0.37[c]	Crenshaw 1981[38]
	Rib	Whole bone	35.6	2.24[c]	Crenshaw 1981[38]
	3MC[b]	Whole bone	37.2	0.22[c]	Crenshaw 1981[38]
Cat	Femur	Whole bone	36 ± 9.47	7.1 ± 0.9	Ayers 1996[39]
	Tibia	Whole bone	60.5 ± 12	11.4 ± 3.2	Ayers 1996[39]
Rabbit	Femur	Whole bone	130 ± 5	13.6 ± 0.4	An 1996[40]
		Whole bone	88 ± 20	10.7 ± 2.5	Ayers 1996[39]
	Tibia	Whole bone	195 ± 6	21.3 ± 0.7	An 1996[40]
		Whole bone	192 ± 47	23.3 ± 7.0	Ayers 1996[39]
	Humerus	Whole bone	167 ± 5	13.3 ± 0.6	An 1996[40]
Rat	Femur	Whole bone	180 ± 6	6.9 ± 0.3	Jørgensen 1991[41]
		Whole bone	134 ± 4	8.0 ± 0.4	Barengolts 1993[42]
		Whole bone	153 ± 45	4.9 ± 4	Ejersted 1993[43]
Mouse	Femur	Whole bone	104–173[a]	8.8–11.4[a]	Simske 1992[44]
		Whole bone	40 ± 13	5.3 ± 1.8	Ayers 1996[39]
	Tibia	Whole bone	78 ± 12	8.9 ± 0.2	Ayers 1996[39]

[a] Range of average values.
[b] Third metatarsus and third metacarpus.
[c] Value is questionable.

TABLE 3.5
Comparison of Mechanical Properties of Whole Long Bones and Cortical Bone Rods or Beams

	Whole Bones	Rods or Beams	Difference	Ratio, %	P Value
Strength (MPa)	125 ± 58 (n = 14[a])	202 ± 40 (n = 13[b])	77	61.8	<0.05
Elastic modulus (GPa)	10.3 ± 5.7 (n = 15[a])	16.5 ± 3.6 (n = 16[b])	6.2	62.4	<0.05

[a] n = the number of strength or elastic modulus values from 14 to 15 studies or experiments chosen from Table 3.4 (the three sets of questionable values are not included).
[b] Number of values taken from Table 3.3.

With the development of modern absorptiometric techniques, BMD and BMC can be measured noninvasively. Such methods include radiographic absorptiometry (RA), single photon absorptiometry (SPA), dual energy absorptiometry (DEA), or dual-energy X-ray absorptiometry (DEXA), quantitative computed tomography (QCT), micro-CT (μCT), peripheral CT (pCT), magnetic resonance imaging (MRI), and ultrasound methods.[53] Extensive studies have been done on the correlation between cortical bone densities measured by above-mentioned methods, such as BMD and BMC, and the mechanical properties of bone.[48,53,54] These methods are commonly used for predicting fracture risk and for the diagnosis of osteoporosis.

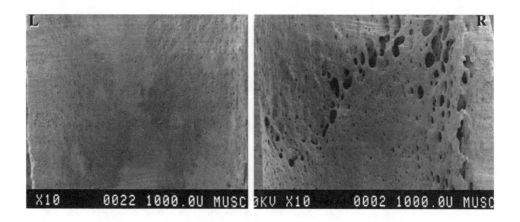

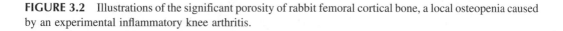

FIGURE 3.2 Illustrations of the significant porosity of rabbit femoral cortical bone, a local osteopenia caused by an experimental inflammatory knee arthritis.

C. POROSITY

The strong effects of porosity of cortical bone on mechanical properties have been well studied.[9] It is easy to understand that a more porous bone has a weaker mechanical strength. Porosity (p) is defined as the ratio of void volume to total volume, which is commonly measured on two dimensional histologic sections (traditionally point counting)[29,46] or X rays.[55] In cortical bone, the mechanical properties are affected by Haversion canals and related resorption cavities and vascular channels. There are reports on the correlations of porosity and mechanical properties, such as the equation proposed by Schaffler and Burr[46] on bovine cortical bone using tensile tests:

$$E = 33.9 \ (1-p)^{10.9} \qquad (3.2)$$

where E is the elastic modulus and $(1-p)$ is the bone volume fraction, and the equation by Currey for cortical bone of a wide variety of species under tension is

$$E = 23.4 \ (1-p)^{5.74} \qquad (3.3)$$

McElhaney et al.[56] found that

$$E = 12.4 \ (1-p)^{3} \qquad (3.4)$$

for compression of human skull bones.

Figure 3.2 shows significant porosity of rabbit femoral cortical bone, a localized osteopenia caused by an experimental inflammatory knee arthritis.[57] The bone loss leads to subendosteal cavitation and conversion of the inner portion of the cortex to a trabecular-like structure. These changes reduced the bending strength of the femur from 97 ± 21 MPa to 80 ± 16 MPa and the elastic modulus from 8.3 ± 1.5 to 7.1 ± 1.4 GPa.

D. ANISOTROPY AND HETEROGENEITY

The meaning of *anisotropic* is nonuniform or unevenly distributed, and is the opposite of isotropic. The structural anisotropy determines the mechanical anisotropy. The mechanical properties of cortical bone depend on loading directions of the testing method. The longitudinal (0° normally

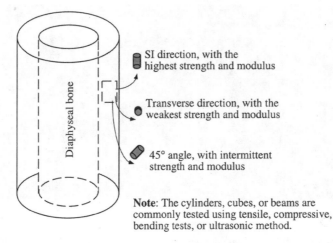

Note: The cylinders, cubes, or beams are commonly tested using tensile, compressive, bending tests, or ultrasonic method.

FIGURE 3.3 Cortical bone cylindrical specimens taken from different directions from the cortex, showing the anisotropic characteristics of cortical bone.

the weight-bearing direction) elastic modulus is the highest, the transverse (90° lateral directions) elastic modulus is the lowest, and the moduli of the specimens taken at any angles in between 0 and 90° have intermittent magnitudes (Figure 3.3).[2,4,58-60] The reason for the anisotropic phenomenon is the longitudinally oriented collagen fibers and osteons.[9,32] Sasaki et al.[61] studied the orientation of hydroxyapatite (HA) crystals in bovine femoral mineral using X-ray pole figure analysis. It was found that the *c*-axis of HA generally orients parallel to the longitudinal axis of bone (bone axis) and a significant amount of *c*-axis was oriented in other directions, in particular, perpendicular to the bone axis. They concluded that the anisotropy in mechanical properties of bone can be well explained by taking account of the nonlongitudinal (off-bone) axial distribution of orientation of bone mineral. Similar findings were also reported by Turner et al.[62]

Cortical bone is mechanically heterogeneous, which had already been documented nearly 50 years ago by Evans and Lebow in 1951.[20] They found that the middle third of the femoral shaft has the highest ultimate strength and elastic modulus and the lower third has the lowest average strength and modulus. The lateral quadrant of the shaft has the highest ultimate tensile strength while the anterior quadrant has the lowest. McAlister and Moyle[35] studied the ultimate compressive strength and modulus of elasticity of femoral cortical bone (femur) from adult geese by sex and by quadrant by compressing small right circular cylinders and the bending strength and elastic modulus by a three-point bending test on small rectangular prisms. They found that both the females and males had a significantly lower modulus and strength in the anterior quadrant as compared with other quadrants by both compression and bending tests. Their data are in accordance with that of Evans and Lebow.[20] Using ultrasonic techniques, Rho[122] measured the elastic properties of eight human tibiae to determine and map the elastic properties of cortical and cancellous bone. The study showed cortical bone to be at least orthotropic in its material symmetry. The mechanical properties of cortical bone are more homogeneous along the length than around the circumference. The variations in the properties around the quadrant of cortical bone are small, less than 10%.

E. SINGLE OSTEONS AND MICROSPECIMENS

The mechanical properties of single osteons or cortical bone microspecimens have been tested by several groups using bending, compression, tensile, and torsional methods (Table 3.6). Based on the angles of the fiber directions of two successive lamellae, Ascenzi et al.[63,64] classified three osteon types: (1) transversal (T) osteon having marked transversal spiral course of fiber bundles in successive lamellae; (2) alternate (A) osteon having fiber bundles in one lamella making an angle

TABLE 3.6
Mechanical Properties of Single Osteons or Microcortical Bone Specimens

Specimen	Test Method	Elastic Modulus (GPa)	Reference
Human tibia	Acoustic speaker (alternate tension and compression)	11.7	Fraska 1981[65]
	Three-point-bending (100 × 170 × 1500 μm beam)	3.07–7.63	Choi 1990[67]
Human femur			
L osteon	Three-point-bending	2.32 ± 1.20	Ascenzi 1990[67]
A osteon	Three-point-bending	2.69 ± 0.93	
L osteon	Tension	11.7 ± 5.8	Ascenzi 1968[66]
A osteon	Tension	5.5 ± 2.6	
L osteon	Compressive	6.3 ± 1.8	Ascenzi 1968[63]
A osteon	Compressive	7.4 ± 1.6	
T osteon	Compressive	9.3 ± 1.6	
Goose femur	Compressive (0.8 × 2.5 mm cylinder)	13.2 ± 34	McAlister 1983[35]

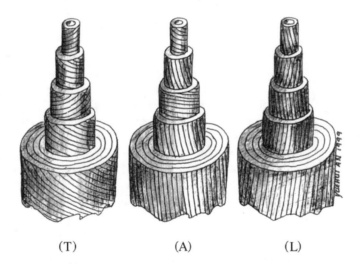

(T)   (A)   (L)

FIGURE 3.4 Illustrations of the three types of osteons — transversal (T) osteon, alternate (A) osteron, and longitudinal (L) osteron — found by Ascenzi et al. (Adapted from Ascenzi, A. and Bonuci, E., The compressive properties of single osteons, *Anat. Rec.,* 161, 377, 1968.)

of nearly 90° with the fiber bundles of the next one; and (3) longitudinal (L) osteon having marked longitudinal spiral course of fiber bundles in successive lamellae (Figure 3.4). They found that the A osteons are more resistant to bending stress. The Type L osteons are stronger in tension and Type A osteons are weaker in tension. Under compressive loading, Type T osteons are stronger than Type A and L osteons. Based on the data included in Table 3.6, most osteonal or microcortical bone specimens have their elastic moduli falling in the range of 2 to 12 GPa. Variations in the mechanical properties of osteons with different collagen fiber directions suggest that they are individually adapted to enhance locally the ability of bone to support a particular type of stress.

Microanisotropy càn be used to describe the uneven distribution of structures at the osteonal level.[62] Based on the study by Turner et al.,[62] the anisotropic elastic symmetry of osteonal bone reflects the ultrastructural organization of collagen fibrils and mineral crystals within the osteons as well as the lamellar microstructure. Turner et al. reported measurements of bone anisotropy using high-precision acoustic microscopy. The elastic properties of canine femoral bone specimens were measured at 10° increments from the long axis of the bone. Half of the bone specimens subsequently were demineralized in EDTA solution, the other half were decollagenized in sodium hypochlorite solution, and the acoustic measurements were repeated. It was found the elastic symmetry of osteonal bone deviates significantly from orthotropic theory, supporting the hypothesis that the lamellar microstructure forms a "rotated plywood."[68] The principal orientation of bone mineral was along the long axis of the bone, while bone collagen appeared to be aligned at a 30° angle to the long axis. The misalignment between the mineral and the collagen suggests that (1) a substantial percentage of the mineral is extrafibrillar, and (2) the alignment of extrafibrillar mineral is governed by external influences, e.g., mechanical stresses.

III. MECHANICAL PROPERTIES OF CANCELLOUS BONE

The porous nature of cancellous bone, with bony trabecular columns and struts and marrow-filled pores or cavities (a two-phase structure)[69-72] lends itself to a mechanical description by both structural and material properties. The mechanical properties of cancellous bone are determined by several major factors, including apparent density and ash density, trabecular connectivity, and location and function.

A. STRUCTURAL PROPERTIES

The structural properties of cancellous bone are commonly measured by compression, tensile, or bending tests. The common phrase "mechanical properties of cancellous bone" means the structural properties. It is known that the strength and elastic modulus by tensile tests are smaller than that by compression tests. For example, the strength by tensile test is approximately 60% of the value by compression test reported by Kaplan et al.,[73] and the elastic modulus by tensile test is approximately 70% of the value by compression test reported by Keaveny et al.[74,75]

According to the selected data from the literature (Table 3.7), the values of strength and elastic moduli of cancellous bone are 1.5 to 38 MPa and 10 to 1570 MPa, respectively. The structural properties of cancellous bone are much smaller than those of cortical bone. The average values of elastic modulus are several hundred mega pascal for cancellous bone,[76] compared with 5 to 21 GPa for cortical bone.[29]

B. BONE DENSITY

There is a strong correlation between the mechanical properties of cancellous bone, both for strength and stiffness, and its apparent density and mineral (or ash) density. The apparent density of cancellous bone ranges from 0.14 to 1.10 g/cm³ (average: 0.62 g/cm³, $n = 16$; see Table 3.7). The compressive strength (σ in MPa) of cancellous bone is related to its apparent density (ρ in g/cm³) by a power law of the form:[13]

$$\sigma = 60\rho^2 \tag{3.5}$$

The compressive modulus (E in MPa) of cancellous bone is related to the apparent density (ρ in g/cm³) by:[13]

$$E = 2915\rho^2 \tag{3.6}$$

Selected data of ash densities of human and animal cancellous bones are also listed in Table 3.2; they range from 0.19 to 0.56 g/cm³ with an average of 0.37 ± 0.10 g/cm³ ($n = 12$), which is about 60% of the value of apparent density as shown in the following equation:

$$\rho_{Ash} \approx 0.6 \times \rho_{Apparent} \tag{3.7}$$

TABLE 3.7
Mechanical Properties and Densities of Cancellous Bone Tissues

Bone	Specimen	Ultimate Strength (MPa)	Elastic Modulus (MPa)	Apparent Density (g/cm³)	Ash Density (g/cm³)	Reference
Human						
Femoral head	8 mm diam. cylinder	9.3 ± 4.5	900 ± 710	—	—	Martens 1983[77]
Proximal femur	8 mm diam. cylinder	6.6 ± 6.3	616 ± 707	—	—	Martens 1983[77]
Distal femur	8 mm cube	5.6 ± 3.8	298 ± 224	0.43 ± 0.15	0.26 ± 0.08	Kuhn 1989[78]
	10.3 mm diam., 5 mm cylinder	1.5–45[a]	10–500[a]	0.24 ± 0.09	—	Carter 1977[69]
	5 mm diam./7.5 mm cylinder	5.96	103–1058[a]	0.46	—	Odgaard 1989[79]
Proximal tibia	7.5:7.5 mm cylinder	5.3 ± 2.9	445 ± 257	—	—	Linde 1989[80]
Vertebral body	Dimensions ? cylinders	—	165 ± 110	0.14 ± 0.06	—	Keaveny 1997[81]
Monkey						
Femoral head	5 mm diam./6 mm cylinder	23.1 ± 5.4	372 ± 54	—	—	Kasra 1994[36]
Cattle						
Distal femur	5.5 mm diam./8 mm cylinder	8.5 ± 4.2	117 ± 61	—	—	Poumarat 1993[82]
Proximal tibia	15 mm cube, ultrasonic method	—	648 ± 430	0.41 ± 0.16	—	Rho 1997[83]
Proximal humerus	Dimensions ? cylinders	—	1570 ± 628	0.71 ± 0.22	—	Keaveny 1997[81]
Vertebral body	6 mm diam./7.5 mm cylinder	7.1 ± 3.0	173 ± 97	0.45 ± 0.09	0.19 ± 0.06	Swartz 1991[84]
Dog						
Femoral head	5 mm cube	12 ± 5.8	435	—	—	Vahey 1987[85]
Distal femur	8 mm cube	7.1 ± 4.6	209 ± 140	0.44 ± 0.16	0.26 ± 0.08	Kuhn 1989[78]
	4 mm diam./5 mm cylinder	13–28[b]	210–394[b]	0.69–0.98	0.40–0.56[b]	Kuhn 1998[86]
Proximal tibia	4 mm diam./5 mm cylinder	5–24[b]	106–426[b]	0.41–0.83b	0.22–0.44[b]	Kuhn 1998[86]
	12.5 mm diam./10 mm cylinder	—	301–850	—	—	Sumner 1994[87]
	5 mm cube	—	344–1278	—	—	Sumner 1994[87]
Humeral head	4 mm diam./5 mm cylinder	18 ± 6	350 ± 171	0.84 ± 0.17	0.43 ± 0.06	Kuhn 1998[86]
Distal humerus	6 mm diam./15 mm cylinder	13 ± 3	1490 ± 300	—	—	Kaneps 1997[37]
Vertebral body	5 mm diam./8 mm cylinder	10.1 ± 2.6	530 ± 40	—	—	Acito 1994[88]
Goat						
Femoral head	4 mm diam./5 mm cylinder	19.2 ± 6.9	502 ± 268	0.91 ± 0.04	0.48 ± 0.03	An 1998[89]
Distal femur	4 mm diam./5 mm cylinder	14.1–23.5[b]	399–429[b]	0.54–0.66[b]	0.32–0.40[b]	An 1998[89]
Proximal tibia	4 mm diam./5 mm cylinder	24.7–26.1[b]	532–566[b]	0.93–1.1b	0.50–0.56b	An 1998[89]
Humeral head	4 mm diam./5 mm cylinder	10.0 ± 1.0	247 ± 20	0.75 ± 0.03	0.36 ± 0.01	An 1998[89]
Sheep						
Femoral neck	8 mm diam./10 mm cylinder	3.2 ± 0.3	2.0 ± 0.2[c]	—	—	Geusens 1996[90]
Vertebral body	7 mm diam./9 mm cylinder	23.6 ± 4.4	—	—	—	Deloffre 1995[91]
	.5 mm diam./9 mm cylinder	22.3 ± 7.1	1510 ± 784	0.60 ± 0.16	0.37 ± 0.11	Mitton 1997[92]
Pig						
Vertebral body	7 mm diam./5 mm cylinder	27.5 ± 3.4	1080 ± 470	—	0.46 ± 0.04	Mosekilde 1987[93]
Rabbit						
Epiphyseal long bones	Ground bone surfaces Indentation test	35–81	—	—	—	An 1996[40]
Rat						
Epiphyseal long bones	Ground bone surfaces Indentation test	38–71	—	—	—	An 1997[94]

[a] Range of values.
[b] Range of average values from different parts.
[c] Value is questionable (too low).

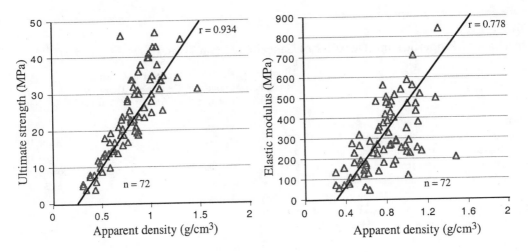

FIGURE 3.5 The correlation between apparent density and properties of cancellous bone.

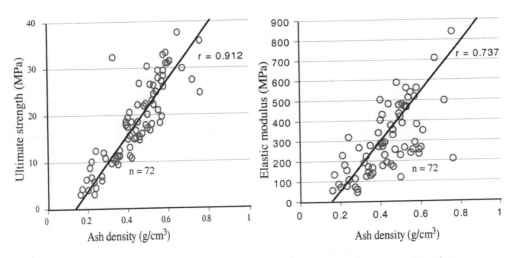

FIGURE 3.6 The correlation between ash density and properties of cancellous bone.

In the author's laboratory, a set of data was generated on the correlations between the mechanical properties and bone densities of canine trabecular bone.[86] Cancellous bone specimens ($n = 72$) were taken from different locations including humeral head, femoral head, femoral condyle, and upper tibia. Figure 3.5 shows the strong correlation between the mechanical properties and their apparent density. Similarly, the mechanical properties of cancellous bone correlate well with their ash density (Figure 3.6).[57]

C. MICROSTRUCTURE

The more commonly used parameters for trabecular bone structures or architecture include (1) BV (bone volume) or TBA (trabecular bone area, which is the trabecular surface area divided by the total area in μm^2); (2) Tb.Th (trabecular thickness, the average thickness of trabeculae in μm); and (3) Tb.Sp (trabecular separation, the average distance between trabeculae, representing the amount of marrow space in μm).[95]

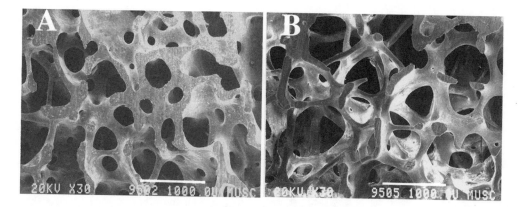

FIGURE 3.7   A scanning electron microscope (SEM) image showing the osteopenic changes of the upper tibial trabecular bone in a rabbit knee inflammatory arthritis model.

Common parameters for trabecular bone spatial connectivity include Tb.N (trabecular number, the average number of continuous trabecular elements encountered per unit area), Ho.N (hole number, the average number of holes per unit area), N.Nd (trabecular node number; nodes: trabecular branch points), N.Tm (trabecular terminus number; termini: trabecular end points), and Nd/Tm ratio. Most of the parameters can be measured using specialized imaging software based on a single histological section (two dimensional), serial sections, or serial image scanning (three dimensional).

In a local osteopenic model reported from the author's laboratory,[57] the significant reduction of cancellous bone strength (26 ± 8 MPa compared with the control side 68 ± 15 MPa using an indentation test) could be explained by the reduction of trabecular BV or TBA and increased perforation and disconnectivity of the trabecular tissue (Figure 3.7). According to morphometrical analysis, the cancellous bones showed obvious perforation and disconnectivity in a very short period of time, as indicated by TBV, Nd, free end (Tm), continuous CTE, Ho.N, Nd/Tm ratio, and Euler number (calculated by deducting Ho.N. from Th.N[96]). These changes may represent a rapid bone loss[97] featuring perforation and disconnection of the trabecular network and increased size of marrow cavities. Significant correlations have been found between the mechanical and morphological parameters (Table 3.8).

Recent development in three-dimensional imaging of cancellous bone has made possible true three-dimensional quantification of trabecular architecture. This provides a significant improvement of the tools available for studying and understanding the mechanical functions of cancellous bone. Goldstein et al.[98] utilized a three-dimensional, microcomputed tomography (μCT) system to measure trabecular plate thickness, trabecular plate separation, trabecular plate number, surface-to-volume ratio, bone volume fraction, anisotropy, and connectivity in isolated specimens of trabecular bone. The results of these studies demonstrate that in normal bone, more than 80% of the variance in its mechanical behavior can be explained by measures of density and orientation.[98] Odgaard et al.[99,100] argued that connectivity and architectural anisotropy (fabric) are of special interest in mechanics–architecture relations. They addressed the possible significance of trabecular connectivity for the mechanical quality of cancellous bone. By using the detailed three-dimensional reconstructions as input for microstructural finite-element models, the complete elastic properties of the trabecular architecture were obtained and maximum and mean stiffness could be calculated. Volume fraction and true three-dimensional architectural measurements of connectivity density and surface density were determined. Connectivity density was determined in an unbiased manner by the Euler number. By using multiple regression analysis it was found that volume fraction explained by far the greatest part (84 to 94%) of the variation in both mean and maximum stiffness. When connectivity density and surface density were included, the correlations increased marginally to 89 to 95%. Recently, Kinney and Ladd[101] used a finite-element model to explore the relationship

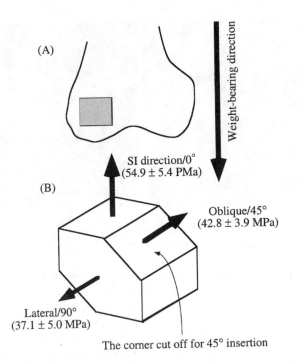

FIGURE 3.8 Illustration of a test for screw-holding powers of bovine cancellous bone from different directions, showing the anisotropic behavior of cancellous bone. (A) The sampling site and orientation. (B) The directions of screw insertion and the average values of pullout strength ($n = 16$).

TABLE 3.8
Correlation Analysis (Pearson Correlation Coefficient) between Mechanical and Morphometric Parameters[a]

	Ultimate Load	Stiffness	Ultimate Strength
TBV (%)	0.796[b]	0.888[c]	0.796
Tb.Th (µm)	0.918[c]	0.869[b]	0.918[c]
Tb.sp	−0.459	0.562	−0.462
Ho.N/mm²	0.823[b]	0.880[b]	0.823[b]
Euler number/mm²	−0.832[b]	−0.892[b]	−0.883[c]
Nd/mm²	0.868[b]	0.950[d]	0.868
Tm/mm²	−0.879[b]	−0.925	−0.881
Nd/Tm ratio	0.940[d]	0.831[c]	0.940[d]

Note: A "–" means a negative correlation.

[a] $n = 6$; degrees of freedom $n' = n − 2 = 4$; one-way (for positive r) or two-way (negative r) analysis.
[b] $P < 0.05$.
[c] $P < 0.01$.
[d] $P < 0.005$.

Adapted from Kang et al., *J. Mater. Sci. Mater. Med.*, 9, 463, 1998.

between connectivity density and the elastic modulus of trabecular bone. Although no functional relationship was found between connectivity and elastic modulus, there was a linear relationship, after a full cycle of atrophy and recovery, between the loss of elastic modulus and the overall loss of connectivity. The results indicate that recovery of mechanical function depends on preserving or restoring trabecular connectivity.

D. ANISOTROPY AND HETEROGENEITY

Cancellous bone is anisotropic based on its trabecular morphology.[102] Several investigations have addressed the orthogonal or anisotropic mechanical properties of cancellous bone of both human and animals.[85,103-107] The strength and elastic modulus of cancellous bone depend on the direction of the load employed, as normally measured at SI (superior-interior), AP (anterior-posterior), or ML (medial-lateral) directions. Ciarelli et al.[106] found the highest overall mean of elastic moduli of human long bone metaphyseal locations to be in the SI direction, which is about 2.5 times the value at the AP direction. The AP direction is higher than the ML direction. An earlier study using vertebral cancellous bone specimens by Galante et al.[103] also showed a similar pattern. In a recent study in the author's laboratory, it was found that the screw pullout strength of bovine cancellous bone also depends on the direction of the screw insertion (loading direction). The strength was the strongest (55 ± 5 MPa) at the SI direction (0°), the weakest (37 ± 5 MPa) at the lateral direction (90°), and intermediate (43 ± 4 MPa) at a direction of 45°.[108] This phenomenon may be explained by a column–strut model proposed by the author's group (see Chapter 21).[109] Figure 3.8 shows the effects of the directions of screw insertion on the pullout strength of cancellous bone in bovine distal femoral cancellous bone.

As stated by Goldstein,[76] nearly 40 years ago Evans and King documented the mechanical properties of trabecular bone from multiple locations in the proximal human femur. Since that time, many investigators have cataloged the distribution of trabecular bone material properties from multiple locations within the human skeleton to include the femur, tibia, humerus, radius, vertebral bodies, calcaneus, and iliac crest. According to the data list summarized by Goldstein (21 sets of data generated using compression tests), the average values of strength and elastic modulus of human cancellous bone from different locations are 6.6 to 36.2 MPa and 130 to 1080 Mpa, respectively.[76] Both linear and power functions have been found to explain the relationship between trabecular bone density and material properties.[76] In the author's laboratory, the strength and elastic modulus of epiphysometaphyseal bones of animals, such as rats,[94] rabbits,[39] dogs,[86,110] and goats,[110] have been investigated using compression and indentation tests. Generally, for both humans and animals, the cancellous bones of lower limbs (hind limbs) are stronger and stiffer than those of upper limbs (front limbs). This heterogeneous mechanical characteristic of cancellous bone is determined by functional adaptation.[76,111]

Cancellous bone is also heterogeneous at a given location. At the metaphysioepiphyseal area of long bones, more trabecular bone material is located at the subchondral bone plate and gradually becomes less concentrated toward the diaphysis (Figure 3.9). This structural pattern determines a decreasing mechanical strength from the subchondral bone plate toward the medullary canal. In our recent study, cylinders (4 mm diam. × 5 mm length) from two levels of cancellous bone from canine medial femoral condyles were measured for strength and elastic modulus using compression tests.[86] The results showed that the distal level (the one close to the joint surface) has a much higher strength and modulus (28 ± 7 vs. 19 ± 5 MPa). A similar finding was also demonstrated in a study on the glenoid.[112]

If a cut is made below the upper tibial joint surface, the mechanical property was found to be very inhomogeneous.[113] Figure 3.10 also shows that the high-strength areas, tested by an indentation test,[114] are where the intimate joint contact occurs. At the peripheral area, the bone is stronger than the immediate neighboring areas, which is caused by the strengthening effect of cortical bone shell.[115] In one of Rho's studies,[122] he found that variations in the properties around the quadrant of tibial cortical

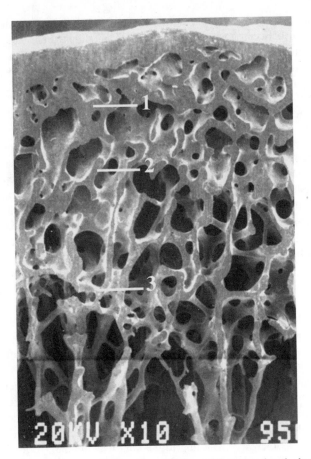

FIGURE 3.9   Rabbit upper tibial cross section at coronal plane (SEM), showing the heterogeneous trabecular structure from the subchondral bone plate toward the medullary canal. Note the dense structure at the subchondral plate (above Line 1) and the loose trabeculae below Line 3.

bone are small, less than 10%, while the differences in the properties around the circumference of cancellous bone are more apparent, approximately five times those of cortical bone. The elastic properties of cancellous bone exhibited inhomogeneity and some consistency pattern along both the length and the circumference. Similar morphology is also seen in the vertebral body. Very inhomogeneous bone structure and mechanical properties are also found in almost every possible location, such as the human glenoid,[112] human proximal and distal femur,[116-118] human upper tibia,[118] canine upper tibia,[87] human patella,[104] vertebrae,[117] calcaneus,[117] and even the pig mandibular condyle.[119]

Table 3.7 lists articles on the mechanical properties of animal cancellous bones, which include studies of bovine, canine, or goat distal femur, proximal tibia, and vertebrae determined by compression test, or of canine, rabbit, or rat epiphysometaphyseal bones examined using indentation test.[57,86,94]

E. MATERIAL PROPERTIES

The material properties of cancellous bone are defined by the intrinsic properties of individual trabeculae, which have been measured by mechanical testing of single trabeculae using methods such as buckling analysis,[120] compression test,[121] microtensile test,[122] cantilever test plus finite-element modeling,[123] finite-element modeling,[124] or ultrasound methods.[122] The elastic modulus of trabecular bone material (individual trabeculae) is about 10 to 30% less than that of cortical bone (Table 3.9). For

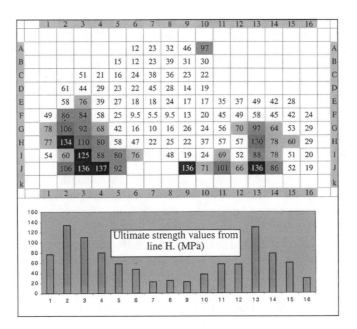

FIGURE 3.10 Illustrations of the heterogeneous distribution of bone strength values. Note the high-strength areas are in the medial and lateral condyles where the tibia and femur articular surfaces contact.

example, the elastic modulus is 14.8 GPa for trabeculae and 20.7 GPa for cortical bone measured by an ultrasonic technique and 10.4 and 18.6 GPa, respectively, using a microtensile test.[122]

TABLE 3.9
Mechanical Properties of Cancellous Bone Material

Bone specimen	Test Method	Elastic modulus (GPa)	Ref.
Human distal femur	Buckling	8.69 ± 3.17 (dry)	Runkle 1975[120]
Human proximal tibia	Buckling	11.38 (wet)	Townsend 1975[121]
Human femur	Ultrasound	12.7 ± 2.0 (wet)	Ashman 1988[125]
Bovine femur	Tensile	10.9 ± 1.6 (wet)	Ashman 1988[125]
Human femur, tibia	Cantilever	8.7 (6.2–11.2)	Menta 1989[123]
Human iliac crest	Tensile	0.8 ± 0.4	Ryan 1989[71]
Human upper tibia	Three-point bending	4.59	Choi 1990[67]
Human tibia	Four-point bending	5.7 ± 1.3	Choi 1990[126]
	Tensile	10.4 ± 3.5	Rho 1993[122]

IV. CONTINUUM ASSUMPTION

Most existing analyses of strength and stiffness of both cortical and cancellous bone assume that it can be modeled as a continuum.[127] One basic requirement of using the continuum assumption is that the minimum dimension of the sample must be significantly larger than the dimension of its structural subunits. Harrigan et al.[128] developed a criterion for the validity of this assumption. The limitations of the continuum assumption appear in two areas: near biologic interfaces and in areas of large stress gradients, such as subchondral bone, the transitional area between cortical shell and cancellous bone, and bone under intimate joint contact areas. These limitations are explored using a probabilistic line-scanning model for density measurements, resulting in an estimate of density accuracy as a function of line length which is experimentally verified. For cancellous bone, within a distance of three to five trabeculae (about 300 to 1500 μm in length), a continuum model is not valid. For compression testing on cancellous bone, Linde[129] suggested that a specimen dimension larger than 5 mm can fulfill the requirement of continuum assumption. For cortical bone, because of its dense structure the limit for continuum assumption can be smaller.

V. SUMMARY

Bone is an elastic, anisotropic, heterogeneous, and composite material. The determinants of bone mechanical properties include (1) its density (apparent density and mineral density); (2) porosity (vascular canals in cortical bone and marrow space in cancellous bone); and (3) microscopic structure, such as cortical bone architecture (primary and secondary osteons), osteonal structure (compositions of lamellae with different collagen fiber arrangement), trabecular structure (trabecular orientation, trabecular bone volume, and trabecular connectivity), and collagen fiber orientation.[127]

Due to the limited scope of this text, only selected mechanical properties of bone obtained using traditional mechanical testing methods and their determinants at macro- or microstructural levels are included in this chapter. This is not enough to understand fully the biomechanics of bone tissues. As mentioned by Rho et al.,[4] detailed descriptions of the structural features of bone abound in the literature; however, the mechanical properties of bone, in particular those at the micro- and nanostructural level (material level), remain poorly understood. Therefore, further investigations of mechanical properties at the "materials level,"[68] in addition to the studies at the "structural level" are needed to fill the gap in our present knowledge and to achieve a complete understanding of the mechanical properties of bone.

Although one should know the limitations of traditional mechanical testing methods (which often underestimate the true values of strength and stiffness of the materials) and also that of noninvasive techniques, such as ultrasound, 3-D imaging, or finite-element analysis, most of the mechanical data of bone obtained by traditional testing methods remains valid and serves as basic data for validating any noninvasive techniques.

Bone is a heterogenous and anisotropic material and cannot be treated simply as a homogeneous material like Daro foam (formed by mixing isocyanate and a resin, polyol) or saw bone. However, certain assumptions can be applied to bone specimens within reason in order to achieve useful data of mechanical properties of bone.

REFERENCES

1. Spatz, H.C., O'Leary, E.J., and Vincent, J.F., Young's moduli and shear moduli in cortical bone, *Proc. R. Soc. Lond. B. Biol. Sci.,* 263, 287, 1996.
2. Ashman, R.B., Experimental techniques, in *Bone Mechanics*, Cowin, S.C., Ed., CRC Press, Boca Raton, FL, 1989, 91.
3. Katz, J.L., The structure and biomechanics of bone, *Symp. Soc. Exp. Biol.,* 34, 137, 1980.
4. Rho, J.Y., Kuhn-Spearing, L., and Zioupos, P., Mechanical properties and the hierarchical structure of bone, *Med. Eng. Phys.,* 20, 92, 1998.
5. Yamada, H., Ed., *Strength of Biological Materials*, Williams & Wilkins, Baltimore, MD, 1970.
6. Evans, F.G., *Mechanical Properties of Bone*, Charles C Thomas, Springfield, IL, 1973.
7. Currey, J., *The Mechanical Adaptations of Bones*, Princeton University Press, Princeton, NJ, 1984.
8. Cowin, S.C., Ed., *Bone Mechanics*, CRC Press, Boca Raton, FL, 1999.
9. Martin, R.B., Burr, D.B., and Sharkey, N.A., *Skeletal Tissue Mechanics*, Springer, New York, 1998.
10. Nordin, M. and Frankel, V.H., Biomechanics of whole bones and bone tissue, in *Basic Biomechanics of Skeletal System*, Frankel, V.H. and Nordin, M., Eds., Lea & Febiger, Philadelphia, 1980, 15.

11. Albright, J.A., Bone: physical properties, in *The Scientific Basis of Orthopaedics*, Albright, J.A. and Brand, R.A., Eds., Appleton & Lange, Norwalk, CT, 1987, 213.

12. Einhorn, T.A., Biomechanics of bone, in *Principles of Bone Biology*, Bilezikian, J.P., Raisz, L.G., and Rodan, G.A., Eds., Academic Press, San Diego, CA, 1996, 25.

13. Hayes, W.C. and Bouxsein, M.L., Biomechanics of cortical and trabecular bone: implications for assessment of fracture risk, in *Basic Orthopaedic Biomechanics*, Mow, V.C. and Hayes, W.C., Eds., Lippincott-Raven, Philadelphia, 1997, Chapter 3.

14. Whiting, W.C. and Zernicke, R.F., Biomechanical concepts, in *Biomechanics of Musculoskeletal Injury*, Whiting, W.C. and Zernicke, R.F., Eds., Human Kinetics, Champaign, IL, 1998, 41.

15. Reilly, D.T., Burstein, A.H., and Frankel, V.H., The elastic modulus for bone, *J. Biomech.,* 7, 271, 1974.

16. Burstein, A.H., Reilly, D.T., and Martens, M., Aging of bone tissue: mechanical properties, *J. Bone Joint Surg. Am.,* Vol. 58, 82, 1976.

17. Cezayirlioglu, H., Bahniuk, E., Davy, D.T., and Heiple, K.G., Anisotropic yield behavior of bone under combined axial force and torque, *J. Biomech.,* 18, 61, 1985.

18. McElhaney, J.H., Fogle, J., Byars, E., and Weaver, G., Effect of embalming on the mechanical properties of beef bone, *J. Appl. Physiol.,* 19, 1234, 1964.

19. Simkin, A. and Robin, G., The mechanical testing of bone in bending, *J. Biomech.,* 6, 31, 1973.

20. Evans, F.G. and Lebow, M., Regional differences in some of the physical properties of the human femur, *J. Appl. Physiol.,* 3, 563, 1951.

21. Vincentelli, R. and Grigorov, M., The effect of Haversian remodeling on the tensile properties of human cortical bone, *J. Biomech.,* 18, 201, 1985.

22. Burstein, A.H., Zika, J.M., Heiple, K.G., and Klein, L., Contribution of collagen and mineral to the elastic-plastic properties of bone, *J. Bone Joint Surg. Am.,* Vol. 57, 956, 1975.

23. Hazama, H., Study on the torsional strength of the compact substance of human beings, *J. Kyoto Pref. Med. Univ.,* 60, 167, 1956.

24. Reilly, D.T. and Burstein, A.H., The elastic and ultimate properties of compact bone tissue, *J. Biomech.,* 8, 393, 1975.

25. Sedlin, E.D. and Hirsch, C., Factors affecting the determination of the physical properties of femoral cortical bone, *Acta Orthop. Scand.,* 37, 29, 1966.

26. Keller, T.S., Mao, Z., and Spengler, D.M., Young's modulus, bending strength, and tissue physical properties of human compact bone [see comments], *J. Orthop. Res.,* 8, 592, 1990.

27. Lotz, J.C., Gerhart, T.N., and Hayes, W.C., Mechanical properties of metaphyseal bone in the proximal femur, *J. Biomech.,* 24, 317, 1991.

28. Currey, J.D., Foreman, J., Laketic, I. et al., Effects of ionizing radiation on the mechanical properties of human bone, *J. Orthop. Res.,* 15, 111, 1997.

29. Currey, J.D., The effect of porosity and mineral content on the Young's modulus of elasticity of compact bone, *J. Biomech.,* 21, 131, 1988.

30. Currey, J.D., The effects of drying and re-wetting on some mechanical properties of cortical bone, *J. Biomech.,* 21, 439, 1988.

31. Currey, J.D., Brear, K., Zioupos, P., and Reilly, G.C., Effect of formaldehyde fixation on some mechanical properties of bovine bone, *Biomaterials,* 16, 1267, 1995.

32. Martin, R.B. and Boardman, D.L., The effects of collagen fiber orientation, porosity, density, and mineralization on bovine cortical bone bending properties, *J. Biomech.,* 26, 1047, 1993.

33. Schryver, H.F., Bending properties of cortical bone of the horse, *Am. J. Vet. Res.,* 39, 25, 1978.

34. Bigot, G., Bouzidi, A., Rumelhart, C., and Martin-Rosset, W., Evolution during growth of the mechanical properties of the cortical bone in equine cannon-bones, *Med. Eng. Phys.,* 18, 79, 1996.

35. McAlister, G.B. and Moyle, D.D., Some mechanical properties of goose femoral cortical bone, *J. Biomech.,* 16, 577, 1983.

36. Kasra, M. and Grynpas, M.D., Effect of long-term ovariectomy on bone mechanical properties in young female cynomolgus monkeys, *Bone,* 15, 557, 1994.

37. Kaneps, A.J., Stover, S.M., and Lane, N.E., Changes in canine cortical and cancellous bone mechanical properties following immobilization and remobilization with exercise, *Bone,* 21, 419, 1997.

38. Crenshaw, T.D., Peo, E.R., Jr., Lewis, A.J., et al., Influence of age, sex and calcium and phosphorus levels on the mechanical properties of various bones in swine, *J. Anim. Sci.,* 52, 1319, 1981.

39. Ayers, R.A., Miller, M.R., Simske, S.J., and Norrdin, R.W., Correlation of flexural structural properties with bone physical properties: a four species survey, *Biomed. Sci. Instrum.,* 32, 251, 1996.

40. An, Y.H., Kang, Q., and Friedman, R.J., Mechanical symmetry of rabbit bones studied by bending and indentation testing, *Am. J. Vet. Res.,* 57, 1786, 1996.

41. Jorgensen, P.H., Bak, B., and Andreassen, T.T., Mechanical properties and biochemical composition of rat cortical femur and tibia after long-term treatment with biosynthetic human growth hormone, *Bone,* 12, 353, 1991.

42. Barengolts, E.I., Lathon, P.V., Curry, D.J., and Kukreja, S.C., Effects of endurance exercise on bone histomorphometric parameters in intact and ovariectomized rats, *Bone Miner.,* 26, 133, 1994.

43. Ejersted, C., Andreassen, T.T., Oxlund, H., et al., Human parathyroid hormone (1-34) and (1-84) increase the mechanical strength and thickness of cortical bone in rats, *J. Bone Miner. Res.,* 8, 1097, 1993.

44. Simske, S.J., Guerra, K.M., Greenberg, A.R., and Luttges, M.W., The physical and mechanical effects of suspension-induced osteopenia on mouse long bones, *J. Biomech.,* 25, 489, 1992.

45. Yeni, Y.N., Brown, C.U., and Norman, T.L., Influence of bone composition and apparent density on fracture toughness of the human femur and tibia, *Bone,* 22, 79, 1998.

46. Schaffler, M.B. and Burr, D.B., Stiffness of compact bone: effects of porosity and density, *J. Biomech.,* 21, 13, 1988.

47. Jurist, J.M. and Foltz, A.S., Human ulnar bending stiffness, mineral content, geometry and strength, *J. Biomech.,* 10, 455, 1977.

48. Stromsoe, K., Hoiseth, A., Alho, A., and Kok, W.L., Bending strength of the femur in relation to noninvasive bone mineral assessment, *J. Biomech.,* 28, 857, 1995.

49. Shah, K.M., Goh, J.C., Karunanithy, R., et al., Effect of decalcification on bone mineral content and bending strength of feline femur, *Calcif. Tissue Int.,* 56, 78, 1995.

50. Currey, J.D., Physical characteristics affecting the tensile failure properties of compact bone, *J. Biomech.,* 23, 837, 1990.

51. Currey, J.D., The mechanical consequences of variation in the mineral content of bone, *J. Biomech.,* 2, 1, 1969.

52. Currey, J.D., The relationship between the stiffness and the mineral content of bone, *J. Biomech.,* 2, 477, 1969.

53. Wong, D.M. and Sartoris, D.J., Noninvasive methods for assessment of bone density, architecture, and biomechanical properties: fundamental concepts, in *Osteoporosis: Diagnosis and Treatment,* Sartoris, D.J., Ed., Marcel Dekker, New York, 1996, 201.

54. Van der Perre, G. and Lowet, G., Physical meaning of bone mineral content parameters and their relation to mechanical properties, *Clin. Rheumatol.,* 13 (Suppl. 1), 33, 1994.

55. Lazenby, R., Porosity–geometry interaction in the conservation of bone strength, *J. Biomech.,* 19, 257, 1986.

56. McElhaney, J.H., Alem, N., and Roberts, V., A porous block model for cancellous bones, ASME Publ., 70-WA1BHF-2, 1970.

57. Kang, Q., An, Y.H., Butehorn, H.F., and Friedman, R.J., Morphological and mechanical study of the effects of experimentally induced inflammatory knee arthritis on rabbit long bones, *J. Mater. Sci. Mater. Med.,* 9, 463, 1998.

58. Hirsch, C. and Silva, O.D., The effect of orientation on some mechanical properties of femoral cortical specimens, *Acta Orthop. Scand.,* 38, 45, 1967.

59. Bonfield, W. and Grynpas, M.D., Anisotropy of the Young's modulus of bone, *Nature.,* 270, 453, 1977.

60. Katz, J.L., Anisotropy of Young's modulus of bone, *Nature,* 283, 106, 1980.

61. Sasaki, N., Matsushima, N., Ikawa, T., et al., Orientation of bone mineral and its role in the anisotropic mechanical properties of bone — transverse anisotropy, *J. Biomech.,* 22, 157, 1989.

62. Turner, C.H., Chandran, A., and Pidaparti, R.M., The anisotropy of osteonal bone and its ultrastructural implications, *Bone,* 17, 85, 1995.

63. Ascenzi, A. and Bonucci, E., The compressive properties of single osteons, *Anat. Rec.,* 161, 377, 1968.

64. Ascenzi, A., Baschieri, P., and Benvenuti, A., The bending properties of single osteons, *J. Biomech.,* 23, 763, 1990.

65. Frasca, P., Jacyna, G., Harper, R., and Katz, J.L., Strain dependence of dynamic Young's modulus for human single osteons, *J. Biomech.,* 14, 691, 1981.

66. Ascenzi, A. and Bonucci, E., The tensile properties of single osteons, *Anat. Rec.,* 158, 375, 1967.

67. Choi, K., Kuhn, J.L., Ciarelli, M.J., and Goldstein, S.A., The elastic moduli of human subchondral, trabecular, and cortical bone tissue and the size-dependency of cortical bone modulus, *J. Biomech.,* 23, 1103, 1990.

68. Weiner, S. and Traub, W., Bone structure: from angstroms to microns, *FASEB J.,* 6, 879, 1992.

69. Carter, D.R. and Hayes, W.C., The compressive behavior of bone as a two-phase porous structure, *J. Bone Joint Surg. Am.,* Vol. 59, 954, 1977.

70. Carter, D.R. and Hayes, W.C., Bone compressive strength: the influence of density and strain rate, *Science,* 194, 1174, 1976.

71. Ryan, S.D. and Williams, J.L., Tensile testing of rodlike trabeculae excised from bovine femoral bone, *J. Biomech.,* 22, 351, 1989.

72. Gibson, L.J., The mechanical behavior of cancellous bone, *J. Biomech.,* 18, 317, 1985.

73. Kaplan, S.J., Hayes, W.C., Stone, J.L., and Beaupre, G.S., Tensile strength of bovine trabecular bone, *J. Biomech.,* 18, 723, 1985.

74. Keaveny, T.M., Wachtel, E.F., Ford, C.M., and Hayes, W.C., Differences between the tensile and compressive strengths of bovine tibial trabecular bone depend on modulus [see comments], *J. Biomech.,* 27, 1137, 1994.

75. Keaveny, T.M., Guo, X.E., Wachtel, E.F., et al., Trabecular bone exhibits fully linear elastic behavior and yields at low strains, *J. Biomech.,* 27, 1127, 1994.

76. Goldstein, S.A., The mechanical properties of trabecular bone: dependence on anatomic location and function, *J. Biomech.,* 20, 1055, 1987.

77. Martens, M., Van Audekercke, R., Delport, P., et al., The mechanical characteristics of cancellous bone at the upper femoral region, *J. Biomech.,* 16, 971, 1983.

78. Kuhn, J.L., Goldstein, S.A., Ciarelli, M.J., and Matthews, L.S., The limitations of canine trabecular bone as a model for human: a biomechanical study, *J. Biomech.,* 22, 95, 1989.

79. Odgaard, A., Hvid, I., and Linde, F., Compressive axial strain distributions in cancellous bone specimens, *J. Biomech.,* 22, 829, 1989.

80. Linde, F., Hvid, I., and Pongsoipetch, B., Energy absorptive properties of human trabecular bone specimens during axial compression, *J. Orthop. Res.,* 7, 432, 1989.

81. Keaveny, T.M., Pinilla, T.P., Crawford, R.P., et al., Systematic and random errors in compression testing of trabecular bone, *J. Orthop. Res.,* 15, 101, 1997.

82. Poumarat, G. and Squire, P., Comparison of mechanical properties of human, bovine bone and a new processed bone xenograft, *Biomaterials,* 14, 337, 1993.

83. Rho, J.Y., Flaitz, D., Swarnakar, V., and Acharya, R.S., The characterization of broadband ultrasound attenuation and fractal analysis by biomechanical properties, *Bone,* 20, 497, 1997.

84. Swartz, D.E., Wittenberg, R.H., Shea, M., et al., Physical and mechanical properties of calf lumbo-sacral trabecular bone, *J. Biomech.,* 24, 1059, 1991.

85. Vahey, J.W., Lewis, J.L., and Vanderby, R., Jr., Elastic moduli, yield stress, and ultimate stress of cancellous bone in the canine proximal femur, *J. Biomech.,* 20, 29, 1987.

86. Kang, Q., An, Y.H., and Friedman, R.J., The mechanical properties and bone densities of canine cancellous bones, *J. Mater. Sci. Mater. Med.,* 9, 1998.

87. Sumner, D.R., Willke, T.L., Berzins, A., and Turner, T.M., Distribution of Young's modulus in the cancellous bone of the proximal canine tibia, *J. Biomech.,* 27, 1095, 1994.

88. Acito, A.J., Kasra, M., Lee, J.M., and Grynpas, M.D., Effects of intermittent administration of pamidronate on the mechanical properties of canine cortical and trabecular bone, *J. Orthop. Res.,* 12, 742, 1994.

89. An, Y.H., Kang, Q., and Friedman, R.J., The mechanical properties and bone densities of goat cancellous bones, unpublished data, 1998.

90. Geusens, P., Boonen, S., Nijs, J., et al., Effect of salmon calcitonin on femoral bone quality in adult ovariectomized ewes, *Calcif. Tissue Int.,* 59, 315, 1996.

91. Deloffre, P., Hans, D., Rumelhart, C., et al., Comparison between bone density and bone strength in glucocorticoid-treated aged ewes, *Bone,* 17, 409S, 1995.

92. Mitton, D., Rumelhart, C., Hans, D., and Meunier, P.J., The effects of density and test conditions on measured compression and shear strength of cancellous bone from the lumbar vertebrae of ewes, *Med. Eng. Phys.,* 19, 464, 1997.

93. Mosekilde, L., Kragstrup, J., and Richards, A., Compressive strength, ash weight, and volume of vertebral trabecular bone in experimental fluorosis in pigs, *Calcif. Tissue Int.,* 40, 318, 1987.

94. An, Y.H., Zhang, J.H., Kang, Q., and Friedman, R.J., Mechanical properties of rat epiphyseal cancellous bones studied by indentation test, *J. Mater. Sci. Mater. Med.,* 8, 493, 1997.

95. Parfitt, A.M., Drezner, M.K., Glorieux, F.H., et al., Bone histomorphometry: standardization of nomenclature, symbols, and units. Report of the ASBMR Histomorphometry Nomenclature Committee, *J. Bone Miner. Res.,* 2, 595, 1987.

96. Compston, J.E., Connectivity of cancellous bone: assessment and mechanical implications [editorial], *Bone,* 15, 463, 1994.

97. Parfitt, A.M., Age-related structural changes in trabecular and cortical bone: cellular mechanisms and biomechanical consequences, *Calcif. Tissue Int.,* 36, S123, 1984.

98. Goldstein, S.A., Goulet, R., and McCubbrey, D., Measurement and significance of three-dimensional architecture to the mechanical integrity of trabecular bone, *Calcif. Tissue Int.,* 53, S127, 1993.

99. Odgaard, A., Three-dimensional methods for quantification of cancellous bone architecture, *Bone,* 20, 315, 1997.

100. Kabel, J., Odgaard, A., van Rietbergen, B., and Huiskes, R., Connectivity and the elastic properties of cancellous bone, *Bone,* 24, 115, 1999.

101. Kinney, J.H. and Ladd, A.J., The relationship between three-dimensional connectivity and the elastic properties of trabecular bone, *J. Bone Miner. Res.,* 13, 839, 1998.

102. Whitehouse, W.J., The quantitative morphology of anisotropic trabecular bone, *J. Microsc.,* 101(2), 153, 1974.

103. Galante, J., Rostoker, W., and Ray, R.D., Physical properties of trabecular bone, *Calcif. Tissue Res.,* 5, 236, 1970.

104. Townsend, P.R., Raux, P., Rose, R.M., et al., The distribution and anisotropy of the stiffness of cancellous bone in the human patella, *J. Biomech.,* 8, 363, 1975.

105. Williams, J.L. and Lewis, J.L., Properties and an anisotropic model of cancellous bone from the proximal tibial epiphysis, *J. Biomech. Eng.,* 104, 50, 1982.

106. Ciarelli, M.J., Goldstein, S.A., Kuhn, J.L., et al., Evaluation of orthogonal mechanical properties and density of human trabecular bone from the major metaphyseal regions with materials testing and computed tomography, *J. Orthop. Res.,* 9, 674, 1991.

107. Njeh, C.F., Hodgskinson, R., Currey, J.D., and Langton, C.M., Orthogonal relationships between ultrasonic velocity and material properties of bovine cancellous bone, *Med. Eng. Phys.,* 18, 373, 1996.

108. An, H.Y., Kang, Q., Friedman, R.J., and Young, F.A., The effect of microstructure of cancellous bone on screw pullout strength, *Trans. Soc. Biomater.,* 20, 385, 1997.

109. An, H.Y. and Draughn, R.A., Mechanical properties and testing methods of bone, in *Animal Models in Orthopaedic Research,* An, Y.H. and Friedman, R.J., Eds., CRC Press, Boca Raton, FL, 1999, Chapter 8.

110. An, Y.H., Kang, Q., and Friedman, R.J., et al., Do mechanical properties of epiphyseal cancellous bones vary?, *J. Invest. Surg.,* 10, 221, 1997.

111. Goldstein, S.A., Wilson, D.L., Sonstegard, D.A., and Matthews, L.S., The mechanical properties of human tibial trabecular bone as a function of metaphyseal location, *J. Biomech.,* 16, 965, 1983.

112. Mansat, P., Barea, C., Hobatho, M.C., et al., Anatomic variation of the mechanical properties of the glenoid, *J. Shoulder Elbow Surg.,* 7, 109, 1998.

113. Ashman, R.B., Rho, J.Y., and Turner, C.H., Anatomical variation of orthotropic elastic moduli of the proximal human tibia, *J. Biomech.,* 22, 895, 1989.

114. Kang, Q., An, Y.H., and Friedman, R.J., Effects of multiple freezing–thawing cycles on ultimate indentation load and stiffness of bovine cancellous bone, *Am. J. Vet. Res.,* 58, 1171, 1997.

115. Hvid, I., Jensen, J., and Nielsen, S., Contribution of the cortex to epiphyseal strength. The upper tibia studied in cadavers, *Acta Orthop. Scand.,* 56, 256, 1985.

116. Brown, T.D. and Ferguson, A.B., Jr., Mechanical property distributions in the cancellous bone of the human proximal femur, *Acta Orthop. Scand.,* 51, 429, 1980.

117. Augat, P., Link, T., Lang, T.F., et al., Anisotropy of the elastic modulus of trabecular bone specimens from different anatomical locations, *Med. Eng. Phys.,* 20, 124, 1998.

118. Behrens, J.C., Walker, P.S., and Shoji, H., Variations in strength and structure of cancellous bone at the knee, *J. Biomech.,* 7, 201, 1974.

119. Teng, S. and Herring, S.W., Anatomic and directional variation in the mechanical properties of the mandibular condyle in pigs, *J. Dent. Res.,* 75, 1842, 1996.

120. Runkle, J.C. and Pugh, J., The micromechanics of cancellous bone. II. Determination of the elastic modulus of individual trabeculae by a buckling analysis, *Bull. Hosp. Joint Dis.,* 36, 2, 1975.

121. Townsend, P.R., Rose, R.M., and Radin, E.L., Buckling studies of single human trabeculae, *J. Biomech.,* 8, 199, 1975.

122. Rho, J.Y., Ashman, R.B., and Turner, C.H., Young's modulus of trabecular and cortical bone material: ultrasonic and microtensile measurements, *J. Biomech.,* 26, 111, 1993.

123. Mente, P.L. and Lewis, J.L., Experimental method for the measurement of the elastic modulus of trabecular bone tissue, *J. Orthop. Res.,* 7, 456, 1989.

124. van Rietbergen, B., Weinans, H., Huiskes, R., and Odgaard, A., A new method to determine trabecular bone elastic properties and loading using micromechanical finite-element models, *J. Biomech.,* 28, 69, 1995.

125. Ashman, R.B. and Rho, J.Y., Elastic modulus of trabecular bone material, *J. Biomech.,* 21, 177, 1988.

126. Choi, K. and Goldstein, S.A., A comparison of the fatigue behavior of human trabecular and cortical bone tissue, *J. Biomech.,* 25, 1371, 1992.

127. Martin, R.B., Determinants of the mechanical properties of bones [published erratum appears in *J. Biomech.* 25, 1251, 1992], *J. Biomech.,* 24, 79, 1991.

128. Harrigan, T.P., Jasty, M., Mann, R.W., and Harris, W.H., Limitations of the continuum assumption in cancellous bone, *J. Biomech.,* 21, 269, 1988.

129. Linde, F., Elastic and viscoelastic properties of trabecular bone by a compression testing approach, *Dan. Med. Bull.,* 41, 119, 1994.

4 Factors Affecting Mechanical Properties of Bone

Peter Zioupos, Chris W. Smith, and Yuehuei H. An

CONTENTS

I. INTRODUCTION

The usual purpose of mechanical testing of bone is to characterize the range of normal mechanical properties and to define abnormalities according to those normal values. In this section and the next, the factors affecting the mechanical properties of bone are discussed, including (1) systemic or *in vivo* factors, such as age, sex, species, function, composition, weightlessness and hypergravity, hormones, steroids, and arthritis, and (2) *in vitro* factors, such as embalming or fixation, boiling and autoclaving, freezing storage, drying and freeze-drying, sterilization methods, holes in bone, sample preparation, and the testing machine.

Bone in this chapter, in agreement with the rest of the book, refers to the structure and properties of the bone–tissue material and not those of the bone as a structure (as in a whole femur or tibia). The distinction is important in this chapter because much of what is defined as *factors* or *determinants* of the mechanical properties of bone are more effective when coupled with changes in the shape, size, and thickness of the whole bone than when simply acting on the bone tissue level. In the same vein, *normal* refers to the majority of bone tissue characteristics while *abnormal* or *pathophysiological* refers to changes caused by the so-called factor.

To begin, one needs a basic appreciation of the general nature of the mechanical characteristics of bone and its intricate microstructure. These two elements may allow one, in most circumstances, to anticipate the likely deviations from normality. For instance, in bone mechanics terms, bone is a (1) viscoelastic, (2) elastic/brittle, (3) anisotropic material. The viscoelastic property means that the applied strain rate during testing is in itself a determinant/factor of the recorded behavior *in vivo* or *in vitro*; the elastic/brittle property describes when the elastic behavior ends and bone develops internal damage when some threshold limits for stress or strain are reached; and anisotropic properties depend on the direction of loading or the direction of preparation of a sample. On the other hand, bone at the nanomicroscale is composed of collagen impregnated by mineral crystallites. The behavior of this bone–tissue matrix will be a function of the individual properties of the two constituents, their degree of association and cohesion, the size and shape of the enclosed crystallites, and their orientation. It is conceivable, therefore, that a disease state which will preferentially affect any of these determinants will directly reflect on the average material properties of the bone itself, often in a somewhat predictable manner.

Provided that due attention is given to these and similar considerations, readers are invited to exercise their own critical faculties to discern whether the conditions of some bone tests reported in the past allow for a great degree of confidence in the results. In general, anything other than physiological temperature, ambient conditions, and loading rates similar to those *in vivo* should be viewed with skepticism. However, it must be stressed that most research on deriving material properties for bone tissue is carried out almost inevitably in quasi-static conditions which are easier to control in the lab and allow easier standardization between labs.

One last word of caution: the factors referred to here can interplay and affect each other. For instance, it is entirely feasible that a certain increase in the degree of porosity caused by osteonal remodeling may cause a change in the degree of anisotropy of the tissue. Similarly, a certain sterilization method or chemical treatment, which is meant to affect, for instance, only the collagen component of bone, may also inadvertently cause demineralization or structural microdamage in the material. The possibility that most factors can, therefore, act in a somewhat "composite" way should not be ignored.

II. SYSTEMIC OR *IN VIVO* FACTORS AFFECTING THE MECHANICAL PROPERTIES OF BONE

A. AGE

Age affects the properties of bone in animals and humans. However, the so-called aging effect is of primary importance to humans who suffer the effects of senescence as they grow and survive into old age. Most animals by comparison do not live long after the end of their child-bearing and child-rearing age. It is questionable, therefore, whether animal models (like rats and baboons) can be used to study "aging" effects, although they may be perfectly acceptable for studies on age alone.[1,2]

TABLE 4.1
Data from Wet Specimens at Room Temperature (Femur/Tibia)[5]

	Age (years)						
	20–30	30–40	40–50	50–60	60–70	70–80	80–90
Elastic Modulus (GPa)							
Tension	17.0/18.9	17.6/27.0	17.7/28.8	16.6/23.1	17.1/19.9	16.3/19.9	15.6/29.2
Compression	18.1/—	18.6/35.3	18.7/30.6	18.2/24.5	15.9/25.1	18.0/26.7	15.4/25.9
Ultimate Strength (MPa)							
Tension	140/161	136/154	139/170	131/164	129/147	129/145	120/156
Compression	209/—	209/213	200/204	192/192	179/183	190/183	180/197
Ultimate Strain (%)							
Tension	3.4/4.0	3.2/3.9	3.0/2.9	2.8/3.1	2.5/2.7	2.5/2.7	2.4/2.3
Compression	—	—	—	—	—	—	—

Source: Burstein, A. H. et al., *J. Bone Joint Surg.*, 58A, 82, 1976.

TABLE 4.2
Data from Relatively Wet Specimens at Room Temperature (Femur)[8]

	Age (years)						
	10–20	20–30	30–40	40–50	50–60	60–70	70–80
Ultimate Strength (MPa)							
Tension	114	123	120	112	93	86	86
Compression	—	167	167	161	155	145	—
Bending	151	173	173	162	154	139	139
Torsion		57	57	52	52	49	49
Ultimate Strain (%)							
Tension	1.5	1.4	1.4	1.3	1.3	1.3	1.3
Compression	—	1.9	1.8	1.8	1.8	1.8	—
Torsion	—	2.8	2.8	2.5	2.5	2.7	2.7

Source: Martin, R.B. and Burr, D.B., *Structure, Function, and Adaptation of Compact Bone,* Raven Press, New York, 1989, 214.

In general, with age there is an increase in the mineral content of the bone tissue, which achieves its best strength and stiffness at maturity. Maturity is set at a nominal age of about 35 years for humans (and varies from animal to animal). Thereafter, the elastic, ultimate, and fracture properties[3] of bone tissue deteriorate in both men and women.[4-7] Early results are summarized in Tables 4.1 and 4.2.

Lindahl and Lindgren[4] tested mixed male/female samples at room temperature and 65% humidity; they observed that the ultimate tensile strength (UTS) fell from about 147 MPa at 30 years of age to about 125 MPa at 90 years; the strain at failure fell from 2.3% at 30 years to about 1.6% at 90 years. Wall et al.,[6] testing samples at body temperature which were sprayed with Hank's solution, found that UTS fell from 102 MPa at 40 years to 73.5 MPa at 90 years. McCalden et al.[7] conducted tensile tests at room temperature on wet specimens at a strain rate of 0.03 s^{-1}; they found

TABLE 4.3
Some Indicative Values for Both Sexes in Humans and Animals

Subject	Bone	Mechanical Property	Male	Female	P Value	Ref.
Human	Femur cortical	Tensile strength (MPa)	138 ± 2	131 ± 3	>0.05	4
		Elastic modulus (GPa)	14.9 ± 0.0	14.7 ± 0.0	>0.05	
	Vertebral cubes	Compressive yield force (lb)	123 ± 62	78 ± 57	0.064	9
		Consolidation force (lb)	165 ± 93	100 ± 51	0.041	
Pigs	Diaphyseal bones	Bending strength (kg cm^{-2})	340	428	<0.01	1
		Bending modulus (kg cm^{-2})	5453	6401	<0.01	

UTS fell from 120 MPa at 30 years to 70 MPa at 100 years of age, ultimate strain fell from 3.3% at 30 years to 1% at 100 years, fracture energy reduced by 90% between 30 and 100 years of age similar to the reduction in the plastic energy stored, and the elastic component was mostly unaffected by age. Zioupos and Currey,[3] testing in three-point bending at 37°C and using Ringer's solution, found that the elastic modulus, 15.2 GPa at 35 years of age, fell by 2.3% of its value per decade in later life; the bending strength fell similarly from 170 MPa by 3.7%; the transverse fracture toughness K_C from 6.4 MPa m$^{1/2}$ by 4.1%; the J-integral from 1.2 kJ m^{-2} by 3% and the work to transverse fracture from 3.4 kJ m^{-2} by 8.7%.

Cancellous bone aging effects are masked by the gross changes in architecture and density of this tissue with age. There is a consensus today that strength and stiffness of bulk cancellous bone change (roughly) as a quadratic power of the apparent density. Two recent review articles also claim that, after consideration of all recent experiments, the material that makes up the trabeculae in cancellous bone is in terms of stiffness and strength within 10 to 20% of that of neighboring cortical bone. Hence, the age effects of cancellous bone are primarily reduced into describing its architecture, connectivity, and level of porosity and, following that, in order to complete the picture it may be assumed that the trabecular tissue material degrades similarly to its cortical neighbor.

B. Sex

Lindahl and Lindgren[4] found that there was no difference between the sexes with respect to the mechanical properties of cortical bone. In general, the differences between male and female bone (Table 4.3) are caused by differences in mass, that is, the quantity of bone not the quality of it. Males have on average bigger and heavier skeletons, not necessarily comprised of denser bone. From birth until menopause, female bone material properties "shadow" those of the males. However, after menopause female bones show accelerated resorption rates which cause increased porosity levels and consequently produce a weaker bone matrix material (internal porosity) as well as a thinning of the structure of the bones (breakdown of bone matrix).

C. Species

The properties of the bone material of the long bones of mammalian animals differ considerably in absolute values. Table 4.4 shows indicative values for a number of mechanical properties from four species.

D. Composition — Porosity, Density, Mineralization

1. Cortical Bone

Cortical bone is compact material with a small degree of internal porosity. The porosity of bone (measured in a small bone specimen) is the fraction of the *actual bone material volume* (usually

TABLE 4.4
Mechanical Property Values[10] for Human, Equine, Bovine, and Porcine Bone Tissue

Mechanical Property	Human	Horses	Cattle	Pigs
Ultimate tensile strength (MPa)	124/174/125/152	121/113/102/120	113/132/101/135	88/108/88/100
Ultimate extension (%)	1.41/1.50/1.43/1.50	0.75/0.70/0.65/0.71	0.88/0.78/0.76/0.79	0.68/0.76/0.70/0.73
Elastic modulus in tension (GPa)	17.6/18.4/17.5/18.9	25.5/23.8/17.8/22.8	25.0/24.5/18.3/25.9	14.9/17.2/14.6/15.8
Ultimate compressive strength (MPa)	170/—/—/—	145/163/154/156	147/159/144/152	100/106/102/107
Ultimate contraction (%)	1.85/—/—/—	2.4/2.2/2.0/2.3	1.7/1.8/1.8/1.8	1.9/1.9/1.9/1.9
Elastic modulus in compression (GPa)	—/—/—/—	9.4/8.5/9.0/8.4	8.7/—/—/—	4.9/5.1/5.0/5.3
Ultimate shear strength (MPa)	54/—/—/—	99/89/90/94	91/95/86/93	65/71/59/64
Elastic modulus in torsion (GPa)	3.2/—/—/—	16.3/19.1/23.5/15.8	16.8/17.1/14.9/14.3	13.5/15.7/15.0/8.4

Note: In each cell the four values are in order for femur/tibia/humerus/radius.

measured by immersion in water and use of the Archimedes principle) over *the total apparent specimen volume*, which can be measured externally by using calipers (provided that the specimen has a regular shape such as a cylinder or cube). Porosity affects the modulus of elasticity of compact bone as a power that ranges between 3 and 5 depending on whether results come from one species or across a range of species.[11,12]

The material density of cortical bone is the wet weight divided by the actual bone material volume and ranges between 1.7 and 2.1 g cm^{-3}. The most commonly used *wet bone density* is simply the wet weight divided by the externally measured apparent specimen volume and this includes a small degree of porosity, which for cortical bone varies between 0 and 5%. It is more or less generally accepted today that apparent density influences[11] the elastic stiffness as a power of 2 and the strength as a power of 3.

The mineral content of bone tissue varies with the species, age, the mechanical function of the bone, the health or pathophysiological condition of the individual, etc. All these factors are interdependent and each one makes bone what it is. The level of mineral mass ranges between 40 and 70% of the total mass, but in some extreme cases it is as high as 80% (for the fin whale, *Tympanic bulla*) or even 98% (for the rostral bone of the whale, *Mesoplodon densirostris*). Figure 4.1 shows in a ternary diagram some variations between species and how the three main components of bone — water, mineral, and collagen — complement each other.[13]

Table 4.5 shows the combined species mineral content effect on the mechanical properties of various bone tissues.[13,14]

The Young's modulus of elasticity can range from 4 to 32 GPa, bending strength from 50 to 300 MPa, and the work of fracture from 200 to 7000 J m^{-2}. It is not possible for any one type of bone to have high values for all three properties. Very high values of mineralization produce high values of Young's modulus but low values of work of fracture (which is a measure of fracture toughness). Rather low values of mineralization are associated with high values of work of fracture but low values of Young's modulus and intermediate values of bending strength. The reason for the high value for Young's modulus associated with high mineralization is intuitively obvious, but has not yet been rigorously modeled. The low fracture toughness associated with high mineralization may be caused by the failure of various crack-stopping mechanisms that act at low mineral contents when the cohesion between the various building blocks of bone (i.e., mineralized bone fibrils, lamellae, osteons, etc.) is low. When the mineral content of the bone is high, an advancing crack "sees" in front of it a rather uniform (it could be said, single-phase) material and advances unhindered, causing rapid failure. The adoption of different degrees of mineralization by different bones, leading to different sets of mechanical properties, is shown to be adaptive in most cases studied, but some puzzles still remain.[15]

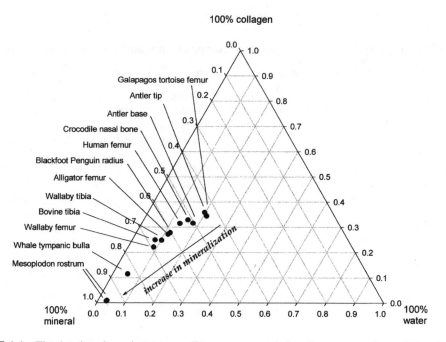

FIGURE 4.1   The drawing shows in a ternary diagram some variations between species and how the three main components of bone — water, mineral, and collagen — complement each other.

Table 4.6 shows the combined effects of species, methods, and direction of testing (anisotropy factor) on the measured toughness of various bones. The antler analogue included in the list helps to illustrate that above and beyond the considerations described in the previous paragraph (which are solely focused on the degree of mineralization), there are other factors such as intricate internal architecture that help to produce some very tough bone tissue examples.[16]

Some researchers[33-35] have attempted to examine the effects of mineralization *in vitro* by controllably dissolving the mineral and demineralizing bone by means of acids and chelating agents (Table 4.7). This approach has one inherent and inevitable disadvantage in that the dissolving medium acts by diffusion from the free surfaces that are in contact with the solution and hence it cannot guarantee a uniform result throughout the whole volume of the test sample at all times. Nevertheless, the results are consistent with the previous *in vivo* patterns.

Walsh et al.[36-38] studied the effects of phosphate and fluoride ions on the compressive properties of cortical bone. Bone tissue is an anisotropic nonhomogeneous composite material composed of inorganic bone mineral fibers (hydroxyapatite) embedded in an organic matrix (type I collagen and noncollagenous proteins). One factor contributing to the overall mechanical behavior is the interfacial bonding interactions between mineral and organic matrix. This interfacial bonding is based, in part, on electrostatic interactions between negatively charged organic domains and the positively charged mineral surface. Phosphate and fluoride ions have been demonstrated to alter mineral–organic interactions, thereby influencing the mechanical properties of bone in tension. It is now accepted that fluoride increases the resistance of bone tissue to chemical attack and degradation, but it impairs the mechanical strength of the material as a result of the previously mentioned altered interactions at the mineral–collagen interface.

2. Cancellous Bone

There are three main contributors to the material properties of cancellous bone: (1) the material characteristics of the trabeculae; (2) the architecture of the trabeculae; and (3) the quantity of the

TABLE 4.5

Mechanical Properties — Young's Modulus (E) Ultimate Tensile Stress (UTS), Ultimate Tensile Strain (ε_f), and Mineral Content (mineral weight/wet bone weight) of Various Bones[13,14]

Species and Tissue	Mineral Content	E (GPa)	UTS (MPa)	ε_f
Red deer, immature antler	0.385	10	250	0.109
Red deer, mature antler	0.393	7.2	158	0.114
Reindeer, antler	0.411	8.1	95	0.051
Polar bear (3 months), femur	0.441	6.7	85	0.044
Narwhal, tusk cement	0.454	5.3	84	0.060
Narwhal, tusk dentine	0.466	10.3	120	0.037
Sarus crane, tarsometatarsus	0.467	23.1	218	0.018
Walrus, humerus	0.482	14.2	105	0.026
Fallow deer, radius	0.493	25.5	213	0.019
Human adult, femur	0.496	16.7	166	0.029
Bovine, tibia	0.499	19.7	146	0.018
Polar bear (9 months), femur	0.501	11.2	137	0.042
Leopard, femur	0.514	21.5	215	0.034
Brown bear, femur	0.517	16.9	152	0.032
Donkey, radius	0.522	15.3	114	0.020
Sarus crane, tibiotarsus	0.523	23.5	254	0.031
Flamingo, tibiotarsus	0.523	28.2	212	0.013
Roe deer, femur	0.525	18.4	150	0.011
Polar bear (3.5 years), femur	0.529	18.5	154	0.022
King penguin, radius	0.540	22.1	195	0.010
Horse, femur	0.541	24.5	152	0.008
Wallaby, tibia	0.551	25.4	184	0.010
Bovine femur	0.562	26.1	148	0.004
King penguin, ulna	0.577	22.9	193	0.011
Axis deer, femur	0.586	31.6	221	0.019
Fallow deer, tibia	0.589	26.8	131	0.006
Wallaby, femur	0.599	21.8	183	0.009
King penguin, humerus	0.621	22.8	175	0.008
Fin whale, *T. bulla*	0.768	34.1, 31.3[a]	—, 33[a]	0.002, 0.0011[a]
Mesoplodon rostrum	0.960	41[a]	60[a]	0.0015[a]

Note: The mineral content was derived from calcium content measurements assuming that the tissues have the same element stoichiometry. Note that the two most mineralized tissues at the bottom of the list are extremely brittle compared to all the rest.

[a] Values are in three-point bending[13] for the last two most brittle bones the ultimate tensile stress is also the stress at yield. The authors believe that the reason for this is that in three-point bending the region of maximum stress is very confined to the outmost fibers and, therefore, when the tissue yields (= microcracks) the failure is catastrophic because the generated macrocrack cannot be stopped effectively.

bone material.[39-41] These features are reflected in the previously mentioned apparent density, expressing mostly the quantity of bone present, and real material density, which may reflect the quality of the trabecular material, (Table 4.8). Theoretical expectations suggest that apparent density should influence stiffness as a power of 2 and strength as a power of 3. However, the most recent studies show both these properties to change roughly as a quadratic power of the apparent density.

TABLE 4.6
Fracture Mechanics Properties and Values from the Literature (in chronological order)

Bone	Orientation	K_c (MPa m$^{1/2}$)	Energy Requirements	Type of Test	Speed	Ref.
Bovine femur	Long	3.21	$G_{IC} = 1.4$–2.6	SENT	Slow	17
	Long	5.05	—	SENT	Fast	17
	Trans	5.6	$G_{IC} = 3.1$–5.5	SENT	Slow	17
	Trans	7.7	—	SENT	Fast	17
	Trans	2.2–4.6	$G_{IC} = 0.78$–1.12	SENT	Slow	18
	Long	3.62	—	CT	Slow	19
	Trans	5.7	—	3–pb	Slow	20
	Long	2.4–5.2	$G_{IC} = 0.9$–2.8	CT	Slow	21
Bovine tibia	Long	2.8	$G_{IC} = 0.63$	CT	Slow	22
	Long	6.3	$G_{IC} = 2.88$	CT	Fast	22
Human tibia	Long	2.4–5.3	—	CT	Slow	23
Bovine tibia	Trans	11.2	$W_f = 7.96$	SENB	Slow	24
	Long	3.2	—	CT (v)	Very slow	25
	Trans	6.5	—	CT (v)	Very slow	25
Human tibia	Long	3.7	$G_{IC} = 0.36$	CT	Slow	26
Bovine tibia	Long	7.2	—	CT	Slow	26
	Long	8.0	$G_{IC} = 0.94$	CT	Very slow	27
Antler	Trans	5.4	—	SENT	Slow	28
Human tibia	Long	4.0–4.3	$G_{IC} = 0.59$–0.83	CT	Slow	29
Bovine tibia	Long	6.2–6.7	$G_{IC} = 0.9$–1.0	CT	Slow	29
Human (75 years), porosity (5%)						
Femur	Long		$G_{IC} = 0.70$, $G_{IIC} = 3.00$	CT	Slow	3
Tibia	Long	$K_{IC} = 2.12$, $K_{IIC} = 8.32$	$G_{IC} = 0.40$, $G_{IIC} = 5.50$			31
Human femur (35 years)	Trans	6.5	$W_f = 3.5$, $J_{int} = 1.2$	SENB	Slow	3
Baboons femurs	Long	2.3	—	CT	Slow	32
Bovine femur	Trans	5.0	$W_f = 3.00$	SENB	Slow	13
Mesoplodon rostrum	Trans	1.3	$W_f = 0.091$	SENB	Slow	13

Note: Orientation is the direction with respect to the bone axis, either longitudinal or transverse. Type of test indicates the test configuration and specimen geometry. CT: compact tension; (v): the specimen has been grooved to force the crack travel in a particular direction; SENT: single-edge notch tension; SENB: single-edge notch bending; W_f: work of fracture; 3-pb: three-point bending with a single notch. The energy requirements are either for W_f, or for the critical energy release rate G_C, or for the J-integral (all in comparable values for kJ m^{-2}). Speed: is the speed of crack growth, in most cases this was for slow, stable crack growth, only two studies reported on the unstable rapid propagation of cracks.

Material density of cancellous bone is measured using the weight of bone material (only trabeculae) divided by the volume of only trabeculae, which is in the 1.6 to 1.9 g cm^3 range and a little smaller than that of cortical bone.

E. FUNCTION

1. Microstructure vs. Function

One extreme example demonstrating the different mechanical properties of bone tissues with greatly differing functions was on the mechanical property differences[43] between deer antler, cow femur, and fin whale, *T. bulla* (Table 4.9). The femur of a cow has to be stiff and relatively strong and shows the

TABLE 4.7
Effects of Mineral Content (Examined by Demineralization)
on Mechanical Properties of Bone

Species	Bone	Treatment	Decalcification (%)	Mechanical Property	Change (%)	Ref.
Cats	Whole bone	EDTA*	20	Bending strength	↓35	35
			40		↓51	
			60		↓68	
			80		↓84	
Cows	Tibial samples	EDTA	3	Bending strength	↓30	33
			5		↓39	
			9		↓52	
			24		↓76	

* Ethylenediaminetetra-acetic acid, disodium salt

TABLE 4.8
Correlation Analysis[42] between the Mechanical Parameters
by Compression Test and Canine Cancellous Bone Densities

Mechanical Parameter	Test Method	Apparent Density	Ash Density
Elastic modulus (GPa)	Compression	0.778	0.737
Stiffness (N/mm)	Compression	0.868	0.853
	Indentation	0.944	0.923
Ultimate load (N)	Compression	0.966	0.966
	Indentation	0.940	0.954
Ultimate strength (MPa)	Compression	0.934	0.912
	Indentation	0.939	0.954

Values are correlation coefficients; $n = 10$, $n' = n - 2$, one-way analysis.

P values are at least <0.05.

TABLE 4.9
Mechanical Property Differences[43] of Bones Due
to Different Functions and Species ($n = 3 - 10$)

Parameter	Deer Antler	Cow Femur	Whale *T. bulla*
Bending strength (MPa)	179.4 ± 6.3	246.7 ± 11.6	33.0 ± 6.6
Bending modulus (GPa)	7.4 ± 0.3	13.5 ± 1.0	31.3 ± 1.0

characteristic behavior of "normal" compact bone tissue. The deer antlers are relatively softer, but extremely tough because in life they are expected to survive high impact loading. The ear bone of *T. bulla* is by comparison very brittle. The mechanical requirements placed upon this bone (like the transfer of loads and moments) are minimal; the crucial factor is the acoustic impedance and the loss of vibration quality through viscoelastic phenomena. Nature's answer to this is a very high mineral content which makes the earbone of *T. bulla* very stiff and very brittle. Another example is the differences between weight-bearing and non-weight-bearing bones (Table 4.10).[44]

TABLE 4.10
Mechanical Properties of Rabbit Bone[44] Due to Different Functions
(all from the right side, n = 17 for each bone or location)

Test	Bone	Ultimate Load (N)	Stiffness (N/mm)	Ultimate Strength (MPa)	Elastic Modulus (GPa)
Flexure	Humerus	284 ± 8	367 ± 17	165 ± 5	13.6 ± 0.7
	Femur	353 ± 13	413 ± 19	137 ± 6	15.1 ± 0.7
	Tibia	320 ± 12	301 ± 15	198 ± 8	21.5 ± 1.1
Indentation	Humeral head	136 ± 5	683 ± 66	32 ± 1	—
	Femoral head	362 ± 22	1531 ± 133	86 ± 5	—
	Medial tibial plateau	244 ± 20	1257 ± 139	55 ± 5	—

TABLE 4.11
Bending Properties of Rat Femur Due to Different Levels of Activity

Parameter	Normal	Immobilization	Exercise	Ref.
Strength (ultimate load)	100% (79.1 N)	—	+23.9% (97.2 N)	56, 57
Elasticity (stiffness)	100% (18.4 N/mm)	–8.7% (16.8 N/mm)	+7.1% (19.7 N/mm)	58

2. Activity Levels

Activity levels have an effect upon the bone mass and the bone material itself.[45-52] The mass of a normal bone is determined essentially by the balance between the two remodeling processes, resorption and deposition of the periosteal and endosteal surfaces.[53] The daily loading/straining pattern experienced by an individual bone strongly influences the two processes; increased loading leading to an increase in bone mass and decreased loading leading to a reduction in bone mass. This has become widely known as Wolff's law.[54] The usual example given of remodeling in response to exercise is that of the greater bone mass in the racket arm of tennis players compared with their contralateral arm. This response is also seen in rat femurs in response to an activity regime (Table 4.11) and in response to hypergravity.[55]

The magnitude of the effect of activity levels is not clearly understood although it seems that any effects are greater in adolescents than in mature individuals. In adults any increase in bone mass brought about by increased activity lasts only as long as that activity level is retained.[45-50]

3. Weightlessness

Weightlessness and reduced gravity are known to have very marked effects upon bone both in humans and animals.[59-61] Both situations drastically reduce the daily loading patterns experienced by the bones and thus affect the remodeling process. Space flight, with zero or near zero gravity, inevitably leads to marked net bone loss, something which even modern exercise regimes cannot completely prevent.[59]

Examples of the converse situation, extreme increased loading, may be seen in people who have suddenly changed their activity patterns, e.g., recent widows/widowers, athletes, ballet dancers, or new army recruits.[62-64] In these cases, the sudden large increase in loading (carrying shopping bags or performing housework, heavy training prior to a championship or a premiere, forced marches carrying heavy packs) may stimulate increased deposition, but this is usually outpaced by the increased rate of fatigue damage accumulation. The normal bone repair processes are not able to cope with the effects of this fatigue loading either, and the result is what is clinically termed a "stress fracture," which is a fracture resulting from a buildup of fatigue damage.

F. HORMONES

1. Sex Hormones

The cessation of estrogen production in the female, either through natural or surgical means, significantly affects bone metabolism, reducing bone mass and thus affecting bone quality.[65-68] Androgen production is also lowered following menopause, which also reduces bone mass.[69] The gradual reduction of endogenous production of male sex hormones with aging also leads to reduced bone mass, and is increasingly being recognized as a clinical problem.[70-74] Hormone replacement therapy (oral administration of estrogen) is the usual treatment option for bone loss in women[65-67] but can result in increased risk of artherosclerosis.[75] During pregnancy and lactation the normal calcium homeostasis is altered to allow for the calcium demands made by the fetus while preventing dangerous bone loss from the mother.[76-79] This process is governed mainly by parathyroid hormone.[76,79]

2. Growth Hormone, Insulin-Like Growth Factor, and Thyroid Hormone

Growth hormone deficiency in adult humans has been shown to lead to reduced bone mass and mineral density.[80-82] Growth hormone replacement is one of the treatment options. The action of growth hormone is mediated by insulin-like growth factors (IGF).[83-86] Thyroxine treatment, e.g., for hypothyroidism, is thought to reduce bone mass and density.[87-90]

3. Parathyroid Hormone and Calcitonin

Parathyroid hormone is the principal regulator of the remodeling process in the skeleton, mostly promoting resorption.[67] Oral administration is one of the treatment options for bone loss.[67,91] Calcitonin has been shown to be successful in increasing bone density.[92,93] Its use has been suggested for reversal of the side effects of long-term treatment with glucocorticoids,[93,94] also in combination with dietary calcium supplements.[66]

4. Steroid Administration

Some anabolic steroids, e.g., nandrolone, are recommended for cases where bone mass is lost and does not respond to other bone-promoting drugs, for instance, in hypogonadal men or those receiving treatment with corticosteroids.[72,75] However, they are thought to be ineffective for eugonadal men.[71] Long-term use of glucocorticoids is common for treatment of noninfectious inflammatory disease but leads to loss of bone mass.[93-96] Glucocorticoids are known to suppress osteoblast activity and thus increase resorption.[72,92-94,96] Hence, glucocorticoids suppress deposition of new bone but their action can be somewhat reversed by calcitonin[92,95] and by vitamin D.[72]

G. ARTHRITIS

Rheumatoid or inflammatory arthritis (RA) is either caused by an infection or by an autoimmune reaction and is seen as a disease of the cartilage, whereas osteoarthritis (OA) is a disease of the bone tissue and occurs due to mechanical factors, e.g., wear or impact injury, to the bone or cartilage.[97-99] Patients with RA are at a much higher risk of femoral neck fractures than patients with OA, and it seems RA acts to reduce bone mass,[97-100] but does not alter the mineral content of the bone tissue. OA, on the other hand, tends to increase the bone mass and apparent density by thickening the trabeculae while also reducing the mineral content of the bone tissue. OA is rarely

TABLE 4.12
Effects of Embalming or Fixation on Mechanical Properties of Bone (MPa)

Species Bone	Treatment	Mechanical Property	Change (%)	Ref.
Bovine cortical	10% formalin mixture[b]	Tensile modulus	No change	115
		Impact strength	↓[a]	
		Compressive strength	↓12%	117
		Compressive modulus	↓6%	

[a] Statistically significant.
[b] A mixture of ethanol, phenol, glycerine, formalin, and water.

seen in patients with osteoporosis.[97-99] In short, RA leads to thinning of the bone and reduction in bone strength and stiffness, whereas OA leads to thickening of bone and an increase in bone strength and stiffness, yet both are pathological.

H. OTHER SYSTEMIC FACTORS

Fluoride has a marked toxic effect upon bone tissue, impairing material properties, especially at a high dosage;[101,102] yet it is also capable, paradoxically, of stimulating an increase in bone mass and improving bone material qualities, and has been suggested as a possible treatment for glucocorticoid-induced bone loss.[95,102-104] This paradox is not well understood.

Biphosphophonates are suggested as possible treatment options for bone loss,[71,72,92,103,104] acting to suppress osteoclast activity.[100] Insufficient Ca intake can result from either low levels in the diet or from absorption problems. In its extreme form it results in osteomalacia where the collagen matrix remains unmineralized. Vitamin D, calcifediol, and calcitriol help to increase absorption of Ca.[95,101]

The absence of both selenium and vitamin E in the diet can lead to Kashin–Beck, a type of degenerative osteoarthritis. Experiments with rabbits have shown that selenium- and vitamin-E-deficient diets reduce both bone strength and elastic modulus.[105]

It is well established that chronic alcohol consumption leads to reduction in bone mass and increase in fracture risk,[92,104,106-112] although its exact pathology is unclear.

Zinc deficiency has been linked to bone disorders and hypogonadism, although these two are in themselves linked. Zinc is important for normal growth hormone and IGF production.[113]

III. *IN VITRO* FACTORS AFFECTING THE MECHANICAL PROPERTIES OF BONE

A. EMBALMING OR FIXATION (TABLE 4.12)

Bone from formalin-embalmed bodies is not appropriate for testing of mechanical properties because of the cross-linking of the collagen protein which alters the mechanical properties.[114,115] It is known that the cross-links between the collagen molecules have a significant influence upon the mechanical properties of bone tissue.[116]

It has been reported[115] that in quasistatic loading, mechanical properties of bovine bone were almost unaffected by a certain formalin fixation protocol, but at the same time a significant decrease in impact strength was found. These results indicated that there may be some interaction between fixation- and strain-rate-dependent effects, and, therefore, some caution is needed when using common biomechanical measurement methods on fixed bone material.

TABLE 4.13
Effects of Boiling and Autoclaving on Mechanical Properties of Bone

Bone	Species	Treatment	Temp. (°C)	Time (min)	Mechanical Property	Change (%)	Ref.
Diaphyseal	Rabbit	Autoclave	110	255	Torsional strength	↓35	121
					Torsional stiffness	↓27	
			121	20	Torsional strength	↓23	
					Torsional stiffness	↓20	
			131	2	Torsional strength	↓ 9	
					Torsional stiffness	↓10	
Cancellous	Porcine	Boiling	60	60	Compressive strength	0	122
			80	60	Compressive strength	↓ ?	
			100	60	Compressive strength	↓40	
Cortical	Bovine	Hot saline	95	120	Flexural strength	0	119
					Flexural modulus	↓12	
		Boiling	100	30	Compressive strength	↓32	118
					Compressive modulus	↓25	
		Autoclave	127	10	Compressive strength	↓48	
					Compressive modulus	↓47	
			132	20	Compressive strength	↓70	120

B. BOILING AND AUTOCLAVING (TABLE 4.13)

Borchers et al.[118] studied the effects of boiling and autoclaving on the compressive modulus and strength of bovine trabecular bone. The results showed 26 and 58% reductions in modulus and strength, respectively. Autoclaving on its own also significantly reduced the compressive modulus (by 59%). Another experiment showed that heating in saline for 2 h at temperatures up to 95°C had no effect upon the strength in three-point bending, but did have a significant effect upon the elastic modulus (a 12% drop after 2 h at 95°C).[119] Viceconti et al.[120] also demonstrated a large reduction in mechanical performance following exposure to high temperatures; only 30% remained of the compressive strength following autoclaving at 132°C for 1 h. It is clear that placing bone in high temperatures leads to changes in its mechanical properties.

C. STORAGE (TABLE 4.14)

Owing to complexity of an experiment or unforeseen circumstances, sometimes a specimen may be thawed and frozen a number of times. The question arises whether multiple freezing and thawing is harmful to the mechanical properties. This question has been partially answered by Linde and Sørensen[123] who found that freezing and thawing up to five times did not alter the compressive properties of cancellous bone. In other recent experiments the proximal portion of the tibia of adult cows was sectioned to produce bone slices. The slices were then subjected to four freezing–thawing cycles: freezing with and without saline solution, then thawing in saline solution or exposed to the air. The mechanical properties of the bone before and after the treatments (five cycles of freezing and thawing) were measured using an indentation test. No significant effect on the ultimate load and stiffness of the bone was found; only a trend of difference was noticed for the specimens frozen without saline soaking and thawed in air.[124] This work supports the widely used practice of freezing and thawing bone specimens in saline solution.

The common method for storing bone specimens is freezing at –20°C. The effects of storage on mechanical properties of bone at –20°C for short periods of time are minor. The maximum

TABLE 4.14

The Effects of Freezing on the Mechanical Properties of Bones

Subject/Bone	Temp (°C)	Time	Saline Saturation	Testing Mode	Change in Strength?	Ref.
Human						
Femur	−20	3–4 wk	Yes	Bending/tension	No[a]	131
Long bones	?	?	?	Bending	No	128
Tibia	−20	Five times in 15 days	?	Compression	No	123
Cattle						
Trabecular	−20, −70	8 days	No	Compression	No	118
	−20	Eight times in 8 days	No	Compression	No	118
	−20	Five times in 5 days	No	Indentation	↓(trend)	124
Dog						
Femur/tibia	−40	2 days	Yes	Torsion	↓ 4.6%	125
Femur	−20	1 wk	No/sealed	Compression	↑	130
	−20	16, 32 wks	No/sealed	Compression	No	130
	−20	1, 16, 32 wks	No/sealed	Screw pullout	No	130
Rat						
Femur	−20	2 wks	?	Torsion	No	132
	−20	2 wks	?	Compression	No	132

[a] No = no statistical difference.

effect reported is a 4.6% reduction in torsional strength of canine long bones.[125] However, after thawing, enzymes such as collagenase and protease may become active and degrade the tissue. Also, enzymatic degradation is not completely arrested at −20°C.[126] With concerns about the effects of enzyme degradation[127] and evaporation,[128] a question arises as to whether there are significant effects of long-term storage at −20°C. Panjabi et al.[129] found no significant effects of freezing for 7 to 8 months on the mechanical properties of human vertebral bone. Roe et al.[130] found that bones frozen at −20°C for 8 months did not become significantly weaker. Because time periods longer than 8 months have not been reported for frozen storage at −20°C, storage at this temperature for more than 8 months is not recommended. Alternatively, −70°C, −80°C, or even lower temperatures or liquid nitrogen are suggested for long-term bone storage, since these temperatures may minimize evaporation[128] and markedly reduce enzyme activity.[127] However, the remote possibility may then arise that at these lower temperatures other kinds of alterations may be inflicted upon bone tissue, either by microcracking or by damaging the collagen moiety of bone.

D. DRYING AND FREEZE-DRYING

It is not uncommon that specimens are sometimes, probably unintentionally, allowed to dry out in air prior to or during a mechanical test. Some specimens may also only be available in the dried state. Early work[133] has shown that the mechanical properties did not change following drying in air and rewetting. Nothing exists in the literature concerning the changes in properties if specimens remain in the dry state for a period of time, perhaps because it is obvious that they are very different from those in the wet state.

Freeze-drying is a very common preservation technique. During this process, water changes from the solid state into the gaseous state without entering the liquid state (sublimation). It is usually felt that this process is better at preserving fine structure. Indeed, there is usually no obvious change with many tissues following freeze-drying and rehydration. However, most studies have shown that there is a reduction in mechanical properties of bone following this process.[119,132,134-136] It is known that freeze-drying has little or no effect in purely collagenous tissues such as tendon,[137-139]

TABLE 4.15
Effect of Transcortical Drill Hole on the Mechanical Strength of Diaphyseal Bone

Subject	Bone	Bone Diam. (mm)	Hole Diam./ Outer Diam. of Bone	Hole Type	Mechanical Test	Strength Reduction (%)	Ref.
Sheep	Femur	?	20	Unicortical	Torsion	34	143
		19.6	50	Unicortical	Torsion	60	144
Dog	Femur	13.76	44	Unicortical	4-pt bend	38	145
		13.76	44	Bicortical	4-pt bend	51	145

so it would appear that the observed effects in bone result from its composite nature, whereby the mineralized collagen matrix contracts differentially and distorts and hence experiences damage (microcracks), which affects its properties.

E. STERILIZATION

Common techniques for sterilization of bone are γ-irradiation and exposure to ethylene oxide gas. It is normal to dry bone prior to exposure to ethylene oxide as toxic residues are produced with water present. Common dosages used for γ-irradiation by Co^{60} are between 1 and 3 MRad (10 to 30 kGy) while the bone is frozen in water or saline. It is not clear from the literature whether bone material suffers significant reductions in its mechanical competence following exposure to irradiation in such circumstances.[140,141] It is probable that the conditions during irradiation determine the changes in properties. It is known that irradiation has two contradictory effects in purely collagenous materials like tendons. On the one hand, it causes direct molecular chain scission and, on the other hand, it promotes crosslinks between molecular chains.[142] The mobility of the molecules influences the cross-linking process, while scission is controlled by the dose. The greater the amount of cross-linking relative to chain scission, the smaller the reduction in mechanical competence. The presence of water, especially as a liquid, during irradiation will most likely be beneficial for mechanical competence.

F. HOLES IN BONE

Holes are introduced in bone during restorative applications, when inserting screws or pins for fixation, etc. These have undoubtedly a detrimental effect[143-145] on the strength of a whole bone as shown in Table 4.15. Bone has two ways of coping with this adversity. In the long term, if the insertion is removed, the bone will fill in the hole and (by repairing) alleviate some of the danger. In the short term, bone benefits from its ability (which is also a material property) to yield around stress concentrating defects (as by microcracking) and thus blunting their deleterious effect.[146]

G. SAMPLE AND MACHINE

Sample preparation, sample size and shape, test conditions, sample–machine interface, and machine compliance are common determining factors for the scattering results of mechanical testing of bone.[147,148] Detailed discussion follows in Chapter 7.

IV. SUMMARY

There are many factors that can potentially influence the mechanical properties of bone. However, unlike anthropogenic composites, bones are able to adapt and change in life (and in disease), and that adds a few extra complications (unknown factors). Composites are what they are as a function of (1) the mixture/combination of a few primary elements; (2) the properties of these elements; and (3) their interaction. In bones mere considerations of mineral content, hydroxyapatite stoichiometry and the collagen condition do not apply simply and in a straightforward manner across species, ages, disease, treatments, etc. To make matters worse, these factors interplay and interdepend on each other. It becomes obvious that examining the mechanical properties of bone is an art in its own right. It requires due care and attention and, it could be said, some "reflection" on what is actually happening, what the knowledge is that is needed to be acquired and how deeply the process/situation at hand is comprehended. None of these should deter ambitious workers from engaging in bone biomechanics research and making their own mark in this field.

REFERENCES

1. Crenshaw, T.D., Peo, E.R., Jr., Lewis, A.J., et al., Influence of age, sex and calcium and phosphorus levels on the mechanical properties of various bones in swine, *J. Anim. Sci.*, 52, 1319, 1981.
2. Lawrence, L.A., Ott, E.A., Miller, G.J., et al., The mechanical properties of equine third metacarpals as affected by age, *J. Anim. Sci.*, 72, 2617, 1994.
3. Zioupos, P. and Currey, J.D., Changes in the stiffness, strength and toughness of human cortical bone with age, *Bone*, 22, 56, 1998.
4. Lindahl, O. and Lindgren, A.G., Cortical bone in man. II. Variation in tensile strength with age and sex, *Acta Orthop. Scand.*, 38, 141, 1967.
5. Burstein, A.H., Reilly, D.T., and Martens, M., Aging of bone tissue: mechanical properties, *J. Bone Joint Surg.*, 58A, 82, 1976.
6. Wall, J.C., Chatterji, S.K., and Jeffery, J.W., Age related changes in the density and tensile strength of human femoral cortical bone, *Calcif. Tissue Int.*, 27, 105, 1979.
7. McCalden, R.W., McGeouch, J.A., Barker, M.B., and Court-Brown, C.M., Age-related changes in the tensile properties of cortical bone, *J. Bone Joint Surg.*, 75A, 1193, 1993.
8. Martin, R.B. and Burr, D.B., Aging effects, in *Structure Function and Adaptation of Compact Bone*, Raven Press, New York, 1989, 214.
9. Oyster, N., Sex differences in cancellous and cortical bone strength, bone mineral content and bone density, *Age Ageing*, 21, 353, 1992.
10. Fung, Y.C., *Biomechanics — Mechanical Properties of Living Tissues*, Springer-Verlag, New York, 1981.
11. Martin, R.B., Determinants of the mechanical properties of bones, *J. Biomech.*, 24, 79, 1991.
12. Currey, J.D., Physical characteristics affecting the tensile failure properties of compact bone, *J. Biomech.*, 23, 837, 1990.
13. Zioupos, P., personal communication, 1999.
14. Currey, J.D., Mechanical properties of vertebrate hard tissues, *Proc. Inst. Mech. Eng.*, 212, 399, 1998.
15. Currey, J.D., Effects of differences in mineralization on the mechanical properties of bone, *Philos. Trans. R. Soc. London B*, 304, 509, 1984.
16. Zioupos, P., Currey, J.D., and Sedman, A.J., An examination of the micromechanics of failure of bone and antler by acoustic emission tests and laser scanning confocal microscopy, *Med. Eng. Phys.*, 16, 203, 1994.
17. Melvin, J.W. and Evans, F.G., Crack propagation in bone, in *Biomech. Symp. ASME*, American Society of Mechanical Engineers, New York, 1973, 87.
18. Bonfield, W. and Datta, P.K., Fracture toughness of compact bone, *J. Biomech.*, 9, 131, 1976.
19. Wright, T.M. and Hayes, W.C., Fracture mechanics parameters for compact bone — effects of density and specimen thickness, *J. Biomech.*, 10, 419, 1977.
20. Robertson, D.M., Robertson, D., and Barret, C.R., Fracture toughness, critical crack length and plastic zone size in bone, *J. Biomech.*, 11, 359, 1978.
21. Bonfield, W., Grynpas, M.D., and Young, R.J., Crack velocity and the fracture of bone, *J. Biomech.*, 11, 473, 1978.
22. Behiri, J.C. and Bonfield, W., Fracture mechanics of bone — the effects of density, specimen thickness and crack velocity on longitudinal fracture, *J. Biomech.*, 17, 25, 1984.

23. Bonfield, W., Behiri, J.C., and Charalambides, B., Orientation and age-related dependence of the fracture toughness of cortical bone, in *Biomechanics: Current Interdisciplinary Research*, Perrin, S.M. and Schneider, E., Eds., Martinus Nijhoff, Dordrecht, the Netherlands, 1984, 185.

24. Moyle, D.D. and Gavens, A.J., Fracture properties of bovine tibial bone, *J. Biomech.*, 19, 919, 1986.

25. Behiri, J.C. and Bonfield, W., Crack velocity dependence of longitudinal fracture in bone, *J. Mater. Sci.*, 15, 1841, 1989.

26. Norman, T.L., Vashishth, D., and Burr, D.B., Mode I fracture toughness of human bone, *Adv. Bioeng.*, 20, 361, 1991.

27. Norman, T.L., Vashishth, D., and Burr, D.B., Effect of groove on bone fracture toughness, *J. Biomech.*, 25, 1849, 1992.

28. Sedman, A.J., Mechanical Failure of Bone and Antler: The Accumulation of Damage, D.Phil. thesis, University of York, U.K., 1993.

29. Norman, T.L., Vashishth, D., and Burr, D.B., Fracture toughness of human bone under tension, *J. Biomech.*, 28, 309, 1995.

30. Norman, T.L., Nivargikar, S.V., and Burr, D.B., Resistance to crack growth in human cortical bone is greater in shear than in tension, *J. Biomech.*, 29, 1023, 1996.

31. Yeni, Y.N., Brown, C.U., Wang, Z., and Norman, T.L., The influence of bone morphology on fracture toughness of human femur and tibia, *Bone*, 21, 453, 1997.

32. Wang, X.D., Masilamani, N.S., Mabrey, J.D., et al., Changes in the fracture toughness of bone may not be reflected in its mineral density, porosity, and tensile reports, *Bone*, 23, 67, 1998.

33. Broz, J.J., Simske, S.J., and Greenberg, A.R., Material and compositional properties of selectively demineralized cortical bone, *J. Biomech.*, 28, 1357, 1995.

34. Guo, M.Z., Xia, Z.S., and Lin, L.B., The mechanical and biological properties of demineralised cortical bone allografts in animals, *J. Bone Joint Surg.*, 73B, 791, 1991.

35. Shah, K.M., Goh, J.C., Karunanithy, R., et al., Effect of decalcification on bone mineral content and bending strength of feline femur, *Calcif. Tissue Int.*, 56, 78, 1995.

36. Walsh, W.R. and Guzelsu, N., The role of ions and mineral–organic interfacial bonding on the compressive properties of cortical bone, *Biomed. Mater. Eng.*, 3, 75, 1993.

37. Walsh, W.R. and Guzelsu, N., Compressive properties of cortical bone: mineral–organic interfacial bonding, *Biomaterial*, 15, 137, 1994.

38. Walsh, W.R., Labrador, D.P., Kim, H.D., and Guzelsu, N., The effect of *in vitro* fluoride ion treatment on the ultrasonic properties of cortical bone, *Ann. Biomed. Eng.*, 22, 404, 1994.

39. Carter, D.R. and Hayes, W.C., The compressive behavior of bone as a two-phase porous structure, *J. Bone Joint Surg.*, 59A, 954, 1977.

40. Ashman, R.B. and Rho, J.Y., Elastic modulus of trabecular bone material, *J. Biomech.*, 21, 177, 1988.

41. Rice, J.C., Cowin, S.C., and Bowman, J.A., On the dependence of the elasticity and strength of cancellous bone on apparent density, *J. Biomech.*, 21, 155, 1988.

42. Kang, Q., An, Y.H., and Friedman, R.J., The mechanical properties and bone densities of canine cancellous bones, *J. Mater. Sci. Mater. Med.*, 9, 463, 1998.

43. Currey, J.D., Mechanical properties of bone tissues with greatly differing functions, *J. Biomech.*, 12, 313, 1979.

44. An, Y.H., Kang, Q., and Friedman, R.J., Mechanical symmetry of rabbit bones studied by bending and indentation testing, *Am. J. Vet. Res.*, 57, 1786, 1996.

45. Chen, M.M., Yeh, J.K., Aloia, J.F., et al., Effect of treadmill exercise in tibial cortical bone in aged female rats — a histomorphometry and dual energy X-ray absorptiometry study, *Bone*, 15, 313, 1994.

46. Lin, B.Y., Jee, W.S., Chen, M.M., et al., Mechanical loading modifies ovariectomy-induced cancellous bone loss, *Bone Miner.*, 25, 199, 1994.

47. Bagi, C.M. and Miller, S.C., Comparison of osteoporotic changes in cancellous bone induced by ovariectomy and/or immobilization in adult rats, *Anat. Rec.*, 239, 243, 1994.

48. Palle, S., Vico, L., Bourrin, S., and Alexandre, C., Bone tissue response to 4 month anti-orthostatic bedrest — a bone histomorphometric study, *Calcif. Tissue Int.*, 51, 189, 1992.

49. Li, K.C., Zernicke, R.F., Barnard, R.J., and Li, A.F., Differential response of rat limb bones to strenuous exercise, *J. Appl. Phys.*, 70, 554, 1991.

50. Forwood, M.R. and Burr, D.B., Physical activity and bone mass — exercises in futility, *Bone Miner.*, 21, 89, 1993.

51. Gordon, K.R., Levy, C., Perl, M., and Weeks, O.I., Adaptive modelling in a mammalian skeletal model system, *Growth Dev. Aging*, 57, 101, 1993.
52. Reilly, G.C., Currey, J.D., and Goodship, A.E., Exercise of young thoroughbred horses increases impact strength of the third metacarpal bone, *J. Orthop. Res.*, 15, 862, 1997.
53. Currey, J.D., *The Mechanical Adaptations of Bone*, Princeton University Press, Princeton, NJ, 1984.
54. Cowin, S.C., *Bone Mechanics*, 1986, CRC Press, Boca Raton, FL, 1986.
55. Kimura, T., Amtmann, E., Doden, E., and Oyama, J., Compressive strength of the rat femur as influenced by hypergravity, *J. Biomech.*, 12, 361, 1979.
56. Barengolts, E.I., Curry, D.J., Bapna, M.S., and Kukreja, S.C., Effects of endurance exercise on bone mass and mechanical properties in intact and ovariectomized rats, *J. Bone Miner. Res.*, 8, 937, 1993.
57. Umemura, Y., Ishiko, T., Yamauchi, T., et al., Five jumps per day increase bone mass and breaking force in rats, *J. Bone Miner. Res.*, 12, 1480, 1997.
58. Nordsletten, L., Kaastad, T.S., Skjeldal, S., et al., Training increases the *in vivo* strength of the lower leg: an experimental study in the rat, *J. Bone Miner. Res.*, 8, 1089, 1993.
59. Johnson, R.B., The bearable lightness of being: bone, muscles and spaceflight, *Anat. Rec.*, 253, 24, 1998.
60. Bikle, D.D., Halloran, B.P., and Morey-Holton, E., Space flight and the skeleton: lessons for the earthbound, *Endocrinologist*, 7, 10, 1997.
61. Sulzman, F.M., Life sciences space missions — overview, *J. Appl. Physiol.*, 81, 3, 1996.
62. Norman, E., Walter, M.D., and Wolf, M.D., Stress fractures in young athletes, *Am. J. Sports Med.*, 5, 165, 1977.
63. Orava, S. and Hulkko, A., Stress fractures of the mid-tibial shaft, *Acta Orthop. Scand.*, 55, 35, 1984.
64. Schneider, H.J., King, A.Y., Bronson, J.L., and Miller, E.H., Stress injuries and developmental change of lower extremities in ballet dancers, *Radiology*, 113, 627, 1974.
65. Notelovitz, M., Estrogen therapy and osteoporosis: principles & practice, *Am. J. Med. Sci.*, 313, 2, 1997.
66. Nieves, J.W., Komar, L., Cosman, F., and Lindsay, R., Calcium potentiates the effect of estrogen and calcitonin on bone mass: review and analysis, *Am. J. Clin. Nutr.*, 67, 18, 1998.
67. Masiukiewicz, U.S. and Insogna, K.L., The role of parathyroid hormone in the pathogenesis, prevention and treatment of postmenopausal osteoporosis, *Aging* (Milan), 10, 232, 1998.
68. Oursler, M.J., Estrogen regulation of gene expression in osteoblasts and osteoclasts, *Crit. Rev. Eukaryotic Gene Expression*, 8, 125, 1998.
69. Abraham, D. and Carpenter, P.C., Issues concerning androgen replacement therapy in postmenopausal women, *Mayo Clin. Proc.*, 72, 1051, 1997.
70. Bennell, K.L., Brukner, P.D., and Malcolm, S.A., Effect of altered reproductive function and lowered testosterone levels on bone density in male endurance athletes, *Br. J. Sports Med.*, 30, 205, 1996.
71. Burns-Cox, N. and Gingell, C., The andropause: fact or fiction? *Postgrad. Med. J.*, 73, 553, 1997.
72. Reid, I.R., Glucocorticoid osteoporosis — mechanisms and management, *Eur. J. Endocrinol.*, 137, 209, 1997.
73. Maas, D., Jochen, A., and Lalande, B., Age-related changes in male gonadal function — implications for therapy, *Drugs Aging*, 11, 45, 1997.
74. Ebeling, P.R., Osteoporosis in men — new insights into aetiology, pathogenesis, prevention and management, *Drugs Aging*, 13, 421, 1998.
75. St. Clair, R.W., Estrogens and atherosclerosis: phytoestrogens and selective estrogen receptor modulators, *Curr. Opinion Lipidol.*, 9, 457, 1998.
76. Hosking, D.J., Calcium homeostasis in pregnancy, *Clin. Endocrinol.*, 45, 1, 1996.
77. Khovidhunkit, W. and Epstein, S., Osteoporosis in pregnancy, *Osteoporosis Int.*, 6, 345, 1996.
78. Koeger, A.C., Timsit, M.A., and Oberlin, F., Calcium metabolism in normal pregnancy and lactation, *Rev. Med. Intern.*, 18, 533, 1997.
79. Koeger, A.C. and Oberlin, F., Calcium and bone disorders during pregnancy and lactation, *Rev. Med. Intern.*, 18, 546, 1997.
80. Meling, T.R. and Nylen, E.S., Growth hormone deficiency in adults: a review, *Am. J. Med. Sci.*, 311, 153, 1996.
81. Russell-Jones, D.L. and Weissberger, A.J., The role of growth hormone in the regulation of body composition in the adult, *Growth Regul.*, 6, 247, 1996.

82. Marcus, R. and Hoffman, A.R., Growth hormone as therapy for older men and women, *Annu. Rev. Pharmacol. Toxicol.*, 38, 45, 1998.

83. Bonjour, J.P., Chevalley, T., Ammann, P., et al., Growth hormone, IGF and bone metabolism in the adult, *Ann. Endocrinol.*, 57, 147, 1996.

84. Eriksen, E.F., Kassem, M., and Langdahl, B., Growth hormone, insulin-like growth factors and bone remodelling, *Eur. J. Clin. Invest.*, 26, 525, 1996.

85. Rosen, C.J. and Donahue, L.R., Insulinlike growth factors: potential therapeutic options for osteoporosis, *Trends Endocrine Metab.*, 6, 235, 1995.

86. Inzucchi, S.E. and Robbins, R.J., Growth hormone and the maintenance of adult bone mineral density, *Clin. Endocrinol.*, 45, 665, 1996.

87. Bartalena, L., Bognzzi, F., and Martino, E., Adverse effects of thyroid hormone preparations and antithyroid drugs, *Drug Saf.*, 15, 53, 1996.

88. Lauwers, A. and Alexandre, C., Impact on bone of thyroid hormone therapy, *Rev. Rhum.*, 64, 112, 1997.

89. Williams, J.B., Adverse effects of thyroid hormones, *Drugs Aging*, 11, 460, 1997.

90. Williams, G.R., Robson, H., and Shalet, S.M., Thyroid hormone actions on cartilage and bone: interactions with other hormones at the epiphyseal plate and effects on linear growth, *J. Endocrinol.*, 157, 391, 1998.

91. Cosman, F. and Lindsay, R., Is parathyroid hormone a therapeutic option for osteoporosis? A review of the clinical evidence, *Calcif. Tissue Int.*, 62, 475, 1998.

92. Picado, C. and Luengo, M., Corticosteroid-induced bone loss — prevention and management, *Drug Saf.*, 15, 347, 1996.

93. Moe, S.M., The treatment of steroid-induced bone loss in transplantation, *Curr. Opinion Nephrol. Hypertension*, 6, 544, 1997.

94. Keenan, G.F., Management of complications of glucocorticoid therapy, *Clin. Chest Med.*, 18, 507, 1997.

95. Schatz, M. and Hamilos, D., Osteoporosis in glucocorticoid-dependent asthmatic patients; literature review and recommendations, *Clin. Immunother.*, 4, 180, 1995.

96. Lane, N.E. and Lukert, B., The science and therapy of glucocorticoid-induced bone loss, *Endocrine Metab. Clin. North Am.*, 27, 465, 1998.

97. Li, B.H. and Aspden, R.M., Mechanical and material properties of the subchondral bone plate from the femoral head of patients with osteoarthritis or osteoporosis, *Ann. Rheum. Dis.*, 56, 247, 1997.

98. Li, B.H. and Aspden, R.M., Composition and mechanical properties of cancellous bone from the femoral head of patients with osteoporosis or osteoarthritis, *J. Bone Miner. Res.*, 12, 641, 1997.

99. Li, B.H. and Aspden, R.M., Material properties of bone from the femoral neck and calcar femorale of patients with osteoporosis or osteoarthritis, *Osteopororis Int.*, 7, 450, 1997.

100. Bellingham, C.M., Lee, J.M., Moran, E.L., and Bogoch, E.R., Bisphosphonate (Pamidronate APD) prevents arthritis-induced loss of fracture toughness in the rabbit femoral diaphysis, *J. Orthop. Res.*, 13, 876, 1995.

101. Wolinskyfriedland, M., Drug induced metabolic bone disease, *Endocrine Metab. Clin. North Am.*, 24, 395, 1995.

102. Kleerekoper, M., Fluoride and the skeleton, *Crit. Rev. Clin. Lab. Sci.*, 33, 139, 1996.

103. Eastell, R., Boyle, I.T., Compston, J., et al., Management of male osteoporosis: report of the U.K. Consensus Group, *Q. J. Med.*, 91, 71, 1998.

104. Anderson, F.H., Osteoporosis in men, *Int. J. Clin. Pract.*, 52, 176, 1998.

105. Turan, B., Balcik, C., and Akkas, N., Effect of dietary selenium and vitamin E on the biomechanical properties of rabbit bones, *Clin. Rheum.*, 16, 441, 1997.

106. Kelepouris, N., Harper, K.D., Gannon, F., et al., Severe osteoporosis in men, *Ann. Intern. Med.*, 123, 452, 1995.

107. Wark, J.D., Osteoporotic fractures: background and prevention strategies, *Maturitas*, 23, 193, 1996.

108. Auquier, P., Manuel, C., and Molines, C., Risk factors of post menopausal osteoporosis. Analysis of the literature 1990–1995, *Rev. Epidem. Sante Publique*, 45, 328, 1997.

109. Preedy, V.R., Peters, T.J., and Why, H., Metabolic consequences of alcohol dependency, *Adverse Drug React. Toxic. Rev.*, 16, 235, 1997.

110. Hachulla, E. and Cortet, B., Prevention of glucocorticoid-induced osteoporosis, *Rev. Med. Intern*, 19, 492, 1998.

111. Gennari, C., Martini, G., and Nuti, R., Secondary osteoporosis, *Aging Clin. Exp. Res.,* 10, 214, 1998.
112. Treves, R., Louer, V., Bonnet, C., et al., Osteoporosis in men, *Presse Med.,* 27, 1647, 1998.
113. Nishi, Y., Zinc and growth, *J. Am. Coll. Nutr.,* 15, 340, 1996.
114. Wilke, H.J., Krischak, S., and Claes, L.E., Formalin fixation strongly influences biomechanical properties of the spine, *J. Biomech.,* 29, 1629, 1996.
115. Currey, J.D., Brear, K., Zioupos, P., and Reilly, G. C., Effect of formaldehyde fixation on some mechanical properties of bovine bone, *Biomaterials,* 16, 1267, 1995.
116. Oxlund, H., Barchman, M., Rotoft, G., and Andreassen, T.T., Reduced concentrations of collagen cross-links are associated with reduced strength of bone, *Bone,* 17, S365, 1995.
117. McElhaney, J.H., Fogle, J., Byars, E., and Weaver, G., Effect of embalming on the mechanical properties of beef bone, *J. Appl. Physiol.,* 19, 1234, 1964.
118. Borchers, R.E., Gibson, L.J., Burchardt, H., and Hayes, W.C., Effects of selected thermal variables on the mechanical properties of trabecular bone, *Biomaterials,* 16, 545, 1995.
119. Smith, C.W., The Mechanical Properties of Biological Materials Stored by Tissue Banks, Ph.D. thesis, University of Leeds, U.K., 1995.
120. Viceconti, M., Toni, A., Brizio, L., et al., The effect of autoclaving on the mechanical properties of bank bovine bone, *Chir. Organi. Mov.,* 81, 63, 1996.
121. Kohler, P., Kreicbergs, A., and Stromberg, L., Physical properties of autoclaved bone. Torsion test of rabbit diaphyseal bone, *Acta Orthop. Scand.,* 57, 141, 1986.
122. Knaepler, H., Haas, H., and Puschel, H.U., [Biomechanical properties of heat and irradiation treated spongiosa], *Unfallchirurgie,* 17, 194, 1991.
123. Linde, F. and Sørensen, H.C., The effect of different storage methods on the mechanical properties of trabecular bone, *J. Biomech.,* 26, 1249, 1993.
124. Kang, Q., An, Y.H., and Friedman, R.J., Effects of multiple freezing–thawing cycles on ultimate indentation load and stiffness of bovine cancellous bone, *Am. J. Vet. Res.,* 58, 1171, 1997.
125. Strömberg, L. and Dalén, N., The influence of freezing on the maximum torque capacity of long bones. An experimental study on dog, *Acta Orthop. Scand.,* 47, 254, 1976.
126. Tomford, W.W., Doppelt, S.H., Mankin, H.J., and Friedlaender, G.E., 1983 bone bank procedures, *Clin. Orthop.,* 174, 15, 1983.
127. Sumner, D.R., Willke, T.L., Berzins, A., and Turner, T.M., Distribution of Young's modulus in the cancellous bone of the proximal canine tibia, *J. Biomech.,* 27, 1095, 1994.
128. Malinin, T.I., Martinez, O.V., and Brown, M.D., Banking of massive osteoarticular and intercalary bone allografts-12 years' experience, *Clin. Orthop.,* 197, 44, 1985.
129. Panjabi, M.M., Krag, M., Summers, D., and Videman, T., Biomechanical time-tolerance of fresh cadaveric human spine specimens, *J. Orthop. Res.,* 3, 292, 1985.
130. Roe, S.C., Pijanowski, G.J., and Johnson, A.L., Biomechanical properties of canine cortical bone allografts: effects of preparation and storage, *Am. J. Vet. Res.,* 49, 873, 1988.
131. Sedlin, E.D. and Hirsch, C., Factors affecting the determination of the physical properties of femoral cortical bone, *Acta Orthop. Scand.,* 37, 29, 1966.
132. Pelker, R.R., Friedlaender, G.E., and Markham, T.C., et al., Effects of freezing and freeze-drying on the biomechanical properties of rat bone, *J. Orthop. Res.,* 1, 405, 1984.
133. Currey, J.D., The effects of drying and re-wetting on some mechanical properties of cortical bone, *J. Biomech.,* 21, 439, 1988.
134. Triantafyllou, N., Sotiropoulos, E., and Triantafyllou, J.N., The mechanical properties of lyophilized and irradiated bone grafts, *Acta Orthop. Belg.,* 41, 35, 1975.
135. Bright, R.W. and Burstein, A.H. Material properties of preserved cortical bone, *Trans. Orthop. Res. Soc.,* 24, 210, 1978.
136. Simonian, P.T., Conrad, E.U., Chapman, J.R., et al., Effect of sterilization and storage treatments on screw pullout strength in human allograft bone, *Clin. Orthop.,* 302, 290, 1994.
137. Webster, D.A. and Werner, F.W., Mechanical and functional properties of implanted freeze-dried flexor tendons, *Clin. Orthop.,* 180, 302, 1983.
138. Jackson, D.W., Grood, E.S., Arnoczky, S.P., et al., Freeze-dried anterior cruciate ligament allografts, *Am. J. Sports Med.,* 15, 295, 1988.
139. Smith, C.W., Young, I.S., and Kearney, J.N., Mechanical properties of tendons: changes with sterilization and preservation, *J. Biomech. Eng.,* 118, 56, 1996.

140. Sugimoto, M., Takahashi, S., Toguchida, J., et al., Changes in bone after high dose irradiation — biomechanics and histomorphology, *J. Bone Joint Surg.*, 73B, 492, 1991.
141. Anderson, M.J., Keyak, J.H., and Skinner, H.B., Compressive mechanical properties of human cancellous bone after gamma irradiation, *J. Bone Joint Surg.*, 74A, 747, 1992.
142. Smith, C.W. and Kearney, J.N., The effects of irradiation and hydration upon the mechanical properties of tendon, *J. Mater. Sci. Mater. Med.*, 7, 645, 1996.
143. Edgerton, B.C., An, K.N., and Morrey, B.F., Torsional strength reduction due to cortical defects in bone, *J. Orthop. Res.*, 8, 851, 1990.
144. Hipp, J.A., Edgerton, B.C., An, K.N., and Hayes, W.C., Structural consequences of transcortical holes in long bones loaded in torsion, *J. Biomech.*, 23, 1261, 1990.
145. An, Y.H. and Bell, T.D., Experimental design, evaluation methods, data analysis, publication, and research ethics, in *Animal Models in Orthopaedic Research*, An, Y.H. and Friedman, R.J., Eds., CRC Press, Boca Raton, FL, 1999.
146. Zioupos, P., Currey, J.D., Mirza, M.S., and Barton, D.C., Experimentally determined microcracking around a circular hole in a flat plate of bone: comparison with predicted stresses, *Philos. Trans. R. Soc. London B*, 347, 383, 1995.
147. Ashman, R.B., Experimental techniques, in *Bone Mechanics*, Cowin, S.C., Ed., CRC Press, Boca Raton, FL, 1989, 91.
148. Wall, J.C., Chatterji, S., and Jeffery, J.W., On the origin of scatter in results of human bone strength tests, *Med. Biol. Eng.*, 8, 171, 1970.

5 Basic Facilities and Instruments for Mechanical Testing of Bone

Christopher V. Bensen and Yuehuei H. An

CONTENTS

I. INTRODUCTION

The biomechanical evaluation of bone, bone implants, and the bone–implant interface has been carried out for many years. Such investigations nearly always employ the use of mechanical testing systems to generate information on the physical properties of these materials. From simple compression and tension failure testing to fatigue analysis of new total joint prostheses, modern computer-driven machines are commonly used to provide analysis and information.

Increased prevalence of debilitating conditions such as degenerative joint disease as well as rising popularity of internal devices for fracture fixation has led to rapid growth of the orthopaedic and biomechanical research communities. Along with this growth has been a commensurate rise in the diversity and production of commercially available testing systems to meet the ever-increasing demand for better and less expensive implants and the specific needs of the modern investigator.

Implementation of a materials testing laboratory is neither an easy nor inexpensive endeavor. However, the utility and potential capabilities of even the most basic laboratory can provide the opportunity to perform numerous experiments and far outweigh the initial difficulties or expenses encountered. In addition to being a useful research platform, a mechanical testing laboratory is a valuable and practical "hands-on" teaching tool for orthopaedic surgery residents, graduate students, and technicians alike.

This chapter reviews the scope of modern mechanical testing systems, both commercial and otherwise, and examines the requirements for implementation of a materials testing laboratory. Finally, the chapter provides information on necessary ancillary materials which facilitate the execution of biomechanical investigations. It is the authors' hope that this information will be useful to both the established and the new investigator attempting to set up a materials testing laboratory.

II. MECHANICAL TESTING MACHINES

Although numerous types of mechanical testing systems are currently in production, the vast majority can be divided into two types based on the methods by which load is applied to the specimen: servohydraulic and electromechanical. Servohydraulic testing machines comprise the majority of systems in use for examination of orthopaedic materials. In these systems, a servovalve is used to transform electrical energy into hydraulic fluid pressure. This pressure is then applied as load to the specimen. Even smaller servohydraulic machines are capable of delivering relatively large loads to test specimens, often exceeding 25 kN. Electromechanical machines provide relatively small loads, usually 1 kN or less. They are suitable for evaluating smaller specimens, such as sutures, bone–tendon complexes, and screw pullout models. There are numerous types of servohydraulic systems currently available and their components and major types along with their potential applications are described below.

A. COMPONENTS OF MECHANICAL TESTING MACHINES

The typical mechanical testing machine has several key components, including the hydraulic power supply (HPS), actuator, controller, load unit, force transducer, fixture devices, and data generator. Each of these integral components is briefly described below.

1. Hydraulic Power Supply Units

The HPS provides the fluid pressure necessary to drive the actuator piston. Hydraulic fluid is circulated at flow rates between 3 gallons per minute (gpm) to over 200 gpm on larger models providing continuous pressures of 1000 to 3000 psi. The regulation of hydraulic fluid flow and pressure is controlled by a servovalve. The servovalve is usually mounted to an actuator and uses changes in voltage to govern direction and flow of hydraulic fluid, which consequently moves the actuator rod. Figure 5.1 illustrates a typical HPS unit. HPS units can be either air cooled or water cooled depending on the size and maximum pressures attained by the system. HPS units are typically protected from overheating and low fluid levels by electronic interlocks that automatically turn off the unit should hazardous conditions exist.

2. Load Units

The load unit of the system employs actuator rods to apply load to the specimen. These actuators can be mounted in linear, rotary, or angular alignment depending on the system. In servohydraulic systems, the actuator operates under control of a servovalve and contains a linear variable differential transducer (LVDT), which provides rod displacement information to the controller. In axial-only load units, there is a single linear mounted actuator rod which can apply compression or tensile forces to a specimen. For torsional forces, a rotary actuator is added to the linear one allowing the application of biaxial forces to the specimen. More complex and specialized load units are also available for a variety of applications.

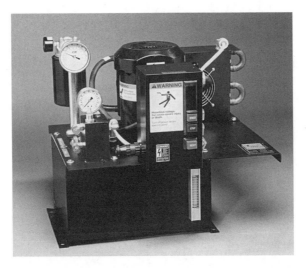

FIGURE 5.1   Typical hydraulic power supply unit for a small mechanical testing machine (MTS Model 512). (Courtesy of MTS Systems, Inc., Eden Prairie, MN.)

3. Force Transducers

Load applied to specimens during testing procedures is measured with a force transducer, commonly called a load cell, which is mounted on the fixed side opposite the load unit. Transducers are available in a variety of load ranges and should be selected based on both the operating limitations of the actuator as well as the intended use of the testing system. Another type of transducer commonly used in mechanical testing of bone is the extensometer. This device measures the displacement and/or strain on a specimen which is typically being tested to loads below the yield point.

4. Controllers

Controllers provide several functions including control of the HPS and servovalve, transducer conditioning, function generation, and data output. The most basic controllers are usually single-channel devices which are suited to uniaxial testing. They typically include function generators which provide waveforms such as sine and square which are commonly used in fatigue testing. The controller is used to set testing variables and parameters including the rate of load application to the specimen, peak load, and maximum displacement of the actuator rod. Tests are based either on displacement control in which displacement is carried out at a constant rate while the load is measured or on displacement control in which displacement is measured during a constant loading rate. Figure 5.2 illustrates a typical controller for basic mechanical testing systems. More powerful controllers have the capability of receiving externally generated command signals and even allow the design and programming of specific testing protocols. Controllers for joint simulation systems are multichannel and are capable of controlling multiaxial motion in a temperature-controlled environment for several testing stations.

5. Sample-Holding Devices

A critical aspect of any testing procedure is mounting the specimen on the mechanical testing system. It is imperative that the specimen be held firmly without slippage and, more importantly, without damage to the specimen itself. Incomplete or irregular gripping of the specimen can cause premature failure at the specimen–clamp interface and can lead to erroneous testing values.

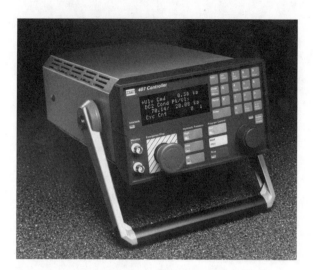

FIGURE 5.2   Single-channel controller useful for all types of single-axis research (MTS Model 407). (Courtesy of MTS Systems, Inc., Eden Prairie, MN.)

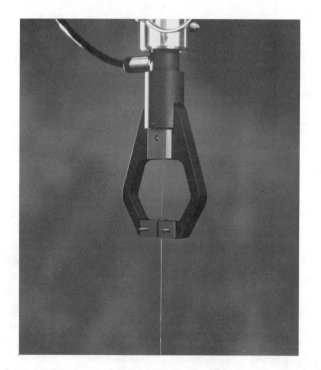

FIGURE 5.3   Typical pneumatic grips used for holding small specimens. (Courtesy of MTS Systems, Inc., Eden Prairie, MN.)

Numerous holding devices and grips are commercially available for this purpose. For bone and bone–tendon complexes, simple screw clamps often will suffice. For testing wires, sutures, small tendons, and similar specimens, specialized grips can facilitate the testing and minimize risk of damage to the specimen (Figure 5.3).

Over the past several years, pneumatically driven holding devices have become the standard method of specimen fixation. These units have interchangeable grips for a variety of testing requirements and have significantly reduced the problems associated with specimen fixation.

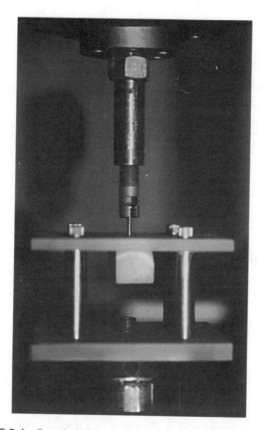

FIGURE 5.4 Sample holding device used for screw pullout testing.

An alternative to these grips and holding devices is available if there is access to a machine shop. Simple, yet useful clamps and grips with screw and wing nut locking mechanisms can be machined from stock aluminum or stainless steel at a fraction of the cost of commercially manufactured ones and will often suffice, especially with durable specimens. In fact, most investigations are carried out with custom-designed grips and fixtures. An example of such a fixture used for testing screw pullout strength is shown in Figure 5.4. This fixture was designed and produced in the authors' laboratory.

6. Data Management Systems

Historically, data acquisition from most mechanical testing systems was achieved by means of a graphic chart recorder. Figure 5.5 shows an older single-axis testing system with a chart recorder in one of the laboratories at the authors' institution.

Load–displacement curves can be easily plotted using such a device; however, meticulous manual measurements and calculations are required to determine biomechanical parameters of the specimen. Consequently, there is additional risk of obtaining errors in data analysis.

In modern testing machines, data are transferred from the controller to a computer where data points can be stored and parameters can be automatically calculated. There are numerous software packages available for mechanical testing system–linked PCs such as LabView (National Instruments Corporation, Austin, TX). These programs can greatly facilitate data acquisition, management, and analysis. Alternatively, the major mechanical testing machine companies also offer software support both for the controller and PC-based systems.

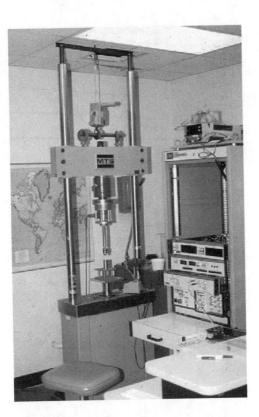

FIGURE 5.5   Older model mechanical testing machine with chart recorder.

B. COMMON TYPES OF MECHANICAL TESTING MACHINES OR DEVICES

1. Single-Axis Machines

Mechanical testing systems with a single linear actuator are suitable for a very large variety of testing procedures and are the systems most widely used today (Figure 5.6). Compression, tensile, bending, and indentation or hardness testing can all be accomplished with single-axis machines. Compression testing is commonly used to determine the mechanical properties of both cortical and cancellous bones.[1] Tensile testing is also very commonly used to measure the elasticity of bones, tendons, ligaments, as well as bone–tendon and bone–ligament–bone complexes. Three-point bending tests may also be performed on either standard-cut cortical specimens or intact bones. Finally, single-axis machines can be used for screw pullout tests to compare various types of screws or screw fixation. Pushout testing is also one of the most common and simplest ways to evaluate the bone–implant interface.[2-4]

2. Multiaxial Machines

The addition of a rotary actuator allows simultaneous testing of two mechanical properties of a specimen. This type of machine is essential for numerous types of testing, including that of the spine (Figure 5.7). Additionally, torsional testing of whole long bones and other materials can be evaluated while an axial load is being applied. This load simulates the body weight of an animal and more closely resembles *in vivo* physiological forces.

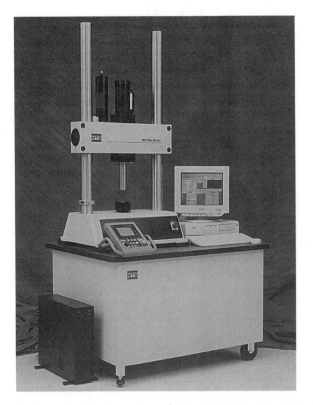

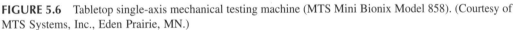

FIGURE 5.6 Tabletop single-axis mechanical testing machine (MTS Mini Bionix Model 858). (Courtesy of MTS Systems, Inc., Eden Prairie, MN.)

3. Micromechanical Testing Machines

Evaluation of the microstructure of bone requires mechanical testing of single osteons or trabeculae. Tension, compression, bending, and torsional tests of single osteons have all been undertaken over the past several decades.[5-9] Highly specialized equipment is required in these investigations, as sample isolation, preparation, and mounting all require a higher degree of precision. Numerous devices have been designed and assembled by investigators themselves and one example of such a machine developed by Mente is shown in Figure 5.8.[10] Another example is the tensile micromechanical testing device developed by Rho (Figure 5.9). Additionally, several of the major mechanical testing machine companies have the capability to custom-design testing platforms to specifications required by the investigator. A few machines are also commercially available (Figure 5.10). Micromechanical testing is covered further in Chapters 18 and 19.

4. Hardness/Indentation Testing Devices

Another specialized mechanical testing system is the hardness or indentation testing machine. Hardness is a common parameter used to compare resistance of materials (including bone) to indentation or abrasion. There are a variety of testing systems based on the size and geometry of the specimens and the loads applied. First, macroindentation testing such as the Brinell method is useful for evaluating the hardness of specimens such as cortical or cancellous bone surfaces using loads of 1 kg or greater (Figure 5.11).[11,12] Microhardness testing using the Knoop and Vickers indenters allows evaluation of resistance of bone to indentation which can reflect biochemical

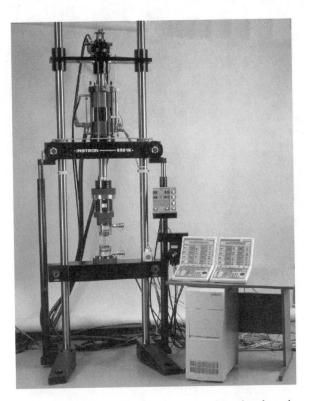

FIGURE 5.7 Multiaxis mechanical testing machine capable of torsional testing. (Courtesy of Instron Corporation, Canton, MA.)

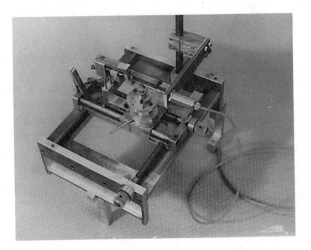

FIGURE 5.8 Micromechanical testing machine. (Courtesy of Dr. Peter Mente.)

properties such as mineral content.[13-15] Finally, over the past decade, the development of nanoindentation testing machines has allowed the testing of mechanical properties of specimens on the order of nanometers, such as individual trabeculae and osteonic lamellae.[16-18] Figure 5.12 shows a typical nanoindentation testing device. There are also combination imaging–testing devices such as the TriboScope© (Figure 5.13, Hysitron, Inc., Minneapolis, MN). This device combines atomic force microscopy with a nanoindenter which allows the investigator to image the sample, choose

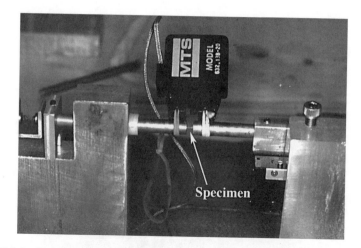

FIGURE 5.9   Tensile micromechanical testing machine. (Courtesy of Dr. Jae-Rong Rho.)

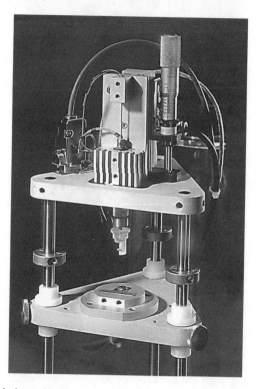

FIGURE 5.10   Latour-Black dynamic micromechanical tester. (Courtesy of Dynatek Delta Scientific Instruments, Galena, MO.)

the test location, indent, scratch, and wear surfaces with a single device. Nanoindentation testing is covered in further detail in Chapter 17.

III. SAMPLE POTTING MATERIALS

Many specimens cannot be mounted directly to the mechanical testing system and must be "potted" in another medium in order to be tested. These may include small and/or irregularly shaped specimens which do not afford adequate purchase to which standard grips can be attached, as well

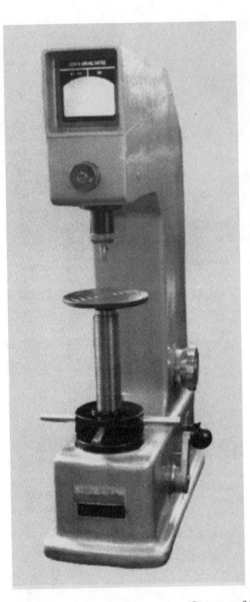

FIGURE 5.11   Brinell-Rockwell-Vickers optical hardness tester. (Courtesy of Nanotek, Inc., Opelika, AL.)

as complex constructs involving several bones. In addition, potting a specimen allows precise alignment and allows testing with minimal risk of damaging the integrity of the specimen.

A variety of materials are available for this purpose including polymethylmethacrylate (PMMA), plaster of paris,[19] epoxy resins,[20] and calcium sulfate-based materials such as dental stone.[21] One such material typically used for creating dental casts from alginate impressions is called Labstone (Heraeus Kulzer, Inc., Dental Products Division, South Bend, IN). This material comes in powder form, is mixed with water in either a disposable or flexible, reuseable container, and has a curing time of approximately 8 to 10 min. This provides ample working time to set the specimen, yet hardens quickly enough such that it can be tested within an hour or so. When dry, it has a compression strength of 8000 psi and volumetric expansion of only 0.12%. The authors have used this material in several investigations without complications. An example of the use of this material in the authors' laboratory is shown in Figure 5.14. In this experiment, the biomechanical properties of various methods of scapulothoracic arthrodesis was examined. Three cadaver ribs

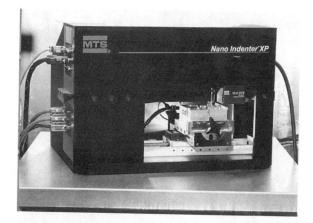

FIGURE 5.12   Nanoindentation machine (Nanindenter XP). (Courtesy of MTS Systems, Inc., Eden Prairie, MN.)

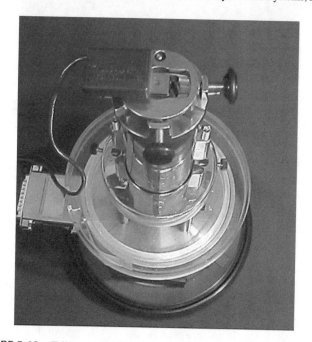

FIGURE 5.13   Triboscope. (Courtesy of Hysitron, Inc., Minneapolis, MN.)

were potted in anatomic position prior to fixation of the scapula. The entire construct could then be mounted on the mechanical testing system using C-clamps at the base of the construct, providing a solid link between the specimen and system.[22]

IV. OTHER BASIC ITEMS

Proper preparation of specimens for mechanical testing requires several key tools. A band saw with a ¼-in. fine-tooth blade is an invaluable general resource for preparing gross bone samples for testing (Figure 5.15). For making small, cylindrical bone specimens for compression testing, a tabletop drill press with a trephine bit is sufficient (Figure 5.16). However, a lathe or milling machine is more appropriate for larger specimens. A wheel grinder/polisher (Figure 5.17) is also a useful tool in final preparation of bone specimens in which specific dimensions must be identical. Electronic calipers also aid in this procedure.

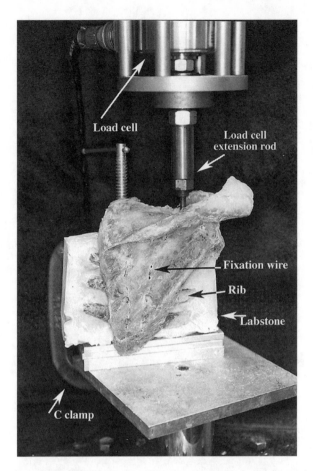

FIGURE 5.14 Illustration of the use of Labstone (Denstone) to embed ribs for testing various methods of scapulothoracic arthrodesis.

One common method of storing bones is freezing at –20°C; however, –70°C is ideal. Numerous investigators have shown that there is little or no detrimental effect on the mechanical properties of bone that is stored at –20°C for periods up to 8 months.[23-25] It is important to freeze bone specimens in an airtight plastic bag containing normal saline. Because it may be impractical to collect all specimens for a single experiment at once, a large-volume freezer is an essential component to a mechanical testing laboratory.

Finally, an operating table and some basic surgical instruments (such as a scalpel, forceps, and scissors), as well as a supply of surgical towels, gloves, plastic bags, saline, etc. should also be readily available in or near the laboratory for proper specimen preparation.

V. SUMMARY

In conclusion, mechanical testing systems offer the orthopaedic researcher the ability to measure numerous properties of a bone specimen or construct. A large variety of machines are commercially available from several companies; it is up to the individual researcher or team to decide which model is appropriate for the research being carried out in the respective laboratory. It is the authors' opinion that a single-axis system affords a relatively inexpensive, yet versatile tool with which mechanical testing of bone can be performed. The vast majority of testing procedures commonly in use, including compression, indentation, and three-point bending, can be achieved

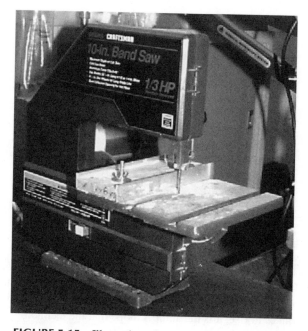

FIGURE 5.15 Illustration of an 8-in. tabletop band saw.

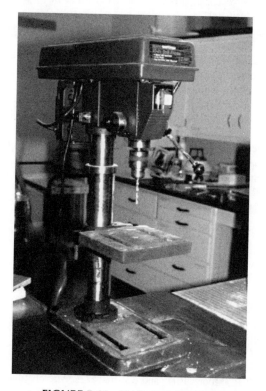

FIGURE 5.16 Tabletop drill press.

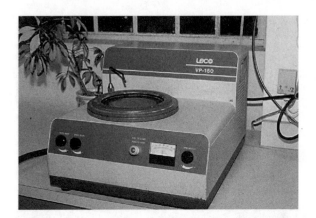

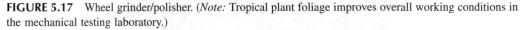

FIGURE 5.17   Wheel grinder/polisher. (*Note:* Tropical plant foliage improves overall working conditions in the mechanical testing laboratory.)

with a single-axis machine. Alternatively, should specialized testing situations demand, multiaxis and even custom-built machines are also available from the major manufacturers.

As the demand for improved implants and devices in the treatment of disorders of the musculoskeletal system continues to rise, it is the authors' hope that the technology of the testing systems designed for their evaluation will continue to improve.

REFERENCES

1. Linde, F., Elastic and viscoelastic properties of trabecular bone by a compression testing approach, *Dan. Med. Bull.,* 41, 119, 1994.
2. Dhert, W.J., Verheyen, C.C., Braak, L.H., et al., A finite-element analysis of the pushout test: influence of test conditions, *J. Biomed. Mater. Res.,* 26, 119, 1992.
3. Friedman, R.J., Bauer, T.W., Garg, K., et al., Histological and mechanical comparison of hydroxyapatite-coated cobalt-chrome and titanium implants in the rabbit femur, *J. Appl. Biomater.,* 6, 231, 1995.
4. An, Y.H., Friedman, R.J., Jiang, M., et al., Bone ingrowth to implant surfaces in an inflammatory arthritis model, *J. Orthop. Res.,* 16, 576, 1998.
5. Ascenzi, A., Baschieri, P., and Benvenuti, A., The bending properties of single osteons, *J. Biomech.,* 23, 763, 1990.
6. Ascenzi, A., Baschieri, P., and Benvenuti, A., The torsional properties of single selected osteons [see comments], *J. Biomech.,* 27, 875, 1994.
7. Ascenzi, A. and Bonucci, E., The compressive properties of single osteons, *Anat. Rec.,* 161, 377, 1968.
8. Frasca, P., Harper, R.A., and Katz, J.L., Micromechanical oscillators and techniques for determining the dynamic moduli of microsamples of human cortical bone at microstrains, *J. Biomech. Eng.,* 103, 146, 1981.
9. Frasca, P., Jacyna, G., Harper, R., and Katz, J.L., Strain dependence of dynamic Young's modulus for human single osteons, *J. Biomech.,* 14, 691, 1981.
10. Mente, P.L. and Lewis, J.L., Experimental method for the measurement of the elastic modulus of trabecular bone tissue, *J. Orthop. Res.,* 7, 456, 1989.
11. Björkstrom, S. and Goldie, I.F., Hardness of the subchondral bone of the patella in the normal state, in chondromalacia, and in osteoarthrosis, *Acta Orthop. Scand.,* 53, 451, 1982.
12. Markel, M.D., Wikenheiser, M.A., and Chao, E.Y., A study of fracture callus material properties: relationship to the torsional strength of bone, *J. Orthop. Res.,* 8, 843, 1990.
13. Knoop, P., Peters, C.G., and Emerson, W.B., A sensitive pyramidal-diamond tool for indentation measurements, *J. Res. Natl. Bur. Stand.,* 23, 39, 1939.
14. Huja, S.S., Katona, T.R., Moore, B.K., and Roberts, W.E., Microhardness and anisotropy of the vital osseous interface and endosseous implant supporting bone, *J. Orthop. Res.,* 16, 54, 1998.

15. Amprino, R., Investigations on some physical properties of bone tissue, *Acta Anat.,* 34, 161, 1958.
16. Lee, F.Y., Rho, J.Y., Harten, R., Jr., et al., Micromechanical properties of epiphyseal trabecular bone and primary spongiosa around the physis: an *in situ* nanoindentation study, *J. Pediatr. Orthop.,* 18, 582, 1998.
17. Rho, J.Y., Tsui, T.Y., and Pharr, G.M., Elastic properties of human cortical and trabecular lamellar bone measured by nanoindentation, *Biomaterials,* 18, 1325, 1997.
18. Zysset, P.K., Guo, X.E., Hoffler, C.E., et al., Mechanical properties of human trabecular bone lamellae quantified by nanoindentation, *Technol. Health Care,* 6, 429, 1998.
19. Davis, P.K., Mazur, J.M., and Coleman, G.N., A torsional strength comparison of vascularized and nonvascularized bone grafts, *J. Biomech.,* 15, 875, 1982.
20. Paavolainen, P., Studies on mechanical strength of bone. I. Torsional strength of normal rabbit tibio-fibular bone, *Acta Orthop. Scand.,* 49, 497, 1978.
21. Lepola, V., Vaananen, K., and Jalovaara, P., The effect of immobilization on the torsional strength of the rat tibia, *Clin. Orthop.,* 55, 1993.
22. Bensen, C.V., Barfield, W.R., Draughn, R.A., and Thompson, J.D., Biomechanical evaluation of methods of scapulothoracic fusion for treatment of FSH muscular dystrophy, *Trans. Orthop. Res. Soc.,* 23, 1147, 1998.
23. Strömberg, L. and Dalén, N., The influence of freezing on the maximum torque capacity of long bones. An experimental study on dogs, *Acta Orthop. Scand.,* 47, 254, 1976.
24. Roe, S.C., Pijanowski, G.J., and Johnson, A.L., Biomechanical properties of canine cortical bone allografts: effects of preparation and storage, *Am. J. Vet. Res.,* 49, 873, 1988.
25. Panjabi, M.M., Krag, M., Summers, D., and Videman, T., Biomechanical time-tolerance of fresh cadaveric human spine specimens, *J. Orthop. Res.,* 3, 292, 1985.

6 Methods of Evaluation for Bone Dimensions, Densities, Contents, Morphology, and Structures

Yuehuei H. An, William R. Barfield, and Ivars Knets

CONTENTS

I. INTRODUCTION

Bone dimensions (such as length, thickness, area, and volume), densities, mineral contents, and structure at both macro- and microlevels, even at the nanolevel, are basic parameters for bone mechanical testing and data analysis. Bone strength and modulus are assessed through determining the macroscopic and microscopic characteristics, which include the size, shape, density, and architecture of the bone, as well as the tested mechanical values. Although simple to execute, the accuracy of these measurements is frequently related to the validity of the methods being used.

II. MACROMEASUREMENTS OF BONE DIMENSIONS

Many methods have been used for measuring length, area, and volume of bone tissues. These methods include direct measurement using a ruler, micrometer, or caliper, measurement based on radiographs, or the use of specially designed devices.[1,2] There may be significant intermethod or interobserver variability.[3,4] Therefore, several observers may be needed to perform the same procedure independently, or more than one method may be used. Caution should be taken when interstudy comparison is made, especially if different measurement techniques are employed. Bone mineral content and the structural properties of femoral cross sections have been calculated from simplifying assumptions based on geometric properties, moduli, and whole-bone strength indexes.[5]

A. DIRECT MEASUREMENTS

Most length and area measurements such as the measurements of long bone dimensions (length, internal and external width) are accomplished reliably by such traditional techniques as a ruler or sliding digital caliper.[3,4] Intraobserver error can result from the use of calipers, but can be lessened with use of an electronic digitizer.[6] A specially designed electronic caliper has also been reported.[7] A magnifying glass to measure radiographs has also been demonstrated as useful. This technique has been reported to provide greater reliability and precision than caliper measurement when measuring bone width and cortical thickness.[7,8]

According to a recent report, a digital coordinatometer-goniometer connected to an optical collimator allows angles and bone lengths to be measured. This new technique allows for location of the bone axis and torsion values using a reference plane and symmetry and tangency criteria. Findings are that angular measures are more precise than through use of traditional instruments.[9]

The archaeological collection of Pecos Pueblo femora and tibiae were examined through use of an electronic digitizer and computer program. Geometric cross sections were determined using a FORTRAN computer program which divided the total bone area of interest into a series of small geometric shapes which were subsequently summed to determine the total composite properties. Cross sections were scaled and electronically digitized with subperiosteal and endosteal boundaries manually traced with a stylus. The geometric data generated from these bone samples pointed to specific *in vivo* loading of the lower limb which served as a natural protective mechanism to manage effectively the stress–strain loadings sustained by the Pecos Pueblo people during this period of history.[10]

B. MEASUREMENTS BASED ON X-RAY IMAGES

Two-dimensional (2D) measurements are often made from X-ray images using a ruler or caliper.[6,8,11,12] The percentage magnification should be considered when using X-ray images for measurements. The amount of magnification depends on the distance between the specimen and the film. A metal bar or strip with known length can be used as a reference. It should be placed at the same distance from the film as the subject. A standard goniometer is effective for measuring angles based on radiographic images. A custom computer program based on X-ray images has been developed in the authors' laboratory. It is capable of evaluating the periosteal and endosteal dimensions of the upper humerus and glenoid. Parameters which may be evaluated include humeral canal width, shaft width, tuberosity offset, head offset, radius of curvature of the head and glenoid, head diameter, canal flare index, glenoid height and depth, arc of enclosure, radius of curvature, and depth of cancellous bone.[13-15]

The length or perimeter of irregular lines or the area of irregular bone or tissue specimens can be measured using computer image analysis. Most image software has the capacity to measure length and area. Images of interest (photographs, radiographs, or prints) can be scanned into the computer, displayed on the screen, outlined, and measured. Careful calibration of the software is necessary before accurate measurements can be made.

Measurement of the torsion angle of long bones (in humans) and the femoral angle of inclination (in dogs) has been reported with the use of computed tomography (CT),[16] a digital coordinator-goniometer,[9] and a symmetric axis-based method.[17]

C. Measurements of Microspecimens

Implicitly, when bone microspecimens are tested, the assumption is that the tissue of interest has homogeneous physical properties microscopically, and thereby represents the entire specimen.[18-21] A dissecting microscope can be used for simple distance measurement, such as thickness of trabeculae or microcortical bone beam.[22] Dissecting microscopy with magnification up to 4× has been used for examining and photographically documenting the surface morphology of bone or implant–tissue interface. Wet specimens should be used, which is an advantage over regular, low-magnification scanning electron microscopy (SEM), because during specimen preparation, using critical point drying, the morphology of the specimen may be changed.

D. In Vivo Measurements

In vivo measurement of bone length or limb length is a challenge. Often, soft tissue landmarks are drawn on the skin and the distance between the marks is measured with a tape measure. A technique called kyniklometry has been reported for measuring the distance between soft tissue landmarks on the lower legs of conscious rabbits. This technique has been demonstrated as comparable to X-ray stereophotogrammetry.[23] A specially designed goniometer has been reported for the measurement of joint angles in clinical practice.[24] Limb circumference measurements are useful for monitoring the progress of a swollen limb or joint, or the growth of a limb. For the quantification of limb circumference, a tape measure is effective. Methods using an electronic digitizer and a mathematical formula for an ellipse (for fetal head and body circumferences) have also been reported.[25]

E. Orientator

The orientator is a technique developed approximately 10 years ago for the estimation of length, surface density, and other stereological parameters using isotropic sections.[26] No special equipment is required. Knowledge of the axis of anisotropy optimizes the efficiency. Random points having uniform probability in space are selected using combinations of simple, stratified, and systematic random sampling. A mapping algorithm ensures isotropic planes, thereby allowing unbiased estimates of surface and length density measurements through classical stereological formulae. The stereological approach randomizes a three-dimensional (3D) polar coordinate system whereby every direction can be defined by a pair of angles and each direction can be graphically represented by a point on the unit sphere.[26]

III. MICROMEASUREMENT OF BONE STRUCTURES

A. Histomorphometry

Paraffin embedding and sectioning remains the most common method for histological study of soft tissues (subcutaneous tissue, muscle, tendon, ligament), cartilage, and also decalcified bone specimens. Undecalcified preparation and sectioning are specialized procedures for the evaluation of osseous tissues (bone, calcified tissues), dental tissues, and especially specimens containing metal implants. In this technique specimens are embedded in plastic media such as methylmethacrylate or Spurr's resin. There are three major sectioning methods for plastic embedded specimens: (1) direct sectioning using heavy-duty microtomes; (2) "sawing-grinding"; and (3) sawing only.[27-29]

Observation and characterization are normally conducted using a light microscope. Descriptive histology and histomorphometry are the two main types of histological study. Depending on the particular situation, either or both may be used. Descriptive histology is used to give a general picture of the tissue of interest, including the morphology, structure, and arrangement of cells, matrix, trabeculae, or marrow space. Scoring systems are often designed in order to semiquantify the components of interest. Care must be observed when comparing control data from other sources, particularly if other techniques are employed. Intermethod and interobserver variation on bone area measurement, osteoid perimeter, and width have been shown to occur; some bone area measurements differ due to inherent sampling variation.[30]

Histomorphometric analysis has been performed using histological sections, microradiographs, and backscattered electron microscopic (BSEM) images (on plastic-embedded surfaces). Standard SEM images of a specimen surface are less favorable for histomorphometric analysis due to the fact that overlying components from adjacent areas are not well demonstrated.[27]

Histomorphometry is a methodology for quantitatively analyzing (1) length (perimeter or boundary), such as the surface perimeter of an implant; (2) distance between points, such as the clearance at the implant–tissue interface or distance between the central lines of two trabeculae; (3) area, such as trabecular bone area or repair tissue area; and (4) the number of components of interest, such as trabecular number.[31] These parameters are the four types of primary measurements which can be made based on 2D images. Three-dimensional parameters or structures can be calculated or reconstructed from 2D measurements according to carefully considered assumptions. Although accurate 3D data are necessary for proper comparison between different specimens (such as treated and control bone structure), it is often very difficult to reconstruct a 3D structure based on a single 2D image because the structures of most biological tissues (such as bone tissue) are anisotropic. This problem has been partially conquered by the introduction of quantitative CT[32,33] and magnetic resonance imaging (MRI),[33] which can easily section and reconstruct the specimen.

In spite of its limitations, 2D histomorphometric analysis remains a common and useful method for analyzing the structural changes in trabecular bone,[33,34] the callus composition in healing fracture sites, the repair tissues of bone or defects, and the bone apposition and ingrowth into implant surfaces.

Standard nomenclature, symbols, and units for bone histomorphometry can be found in the review by Parfitt et al.[31] The more commonly used terms for trabecular bone structures include BV (bone volume) or TBA (trabecular bone area, which is the trabecular surface area divided by the total area in mm^2); Tb.Th (trabecular thickness, the average thickness of trabeculae in μm); and Tb.Sp (trabecular separation, the average distance between trabeculae, representing the amount of marrow space in μm). Common parameters for trabecular bone spatial connectivity include Tb.N (trabecular number, the average number of continuous trabecular elements encountered per unit area); Ho.N (hole number, the average number of holes per unit area); N.Nd (trabecular node number; nodes: trabecular branch points); N.Tm (trabecular terminus number; termini: trabecular end points); and Nd/Tm ratio. Most of the parameters can be measured using specialized imaging software.

In the histomorphometric analysis of implant–bone interfaces, the useful parameters are (1) bone apposition (or ongrowth), which is the fractional linear extent of bone apposed to implant surface divided by the total surface perimeter of the implant (i.e., the surface potentially available for apposition)[35,36] and (2) bone ingrowth, which represents the amount of ingrown bone per unit of available surface area, porous space, and ingrowth depth.[35,37,38] In the case of bone ingrowth within an osteopenic bone bed, the structure of the bone, represented by TBA, Tb.Th, Tb.N, and Tb.Sp, should be also analyzed.[35,38]

B. Scanning Electron Microscopy

SEM and BSEM are important methods for evaluation of the structure and morphology of bone structures[34,39] and bone–implant interfaces.[40,41] The shortcomings of SEM are that the specimen must be dried before observation, causing distortion of the original spatial structure and morphology,[42] and in some instruments specimen size is limited. The first problem seems to have been solved by the new low-temperature or cryo-SEM system.[43] BSEM provides better resolution than microradiography with demonstrated consistency and is not affected by projection-effect errors. BSEM also accurately images despite bone and mineral variations.[44]

C. Confocal Microscopy

Confocal laser scanning microscopy (CLSM) utilizes a laser beam that can penetrate tissue to a depth of 300 to 500 μm and thus reflects images beneath the surface of a specimen. CLSM records the intensity of light from a very narrow aperture, excluding light from out-of-focal planes. Stepwise movement permits an artifact-free, topographic image to be obtained in a nondestructive approach without the use of special staining.[45] Stored multilayer 2D images can then be reorganized to show 3D or cross-sectional pictures. CLSM has been used for viewing the structures at the implant–tissue interface, such as unmineralized bone matrix or mineralized bone.[46,47] Using CLSM, Piattelli et al.[46] found that a layer of unmineralized bone matrix lies between mineralized bone and the titanium screw interface in a rabbit tibial model. Their study revealed that while 40% of the titanium surface contained bone apposition, only 10% of the bone was in direct contact with the screw surface while the other 30% was separated from the surface by an unmineralized tissue layer.

D. Ridge Number Density

Quantitative CT (QCT) and MRI have been shown to be effective methods for measurement of the microarchitecture of cancellous bone in addition to its density. Both, however, lack the spatial resolution to image the individual trabeculae with real precision. Ridge number density (RND) is a process whereby number of trabeculae can be determined from high-resolution QCT 3D images. In the data process step, ridges that correspond to the center points of the trabeculae are extracted from the 3D image. High spatial resolution and low doses of radiation lead to image noise which is managed with a 3D algorithm based on directional derivatives of approximated fit functions. The advantages of RND measurement of bone strength are (1) reproducibility and (2) low dosages of radiation allowing for longitudinal and cross-sectional studies.[48]

IV. BONE APPARENT DENSITY, MATERIAL DENSITY, MINERAL CONTENT, AND MINERAL DENSITY

A. Definitions and Methods of Evaluation

The meanings of bone apparent density, material density, bone mineral content (BMC), and bone mineral density (BMD) should be clearly defined (Table 6.1). Although it looks simple and straightforward, it is a difficult task to define them, especially for BMC and BMD. Based on the methods of evaluation and investigators' preferences, the expressions of BMC and BMD can be mass/unit length, area, or volume, percentage, image gray level, or a number.

For cortical bone, apparent density and material density are basically the same as there is no marrow space in compact bone. Therefore, "cortical bone density" is commonly used to describe the density of cortical bone. For cancellous bone there are different material characteristics arising from the two-phase structure (trabeculae and marrow).[52] Based on their structural (apparent) density and material density, respectively, two mechanical properties are generally considered, the structural and material properties.

TABLE 6.1
Definitions of BMC and BMD (only selected references are included)

	Method of Evaluation	Unit	Definition
Apparent density	Weight	g/cm^3	Wet weight per unit structural volume including bone (such as trabeculae) and marrow space, not including marrow
Material density	Weight	g/cm^3	Wet weight per unit material volume
BMD	Weight	g/cm^3	Bone mineral mass/unit bone volume, or named "ash density" if an ashing (or burning) method is used.
	2D imaging	Gray scale	The intensity of the image portion due to the mineral content to a defined sample thickness; example: X-ray images
	RA	Gray scale	Percentage difference to a normal or standard number[49]
	SPA	g/cm^2	Bone mass/(unit of length × width)[50]
	DEXA	g/cm^2	Bone mass/measured area[50]
	QCT	g/cm^3	Bone mass/measured volume[50]
BMC	Weight	%	The ratio of unit weight of the mineral portion to dry bone unit weight and is frequently reported as a percentage[51]
	SPA	g/cm^2	Bone mass[50]
	DXA	g/cm^2	Bone mass/unit length[50]
	QCT	g/cm^3	Bone mass/measured length[50]

Cortical bone material density is between 1.7 and 2.0 g/cm^3 and cancellous bone material density is between 1.6 and 1.9 g/cm^3. One of the simplest methods for measurement of cortical bone density is based on Archimedes' principle. Alternative approaches include (1) if the specimen is a simple geometric shape, the volume can be calculated via direct measurement; (2) use of preparations of methylene iodine and xylene based on different specific gravity which cause bone specimens to exhibit neutral buoyancy in the solution closest to its own density.

The measurement of structural (apparent) density (ρ_a) is achieved by weighing the cancellous structure without free water in its marrow cavities (wet weight, w_b) and dividing the wet weight by the structural volume (including both trabeculae and marrow cavities):

$$\rho_a = w_b/(\pi d^2 h/4) \tag{6.1}$$

where d and h represent diameter and height of a cylindrical specimen. Other specimen shapes, such as cubic, can be used, but they are technically more demanding and have more sharp corners than cylinders, which may cause bone materials to fracture from the specimen during the processes of defatting or marrow removing. Just as in cortical bone measurement an accurate method for cancellous bone volume is through use of a gravity bottle, based on Archimedes' principle (before marrow removal).

Many methods have been reported for removing bone marrow, including boiling in water with detergent, high-pressure water jet, or chemical solvent. Depending on the size and shape of the specimen, an individualized combination of the above-mentioned methods is appropriate. In the authors' laboratory the following procedure has been used for small specimens (e.g., 4-mm-diam., 5-mm-length cylinder): (1) defatting in 50/50 acetone/ethanol mixture with agitation for 24 h; (2) removing marrow in low concentration bleach (1.0 to 1.5% sodium hypochlorite) with agitation for 12 h; and (3) removing marrow residues with a high-pressure water jet (using a syringe).

For *in vitro* measuring of bone mineral density, the traditional method is burning bone specimens in air in a 500°C furnace and weighing the ash.[53] Instead of "ash weight" or "ash fraction," the authors prefer to use ash density, which is defined as ash weight per unit bone volume (including trabeculae and marrow space for cancellous bone). It is suggested that the crucibles be dried at 500°C overnight, weighed, loaded with the bone specimen, and heated at

500°C for 18 h to remove the organic phase. Then, the crucible containing the ash is weighed to determine the weight of ash.

Image-based BMDs using radiographic absorptiometry (RA), single-photon absorptiometry (SPA), dual-energy X-ray absorptiometry (DEXA), or QCT are used as predictors of the breaking strength of bone.[49] Caution must be exercised, however, since inaccuracies in BMD, which is proportional to the square of the apparent density, can cause large errors in predicted bone strength. When several methods for determination of bone strength, including bone mineral content, areal BMD, volumetric BMD, and bone apparent density were assessed *in vitro*, in spite of measurement errors, bone mass, areal, and volumetric bone density were found to be equally accurate, sensitive and specific surrogates of the breaking strength of bone strength *in vitro*.[11]

Less frequently used methods for determining bone mineral content include the use of decalcifying solution or measuring the radiographic density of whole bone or bone sections. The latter is more suitable for *in vivo* conditions. Other indirect methods for bone mineral content include radiographic and spectrographic methods.[51] One method for the assessment of bone density utilizes cutting resistance measures at low speeds for the identification of various bone densities. By using porcine rib specimens, the outcome of cutting resistance measures were compared with that of radiographic technique. The two procedures demonstrated agreement in the ability to identify bone density.[54]

B. BONE DENSITY VALUES MEASURED BY *IN VITRO* METHODS

The material density of cortical bone is the wet weight divided by the specimen volume. Cortical bone has an average density of approximately 1.9 g/cm^3.[51,55] The common ways to measure the volume of a cortical bone specimen include the use of a gravity bottle based on Archimedes' principle, and directly measuring the dimensions of the specimen. The latter requires that the specimen have a regular shape, such as cylindrical.

Selected reports on apparent densities of human and animal cancellous bones are listed in Table 6.2. The apparent density of cancellous bone ranges from 0.14 to 1.10 g/cm^3 (average: 0.62 g/cm^3, $n = 16$). The compressive strength (σ in MPa) of cancellous bone is related to its apparent density (ρ in g/cm^3) by a power law of the form:

$$\sigma = 60\rho^2 \tag{6.2}$$

Similarly, the compressive modulus (E in MPa) of cancellous bone is related to the apparent density (ρ in g/cm^3) by

$$E = 2915\rho^2 \tag{6.3}$$

Material density of cancellous bone is measured using the weight of bone material (only trabeculae) divided by the volume of only trabeculae. The density is a little lower than that of cortical bone, being 1.6 to 1.9 g/cm^3.[51] The principle is again that the marrow needs to be cleaned thoroughly before the measurements of weight and volume. Using a gravity bottle based on Archimedes' principle is the common way to measure both the weight and volume of the bone specimen. To make the measurement, the marrow is removed so no air bubbles or water will be trapped inside the marrow cavities.

Selected data of ash densities of human and animal cancellous bones are also listed in Table 6.2, ranging from 0.19 to 0.56 g/cm^3 with an average of 0.37±0.10 g/cm^3 ($n = 12$), which is about 60% of the value of apparent density as shown in the following equation:

$$\rho_{Ash} \approx 0.6 \times \rho_{Apparent} \tag{6.4}$$

The latter is calculated from the 11 data sets containing both values of apparent density and ash density.

TABLE 6.2
Apparent and Ash Densities of Cancellous Bones (selected data from the literature)

Species	Bone	Apparent density (g/cm³)	Ash density (g/cm³)	Ref.
Human	Distal femur	0.43 ± 0.15	0.26 ± 0.08	57
		0.46	—	58
	Vertebral body	0.14 ± 0.06	—	59
Cattle	Vertebral body	0.45 ± 0.09	0.19 ± 0.06	60
Dog	Distal femur	0.44 ± 0.16	0.26 ± 0.08	57
		0.69–0.98	0.40–0.56[a]	53
	Proximal tibia	0.41–0.83[a]	0.22–0.44[a]	53
	Humeral	0.84 ± 0.17	0.43 ± 0.06	53
Goat	Femoral head	0.91 ± 0.04	0.48 ± 0.03	61
	Distal femur	0.54–0.66[a]	0.32–0.40[a]	61
	Proximal tibia	0.93–1.1[a]	0.50–0.56[a]	61
	Humeral	0.75 ± 0.03	0.36 ± 0.01	61
Sheep	Vertebral body	0.60 ± 0.16	0.37 ± 0.11	62
Pig	Vertebral body	—	0.46 ± 0.04	63
Mean ± SEM		0.62	0.37	

[a] Range of average values from different locations.

V. SPECIAL TECHNIQUES

A. COMPUTED TOMOGRAPHY

CT has been used for examining bone structure and geometry, bone destruction, new bone formation during fracture healing, bone lengthening in animal models, and dimensions of human bone with regard to the femoral component cortical bone ingrowth.[16,49,64-67] CT is a nondestructive method for determining the cross-sectional contours of various anatomical structures, including bone. Based on a 2D array, Feldkamp et al.[68] developed what has become known as the μ-CT scanner for 3D reconstruction of bone. μ-CT, initially developed for detection of ceramic material defects, operates similarly to commercial CT scanners except with μ-CT the specimen is rotated rather than rotating the source. The specimen is limited in size, and a 2D detector instead of a linear array is used to create a 3D image. The findings are that μ-CT images are not significantly different from sections measured histologically.[18]

Sumner and colleagues[69] have reported that separate CT thresholds need to be used to distinguish endosteal and periosteal surfaces. The absence of such can result in errors up to 30% for cortical area estimates. QCT is capable of analyzing bone structure, even in small rat bones, and is believed to be more sensitive than DEXA.[70] The spatial resolution of CT on cancellous specimens can reach 8 to 80 μm.[71,72] The recent development of QCT has resulted in images with high 3D resolution, which may be used for 3D reconstruction of cancellous bone.[33,73] Another CT method for 3D reconstruction is the X-ray tomographic microscope (XTM), which allows *in vivo* evaluation of cancellous bone.[32]

QCT has also been used for evaluating the density and mechanical properties of bone. It can be applied *in vivo* or on excised bone specimens.[74] CT numbers, image intensity, or CT density values (such as Hounsfield units: HU) are measured in the areas of interest. CT density is based on relative attenuation of X rays by a scanned body as compared with attenuation by water. In general, zero HU equals the density of water and –1000 HU corresponds to the relative density of air. Cortical bone has CT density greater than +1000 HU and cancellous bone has values ranging from −25 to 714 HU. An average CT value of water is determined for each scan to adjust the systematic error of the machine.[74] By correlation analysis, power functions between CT density and mechanical values (such as strength or elastic modulus), apparent density and ash density of bone can be formulated. Therefore, mechanical values and densities of bone can be predicted by CT values.[64,74,75] The advantage of QCT is that it can be applied noninvasively and *in vivo*.

B. Magnetic Resonance Imaging

Recent studies have shown that MRI may also provide high-resolution 3D images of trabecular architecture.[33,49,71,76,77] The technique can add to the quantification of trabecular architecture, anisotropy, and connectivity, factors which provide important contributions to the biomechanical properties of trabecular bone.[78] MRI is believed to be superior to CT and ultrasound methods for this purpose due to its ability to distinguish the boundary between muscle and bone and even between the cortical and cancellous regions within the bone.[71] MRI has also been used for evaluating BMD[79-81] and predicting bone elastic modulus (needs further study),[82] which is very significant for the diagnosis and monitoring of osteoporosis. MR-derived measures can replicate trends that have been previously established and may have future uses to resolve prior issues in *in vitro* and *in vivo* studies.[78]

C. Single-Photon, Single X-ray, and Dual-Energy Absorptiometry

SPA and dual energy absorptiometry (DEA) are two noninvasive methods for measuring BMC, BMD, and cross-sectional geometry.[49,67,83] They are most commonly applied to the appendicular skeleton.[64] DEXA measures the mineral mass rather than bone mass. Therefore, absorptiometry measures the physical definition and material density of bones differently, which may account for observed differences.[84]

The radioactive sources used for SPA are ^{125}I and [241]Am. SPA has commonly been used for measuring the mineral density of the distal radius, ulna, calcaneus and femoral neck. By using formulas generated by regression analysis, SPA can also be used to estimate the mechanical properties of healing bone.[85-87] A new method for measurement of bone mass, reported by Borg et al.,[88] is single X-ray absorptiometry (SXA). The SXA device has an X-ray tube which emits X rays at an energy level of 40 kVp and 0.2 mA. It has been used to measure the BMC and BMD of forearm bones, and the results have shown a positive correlation with the more traditional SPA method.[88]

DEA can be performed with either radioisotopes or X rays. When the dual-energy source is derived from X-rays, the technique is termed DEXA. A high correlation has been found between DEXA and traditional methods for measuring bone density.[88] DEXA has been demonstrated to measure accurately the BMC and BMD of very small areas of interest,[89] such as in rat bone.[90-92] Like SPA, DEXA has been commonly used to evaluate BMC/BMD (even for small bones), and mechanical properties of normal bone,[84] healing bone,[64,85,93] and osteoporotic bone[92,94,95] in animal models.

DEXA is also an accurate and precise method to measure the dimensions of human long bones. Sievanen et al.[83] found that the standard DEXA technique provides a reliable measurement of the width and length in human humerus and femur *in vivo*, and thus may be useful in evaluating the properties of these bones in conjunction with the standard bone mineral measurements.

D. Ultrasound

Quantitative ultrasound (QUS) parameters, such as broadband ultrasound attenuation, ultrasound velocity, and ultrasound attenuation, have been demonstrated to measure densitometric and geometric properties of human bones effectively.[49,88,96,97] In an *in vitro* study on trabecular bone cubes,

TABLE 6.3
Method Selection for Measuring Bone Dimensions, Structure, BMC, BMD, and Mechanical Properties (only selected new or rare references are cited)

Level	Elements	Methods for Specimen Dimensions	Methods for Bone Structures	Methods for Material Densities or BMD	Methods for BMC	Methods for Bone Mechanical Properties
Macrostructure (whole bone)	Femur, humerus, vertebrae, frontal bone, phalangeal bones, calcaneus	Ruler, caliper, X-ray, CT, DEXA, MRI	Macrophotography, X-ray, CT, DEXA, MRI	RA, SPA, DEXA, QCT, MRI, ultrasound	SPA, DEXA	Regular material testing systems, ultrasound
Architecture (tissue level)	Compact bone or cancellous bone blocks, cylinders, cubes, or beams	Ruler, caliper, X-ray, CT, MRI	Microphotography, histology, histomorphometry, SEM, CLSM,[106-109] X-ray, μCT, MRI, AFM[#110]	Archimedes' method, ashing, ultrasound, μCT	Ashing, SPA, DEXA	Regular material testing systems, ultrasound, macroindentation, laser speckle strain measurement[111]
Microstructure (osteonal or trabecular level)	Osteons, trabeculae, or microbeams or cylinders	Microscopy, SEM, CLSM	Microphotography, histology, histomorphometry, SEM, TEM, CLSM[112]	Archimedes' method, ashing, microradiography[113]	Decalcification + atomic absorption spectrophotometry[114]	Micromechanical tests using investigator designed microtesters or small-scale material testing systems, micro- or nanoindentation, FEA,[115] acoustic microscopy[116,117]
Submicrostructure (lamellar level)	Lamella, large collagen fibers	Microscopy, SEM, TEM, CLSM	Microphotography, histology, histomorphometry, SEM, TEM, X-ray diffraction,[118] CLSM, AFM	NA	NA	Nanoindentation,[119] microwave extensometer,[120] acoustic microscopy[116,117]
Ultrastructure (nanostructure)	Collagen fibril and molecule, mineral components	SEM, TEM, AFM	AFM,[121] SEM, TEM, X-ray diffraction[118,122]	NA	NA	AFM,[123] acoustic microscopy[124]

AFM = atomic force microscopy; FEA = finite-element analysis; NA = unknown to the authors.

ultrasound parameters were shown to be significantly associated with bone structural indexes, such as Tb.Sp or trabecular connectivity.[88] However, when ultrasound was used as an independent predictor of femoral strength when combined with femoral or calcaneal BMD, the findings did not improve the prediction of femoral strength. Contributing factors to this weak relationship are likely based on differences in the material properties of the calcaneus and the femur.[98] QUS is becoming an alternative to photon absorptiometry in assessing bone density. This has been useful in the diagnosis and management of osteoporosis.[99-101] The diagnostic sensitivity of QUS on BMD is similar to that of DEXA, even on small rat bones.[99]

Ultrasound is also a very important tool for measuring mechanical properties of bone. Ultrasonic techniques offer some advantages over direct mechanical tests for measuring the elastic modulus of bone.[51] Specifically, the specimens can be smaller, with less-complicated shapes (cylinder or cube), and several anisotropic properties can be tested using one specimen.[102] Recently, with the combination of vibration analysis and ultrasound velocity measurements, whole bone mechanical characteristics have been be assessed *in vivo*.[103]

VI. SUMMARY

Bone has a sophisticated hierarchical structure ranging from macro- to nanoscales,[104] or from whole bone to ultrastructural level (see Chapter 8). Investigations of mechanical properties of bone at all levels are essential for complete understanding of the mechanical properties of bone.[104,105] One should choose the appropriate methods for measuring bone dimensions and evaluating bone structure based on the scale of the specimen (Table 6.3). Attention has been paid to several new technologies, including nanoindentation, acoustic microscopy, CLSM, and atomic force microscopy.

REFERENCES

1. Pensler, J. and McCarthy, J.G., The calvarial donor site: an anatomic study in cadavers, *Plast. Reconstr. Surg.*, 75, 648, 1985.
2. Kim, Y.J. and Kim, C.H., A survey on thickness of the Korean calvarium, *J. Korean Soc. Plast. Reconstr. Surg.*, 13, 147, 1986.
3. Horsman, A. and Leach, A.E., The estimation of the cross-sectional area of ulna and radius, *Am. J. Phys. Anthropol.*, 40, 173, 1963.
4. An, Y.H., Kang, Q., and Friedman, R.J., Mechanical symmetry of rabbit bones studied by bending and indentation testing, *Am. J. Vet. Res.*, 57, 1786, 1996.
5. van der Meulen, M.C., Ashford, M.W., Jr., Kiratli, B.J., et al., Determinants of femoral geometry and structure during adolescent growth, *J. Orthop. Res.*, 14, 22, 1996.
6. Chumlea, W.C., Mukherjee, D., and Roche, A.F., A comparison of methods for measuring cortical bone thickness, *Am. J. Phys. Anthropol.*, 65, 83, 1984.
7. Ross, W.D., Rempel, R.D., Quibell, R.W., et al., Technical note: an electronic caliper designed for measuring bone breadths in living subjects, *Am. J. Phys. Anthropol.*, 90, 373, 1993.
8. Rico, H. and Hernandez, E.R., Bone radiogrametry: caliper vs. magnifying glass, *Calcif. Tissue Int.*, 45, 285, 1989.
9. Gualdi-Russo, E. and Russo, P., A new technique for measurements on long bones: development of a new instrument and techniques comparison, *Anthropol. Anz.*, 53, 153, 1995.
10. Ruff, C.B. and Hayes, W.C., Cross-sectional geometry of Pecos Pueblo femora and tibiae — a biomechanical investigation: I. Method and general patterns of variation, *Am. J. Phys. Anthropol.*, 60, 359, 1983.
11. Tabensky, A.D., Williams, J., DeLuca, V., et al., Bone mass, areal, and volumetric bone density are equally accurate, sensitive, and specific surrogates of the breaking strength of the vertebral body: an *in vitro* study, *J. Bone Miner. Res.*, 11, 1981, 1996.
12. Horsman, A. and Simpson, M., The measurement of sequential changes in cortical bone geometry, *Br. J. Radiol.*, 48, 471, 1975.

13. McPherson, E.J., Friedman, R.J., An, Y.H., et al., Anthropometric study of normal glenohumeral relationships, *J. Shoulder Elbow Surg.*, 6, 105, 1997.

14. Fox, K.M., Kimura, S., Powell-Threets, K., and Plato, C.C., Radial and ulnar cortical thickness of the second metacarpal, *J. Bone Miner. Res.*, 10, 1930, 1995.

15. Hanson, P.D. and Markel, M.D., Radiographic geometric variation of equine long bones, *Am. J. Vet. Res.*, 55, 1220, 1994.

16. Pfeifer, T., Mahlo, R., Franzreb, M., et al., Computed tomography in the determination of leg geometry, *In Vivo*, 9, 257, 1995.

17. Rumph, P.F. and Hathcock, J.T., A symmetric axis-based method for measuring the projected femoral angle of inclination in dogs, *Vet. Surg.*, 19, 328, 1990.

18. Kuhn, J.L., Goldstein, S.A., Feldkamp, L.A., et al., Evaluation of a microcomputed tomography system to study trabecular bone structure, *J. Orthop. Res.*, 8, 833, 1990.

19. Ashman, R.B. and Rho, J.Y., Elastic modulus of trabecular bone material, *J. Biomech.*, 21, 177, 1988.

20. Pugh, J.W., Rose, R.M., and Radin, E.L., A structural model for the mechanical behavior of trabecular bone, *J. Biomech.*, 6, 657, 1973.

21. Townsend, P.R., Raux, P., Rose, R.M., et al., The distribution and anisotropy of the stiffness of cancellous bone in the human patella, *J. Biomech.*, 8, 363, 1975.

22. Kuhn, J.L., Goldstein, S.A., Choi, K., et al., Comparison of the trabecular and cortical tissue moduli from human iliac crests, *J. Orthop. Res.*, 7, 876, 1989.

23. Hermanussen, M., Bugiel, S., Aronson, S., and Moell, C., A noninvasive technique for the accurate measurement of leg length in animals, *Growth Dev. Aging*, 56, 129, 1992.

24. Yang, R.S., A new goniometer, *Orthop. Rev.*, 21, 877, 1992.

25. Hadlock, F.P., Kent, W.R., Loyd, J.L., et al., An evaluation of two methods for measuring fetal head and body circumferences, *J. Ultrasound Med.*, 1, 359, 1982.

26. Mattfeldt, T., Mall, G., Gharehbaghi, H., and Moller, P., Estimation of surface area and length with the orientator, *J. Microsc.*, 159, 301, 1990.

27. An, Y.H., Methods of evaluation in orthopaedic animal research, in *Animal Models in Orthopaedic Research*, An, Y.H. and Friedman, R.J., Eds., CRC Press, Boca Raton, FL, 1999, 85.

28. Gruber, H.E. and Stasky, A.A., Histological study in orthopaedic animal research, in *Animal Models in Orthopaedic Research*, An, Y.H. and Friedman, R.J., Eds., CRC Press, Boca Raton, FL, 1999, 115.

29. Jansen, J.A., Animal models for studying soft tissue biocompatibility of biomaterials, in *Animal Models in Orthopaedic Research*, An, Y.H. and Friedman, R.J., Eds., CRC Press, Boca Raton, FL, 1999, 393.

30. Wright, C.D., Vedi, S., Garrahan, N.J., et al., Combined inter-observer and inter-method variation in bone histomorphometry, *Bone*, 13, 205, 1992.

31. Parfitt, A.M., Drezner, M.K., Glorieux, F.H., et al., Bone histomorphometry: standardization of nomenclature, symbols, and units. Report of the ASBMR Histomorphometry Nomenclature Committee, *J. Bone Miner. Res.*, 2, 595, 1987.

32. Kinney, J.H., Lane, N.E., and Haupt, D.L., *In vivo*, three-dimensional microscopy of trabecular bone, *J. Bone Miner. Res.*, 10, 264, 1995.

33. Odgaard, A., Three-dimensional methods for quantification of cancellous bone architecture, *Bone*, 20, 315, 1997.

34. Kang, Q., An, Y.H., Butehorn, H.F., and Friedman, R.J., Morphological and mechanical study of the effects of experimentally induced inflammatory knee arthritis on rabbit long bones, *J. Mater. Sci. Mater. Med.*, 9, 463, 1998.

35. An, Y.H., Friedman, R.J., Jiang, M., et al., Bone ingrowth to implant surfaces in an inflammatory arthritis model, *J. Orthop. Res.*, 16, 576, 1998.

36. Friedman, R.J., An, Y.H., Ming, J., et al., Influence of biomaterial surface texture on bone ingrowth in the rabbit femur, *J. Orthop. Res.*, 14, 455, 1996.

37. Vigorita, V.J., Minkowitz, B., Dichiara, J.F., and Higham, P.A., A histomorphometric and histologic analysis of the implant interface in five successful, autopsy-retrieved, noncemented porous-coated knee arthroplasties, *Clin. Orthop.*, 293, 211, 1993.

38. Moroni, A., Caja, V.L., Egger, E.L., et al., Histomorphometry of hydroxyapatite coated and uncoated porous titanium bone implants, *Biomaterials*, 15, 926, 1994.

39. Whitehouse, W.J., Dyson, E.D., and Jackson, C.K., The scanning electron microscope in studies of trabecular bone from a human vertebral body, *J. Anat.*, 108, 481, 1971.

40. McNamara, A. and Williams, D.F., Scanning electron microscopy of the metal–tissue interface. II. Observations with lead, copper, nickel, aluminium, and cobalt, *Biomaterials*, 3, 165, 1982.

41. Orr, R.D., de Bruijn, J.D., and Davies, J.E., Scanning electron microscopy of the bone interface with titanium, titanium alloy and hydroxyapatite, *Cells Mater.*, 2, 241, 1992.

42. Kobayashi, S., Yonekubo, S., and Kurogouchi, Y., Cryoscanning electron microscopic study of the surface amorphous layer of articular cartilage, *J. Anat.*, 187, 429, 1995.

43. Kobayashi, S., Yonekubo, S., and Kurogouchi, Y., Cryoscanning electron microscopy of loaded articular cartilage with special reference to the surface amorphous layer, *J. Anat.*, 188, 311, 1996.

44. Bloebaum, R.D., Skedros, J.G., Vajda, E.G., et al., Determining mineral content variations in bone using backscattered electron imaging, *Bone*, 20, 485, 1997.

45. Grotz, K.A., Piepkorn, B., Bittinger, F., et al. [Confocal laser scanning microscopy (CLSM) for validation of nondestructive histotomography of healthy bone tissue], *Mund. Kiefer Gesichtschir.*, 2, 141, 1998.

46. Piattelli, A., Trisi, P., Passi, P., et al., Histochemical and confocal laser scanning microscopy study of the bone–titanium interface: an experimental study in rabbits, *Biomaterials*, 15, 194, 1994.

47. Takeshita, F., Iyama, S., Ayukawa, Y., et al., Study of bone formation around dense hydroxyapatite implants using light microscopy, image processing and confocal laser scanning microscopy, *Biomaterials*, 18, 317, 1997.

48. Laib, A., Hildebrand, T., Hauselmann, H.J., and Ruegsegger, P., Ridge number density: a new parameter for *in vivo* bone structure analysis, *Bone*, 21, 541, 1997.

49. Wong, D.M. and Sartoris, D.J., Noninvasive methods for assesment of bone density, architecture, and biomechanical properties: fundamental concepts, in *Osteoporosis: Diagnosis and Treatment*, Sartoris, D.J., Ed., Marcel Dekker, New York, 1996, 201.

50. Van der Perre, G. and Lowet, G., Physical meaning of bone mineral content parameters and their relation to mechanical properties, *Clin. Rheumatol.*, 3 (Suppl. 1), 33, 1994.

51. Ashman, R.B., Experimental techniques, in *Bone Mechanics*, Cowin, S.C., Ed., CRC Press, Boca Raton, FL, 1989, 91.

52. Carter, D.R. and Hayes, W.C., The compressive behavior of bone as a two-phase porous structure, *J. Bone Joint Surg.*, 59A, 954, 1977.

53. Kang, Q., An, Y.H., and Friedman, R.J., The mechanical properties and bone densities of canine cancellous bones, *J. Mater. Sci. Mater. Med.*, 9, 263, 1998.

54. Friberg, B., Sennerby, L., Roos, J., et al., Evaluation of bone density using cutting resistance measurements and microradiography: an *in vitro* study in pig ribs, *Clin. Oral Implants Res.*, 6, 164, 1995.

55. Spatz, H.C., O'Leary, E.J., and Vincent, J.F., Young's moduli and shear moduli in cortical bone, *Proc. R. Soc. London B Biol. Sci.*, 263, 287, 1996.

56. Hayes, W.C. and Bouxsein, M.L., Biomechanics of cortical and trabecular bone: implications for assessment of fracture risk, in *Basic Orthopaedic Biomechanics*, Mow, V.C. and Hayes, W.C., Eds., Lippincott-Raven, Philadelphia, PA, 1997, Chap. 3.

57. Kuhn, J.L., Goldstein, S.A., Ciarelli, M.J., and Matthews, L.S., The limitations of canine trabecular bone as a model for human: a biomechanical study, *J. Biomech.*, 22, 95, 1989.

58. Odgaard, A., Hvid, I., and Linde, F., Compressive axial strain distributions in cancellous bone specimens, *J. Biomech.*, 22, 829, 1989.

59. Keaveny, T.M., Pinilla, T.P., Crawford, R.P., et al., Systematic and random errors in compression testing of trabecular bone, *J. Orthop. Res.*, 15, 101, 1997.

60. Swartz, D.E., Wittenberg, R.H., Shea, M., et al., Physical and mechanical properties of calf lumbosacral trabecular bone, *J. Biomech.*, 24, 1059, 1991.

61. An, Y.H., Kang, Q., and Friedman, R.J., The mechanical properties and bone densities of goat cancellous bones, unpublished data, 1998.

62. Mitton, D., Rumelhart, C., Hans, D., and Meunier, P.J., The effects of density and test conditions on measured compression and shear strength of cancellous bone from the lumbar vertebrae of ewes, *Med. Eng. Phys.*, 19, 464, 1997.

63. Mosekilde, L., Kragstrup, J., and Richards, A., Compressive strength, ash weight, and volume of vertebral trabecular bone in experimental fluorosis in pigs, *Calcif. Tissue Int.*, 40, 318, 1987.

64. Markel, M.D., Wikenheiser, M.A., Morin, R.L., et al., The determination of bone fracture properties by dual-energy X-ray absorptiometry and single-photon absorptiometry: a comparative study, *Calcif. Tissue Int.*, 48, 392, 1991.

65. Schumacher, B., Albrechtsen, J., Keller, J., et al., Periosteal insulin-like growth factor I and bone formation. Changes during tibial lengthening in rabbits, *Acta Orthop. Scand.*, 67, 237, 1996.
66. Feng, Z., Ziv, I., and Rho, J., The accuracy of computed tomography-based linear measurements of human femora and titanium stem, *Invest. Radiol.*, 31, 333, 1996.
67. Bouxsein, M.L., Myburgh, K.H., van der Meulen, M.C., et al., Age-related differences in cross-sectional geometry of the forearm bones in healthy women, *Calcif. Tissue Int.*, 54, 113, 1994.
68. Feldkamp, L.A., Goldstein, S.A., Parfitt, A.M., et al., The direct examination of three-dimensional bone architecture *in vitro* by computed tomography, *J. Bone Miner. Res.*, 4, 3, 1989.
69. Sumner, D.R., Olson, C.L., Freeman, P.M., et al., Computed tomographic measurement of cortical bone geometry, *J. Biomech.*, 22, 649, 1989.
70. Gasser, J.A., Assessing bone quantity by pQCT, *Bone*, 17, 145S, 1995.
71. Mehta, B.V., Rajani, S., and Sinha, G., Comparison of image processing techniques (magnetic resonance imaging, computed tomography scan and ultrasound) for 3D modeling and analysis of the human bones, *J. Digit. Imaging*, 10, 203, 1997.
72. Gluer, C.C., Wu, C.Y., Jergas, M., et al., Three quantitative ultrasound parameters reflect bone structure, *Calcif. Tissue Int.*, 55, 46, 1994.
73. Muller, R., Hildebrand, T., Hauselmann, H.J., and Ruegsegger, P., in *vivo* reproducibility of three-dimensional structural properties of noninvasive bone biopsies using 3D-pQCT, *J. Bone Miner. Res.*, 11, 1745, 1996.
74. Ciarelli, M.J., Goldstein, S.A., Kuhn, J.L., et al., Evaluation of orthogonal mechanical properties and density of human trabecular bone from the major metaphyseal regions with materials testing and computed tomography, *J. Orthop. Res.*, 9, 674, 1991.
75. Ferretti, J.L., Capozza, R.F., and Zanchetta, J.R., Mechanical validation of a tomographic (pQCT) index for noninvasive estimation of rat femur bending strength, *Bone*, 18, 97, 1996.
76. Jara, H., Wehrli, F.W., Chung, H., and Ford, J.C., High-resolution variable flip angle 3D MR imaging of trabecular microstructure *in vivo*, *Magn. Reson. Med.*, 29, 528, 1993.
77. Chung, H.W., Wehrli, F.W., Williams, J.L., and Wehrli, S.L., Three-dimensional nuclear magnetic resonance microimaging of trabecular bone, *J. Bone Miner. Res.*, 10, 1452, 1995.
78. Majumdar, S., Kothari, M., Augat, P., et al., High-resolution magnetic resonance imaging: three-dimensional trabecular bone architecture and biomechanical properties, *Bone*, 22, 445, 1998.
79. Ito, M., Hayashi, K., Uetani, M., et al., Bone mineral and other bone components in vertebrae evaluated by QCT and MRI, *Skeletal Radiol.*, 22, 109, 1993.
80. Kroger, H., Vainio, P., Nieminen, J., and Kotaniemi, A., Comparison of different models for interpreting bone mineral density measurements using DXA and MRI technology, *Bone*, 17, 157, 1995.
81. Bradbeer, J.N., Kapadia, R.D., Sarkar, S.K., et al., Disease-modifying activity of SK&F 106615 in rat adjuvant-induced arthritis. Multiparameter analysis of disease magnetic resonance imaging and bone mineral density measurements, *Arthritis Rheum.*, 39, 504, 1996.
82. Jergas, M.D., Majumdar, S., Keyak, J.H., et al., Relationships between Young's modulus of elasticity, ash density, and MRI derived effective transverse relaxation T2* in tibial specimens, *J. Comput. Assist. Tomogr.*, 19, 472, 1995.
83. Sievanen, H., Kannus, P., Oja, P., and Vuori, I., Dual energy X-ray absorptiometry is also an accurate and precise method to measure the dimensions of human long bones, *Calcif. Tissue Int.*, 54, 101, 1994.
84. Sievanen, H., Kannus, P., Nieminen, V., et al., Estimation of various mechanical characteristics of human bones using dual energy X-ray absorptiometry: methodology and precision, *Bone*, 18, 17S, 1996.
85. Markel, M.D., Wikenheiser, M.A., Morin, R.L., et al., Quantification of bone healing. Comparison of QCT, SPA, MRI, and DEXA in dog osteotomies, *Acta Orthop. Scand.*, 61, 487, 1990.
86. Aro, H.T., Wippermann, B.W., Hodgson, S.F., et al., Prediction of properties of fracture callus by measurement of mineral density using micro-bone densitometry, *J. Bone Joint Surg.*, 71A, 1020, 1989.
87. Nordsletten, L., Kaastad, T.S., Skjeldal, S., et al., Fracture strength prediction in rat femoral shaft and neck by single photon absorptiometry of the femoral shaft, *Bone Miner.*, 25, 39, 1994.
88. Borg, J., Mollgaard, A., and Riis, B.J., Single X-ray absorptiometry: performance characteristics and comparison with single photon absorptiometry, *Osteoporosis Int.*, 5, 377, 1995.
89. Markel, M.D., Sielman, E., and Bodganske, J.J., Densitometric properties of long bones in dogs, as determined by use of dual-energy X-ray absorptiometry, *Am. J. Vet. Res.*, 55, 1750, 1994.

90. Mosheiff, R., Klein, B.Y., Leichter, I., et al., Use of dual-energy X-ray absorptiometry (DEXA) to follow mineral content changes in small ceramic implants in rats, *Biomaterials*, 13, 462, 1992.

91. Lu, P.W., Briody, J.N., Howman-Giles, R., et al., DXA for bone density measurement in small rats weighing 150–250 grams, *Bone*, 15, 199, 1994.

92. Bagi, C.M., Ammann, P., Rizzoli, R., and Miller, S.C., Effect of estrogen deficiency on cancellous and cortical bone structure and strength of the femoral neck in rats, *Calcif. Tissue Int.*, 61, 336, 1997.

93. Markel, M.D., Bogdanske, J.J., Xiang, Z., and Klohnen, A., Atrophic nonunion can be predicted with dual energy X-ray absorptiometry in a canine ostectomy model, *J. Orthop. Res.*, 13, 869, 1995.

94. Vanderschueren, D., Van Herck, E., Schot, P., et al., The aged male rat as a model for human osteoporosis: evaluation by nondestructive measurements and biomechanical testing, *Calcif. Tissue Int.*, 53, 342, 1993.

95. Turner, A.S., Alvis, M., Myers, W., et al., Changes in bone mineral density and bone-specific alkaline phosphatase in ovariectomized ewes, *Bone*, 17, 395S, 1995.

96. Augat, P., Reeb, H., and Claes, L.E., Prediction of fracture load at different skeletal sites by geometric properties of the cortical shell, *J. Bone Miner. Res.*, 11, 1356, 1996.

97. Louis, O., Soykens, S., Willnecker, J., et al., Cortical and total bone mineral content of the radius: accuracy of peripheral computed tomography, *Bone*, 18, 467, 1996.

98. Nicholson, P.H., Lowet, G., Cheng, X.G., et al., Assessment of the strength of the proximal femur *in vitro*: relationship with ultrasonic measurements of the calcaneus, *Bone*, 20, 219, 1997.

99. Amo, C., Revilla, M., Hernandez, E.R., et al., Correlation of ultrasound bone velocity with dual-energy X-ray bone absorptiometry in rat bone specimens, *Invest. Radiol.*, 31, 114, 1996.

100. Njeh, C.F., Boivin, C.M., and Langton, C.M., The role of ultrasound in the assessment of osteoporosis: a review, *Osteoporosis Int.*, 7, 7, 1997.

101. Gregg, E.W., Kriska, A.M., Salamone, L.M., et al., The epidemiology of quantitative ultrasound: a review of the relationships with bone mass, osteoporosis and fracture risk, *Osteoporosis Int.*, 7, 89, 1997.

102. Ashman, R.B., Rho, J.Y., and Turner, C.H., Anatomical variation of orthotropic elastic moduli of the proximal human tibia, *J. Biomech.*, 22, 895, 1989.

103. Van der Perre, G. and Lowet, G., in *vivo* assessment of bone mechanical properties by vibration and ultrasonic wave propagation analysis, *Bone*, 18, 29S, 1996.

104. Rho, J.Y., Kuhn-Spearing, L., and Zioupos, P., Mechanical properties and the hierarchical structure of bone, *Med. Eng. Phys.*, 20, 92, 1998.

105. Ascenzi, A., The micromechanics vs. the macromechanics of cortical bone — a comprehensive presentation, *J. Biomech. Eng.*, 110, 357, 1988.

106. Boyde, A., Hendel, P., Hendel, R., et al., Human cranial bone structure and the healing of cranial bone grafts: a study using backscattered electron imaging and confocal microscopy, *Anat. Embryol.*, 181, 235, 1990.

107. Zioupos, P., Currey, J.D., and Sedman, A.J., An examination of the micromechanics of failure of bone and antler by acoustic emission tests and laser scanning confocal microscopy, *Med. Eng. Phys.*, 16, 203, 1994.

108. Hein, H.J., Czurratis, P., Schroth, D., and Bernstein, A., A comparative study of the application of scanning acoustic microscopy and confocal laser scanning microscopy to the structural assessment of human bones, *Anat. Anz.*, 177, 427, 1995.

109. Boyde, A., Wolfe, L.A., Maly, M., and Jones, S.J., Vital confocal microscopy in bone, *Scanning*, 17, 72, 1995.

110. Lekka, M., Lekki, J., Shoulyarenko, A.P., et al., Scanning force microscopy of biological samples, *Pol. J. Pathol.*, 47, 51, 1996.

111. Kirkpatrick, S.J. and Brooks, B.W., Micromechanical behavior of cortical bone as inferred from laser speckle data, *J. Biomed. Mater. Res.*, 39, 373, 1998.

112. Kabasawa, M., Ejiri, S., Hanada, K., and Ozawa, H., Histological observations of dental tissues using the confocal laser scanning microscope, *Biotech. Histochem.*, 70, 66, 1995.

113. Feldkamp, L.A. and Jesion, G., 3D X-ray computed tomography, in *Review of Progress in Quantitative Non-destructive Evaluation*, Thompson, D.O. and Chimenti, D.E., Eds., Plenum Press, New York, 1986.

114. McAlister, G.B. and Moyle, D.D., Some mechanical properties of goose femoral cortical bone, *J. Biomech.*, 16, 577, 1983.

115. Hogan, H.A., Micromechanics modeling of Haversian cortical bone properties, *J. Biomech.*, 25, 549, 1992.
116. Turner, C.H., Chandran, A., and Pidaparti, R.M., The anisotropy of osteonal bone and its ultrastructural implications, *Bone*, 17, 85, 1995.
117. Katz, J.L. and Meunier, A., Scanning acoustic microscope studies of the elastic properties of osteons and osteon lamellae, *J. Biomech. Eng.*, 115, 543, 1993.
118. Ascenzi, A., Bigi, A., Ripamonti, A., and Roveri, N., X-ray diffraction analysis of transversal osteonic lamellae, *Calcif. Tissue Int.*, 35, 279, 1983.
119. Rho, J.Y., Tsui, T.Y., and Pharr, G.M., Elastic properties of human cortical and trabecular lamellar bone measured by nanoindentation, *Biomaterials*, 18, 1325, 1997.
120. Ascenzi, A., Benvenuti, A., and Bonucci, E., The tensile properties of single osteonic lamellae: technical problems and preliminary results, *J. Biomech.*, 15, 29, 1982.
121. Wiesmann, H.P., Chi, L., Stratmann, U., et al., Sutural mineralization of rat calvaria characterized by atomic-force microscopy and transmission electron microscopy, *Cell Tissue Res.*, 294, 93, 1998.
122. Ascenzi, A., Benvenuti, A., Bigi, A., et al., X-ray diffraction on cyclically loaded osteons, *Calcif. Tissue Int.*, 62, 266, 1998.
123. Tao, N.J., Lindsay, S.M., and Lees, S., Measuring the microelastic properties of biological material, *Biophys. J.*, 63, 1165, 1992.
124. Gardner, T.N., Elliott, J.C., Sklar, Z., and Briggs, G.A., Acoustic microscope study of the elastic properties of fluorapatite and hydroxyapatite, tooth enamel and bone, *J. Biomech.*, 25, 1265, 1992.

7 General Considerations of Mechanical Testing

Yuehuei H. An and Christopher V. Bensen

CONTENTS

I. INTRODUCTION

Before the start of testing, each researcher has to understand clearly what kind of bone material will be tested and what mechanical properties are to be determined. The best results can only be obtained if the researcher plans his or her research project carefully, with a detailed protocol. The protocol should include the sources of bone specimens, the harvesting procedures, methods of storage, preparation of bone specimens for testing, testing procedures (testing conditions, testing, data collection, and analysis), and potential factors which may affect the test results.

II. SOURCES OF BONE

Depending on the source of the bone specimens, considerations should be paid to the timing, harvesting technique, and the methods to prevent the bone from postmortem autolysis.

There are several major sources of bone which can be used in mechanical testing. First, bone specimens can be obtained from a patient during surgery. Because of the functional need and limited volume in the human body, precision of the procedure is essential. It is essential that a consent form be filled out when a bone specimen is taken from or an experimental procedure is performed on a volunteer patient.[1,2]

Bone specimens can also be obtained at necropsy. In order to avoid artifacts caused by autolysis (especially obvious in small animals),[2] a necropsy should be done immediately after the subject, human or animal, has died. If this is not possible, the body should be placed in a leakproof plastic bag and put in a refrigerator until the necropsy is performed. If bone specimens are taken within several days (up to 3 to 4 days) of death or euthanasia (for animals), there will be no significant change on the mechanical properties of the bone.[3] The body should never be frozen if histopathological examination of the tissues is also needed, because ice crystals form inside the cells, and when thawing ocurrs, the cells rupture making histological evaluation difficult or impossible.

When harvesting bones from human cadavers, bone specimens should be taken immediately after death. However, most available cadavers are fresh-frozen, which is acceptable for most mechanical testing purposes. Formalin-embalmed bodies are not appropriate for testing for mechanical properties of bone, because the bone is also fixed by formalin and the mechanical properties have been partially or completely changed.[4-6]

Another source of bone is the animal slaughterhouse. Most animals are euthanized and stored in a cold room for several days before the meat is removed. Arrangement should be made with the owner on the day of harvesting, so adequate procedures can be observed. Ideally, bone should be harvested immediately after the animal is euthanized.

III. HARVESTING OF BONE

When dissecting soft tissues, caution is needed to avoid cutting the bone surface, which will cause stress concentrations. This is especially important when the bone is harvested for whole-bone testing and especially significant for small animal bones. Bone specimens to be used for mechanical testing should be harvested with sufficient extra tissues around the area of interest (not applicable for sampling in patient surgery). A handsaw or wire saw is efficient for cutting bone. Keeping the surrounding soft tissue (muscle, fascia, or skin) intact is very helpful for protecting the bone from drying.

When harvesting large bone specimens, which requires an electric autopsy saw, wire saw, or bow saw, it is important to keep the site irrigated with saline. If only a portion of the bone is needed, a surgical marking pen is helpful for maintaining the size of the desired specimen. Subdivision or trimming with a small bench saw or other saw unit is sometimes necessary before mechanical testing or storage in a freezer.

Before testing or storage, it is good practice to obtain radiographs and photographs of the bone specimens which are useful as documentation or as a guide for further preparation in the future. For harvesting pathological bone specimens, attention should be paid to the size of fracture callus, the alignment of the diaphysis, the positions of the implants or fixation devices, and the surrounding tissues. For conditions involving joints, the morphology of the articular cartilage is another important consideration. Pathological findings include roughened areas caused by arthritis, cartilage defects, fracture lines, or osteophytes. Also, the size of the joint, joint capsule and synovium, the amount and characteristics of the joint fluid, and the appearance of ligaments, menisci, and the soft tissues around the joint should be observed and recorded.

Another good practice is proper labeling of the harvested specimens. Laboratory personnel should be ensured that the patient's information (or animal number), the date of harvesting, the name of the bone, right or left side, and biohazard status are properly labeled on the plastic bag and recorded in the laboratory logbook. Often, some bone specimens in the freezer are found useless for certain projects (which need certain sex, age, and pathological conditions of the bone) simply because the specimens were not properly labeled when they were harvested.

IV. PRESERVATION OF BONE

Regarding the storage conditions for bone specimens, several factors should be considered including the temperature, moisture, use of preservation solutions (such as normal saline or fixatives), and the pretreatment (such as sterilization methods).

Melnis and Knets[3] found that different conditions for the storage of bone tissue play an important role in their mechanical properties. They evaluated five different storage conditions:

1. Stored in room conditions (18°C, moisture: 65%) and also tested in these conditions;
2. Stored for 30 days in polyethelene packages at –4° to –7°C and tested at 37°C and moisture 90%;
3. Stored for 30 days in 0.9% NaCl at –4 to –7°C and tested at 37°C and moisture 90%;
4. Same as 3, plus during testing the samples were wrapped in soft material saturated with saline; and
5. Stored at 18°C and moisture 65% and two days before testing they were kept in saline.

Testing was carried out at 37°C and moisture 90%. During testing the samples were wrapped in soft material saturated with saline. It was found that the largest tensile creep strain arose from those specimens that were stored and tested at room temperature (18°C) and moisture (65%) and the overall results demonstrated the effects of temperature and moisture on mechanical properties of bone.

Roe et al.[4] studied the effects of various preparation and storage procedures and of different storage times on structural properties of canine cortical bone. Preparation and storage procedures evaluated were (1) sterile collection and storage at –20°C; (2) ethylene oxide sterilization and storage at 22°C; (3) chemical sterilization (methanol and chloroform, then iodoacetic acid) and storage at –20°C; and (4) chemical sterilization, partial decalcification, and storage at –20°C. The results revealed that chemically sterilized bone had not changed after 1 week of storage, whereas chemically sterilized and partially decalcified bone had a 40 to 60% decrease in compressive load to failure, pullout load, and screw-stripping torque. Chemically sterilized and partially decalcified bone remained weak after 16 and 32 weeks of storage. Significant structural alterations were not detected in aseptically collected bone after 16 or 32 weeks of storage. Ethylene oxide–sterilized bone had a reduced pullout load after 32 weeks of storage. Chemically sterilized and partially decalcified bone specimens had significantly reduced mechanical strength.

Refrigeration is appropriate for short periods of time, i.e., several days, which has been partially verified by Kaab et al.[5] The only adequate method for the long-term storing of bone specimens for mechanical testing is freezing. Because of the evidence of damage to soft tissues, such as cartilage,[6] tendon,[7] or skin,[8] due to the freezing procedure, there are some questions on the appropriateness of freezing preservation of bone specimens. Owing to the complexity of an experiment or unforeseen circumstances, sometimes a specimen must be thawed and frozen multiple times. The question arises whether multiple freezing and thawing is harmful to the mechanical properties. This question has been partially answered by Linde and Sørensen,[9] who found that freezing and thawing five times did not alter the compressive properties of cancellous bones. In our recent study, the proximal portion of the tibia of adult cows was sectioned to produce bone slices. They were then subjected to four freezing–thawing conditions: freezing with and without saline solution, then thawing in saline solution or exposed to air. The mechanical properties of the bone before and after the treatments (five cycles of freezing and thawing) were measured using an indentation test. It was found that there is no significant effect on the ultimate load and stiffness of the bone. Only a trend of difference was noticed for the specimens frozen without saline soaking and thawed in air.[10] This work supports the practice of freezing and thawing bone specimens in saline solution.

The common method for storing bone specimens is freezing at –20°C. The bones should always be frozen in saline to prevent dehydration. The effects of storage on mechanical properties of bone at –20°C for short periods of time are minor.[10] The maximum effect reported is a 4.6% reduction of torsional strength of canine long bones.[11] However, after thawing, enzymes such as collagenases and proteases may become active and degrade the tissue. Also, enzymatic degradation is not completely arrested at –20°C.[12] With concerns about the effects of enzyme degradation[13] and evaporation,[14] a question arises as to whether there are significant effects of long-term storage at

–20°C. Panjabi et al.[15] found no significant effects of freezing for 7 to 8 months on the mechanical properties of human vertebral bone. Roe et al.[4] found that bones frozen at –20°C for 8 months did not become significantly weaker. Because time periods longer than 8 months have not been reported for frozen storage at –20°C, storage at this temperature for more than 8 months is not recommended. Alternatively, –70°C, –80°C, or even lower temperatures or liquid nitrogen are suggested for long-term bone storage, since these temperatures may minimize evaporation[14] and markedly reduce enzyme activity.[13]

Based on previous investigations, bone specimens should be soaked in saline or phosphate buffered saline (PBS) and frozen at –20°C (a –70°C freezer is ideal if available) in an airtight plastic bag until testing.[10] Before testing, bone specimens should be thawed in saline at room temperature for at least 3 h. If testing cannot be conducted after samples have been prepared and the procedure is expected to be done within 1 or 2 days, the samples should be stored in a –4°C refrigerator until testing. Otherwise, the samples should be put back into saline and frozen. One may encounter a situation where specimens consisting of bone–implant interface have been harvested according to the protocol and there is an unexpected problem with the mechanical testing machine. The specimens should be stored in a refrigerator and effort made to conduct the testing as soon as possible, because the potential effects of freezing on the bone–implant interface has not been documented.

V. PREPARATION OF BONE SPECIMENS FOR MECHANICAL TESTING

Before preparation of specimens, it has to be clear what structural level of the bone is going to be tested. If the purpose is to determine the properties of bone tissue or organ (whole bone), there exists the minimum dimension of the cross section of specimen.[16] This dimension is determined by analysis of the structural levels existing in the composite bone structure and is recommended to be no less than 2 mm. In the case of testing thinner specimens (micromechanical testing), one would expect to get the properties of structural elements of the bone tissue, such as a single osteon, lamellae, or individual trabeculae. Their mechanical behaviors, certainly, may not represent that of bone tissue in general, or whole-bone structural properties.

Rough cuts can be made with a regular bandsaw equipped with a ¼-in. fine-tooth saw blade. For parallel cuts, a bandsaw installed with a customized guide is sufficient for most purposes. To prevent burning, a relatively low speed should be used with sufficient saline irrigation. This kind of cutting may only affect a 1 mm depth of bone at the surface, which can be ground off using a polishing wheel.

Fine cuts can be made using a diamond wafering saw (such as the Buehler Isomet 1000, Leco VC-50, or Struers Accutome-5) (Figure 7.1) or a diamond wire saw (Histosaw, Delaware Diamond Knives, Wilmington, DE) (Figure 7.2) which is particularly good for making smooth, parallel cuts.

For fabrication of cylindrical samples, a tabletop drill press is sufficient for relatively large samples (>5 mm diam.). To prevent the adverse effects of vibration, C-clamps may be used to secure the bone to the machine platform. For 4 to 5 mm diam. samples or less, a lathe or milling machine is recommended. Although electric hand drills can be used, they are not ideal for making cylindrical samples. When drilling holes in the bone for screw pullout tests, a drill press also functions better than a hand drill.

Grinding or polishing is often used to adjust uneven cut surfaces. This is especially important in fracture tests because the imperfections on the surface of the specimen may serve as the initiators of cracks. The commonly used commercially available grinding machines include the Buehler Ecomet 3, Struers Dap-V, or Leco VP-160.

By using a coring bit made from a hypodermic needle on a miniature drill press, small cylindrical specimens, measuring 2 to 3 mm in length and less than 1 mm in diameter, can be obtained.[17] With a low-speed diamond wafering saw and a specially designed miniature milling machine, 100-µm-thick and less than 200-µm-rectangular beams can be made.[18,19]

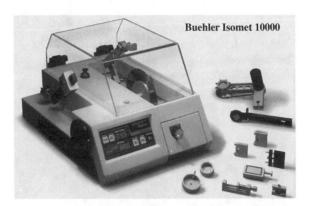

FIGURE 7.1 Fine cuts can be made using a diamond wafering saw (Buehler Isomet 1000, Buehler, Lake Bluff, IL).

To harvest single osteons for micromechanical testing, two methods have been reported. The first one was reported by Ascenzi and Bonucci[20] using a "turning needle" method. Briefly, the device consists of a fine and well-sharpened steel needle which is eccentrically inserted on a dental drill. While the drill is turning, the tip of the needle describes a circle whose diameter corresponds to the average diameter of osteons. By using this method, cylindrical samples measuring 200 μm diam. × 500 μm length can be made. The second method for harvesting single osteons was reported by Frasca et al.[21] using a "splitting and scraping" method.[21-23] Under a 30× stereoscopic microscope, single osteons are isolated by propagating fractures along their natural boundaries using a pair of fine tweezers and a scalpel. They stated that osteons up to 1 or 2 cm can be obtained using their method. Also of note, a more technically demanding method for isolating single osteonic lamellae is also available in the literature reported by Ascenzi's group.[24,25]

Also under a stereoscopic microscope and using microsurgical instruments, single trabeculae can be obtained.[26,27] A common method to mount a trabeculae to the microtester is embedding in polymethylmethacrylate (PMMA)[28] or epoxy.[27,29] A method using cyanoacrylate glue with tube-shaped grips has also been reported.[30] These methods have been reported to study individual trabeculae include the buckling,[26,27] compressive,[28] tensile,[28,30] torsional,[22] cantilever,[29] and bending tests.[31] Also, the tests can be nondestructive.[28]

For a macroindentation test, a cut surface should be further polished using SiC papers (a final 400 grit is good enough). Small bone specimens need to be potted in dental stone or PMMA to facilitate grinding and testing. For micro- and nanoindentation tests, the bone specimens must be mounted in a resin or PMMA block to provide support for polishing and testing. For nanoindentation tests, bone specimens can to be dehydrated and embedded in PMMA to provide support for the porous network.[32,33] Dry bone can also be used without infiltration and embedding.[34] After polishing with successive 400-, 800-, and 1200-grit SiC papers, at least 1.0 μm aluminum oxide paste (Buehler Micropolish C alpha Alumina, Lake Bluff, IL) should be used to finalize the surface for micro-indentation testing. For nanoindentation, 0.3 to 0.05 μm particle size aluminum oxide paste should be used after the polishing with 1200-grit SiC paper or 1.0-μm polishing paste.[33,34]

VI. TESTING PROCEDURES

The temperature and moisture of the laboratory should be controlled as much as possible. If there are no specific requirements, most experiments can be done at room temperature (24°C) and relative moisture (40 to 90%). The specimens should be kept moist with periodic application of normal saline.

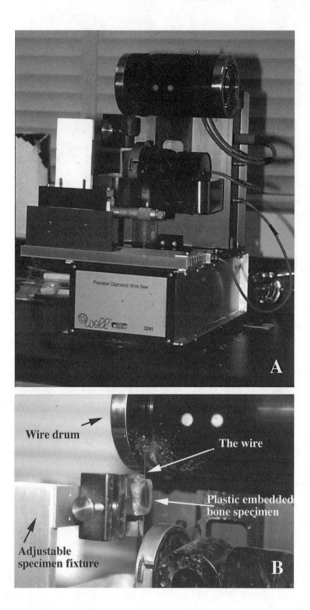

FIGURE 7.2   The Histosaw, by Delaware Diamond Knives, Wilmington, DE, is particularly good for making smooth, parallel cuts.

    Specimens are directly placed on the platform in the case of compression tests or on the two supporting fulcra in the case of bending tests. Bone ends need to be potted in dental stone or resin in tensile tests or torsional tests. The use of screws, wires, or rods for the fixation of specimens to the testing machine or the use of potting procedures for stronger fixation has also been reported.

    The mechanical testing machine is operated in displacement control for most tests. The machine linear variable displacement transducer (LVDT) should be periodically calibrated using an exten-someter. Loading is commonly conducted at a constant slow rate (1 mm/min is the rate used in the authors' laboratory). Load at the peak point of the load–displacement curve is taken as the ultimate load (Figure 7.3). A stiffness measure is obtained by measuring the slope of the linear portion of the curve. If the test machine is controlled with a linear displacement rate and the specimen fixture is very rigid, the time base of the recorder can be converted to specimen

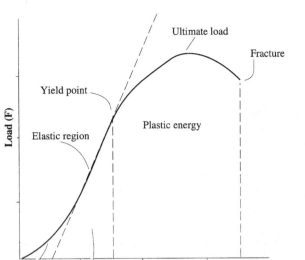

FIGURE 7.3 A typical load–displacement curve.

deformation. An extensometer is recommended when a tensile test is conducted or for other tests when a complicated or less rigid specimen fixture is employed. The deformation measured by a built-in LVDT includes the deformation of the specimen and potential displacements within the specimen fixture or at the specimen–fixture interface. An extensometer attached to the specimen provides a direct measurement of specimen strain without the complications of machine or fixture deformation. Load control mode is often used for fatigue tests. Normally, a small or physiological load or stress (much smaller than the ultimate load or strength of the material) is applied to the specimen repeatedly at certain frequencies until it fails. Both macro- and microspecimens[31,35] can be tested using cyclic loading.

Mechanical testing of materials involves the application of measurable loads to specimens of uniform dimensions. The applied stress is calculated by dividing the applied force by the area over which the force acts. Change in a specimen dimension divided by the original specimen dimension defines strain. Dependent upon the direction in which the force is applied, the test may be tensile, compression, or bending. A simple way to record the data is a load–displacement curve from which the ultimate load, stiffness, and displacement can be obtained. A stress–strain curve is not always plotted. Ultimate strength and elastic modulus (if applicable) are often calculated using the recorded loads, ultimate load and displacements, and dimensions of the specimen.

VII. FACTORS AFFECTING THE TEST RESULTS

A. MACHINE COMPLIANCE

If several fixture parts are used in the testing assembly, significant machine compliance can exist. Routine testing for machine compliance is recommended by testing the fixture column without the specimen in place.[1,2] If the machine and fixture deformation is found to be significant (more than 10% of the specimen value), it should be accounted for in the data analysis.[1] Because the testing gear should be the same for each specimen, only the mean machine compliance (or machine stiffness, S_m) is needed. The stiffness of the bone sample (S_b) is calculated using the following equations:

$$S_b = P/(d_{b+m} - d_m)$$
(7.1)

$$= P/(P/S_{b+m} - P/S_m)$$
(7.2)

$$= S_{b+m}S_m/(S_m - S_{b+m})$$
(7.3)

where P is the load where deformation of the testing machine (d_m) or deformation of the machine plus bone specimen (d_{b+m}) are taken. S_{b+m} is the tested stiffness value (the stiffness of the machine plus bone specimen).

One does not have to worry about the rigidity of the machine frame, which is very rigid such that minimal or no deformation within the allowed loading range will exist. If a significant compliance is observed, the sources are more likely the specimen fixture (made of weak materials) and/or the fixture–machine interface (loose connection, such as loose screw connection). To reduce the effects of machine compliance, specimen fixtures should be firmly machined using rigid materials, should be as simple as possible, and should be firmly connected to the machine. The more connections within the specimen–fixture assembly, the more machine compliance.

B. Specimen–Fixture Interface

When a compression test is used, friction at the specimen and platens should be considered. There can be two completely different forms of fracture depending upon conditions of specimen-machine interface. If this interface is dry leading to strong friction between the bone specimen and loading plate, then fracture of specimen will be caused by maximum shear stresses. The fracture surfaces in the specimen in this case will be oriented at the angle of 45° to the axes of loading. If the specimen–machine interface is oily or wet allowing some sliding along the interface in the transverse direction, then a fracture will be caused by transverse strains arising during loading. The fracture lines in the specimen will be oriented parallel to the axes of loading. Figure 7.4 illustrates a load–displacement curve with microfractures occurring during specimen loading. A similar pattern can also be observed with slippage at the specimen–fixture interface.

An uneven specimen surface causes a triaxial stress field, leading to overestimation of the specimen stiffness. This effect can be limited by using a more accurate procedure for specimen fabrication to achieve parallel end surfaces. An overestimation of specimen stiffness can also be caused by the horizontal friction between the surfaces of the specimen and the platens. It is known that both the axial and lateral deformations of a specimen between the upper and lower platen are larger at the ends of the specimen than in the central part of the specimen (end phenomenon or end effect). Any restrictions to the lateral expansion, such as a rough platen surface, will cause an overestimation of the true specimen stiffness. Common methods for reducing this kind of friction include the use of grease at the interface and using low-friction stainless steel platen surfaces (polished "mirror" surfaces).

When a tensile test is employed, the effect of the specimen–fixture interface should be considered. Any loosening or low rigidity at the interface will lead to an underestimation of the true specimen values. Therefore, a rigid connection between the specimen and the fixture is essential. Using a dumbbell-shaped specimen or a PMMA end-coated specimen are two common strategies to achieve good bonding between the specimen and fixture.[36,37] An external extensometer should be used in these situations to measure the specimen deformation accurately. Slipping out of the ends of the specimen from the grips of the testing machine may cause the most undesirable effect in a tensile test. In this case, when the displacement between the ends of grips is measured automatically by the test machine during testing, then this aforementioned slipping will give an incorrect result. This, consequently, will lead to a distorted stress–strain curve and, further, to incorrectly calculated material parameters, such as strength or modulus of elasticity. Therefore, it is recommended to measure the displacements by special strain gauges attached to the surface of

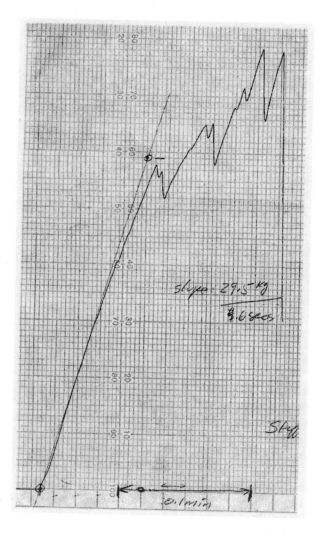

FIGURE 7.4 An actual load–displacement curve illustrating microfractures during specimen loading.

specimen in the middle fifth of the length of the specimen. For very short tensile specimens, there could also be the negative influence of the nonuniform stress distribution at the grip–specimen contact line.

For compressive and tensile testing and most other mechanical testing procedures, preloading with a small load is useful for "tightening" the specimen–fixture interface to further limit the effect of the interface.

C. Specimen Size and Geometry

The size and geometric dimensions of a specimen have significant influence on the outcome of mechanical testing. In the case of whole-bone testing, it is imperative that bones be of uniform size. If procedures or treatments on whole bones are being compared against one another, different sized specimens must be equally distributed among the different groups. This can be achieved by using right and left bones of the same individual and/or by measuring and weighing the specimens. It must be emphasized that significant differences in bone mineral density may exist between individuals and must be considered in these investigations.

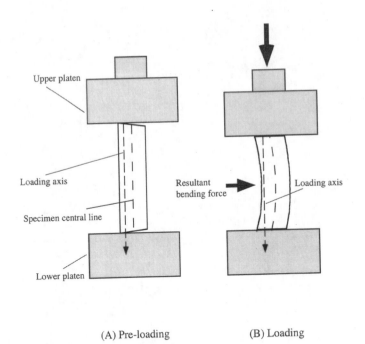

(A) Pre-loading   (B) Loading

FIGURE 7.5   Off-center loading on cylindrical bone specimen. (A) Pre-loading; (B) Loading.

When smaller specimens, i.e., cut bone sections or blocks, are being tested, the question arises in which shape the specimen should be prepared. The most common specimen geometry is that of a cube or cylinder. These specimens are the easiest to prepare and/or machine and are the most reproducible. One important concept in the production of these samples for testing is the length to diameter (L/D) ratio of the specimen. Various ratios have been reported in the literature ranging from 2[38] to 0.25[39] with diameters between 5[40,41] and 20 mm.[39] Wixson et al.[42] compared the strength and stiffness of human bone samples of various length obtained at total knee arthroplasty. They found these parameters to be directly proportional to the length of the specimen. Longer specimens (L/D ratio > 5) have a tendency to "buckle" during testing and should be avoided. Conversely, shorter specimens (L/D < 1) will exhibit a significant friction effect between the specimen and the platens leading to overestimation of stiffness. Consequently, most investigators have recommended an L/D ratio of between 1 and 2 for typical compression testing. Keaveny et al.[43] compared parameters of specimens using an accurate nondestructive method and the platens compression test and found a significant influence of aspect ratio. Specimens with an L/D ratio of 2 had the least differences between the two methods.

Numerous investigators have also employed a "dumbell"-shaped specimen for compression, tensile, and torsional testing of human and animal bones. These specimens allow improved grip holding and rigidity at the specimen–machine interface. However, they are more difficult to machine than standard cylindrical or beam specimens.

The surfaces of specimens should be smooth and without indentations or defects. Such imperfections cause stress concentrations which are especially significant in bending and torsional testing.

The two surfaces of cylindrical or cubic specimens to be tested should be parallel to each other. Unparallel specimens make the loading uneven or off-center, which generates a bending moment to the cylinder and leads to inaccurate data (Figure 7.5).

When preparing a specimen containing a cylindrical implant for a pushout or pullout test, it is important that the two cut surfaces be made perpendicular to the implant followed by precise fine cuts and grinding. If this is not done properly, it will not be possible to align the implant accurately,

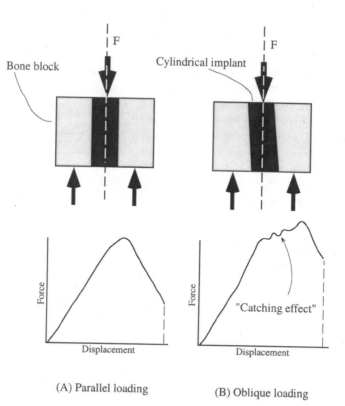

(A) Parallel loading   (B) Oblique loading

FIGURE 7.6 (A) Force transmitted in line with the implant yields reproducible results with a smooth load–displacement curve. (B) If the force is applied obliquely, an irregular curve ("catching effects") results, making the data reduction difficult.

resulting in off-axis load application. If the load applied to the implant is oblique, then erroneous data will be obtained as a result in "catching effects" (Figure 7.6B).

D. SPECIMEN END EFFECTS

In compression testing of bone specimens, attention must be given to the effects of the interface between the specimen and the test platen. One such effect is the "structural end phenomenon." First described by Linde and Hvid in 1989,[50] this occurs when vertically oriented and unsupported trabeculae in a cut-out specimen slide along the surface of the test platen. Consequently, strain inhomogeneity occurs in the specimen, leading to underestimation of stiffness and overestimation of ultimate strain. The magnitude of these errors is dependent on the length and L/D ratio of the specimen.[38] One method of correcting for this effect is embedding the ends of the specimen in PMMA bone cement. One study showed a 40% increase in stiffness with the use of embedded specimens.[50]

E. STRAIN RATES

When performing a mechanical testing procedure, one of the most important considerations in testing parameters is that of strain rate. One of the first investigations of the effect of loading rate on the mechanical properties of bone during compression testing was that of McElhaney and Byars.[44] They studied cortical bone from human and bovine femurs and determined that both ultimate load and modulus of elasticity increased with increased strain rate. For example, a bovine femur specimen loaded at a rate of 0.001 in./in./s yielded an ultimate compressive strength of 17.93 kgf/mm^2 and an elastic modulus of 1898 kgf/mm^2. However, when the strain rate was increased to 1500 in./in./s, those values increased to 37.26 and 4288 kgf/mm^2, respectively. Conversely, the energy absorption capacity (kg-cm/cm^3), maximum strain to failure (%), and Poisson's ratio all decreased with increasing rate of loading. Several other investigators have also demonstrated load rate sensitivity with human calvarial bone plugs.[45-47]

Compression testing studies on human and bovine trabecular bone have also shown that both stiffness and ultimate strength are directly proportional to strain rate.[39,48,49] Linde also found a positive correlation between strain rate and ultimate strength, a finding opposite that of McElhany's results using cortical bone.

These data are of particular interest in the evaluation of fracture models insofar as the properties of specimens in a fatigue test subjected to repetitive, low strain loading may be quite different from those of a traumatic fracture model.

F. Testing Conditions

There has been considerable difference of opinion in the literature whether to conduct testing procedures on wet or dry bone specimens. Several investigations comparing mechanical parameters of both wet and dry specimens suggest that dry specimens will exhibit a higher ultimate tensile strength.[54,55] The specimens should be kept moist with periodic application of normal saline.

The effect of temperature on variations in results of mechanical testing has been well studied. Brear et al.[51] demonstrated that strength, ultimate strain, and Young's modulus parameters of trabecular bone specimens were all lower at body temperature (37°C) than at room temperature (20 to 24°C). Recently, Mitton et al.[2] conducted compression and shear tests on ewe vertebral trabecular bone under two different conditions: room temperature in air ("standard" test conditions) and in a physiological saline bath regulated at 37°C. Testing of the specimens in a 37°C physiological saline bath induced a decrease in the shear strength from 32.5% ($p = 0.0005$) to 37.3% ($p = 0.0001$) of those measured under "standard" test conditions. Similar studies have confirmed this effect in cortical bone as well.[52,53] Although modern investigations of the bone–implant interface, such as total joint replacement simulation, are conducted at 37°C, most mechanical testing of bone is performed at room temperature in air. If there are no specific testing requirements, it is the authors' opinion that most experiments could be done at room temperature (20 to 24°C) at a relative humidity of 40 to 90%.

VIII. SUMMARY

In summary, obtaining accurate and reproducible data in the mechanical testing laboratory requires attention to detail at several important key points in the study. First, specimen collection must be performed carefully in order to avoid damage to the specimen at the time of harvest. This should be carried out immediately prior to the testing procedures if at all possible. However, soaking the specimens in saline and freezing at –20°C is adequate for relatively long-term storage up to 8 months. Preparation of the specimens should be carried out methodically, keeping in mind the effects of heat generation from sawing and/or drilling as well as drying from prolonged exposure to air. Most researchers conduct mechanical testing at room temperature and humidity. However, the specimens should be kept moist during the periods of both preparation and testing. During testing procedures, the investigator must consider the possibility of machine compliance and, perhaps most importantly, the stability and rigidity of the specimen–fixture interface. It is the authors' opinion that more errors are generated in the latter than in any other components of mechanical testing procedures.

REFERENCES

1. An, Y.H., Kang, Q., and Friedman, R.J., Mechanical symmetry of rabbit bones studied by bending and indentation testing, *Am. J. Vet. Res.,* 57, 1786, 1996.
2. Mitton, D., Rumelhart, C., Hans, D., and Meunier, P.J., The effects of density and test conditions on measured compression and shear strength of cancellous bone from the lumbar vertebrae of ewes, *Med. Eng. Phys.,* 19, 464, 1997.
3. Melnis, A. and Knets, I., Viscoelastic properties of compact bone tissue [in Russian], in *Modern Problems of Biomechanics,* Vol. 2, Knets, I., Ed., Zinatne, Riga, 1985, 38.
4. Roe, S.C., Pijanowski, G.J., and Johnson, A.L., Biomechanical properties of canine cortical bone allografts: effects of preparation and storage, *Am. J. Vet. Res.,* 49, 873, 1988.
5. Kaab, M.J., Putz, R., Gebauer, D., and Plitz, W., Changes in cadaveric cancellous vertebral bone strength in relation to time. A biomechanical investigation, *Spine,* 23, 1215, 1998.
6. Bass, E.C., Duncan, N.A., Hariharan, J.S., et al., Frozen storage affects the compressive creep behavior of the porcine intervertebral disc, *Spine,* 22, 2867, 1997.
7. Smith, C.W., Young, I.S., and Kearney, J.N., Mechanical properties of tendons: changes with sterilization and preservation, *J. Biomech. Eng.,* 118, 56, 1996.
8. Quirinia, A. and Viidik, A., Freezing for postmortal storage influences the biomechanical properties of linear skin wounds, *J. Biomech.,* 24, 819, 1991.
9. Linde, F. and Sørensen, H.C., The effect of different storage methods on the mechanical properties of trabecular bone, *J. Biomech.,* 26, 1249, 1993.
10. Kang, Q., An, Y.H., and Friedman, R.J., Effects of multiple freezing–thawing cycles on ultimate indentation load and stiffness of bovine cancellous bone, *Am. J. Vet. Res.,* 58, 1171, 1997.
11. Strömberg, L. and Dalén, N., The influence of freezing on the maximum torque capacity of long bones. An experimental study on dogs, *Acta Orthop. Scand.,* 47, 254, 1976.
12. Tomford, W.W., Doppelt, S.H., Mankin, H.J., and Friedlaender, G.E., 1983 bone bank procedures, *Clin. Orthop.,* 15, 1983.
13. Sumner, D.R., Willke, T.L., Berzins, A., and Turner, T.M., Distribution of Young's modulus in the cancellous bone of the proximal canine tibia, *J. Biomech.,* 27, 1095, 1994.
14. Malinin, T.I., Martinez, O.V., and Brown, M.D., Banking of massive osteoarticular and intercalary bone allografts — 12 years' experience, *Clin. Orthop.,* 44, 1985.
15. Panjabi, M.M., Krag, M., Summers, D., and Videman, T., Biomechanical time-tolerance of fresh cadaveric human spine specimens, *J. Orthop. Res.,* 3, 292, 1985.
16. Knets, I., Pfafrods, G., and Saulgozis, J., *Deformation and Fracture of Hard Biological Tissue* [in Russian], Zinatne, Riga, 1980.
17. McAlister, G.B. and Moyle, D.D., Some mechanical properties of goose femoral cortical bone, *J. Biomech.,* 16, 577, 1983.
18. Choi, K., Kuhn, J.L., Ciarelli, M.J., and Goldstein, S.A., The elastic moduli of human subchondral, trabecular, and cortical bone tissue and the size-dependency of cortical bone modulus, *J. Biomech.,* 23, 1103, 1990.
19. Kuhn, J.L., Goldstein, S.A., Choi, K., et al., Comparison of the trabecular and cortical tissue moduli from human iliac crests, *J. Orthop. Res.,* 7, 876, 1989.
20. Ascenzi, A. and Bonucci, E., The compressive properties of single osteons, *Anat. Rec.,* 161, 377, 1968.
21. Frasca, P., Harper, R.A., and Katz, J.L., Isolation of single osteons and osteon lamellae, *Acta Anat.,* 95, 122, 1976.
22. Ascenzi, A., Baschieri, P., and Benvenuti, A., The torsional properties of single selected osteons [see comments], *J. Biomech.,* 27, 875, 1994.
23. Ascenzi, A., Baschieri, P., and Benvenuti, A., The bending properties of single osteons, *J. Biomech.,* 23, 763, 1990.
24. Ascenzi, A., Bonucci, E., and Simkin, A., An approach to the mechanical properties of single osteonic lamellae, *J. Biomech.,* 6, 227, 1973.
25. Ascenzi, A. and Benvenuti, A., Evidence of a state of initial stress in osteonic lamellae, *J. Biomech.,* 10, 447, 1977.
26. Runkle, J.C. and Pugh, J., The micromechanics of cancellous bone. II. Determination of the elastic modulus of individual trabeculae by a buckling analysis, *Bull. Hosp. Joint Dis.,* 36, 2, 1975.

27. Townsend, P.R., Rose, R.M., and Radin, E.L., Buckling studies of single human trabeculae, *J. Biomech.*, 8, 199, 1975.

28. Samelin, N., Koller, W., Ascherl, R., and Gradinger, R., [A method for determining the biomechanical properties of trabecular and spongiosa bone tissue], *Biomed. Tech (Berlin)*, 41, 203, 1996.

29. Mente, P.L. and Lewis, J.L., Experimental method for the measurement of the elastic modulus of trabecular bone tissue, *J. Orthop. Res.*, 7, 456, 1989.

30. Rho, J.Y., Ashman, R.B., and Turner, C.H., Young's modulus of trabecular and cortical bone material: ultrasonic and microtensile measurements, *J. Biomech.*, 26, 111, 1993.

31. Choi, K. and Goldstein, S.A., A comparison of the fatigue behavior of human trabecular and cortical bone tissue, *J. Biomech.*, 25, 1371, 1992.

32. Hodgskinson, R., Currey, J.D., and Evans, G.P., Hardness, an indicator of the mechanical competence of cancellous bone, *J. Orthop. Res.*, 7, 754, 1989.

33. Lee, F.Y., Rho, J.Y., Harten, R., Jr., et al., Micromechanical properties of epiphyseal trabecular bone and primary spongiosa around the physis: an *in situ* nanoindentation study, *J. Pediatr. Orthop.*, 18, 582, 1998.

34. Rho, J.Y., Tsui, T.Y., and Pharr, G.M., Elastic properties of human cortical and trabecular lamellar bone measured by nanoindentation, *Biomaterials,* 18, 1325, 1997.

35. Ascenzi, A., Ascenzi, M.G., Benvenuti, A., and Mango, F., Pinching in longitudinal and alternate osteons during cyclic loading, *J. Biomech.*, 30, 689, 1997.

36. Reilly, D.T., Burstein, A.H., and Frankel, V.H., The elastic modulus for bone, *J. Biomech.*, 7, 271, 1974.

37. Ashman, R.B. and Rho, J.Y., Elastic modulus of trabecular bone material, *J. Biomech.*, 21, 177, 1988.

38. Linde, F., Hvid, I., and Madsen, F., The effect of specimen geometry on the mechanical behavior of trabecular bone specimens, *J. Biomech.*, 25, 359, 1992.

39. Carter, D.R. and Hayes, W.C., The compressive behavior of bone as a two-phase porous structure, *J. Bone Joint Surg. Am.*, Vol. 59, 954, 1977.

40. Ducheyne, P., Heymans, L., Martens, M., et al., The mechanical behavior of intracondylar cancellous bone of the femur at different loading rates, *J. Biomech.*, 10, 747, 1977.

41. Odgaard, A., Hvid, I., and Linde, F., Compressive axial strain distributions in cancellous bone specimens, *J. Biomech.*, 22, 829, 1989.

42. Wixson, R.L., Elasky, N., and Lewis, J., Cancellous bone material properties in osteoarthritic and rheumatoid total knee patients, *J. Orthop. Res.*, 7, 885, 1989.

43. Keaveny, T.M., Borchers, R.E., Gibson, L.J., and Hayes, W.C., Theoretical analysis of the experimental artifact in trabecular bone compressive modulus [published erratum appears in *J. Biomech.* 26(9), 1143, 1993], *J. Biomech.*, 26, 599, 1993.

44. McElhaney, J.H. and Byars, E.F., Dynamic Response of Biological Materials, ASME Publ., 65-WA/HUF-9, 1, 1965.

45. Roberts, V.L. and Melvin, J.W., The measurement of the dynamic mechanical properties of human skull bone, *Appl. Polym. Symp.*, 12, 235, 1969.

46. Carter, D.R. and Hayes, W.C., Bone compressive strength: the influence of density and strain rate, *Science*, 194, 1174, 1976.

47. Wood, J.L., Dynamic response of human cranial bone, *J. Biomech.*, 4, 1, 1971.

48. Galante, J., Rostoker, W., and Ray, R.D., Physical properties of trabecular bone, *Calcif. Tissue Res.*, 5, 236, 1970.

49. Linde, F., Norgaard, P., Hvid, I., et al., Mechanical properties of trabecular bone. Dependency on strain rate, *J. Biomech.*, 24, 803, 1991.

50. Linde, F. and Hvid, I., The effect of constraint on the mechanical behavior of trabecular bone specimens [see comments], *J. Biomech.*, 22, 485, 1989.

51. Brear, K., Currey, J.D., Raines, S., and Smith, K.J., Density and temperature effects on some mechanical properties of cancellous bone, *Eng. Med.*, 17, 163, 1988.

52. Sedlin, E.D. and Hirsch, C., Factors affecting the determination of the physical properties of femoral cortical bone, *Acta Orthop. Scand.*, 37, 29, 1966.

53. Smith, J.W. and Walmsley, R., Factors affecting the elasticity of bone, *J. Anat.*, 93, 503, 1959.

54. Evans, F.G. and Lebow, M., Regional differences in some of the physical properties of the human femur, *J. Appl. Physiol.*, 3, 563, 1951.

55. Dempster, W.T. and Coleman, R.F., Tensile strength of bone along and across the grain, *J. Appl. Physiol.*, 16, 355, 1960.

8 A Hierarchical Approach to Exploring Bone Mechanical Properties

C. Edward Hoffler, Barbara R. McCreadie, Erica A. Smith, and Steven A. Goldstein

CONTENTS

I. INTRODUCTION

The skeleton, as an organ system, dually functions to perform a variety of mechanical and metabolic activities. It provides the supportive framework enabling locomotion, protects other organs, and participates in mineral homeostasis. All of these functions require the maintenance of mechanical integrity, and compromises in this integrity may impact substantially on an individual's quality of life.

Like any other organ system, functional evaluations of its components are useful for clinical diagnoses and for addressing hypotheses concerning fundamental operational mechanisms. In bone, there are at least four primary motives for mechanical testing. First, structure–function studies may detail specific structural characteristics of bone to resolve the functional consequences of their variation. The second reason is to determine the etiology and pathogenesis of disease to guide clinical therapy and prevention. Typically, the functional consequences (i.e., bone fragility) are clearer than the mechanisms that compromise mechanical integrity. The first and second motives are really complementary approaches to investigating bone mechanical properties. One recognizes a functional deficit and searches for the responsible characteristics. The other approach details variations in bone mechanical properties to understand their functional implications. A third objective is to evaluate bone responses functionally to arthroplasty, fracture fixation techniques, or other

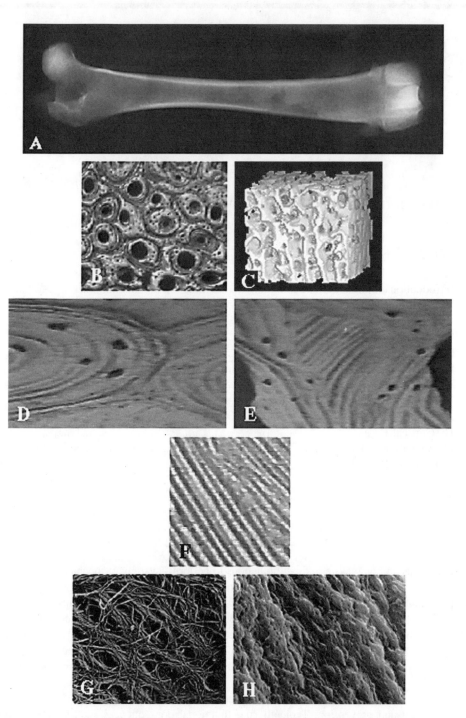

FIGURE 8.1 The hierarchical organization of bone is illustrated. Both the measurement of mechanical properties and the interpretation of their values need to be considered within the context of structural scale. (A) A radiograph of a whole rat femur. (B) Haversian bone light micrograph and (C) trabecular bone μ-CT image at the architectural level. (Courtesy of Nancy J. Caldwell.) (D) Haversian bone and (E) trabecular bone light micrographs at the tissue level. (F) Light micrograph of several bone lamellae. (G) Scanning electron microscopy images of collagen fibers. (Modified from Marotti, G., *Calcif. Tissue Int.*, 53S1, S47, 1993. With permission.) (H) bone mineral at the ultrastructural level. (Modified from Mackie, I.G., Green, M., Clarke, H. and Isaac, D.H., *J. Bone Joint Surg.*, 71B, 509, 1989. With permission.)

reconstruction procedures. Last, mechanical tests provide input for computational models of bone mechanics, adaptation, and repair. These categories are not mutually exclusive or exhaustive, but provide a framework for the overwhelming diversity of investigations that rely on bone mechanical measurements.

II. HIERARCHY OF BONE ARCHITECTURE

From a mechanical perspective, the most striking feature of bone is the hierarchical organization of its architecture (Figure 8.1). Bone structural heterogeneity varies precisely with the scale of magnification employed in its study. Based on the theory of continuous materials, bone hierarchy can be arranged into (1) a whole-bone level (Figure 8.1A); (2) an architectural level, referring to large volumes of cortical or trabecular bone tissue (Figure 8.1B and C); (3) a tissue level, largely containing single trabeculae, single osteons, and cortical microbeams (Figure 8.1D and E); (4) a lamellar level (Figure 8.1F); and (5) an ultrastructural level containing isolated molecular and mineral components of bone (Figure 8.1G). The authors believe that bone mechanical properties at any scale of organization are prescribed by the inherent properties of more microscopic scales. Most importantly, this architectural paradigm shapes the way one thinks about bone mechanical testing and properties.

The hierarchical structure of bone must be considered whenever one decides to evaluate bone mechanically. The different hierarchical, structural elements contribute distinct characteristics to mechanical properties measured at the more global level. These relationships must be considered when an investigation employs bone mechanical testing.

Separation of the various levels of organization is a precarious endeavor and can best be approached through continuous materials theory. Without resorting to mathematical rigor, a continuum is defined to have continuously distributed material properties without discrete local variations. This definition can be consistently applied to resolve levels of bone architecture. Two scales can be distinguished if the global scale properties are independent of local variations in the properties of the more microscopic scale. The structural difference must allow the microscopic scale to approximate continuum properties when observed from the more global level. Discontinuities in structure or material properties are not permitted. Specifically, the microscopic scale must appear to fill completely the volume of the global scale and to have continuously distributed properties.

Compression testing of trabecular bone cubes illustrates an application of these continuum principles. One may measure the stiffness and use it to compute an apparent (or effective) modulus of the cube. By omitting the effect of trabecular architecture in the apparent modulus calculation, the cube is modeled as a single solid continuous material. This is appropriate when the cube scale is much larger than the scale of structural variations. Alternatively, one may use the detailed trabecular structure to generate a finite-element model (assuming homogeneous tissue properties) and calculate the elastic modulus of the trabecular tissue. This approach accounts for the trabecular architecture, but assumes that microstructural tissue features like trabecular packets are sufficiently small that the tissue approximates a continuous material. Note that in each case, the results will be very different because the characteristics which were estimated as continuous are different.

Clearly, the continuum concept has practical implications for bone mechanical testing. For example, as increasingly smaller volumes of cortical bone beams are tested in four-point bending, a threshold can be crossed where the measured modulus begins to vary with the size of the sample.[1] Hence, a practical limit can be defined where cortical bone no longer behaves as a continuum, which allows a more microscopic level of organization to be explored. At a specific hierarchical level, specimens are not typically tested at the upper threshold, but rather using a structural unit that allows one to isolate specific properties of that level. For example, in cortical bone tissue, single osteons and microbeams devoid of Haversian canals are often used; yet larger specimens including few Haversian systems are still considered to be at this level.

Most importantly, the specific hypothesis in question dictates the appropriate hierarchical levels at which to evaluate bone mechanical integrity. Consider two osteogenesis imperfecta (OI) variants: (1) a quantitative defect where normal collagen is produced, but in reduced amounts; (2) a qualitative defect where the triple helix is kinked due to an amino acid substitution in one alpha chain.[2] Bending tests of whole femurs, along with geometric measures, would reveal that the material properties were compromised in both variants, possibly leading to increased fragility. Ultrastructural tensile testing of individual collagen molecules would distinguish the mechanisms responsible for the decreased properties. Therefore, the two scales of testing are appropriate for addressing different hypotheses.

The purpose of this chapter is to emphasize the importance and relevance of a hierarchical approach to the mechanical evaluation of bone. While several investigators have taken a hierarchical approach to testing bone mechanically, the authors have selected a sample of studies from their laboratory which have broadened our understanding of bone structural hierarchy and mechanical integrity. The illustrations are organized as a function of structural scale.

III. WHOLE-BONE LEVEL

Mechanical testing at the whole-bone level measures properties of the entire bone as a structure, which incorporates the properties of the materials that compose the whole bone, as well as its internal and external geometry. At this hierarchical level, most specimens include both cortical and trabecular bone, and therefore contain multiple architectures. These specimens can be either entire excised bones (i.e., a whole femur) or large portions of an entire bone (i.e., a proximal femur). The mechanical behavior of whole-bone specimens most closely approximates the behavior of these structures *in vivo*. In testing whole-bone specimens, it is assumed that the various architectural features are insignificant as individual entities. Hypotheses regarding the structural mechanical behavior of an intact bone, as well as how this may be altered due to aging, various therapies, or genetic mutations, may be addressed at the whole-bone level of hierarchy.

Mechanical testing of whole vertebral bodies has been used in conjunction with quantitative computed tomography (QCT) images in an effort to understand mechanisms of localized trabecular failure and ultimately vertebral fracture. This approach is potentially useful for improving prediction of vertebral fracture risk. Cody et al.[3] found strong correlations between regional bone mineral density (rBMD) measurements from QCT and whole vertebrae failure load. McCubbrey et al.[4] determined a relationship between rBMD measurements and whole vertebral static and fatigue properties.

Mechanical testing of whole femora has proved to be a valuable technique for quantifying alterations in mechanical integrity of cortical bone caused by genetic mutations or drug treatments. These experiments can provide insight regarding how the components of bone extracellular matrix contribute to its functional capacity. Evaluation of whole-bone mechanical properties should be accompanied by characterization of the bone geometry, so deductions regarding potential mechanisms can be made. In the authors' laboratory, mechanical testing of whole femora from transgenic mice is typically performed in four-point bending, and three-dimensional specimen geometry is quantified using digital three-dimensional micro-CT (μ-CT) images. For example, Tseng et al.[5] determined that local production of human growth hormone in transgenic mice stimulated increased femoral bone formation, as indicated by increased cross-sectional geometry (cross-sectional area and moment of inertia), without an associated increase in whole bone mechanical properties. This suggested that the material properties of the bone matrix were decreased due to the local growth hormone production. In addition, interleukin-4 (IL-4) overexpression was demonstrated to cause significant decrease in both mechanical parameters and cortical thickness, as well as an overall shape change, in the middiaphysis of femurs from lck-IL-4 transgenic mice.[6] Ovariectomy was found to have a significant effect on structural properties of whole femurs from osteocalcin-deficient mice, but not wild-type controls.[7]

Mechanical testing on the whole-bone level is also a useful tool to analyze the performance of various joint replacement or fracture fixation techniques, hardware, or cements. The fixation integrity of five commercially available cannulated screw systems were evaluated by Rouleau et al.[8] through mechanical testing of the screws in a femoral head. Moore et al.[9] analyzed the mechanical integrity of a novel *in situ*-setting calcium phosphate cement system to reinforce compression screw fixation of unstable intertrochanteric fractures. In a similar study, Norian SRS® cement (Norian Corp., Cupertino, CA) was evaluated for improvement in strength and stability of femoral neck fracture fixation.[10] In this study, experimental fractures were fixed with cannulated cancellous screws with or without Norian SRS, and were then mechanically tested in fatigue.

Mechanical testing on the whole-bone level of bone hierarchy can be used to determine properties of the complete structural component, which are most directly related to the functional capacity of the specific bone *in vivo*. This technique has been successful in determining the effects of various factors such as aging, pharmacological treatments, genetic mutations, or surgical techniques on the mechanical behavior of whole bones. Due to the complex geometric and material characteristics of whole bones, however, it is not reasonable to calculate directly material-level parameters such as modulus, strength, or stresses in the bone matrix. Mechanical testing solely at the whole-bone level cannot identify particular alterations of bone architecture or extracellular matrix; therefore, specific mechanisms of alterations in mechanical properties must be addressed at more microscopic levels. Similarly, hypotheses regarding damage or fracture initiation, mechanical stimuli to bone cells, or integrity of bone matrix must be investigated at lower levels of bone hierarchy. On the other hand, adaptations to disorders at the cellular or extracellular matrix level may best be evaluated by whole-bone tests. This rationale is based on the possibility that the objective function of the adaptation is to restore whole-bone functional properties.

IV. ARCHITECTURAL LEVEL

The architectural level of bone hierarchy represents specimens dominated by a single type of internal architecture (e.g., trabecular, Haversian/interstitial, circumferential, etc.). In this case, the mechanical properties of a test specimen depend on the arrangement of the dominant type of architecture, as well as the properties of the bone material. The upper limit on specimen size is dictated by the geometry of the bone region from which it is extracted. The lower limit on specimen size is more difficult to define, and is likely different for cortical and trabecular bone. This threshold is defined as the minimum specimen size where the local variations in microstructural properties do not create large variations in properties at the more macroscopic level, as stated by continuum theory. In other words, the specimen must be sufficiently large that the microstructural component does not cause large, discrete fluctuations in mechanical properties. This question was addressed analytically for trabecular bone by Harrigan et al.[11] who concluded that in three dimensions a specimen must contain five intertrabecular lengths to be considered a continuum.

Mechanical testing of trabecular bone specimens on the architectural level is commonly performed using cubes or cylinders of an appropriate size to be considered a continuum. Analogous specimens of cortical bone at the architectural level would be large portions of cortical bone containing many Haversian systems and interstitial regions. In this case, the lower limit on cortical bone specimens is derived from local fluctuations in properties due to the Haversian and interstitial systems. As specimens become smaller, the size of Haversian and interstitial structures relative to specimen size increases, resulting in discontinuities which are too large to be neglected. The continuum assumption, therefore, is only valid if a sufficient number of osteons or interstitial systems are included in the specimen, although this threshold has not been precisely defined. Architectural-level testing of Haversian bone has not been the focus of the authors' laboratory, although others have studied these properties.[12-14]

The primary advantage of testing bone specimens at the architectural level, as compared with the whole-bone level, is the capability of isolating effective properties of a single type of architecture.

Mechanical characterization of these specimens allows one to estimate of the contribution of each architectural type to whole-bone behavior, and a description of how this relationship may be altered due to aging and disease.

At the architectural level of bone hierarchy, many fundamental questions regarding variations in mechanical behavior of trabecular bone due to age, disease, gender, and anatomic location have been addressed. For example, Goldstein et al.[15] tested cylinders of human tibial metaphyseal trabecular bone in compression, and demonstrated strengthening and stiffening of bone in areas of maximum load bearing. Ciarelli et al.[16] tested trabecular bone cubes from various metaphyseal locations in compression in three orthogonal directions. These results showed great variability in properties within each metaphysis, as well as between metaphyseal regions. These data were compared to specimens from canine distal tibiae in a study by Kuhn et al.[17] Results indicated that canine bone displays a lower modulus but higher ultimate strains when compared with human bone, and defines limitations in using canine bone to model the mechanical behavior of human tissue.

There has also been a large research effort in the authors' laboratory to define a strategy to predict fracture risk using various imaging modalities. This has involved searching for relationships between mechanical properties of trabecular bone and measures of density or microstructure. Ciarelli et al.[16] found varying correlations between QCT data from whole metaphyseal regions and orthogonal mechanical properties of trabecular bone cubes. Cody et al.[18] investigated the usefulness of dual-energy X-ray absorptiometry (DEXA) and QCT in predicting local mechanical properties of trabecular bone cubes. This study found that either density measurement could explain 30 to 40% of variance in modulus, and 50 to 60% of the variance in ultimate strength. Goulet et al.[19] tested trabecular bone cubes from human metaphyses in three orthogonal directions and compared these results with morphological measurements obtained from μ-CT. This study determined that bone volume fraction or mean-intercept length measurements alone could only predict about 50 to 60% of variation in mechanical properties, while combining these parameters improved predictions to explain about 90% of mechanical property variations. Taken together, these studies demonstrate that scalar measurements of density alone have some capability in predicting the mechanical behavior of trabecular bone, but indicate that directional measurements of architecture are necessary for more complete characterizations.

Mechanical testing of trabecular bone specimens at the architectural level has provided valuable insight into the behavior of trabecular bone as a function of age, gender, disease, and location. This information can be applied to results from the whole-bone level, and assists in understanding of the contributions of each particular type of architecture to behaviors and pathologies observed *in vivo*. Data derived from studies at the architectural level also indicate that the organization of trabecular bone significantly impacts its mechanical properties. Unfortunately, these studies cannot address the contributions of bone tissue properties to mechanical integrity at either this level or the whole-bone level. However, it is conceivable that these properties may be altered in specific disease states or throughout life. It is therefore necessary to quantify bone properties at lower levels of hierarchy, in order to provide a more complete characterization of its behavior.

V. TISSUE LEVEL

The tissue level describes the properties of bone matrix independent of cortical and trabecular architecture. Tissue-level specimens always include lacunae, and may also include lamellae, cement lines, or Haversian canals, depending on how the specimen is selected. Creating equivalent descriptions of cortical and trabecular tissue-level specimens is difficult, although analogous definitions can be formulated. Trabecular bone tissue includes a number of trabecular packets, but does incorporate the distinctive porous architecture generally associated with trabecular bone. The geometry of trabecular bone places a practical upper limit on the size of specimens, which should not be larger than a single trabecular strut. Once the specimen becomes any larger, its structural organization plays a role, and isolating tissue-level properties becomes mathematically complex.

In cortical bone, a specimen at the tissue level generally incorporates several portions of interstitial regions or osteons, or maybe a single osteon. Inclusion of more than one Haversian canal makes direct evaluation of tissue properties difficult without complicated calculations.

All tissue-level specimens include lacunae and extracellular matrix, which may or may not be in the form of lamellae. Cement lines are generally included in trabecular specimens. Depending on the methods used, Haversian canals and/or cement lines may be contained in cortical test samples. When Haversian canals are included, the calculations should account for the canal and therefore measure the properties of the matrix excluding the canal. The cement lines, if included, are generally the feature which determines the minimum size of specimens. In this case, specimens must contain several cement lines, and therefore several trabecular packets, interstitial packets, or osteons. However, in the case of woven bone tissue or specimens which are obtained without cement lines, the lacunae and their associated cells are the features which will first contradict the continuum assumption. In these cases, it is reasonable to assume that a specimen must only be large enough to contain several lacunae in each direction. When designing experiments or evaluating results, it is particularly important at this level to understand exactly which features are included in the test specimens. In addition, conclusions at this level must be made with the understanding that there are many components of the tissue, such as lacunae geometry and number, lamellar thickness, collagen fibril organization, mineral crystal aggregates, etc., which influence the tissue-level properties.

Several research questions have been addressed at this level. It has been used to explain differences in observed properties at the architectural or whole-bone levels. Specifically, these experiments were designed to determine whether the tissue properties contribute to differences seen in trabecular bone cube (architectural level) or whole-bone mechanical tests. Experimental studies have also been conducted to examine the microstructural level specifically for differences resulting from age, gender, and disease.

Most of the work in the authors' laboratory at this level has involved testing microbeams, bone tissue specimens cut into approximately $120 \times 120 \times 1200$ μm parallelopipeds. Custom-made micromilling and micro-testing machines were developed specifically for these experiments. Early testing relied on three-point bending,[1,17] while later experiments employed four-point bending.[5,20-25] Several studies investigated various properties using monotonic tests,[1,5,17,23] while Jepsen et al.[22] included yield, failure strength, and measures of fatigue. Trabecular and cortical tissues from humans, animals, and transgenic animals have been tested. Limitations of this particular method of testing bone tissue include machining artifacts with both trabecular and cortical specimens, and the required removal of the outer layers of tissue (likely less mineralized) from trabeculae to obtain regularly shaped test specimens.

Several significant results were found for a wide range of research questions. Kuhn et al.[17] found that cortical tissue had a higher modulus than trabecular tissue in humans. Choi and Goldstein[21] confirmed that human cortical tissue had a higher modulus than trabecular tissue, and found that the trabecular tissue had a lower fatigue strength. Choi et al.[1] found a correlation between modulus and specimen size. Wong et al.,[20] Tseng et al.,[5] Jepsen et al.,[22] and Tseng and Goldstein[23] have shown that alterations in gene expression affect the mechanical properties of bone at the tissue level.

There are several other methods which have been utilized to determine properties at the tissue level in both trabecular and cortical bone. Townsend et al.[26] conducted buckling tests of single whole trabeculae from human subchondral bone, without machining a regularly shaped specimen. Rho et al.[27] used single trabeculae and machined cortical bone of similar size, tested them mechanically in tension, and incorporated ultrasonic measurement of properties. Mente and Lewis[28] subjected single trabeculae to cantilever tests, and with the aid of finite-element models of the trabeculae, calculated the modulus of the tissue. Ascenzi and co-workers[29,30] utilized single osteons machined from cortical bone to investigate cortical tissue properties in a variety of testing modalities, including tensile[29] and bending.[30] To the authors' knowledge, these single-osteon studies are the only tissue-level experiments that have not included cement lines in the test specimens.

Regardless of the methods used, specimen preparation and testing is extremely difficult at the tissue level due to the size and delicacy of the specimens. It is important to understand thoroughly the limitations imposed by the methods, the accuracy of any measuring techniques, and any artifacts that may result from creating the specimens. Specimen size has been found to have a significant impact on the calculated modulus, so it is important to use similarly sized specimens throughout the study and clearly state the sizes used.

Despite the limitations, many conclusions have been drawn from the wide range of studies conducted at this level. Many studies have been able to deduce the contribution of specific extracellular matrix proteins to the tissue properties of bone, separating the effects on the tissue properties from compensatory modifications at the architecture or whole-bone level. Several studies suggest that trabecular bone tissue is less stiff than cortical bone tissue. Throughout testing at this level, the properties of bone tissue and reasons for their variation have been clarified.

The specific features that influence tissue properties are still unknown. These may include the geometry and properties of the lamellae, geometry of the lacunae, and the geometry and properties of cement lines. In addition, the structure and properties of the components of the lamellae, including the collagen fibril stiffness and orientation, the mineral aggregate size and location, and the number and orientation of the canaliculi are likely to influence properties obtained at the tissue level. In particular, the observed difference between trabecular and cortical bone tissue suggests that there is a fundamental difference in one or more of these features. Explanations for the differences found at the tissue level are, therefore, sought at more microstructural levels.

VI. LAMELLAR LEVEL

The lamellar level of bone resolves mechanical properties independent of osteocyte lacunae and all microstructural features of remodeling except the lamellae themselves. The upper limit of this scale is defined by the maximum tissue interval that does not incorporate one of the aforementioned structural discontinuities. The lower threshold depends on the scale of bone mineral crystal aggregates, collagen fibrils, and canaliculi. These limits were created for secondary tissue, but can also describe other bone tissues if the upper boundaries are adjusted for the absence of secondary microstructures.

As with other levels, a wealth of research questions can be approached through the lamellar scale. The most fundamental concerns are the property values at this level as a function of age, gender, anatomical location, and disease. One can explore the matrix mechanical consequences of a bone protein deletion or alteration in a transgenic animal. One can also compare primary and lamellar bone properties to determine if remodeling may alter the physical environment of the cell. The strength of lamellar-level measured mechanical properties is their independence from the contributions of bone microstructure. Importantly, lamellar-level studies have direct implications for cell behavior because the mechanical properties are evaluated in the neighborhood of the cell. These extracellular matrix properties can be used for predictive models of tissue behavior in adaptation and remodeling.

The authors' laboratory has been characterizing bone tissue as the medium through which cells receive mechanical signals. The desire is to understand how structure and material properties prescribe bone mechanical integrity and transduce mechanical signals to elicit a bone cell response. To begin addressing these issues, a unique tool called nanoindentation has been used to test hypotheses of bone structure–function at the lamellar level. Nanoindentation uses depth-sensing technology to measure elastic modulus with submicron precision. Recently, the technique has been validated for in vitro bone lamellae measurements at 5 μm resolution.[31] Equipment constraints and the scale of the ultrastructure limit one to measuring the properties of several lamellae at once.

Nanoindentation has permitted testing of hypotheses that were previously unapproachable with direct experiments. Initially, the authors investigated the relationship between microstructural heterogeneity and lamellar mechanical properties.[32] Next, they quantified elastic modulus differences between osteonal, interstitial, and trabecular tissue in four areas of high fracture incidence.[33] Finally, they measured the elastic modulus variation with age and gender at the lamellar level in order to identify microstructural properties possibly responsible for age- and gender-related reductions in mechanical integrity.[34]

The results of these investigations have provided a host of new insights into bone mechanical integrity. Differences in properties between microstructures are consistent with known patterns of homeostatic tissue turnover and greater mineralization, reflecting increased tissue age.[32] Elastic modulus was found to vary with location, suggesting that the local response to the mechanical or metabolic environment determines the elastic properties.[33] The measured trabecular lamellar properties were also inconsistent with whole-bone fragility fracture patterns,[35] suggesting that other mechanical parameters are more important in these maladies. Elastic modulus and hardness did not correlate with age or gender. If lamellar post-yield, fracture, and fatigue properties are also found to be independent of age and gender, these data would suggest that age- and gender-related fragility increases involve the regulation of tissue mass and organization and not the inherent properties of the extracellular matrix.[34]

Whereas nanoindentation has recently emerged as a technique to test human bone mechanically,[36-39] microhardness[40,41] and scanning acoustic microscopy (SAM)[42] have traditionally been used to explore properties at the lamellar level. Microhardness integrates several complex material behaviors and is not a true material property. Therefore, it is qualitatively distinct from elastic modulus and difficult to interpret. SAM measures acoustic reflectivity which is related to the acoustic impedance and the elasticity coefficient of the same direction. Hence, tissue anisotropy can be characterized more completely. SAM also provides a continuous array of data across a surface compared with the discrete sampling required by indentation techniques. Unfortunately, theoretically based elastic modulus measures have been elusive.[42] Empirically based SAM and nanoindentation elastic modulus measurements do not correlate strongly at the lamellar level.[43] Ascenzi and co-workers[44] have admirably attempted to isolate single lamellae and test them in tension, but the experiment has proved technically challenging.

Lamellar-level properties have been shown not to vary consistently with age and gender, suggesting that age- and gender-associated fragilities are more heavily determined by bone mass and organization. However, lamellar properties do vary with anatomical location, possibly indicating different mechanical or metabolic demands. Equally important, bone lamellar properties may reflect mineral content and tissue maturity and are likely influenced by remodeling rate.

As bone is characterized at increasing microscopic levels, one must begin to understand the contributions of matrix protein and mineral to anatomical variations in lamellar properties. One may also explore whether there are components of the extracellular matrix that define a cellular mechanical environment which predispose the bone cell to specific remodeling behaviors. Do collagen fibril properties change with anatomical location and increase cell sensitivity to cyclic loading? Do variations in proteoglycan (PG) flexibility ultimately change the fluid shear environment within canaliculi and lacunae? These are the questions for the next hierarchical level. One must begin to understand the relationship between chemical and mechanical properties of bone matrix molecules and the resulting mechanotransduction consequences for the cell.

VII. ULTRASTRUCTURAL LEVEL

Ultrastructural level describes the molecular network of proteins, glycoproteins, and minerals. It is important to emphasize that the extracellular matrix is no longer characterized as continuous, but rather as a diverse group of mechanical elements interacting with each other and the surface of the cell. At this level, it is appropriate to test the mechanical properties of matrix constituents like collagen fibrils and bone mineral spheroids. Additionally, the interaction between components can be measured. The upper threshold of the ultrastructural level is practically limited by the scales of mineral aggregates, molecules, and macromolecules like a type I collagen fibril. The lower limit is defined by the scale at which these macromolecules and mineral clusters fail to behave as continuous elements. It is difficult to specify a lower threshold for this level as much of the information about architectural and mechanical property variations remains unknown. Moreover, the structural heterogeneity of matrix constituents implies that different components will no longer approximate continuum behavior at different scales of testing. Currently, all molecular studies are grouped as ultrastructural, and attempts to distinguish more microscopic scales should await more detailed characterizations of this level.

Bone ultrastructural components are subcellular in scale and provide the final interface between the external mechanical environment and the cell. Characteristics of more global levels are derived from the molecular properties intrinsic to this scale. However, the ultrastructural level concerns mechanical characteristic of molecules, which are by definition chemical characteristics. Therefore, the hypotheses generated at this scale must describe molecular mechanical behavior as a function of fundamental chemical phenomena. Hydration, salt bridging, homophilic association, and covalent modification are just some of the interactions that will influence molecular mechanics.

Ultrastructural evaluation refers to the direct mechanical characterization of bone components specific to this scale. As defined in this architectural framework, ultrastructural mechanical testing does not include investigations that quantify the contributions of ultrastructural features (i.e., collagen fiber orientation, mineral content, canaliculi volume) to higher-order mechanical properties. Reconsider the OI variant with reduced collagen synthesis. Whole-bone testing is a higher-order test which may reveal that OI bones have weaker material properties when collagen content is reduced. Tensile testing of collagen fibrils would reveal that ultrastructural mechanical properties were unaffected. Again, the two scales of testing are appropriate for addressing different hypotheses. Nonetheless, higher-order studies have provided valuable insights into the effect of collagen fiber orientation on osteonal elastic properties,[45] cross-linking concentration on whole-bone strength[46] and the contributions of collagen and mineral to both elastic-plastic behavior[47] and tissue anisotropy.[48,49]

Basic investigations may quantify the elastic properties of mineral aggregates and type I collagen fibrils. Additionally, one may begin to understand the relative effects of covalent cross-links and collagen-binding proteins on collagen fibril stiffness. Other questions involve noncollagenous matrix constituents. Can hydration alter the ability of PGs to transmit hydrostatic or dilational strains? Ultimately, the hope is to understand the cell mechanical environment as a function of these molecular properties and determine their influence on metabolism and gene expression.

Unfortunately, technology cannot maintain the pace of investigator creativity, and the ability to test hypotheses is often limited by the inadequacy of available experimental techniques. As a result, mechanical testing at the ultrastructural level has been rudimentary at best. To date, the most compelling example of ultrastructural mechanical experiments is single-collagen-molecule tensile testing performed by Luo and colleagues[50] using optical tweezers. Measuring the stiffness of a single collagen molecule is a technical tour de force, and represents the promise of technological advances that will aid understanding of the biophysical issues critical at this level of magnification.

VIII. EXAMPLES OF MULTILEVEL INVESTIGATIONS

A. TRABECULAR BONE

In some studies, the combination of several levels of experimental analysis can explain relationships among the properties at various levels. Often, an investigator will find a difference in properties at one level, and examine a more microscopic level to explain the difference. Other times, one study will be designed *a priori* to evaluate the properties at various levels of hierarchy and discover many relationships between the levels.

One of the authors' current research programs has used both of these methods. It is a series of studies focused on the mechanical properties of human trabecular bone at various hierarchical levels, emphasizing how the properties change with age or differ between males and females. The following summary will describe a subset of these experiments, looking at mechanical tests from the architectural, tissue, and lamellar levels.

Coordinated experiments at the architectural and tissue levels have been reported in part.[24,25] Using the same specimens for both levels allowed comparisons between age and gender groups, as well as analysis of the contribution of the tissue-level properties to the architectural level. Instead of simply comparing the trends observed at various levels as one could do with any set of studies, the authors were able to calculate correlations in the properties between the two levels and directly calculate the contribution of the tissue properties to the architecture level properties. However, it also placed additional requirements on the testing, such as the need for nondestructive testing so the same tissue could be used at multiple levels.

The more macroscopic testing was conducted on trabecular bone cubes, loaded in compression to nondestructive strain levels. Then microbeams were created from trabecular struts obtained from the same cubes, and tested to failure in four-point bending. Although the trends showed that the tissue modulus increased from the 55- to 65- to the 75- to 85-year-old groups, the trend in the cube modulus was to decrease with age. Further analysis showed no correlation between the tissue modulus and the cube modulus, when including males and females in the same two age groups (unpublished analysis). These results led to the conclusion that the fragility seen in osteoporosis and aging is more related to changes in bone mass and organization than it is to the fundamental properties of the bone tissue.

Following testing at the architectural and tissue levels, a large unexplained variation in the properties of the trabecular bone tissue remained. Therefore, the authors attempted to explain these variations by exploring the lamellar level. This encouraged development of nanoindentation techniques for bone tissue, using specimens from the proximal femur. These studies revealed that the lamellar elastic modulus and hardness did not differ with age or gender.[34] Unfortunately, the authors were unable to use the same specimens as those used in the studies previously described, and therefore, could not make direct correlations between the various levels of microstructure.

This research program demonstrates a series of experiments at increasingly microscopic levels designed to explore the etiology of bone fragility associated with osteoporosis and aging. The strength of evaluating mechanical properties on two levels in succession is that direct relationships can be established between properties of the two levels. The clarity of these relationships are further enhanced by conducting these bi-level experiments on the same tissue samples. Combined results of testing at two levels demonstrate that tissue modulus does not significantly influence architectural-level modulus. Since lamellar-level properties do not differ with age and gender, while the whole-bone fracture incidence does, the authors also suggest that the lamellar-level changes may not play a primary role in age- and gender-related bone fragility. Interestingly, material properties at tissue and lamellar levels were unable to explain whole-bone fragility increases. The same specimens for both the tissue and lamellar levels were not used, so the specific relationship between tissue- and lamellar-level properties remains unknown. However, the results as a whole suggest that the distribution and organization of trabecular bone architecture are responsible for increases in bone fragility associated with age and gender. Using a multilevel approach, the authors have refined understanding of fragility increases associated with age and gender by learning that bone mechanical integrity is compromised at a specific hierarchical level. Future investigations into mechanisms of increased bone fragility should focus on trabecular architecture.

B. CORTICAL BONE

Analysis of cortical bone on multiple hierarchical levels is capable of providing specific information on how bone properties are altered by disease, and how this translates into decreased functional capacity at the whole-bone level. An example of this type of analysis was performed using Mov13 mice, which serve as a model of human osteogenesis imperfecta type I. Heterozygous Mov13 mice produce as much as 50% less type I collagen than littermate controls.[51] Although less collagen is produced by these mice, the collagen is still normal in structure. Characterization of mechanical properties of bone from these animals was performed at the whole-bone and tissue levels.

Initially, whole-bone four-point bending tests were performed to failure using femora from Mov13 mice and littermate controls at 8 and 15 weeks of age.[52] The bones were also scanned on the μ-CT system, and diaphyseal cross-sectional geometry was measured. Results indicated that the genetic mutation associated with Mov13 caused significant decreases in stiffness and postyield deformation, and significant increases in failure load and cross-sectional geometry at 15 weeks of age. It is important to note the progressive decrease in stiffness and postyield deformation despite an increase in cross-sectional geometry, which indicates changes in tissue-level properties. This study identified a potential adaptive response to these tissue-level alterations, in which an increase in cross-sectional geometry substantially improved failure properties.

Jepsen et al.[53] investigated potential mechanisms responsible for alterations in postyield behavior of Mov13 whole bones. Whole femora were again tested in four-point bending, and ash density, tissue porosity, collagen fiber orientation, and tissue structure were measured. Although whole-bone mechanical test results showed no significant differences in yield and failure load at 8 weeks of age, postyield deformation was significantly decreased in specimens from Mov13 animals. Visualization of fracture surfaces demonstrated that control bones appeared to fail by cleavage between lamellae, while this mechanism was not effective in Mov13 tissue. Mov13 animals also exhibited a 22% decrease in total collagen content, a two-fold increase in tissue porosity, and an 80% increase in area fractions of woven bone when compared with littermate controls. Taken together, these data indicate that energy absorption mechanisms of various components of the architecture, and maybe even the extracellular matrix, were not functional, resulting in decreased resistance to crack propagation. These findings demonstrate important relationships between whole-bone mechanical integrity and features at the tissue and lamellar levels.

Hypotheses regarding alterations in mechanical properties at the tissue level due to the Mov13 genetic mutation were then addressed by Jepsen et al.[22] In this study, microbeams were milled from the femoral middiaphysis, and then tested either monotonically to failure or cyclically in four-point bending. Monotonic testing revealed that the mechanical integrity of Mov13 tissue was significantly decreased when compared with controls. Similar reductions in fatigue properties were exhibited by Mov13 tissue, but this was possibly related to the decrease in strength of these specimens. In addition, fatigue testing data showed that Mov13 bone tissue began accumulating damage earlier than control tissue. These alterations in tissue properties from Mov13 specimens may be due, in part, to increased woven bone fractions. In general, these findings at the tissue level corroborate suggestions of decreased resistance to fracture made by previous results on the whole-bone level.

These studies, taken together, begin to address mechanisms of bone quality alteration due to a genetic alteration that mimics one form of the disease osteogenesis imperfecta, and may lead to improved strategies for treatment. Use of the Mov13 mouse model also provides valuable insight into the contributions and function of type I collagen in long bones. This series of experiments emphasizes a complementary approach to understanding bone structure–function relationships, as well as the etiology and pathogenesis of disease. These investigations explore a type I collagen mutation that translates into alterations in tissue-level properties, which leads to whole-bone functional deficits. Results of studies conducted at the whole-bone level directed hypotheses for more microscopic levels. This systematic progression through the scales of bone hierarchy allowed a more complete characterization of the role of type I collagen in bone mechanical integrity.

IX. COMPUTATIONAL METHODS

Computational methods play an important role in the analysis of bone properties. Investigations with a large number of parameters can first be conducted using a computer model, and the analytical results used to determine an experimental design including only the most promising treatment groups. In other instances, experiments are difficult or impossible to conduct, or the cost is prohibitive.

Computational analyses can allow greater consistency, since an identical model, free from experimental and interindividual variation, can test various experimental treatments. If feasible, experimental results are generally preferred to computer-generated analyses because fewer assumptions and simplifications are required. However, analytical models are critical tools in the study of bone mechanics. This section will focus on the use of computational methods which have improved understanding of structure–function relationship in bone.

Material properties of bone can be estimated at many hierarchical levels using a variety of computational techniques. There are two basic methods that employ a combination of computational and experimental analyses to evaluate these properties. The first method evaluates material properties at a single hierarchical level based on a mechanical test and a mathematical model of the experiment. In this case, the mechanical test by itself is not enough to determine material properties directly because the test specimen is nonuniform in shape and/or contains inherent architecture. By assuming that the material properties of the specimen are homogeneous and uniform, and by obtaining the geometry of the test specimen by some imaging means, a finite-element model is produced with a preliminary set of material properties. The model is generally linear, resulting in a linear relationship between the property to be measured and the experimental result. The finite-element model is solved using experimental loads to obtain deformation, or vice versa. The preliminary properties are then scaled so the computational model results match the experimental results. Although some experimental artifacts are avoided (such as those induced in the machining process) using this approach, there are additional imaging errors in acquiring the geometry needed to build the model.

Mente and Lewis[28] used this method to calculate tissue properties from mechanical tests of single trabeculae. They dissected individual trabecular struts from human bone, which were tested as cantilever beams. Geometry of the specimen was obtained by a serial grinding and imaging technique. A finite-element model was then created for each trabecular specimen. The experimental displacement results were compared with the results of the finite-element analysis using the experimentally applied loads, and the properties of the trabecular bone tissue were calculated.

Second, it is also possible to calculate mechanical properties at a given hierarchical level from the properties at another level and known geometry. In this case, which will be called the bi-level method, the properties at either the more macroscopic or more microscopic level may be known, but the geometry must be from the more macroscopic level. For example, if one wanted to calculate the properties of trabecular bone tissue based on a trabecular bone cube test (architectural level), the geometry of the trabecular bone cube must be available. In analyses using this method, there are many assumptions that must be acknowledged. First, one assumes that the properties of the more microscopic level are homogeneous and uniform throughout the region of the more macroscopic level analyzed. Second, the analysis is generally linear, so errors associated with the experimental determination of properties at one level will propagate to the other level. Finally, inaccurate geometry will result in inaccurate material properties.

One example of this bi-level method is a study by Guldberg et al.[54] using biopsied tissue from a hydraulic bone chamber in dogs. Finite-element models were constructed based on geometries obtained from μ-CT. They then compared the experimental results from mechanical tests of trabecular bone cubes with the finite-element results in an effort to calculate tissue modulus. Another example is Ladd et al.,[55] who calculated the tissue modulus of human vertebral trabecular bone. Finite-element models were created from synchrotron tomography images. Experimental results from mechanical testing of the trabecular bone cubes were compared with the finite-element results, which again allowed calculation of the tissue properties.

A variation of the bi-level method is to develop mathematical expressions of the properties at one level based on measures of the structure and knowledge of the properties at the next most microscopic level. An example of this method is a study by Zysset et al.[56] Mean intercept length and average bone length, measures of the structure at the architectural level, were obtained from μ-CT images of trabecular bone cubes. They calculated an elastic tensor for the bone specimen using the homogenization method, and then the closest orthotropic tensor using an optimization procedure. There was a strong relationship between the structural measures (mean intercept length and average bone length) and the orthotropic elastic tensor. These results suggest that the properties of bone at the architectural level can be estimated based on measures of the structure, values of the tissue properties, and the relations they reported.

A second variation of the bi-level approach is to assume a simple geometric structure for the architecture of trabecular bone. Finite-element models can be developed based on the idealized structure and used to estimate the properties of the bone at the architectural level. Again, properties of the bone at the tissue level must be assumed. This method is often used to determine how changes in the structural organization of bone trabeculae will affect the properties at the architectural level. One example is a study by Gibson[57] in which trabecular bone is modeled as a cellular material similar to foam. Using different models for the unit cell, which represent the different possible trabecular architectures, Gibson was able to simulate the compressive behavior of the bone. In fact, the asymmetric models were able to match the experimental results from previous studies. Hollister et al.[58] investigated the use of regularly shaped unit cells to model trabecular architecture. Using a strut model and a spherical void model, they found that the tissue strain results were very dependent on the geometry of the model, particularly at low tissue volume fractions. Therefore, they suggested that a single model cannot be used to estimate the properties of all regions of trabecular bone. Instead, separate microstructural models may be required for each location. Trabecular bone architecture has also been modeled using tetrakaidecahedral cells, with struts or plates to create open or closed cells, respectively. This method has been used to model failure of trabecular bone, showing that localized plastic collapse is a probable failure mode, while elastic buckling is unlikely.[59] A similar model, restricted to two dimensions, examined the effects of damage accumulation. Guo et al.[60] modeled the trabecular architecture as repeating hexagonal cells and removed elements when they were determined to be damaged. By applying cyclic compressive loading, they were able to demonstrate that fracture of a few trabecular struts can result in a significant decrease in overall stiffness of the structure. They conclude that the model accurately predicts fatigue behavior of trabecular bone under low-stress, high-cycle loading conditions.

Although a wide variety of computational studies have been described, this section has not come close to describing the breadth of possible uses of these techniques. The main limitation of these methods is that one cannot model the true complexity of bone. Instead, one must apply simplifying assumptions for the structure and material properties. Nonetheless, computational analyses are critically important in advancing understanding of bone properties and function. Obviously, only computational analyses can be conclusive. However, computational approaches provide the advantages of repeatability and inexpensive parametric testing which are required to address a wide variety of research questions.

X. CONCLUDING REMARKS

The purpose of this chapter was to outline methods of mechanically testing bone within the context of a hierarchically based paradigm. Specific methods or approaches chosen by investigators should be applied at a scale consistent with the hypotheses being tested. The interpretation of (or inferences from) the results, however, may transcend more than one hierarchical level. The remaining chapters in this text provide detailed methodological descriptions of biomechanical test methods. Choosing a protocol for any study should be done only after careful consideration of the scale of the research question.

ACKNOWLEDGMENTS

The authors would like to acknowledge the help of Peggy Piech in the preparation of this chapter, and Nancy Caldwell for the trabecular bone architecture image. Bone structure–function studies were primarily funded by the National Institutes of Health (AR 34399).

REFERENCES

1. Choi, K., Kuhn, J.L., Ciarelli, M.J., and Goldstein, S.A., The elastic moduli of human subchondral, trabecular, and cortical bone tissue and the size-dependency of cortical bone modulus, *J. Biomech.*, 23, 1103, 1990.
2. Prockop, D.J., Kuivaniemi, H., and Tromp, G., Molecular basis of osteogenesis imperfecta and related disorders of bone, *Clin. Plast. Surg.*, 21, 407, 1994.
3. Cody, D.D., Goldstein, S.A., Flynn, M.J., and Brown, E.B., Correlations between vertebral regional bone mineral density (rBMD) and whole bone fracture load, *Spine*, 16, 146, 1991.
4. McCubbrey, D.A., Cody, D.D., Peterson, E.L., et al., Static and fatigue failure properties of thoracic and lumbar vertebral bodies and their relation to regional density, *J. Biomech.*, 28, 891, 1995.
5. Tseng, K.F., Bonadio, J.F., Stewart, T.A., et al., Local expression of human growth hormone in bone results in impaired mechanical integrity in the skeletal tissue of transgenic mice, *J. Orthop. Res.*, 14, 598, 1996.
6. Lewis, D.B., Liggitt, H.D., Effmann, E.L., et al., Osteoporosis induced in mice by overproduction of interleukin 4, *Proc. Natl. Acad. Sci. U.S.A.*, 90, 11618, 1993.
7. Ducy, P., Desbois, C., Boyce, B., et al., Increased bone formation in osteocalcin-deficient mice, *Nature*, 382, 448, 1996.
8. Rouleau, J.P., Blasier, R.B., Tsai, E., and Goldstein, S. A., Cannulated hip screws: a study of fixation integrity, cut-out resistance, and high-cycle bending fatigue performance, *J. Orthop. Trauma*, 8, 293, 1994.
9. Moore, D.C., Frankenburg, E.P., Goulet, J.A., and Goldstein, S.A., Hip screw augmentation with an *in situ*-setting calcium phosphate cement: an *in vitro* biomechanical analysis, *J. Orthop. Trauma*, 11, 577, 1997.
10. Goodman, S.B., Bauer, T.W., Carter, D., et al., Norian SRS cement augmentation in hip fracture treatment. Laboratory and initial clinical results, *Clin. Orthop.*, 348, 42, 1998.
11. Harrigan, T.P., Jasty, M., Mann, R.W., and Harris, W.H., Limitations of the continuum assumption in cancellous bone, *J. Biomech.*, 21, 269, 1988.
12. Burstein, A.H., Reilly, D.T., and Martens, M., Aging of bone tissue: mechanical properties, *J. Bone Joint Surg.*, 58A, 82, 1976.
13. Carter, D.R., Hayes, W.C., and Schurman, D.J., Fatigue life of compact bone — II. Effects of microstructure and density, *J. Biomech.*, 9, 211, 1976.
14. Schaffler, M.B., Radin, E.L., and Burr, D.B., Mechanical and morphological effects of strain rate on fatigue of compact bone, *Bone*, 10, 207, 1989.
15. Goldstein, S.A., Wilson, D.L., Sonstegard, D.A., and Matthews, L.S., The mechanical properties of human tibial trabecular bone as a function of metaphyseal location, *J. Biomech.*, 16, 965, 1983.
16. Ciarelli, M.J., Goldstein, S.A., Kuhn, J.L., et al., Evaluation of orthogonal mechanical properties and density of human trabecular bone from the major metaphyseal regions with materials testing and computed tomography, *J. Orthop. Res.*, 9, 674, 1991.
17. Kuhn, J.L., Goldstein, S.A., Ciarelli, M.J., and Matthews, L.S., The limitations of canine trabecular bone as a model for human: a biomechanical study, *J. Biomech.*, 22, 95, 1989.
18. Cody, D.D., McCubbrey, D.A., Divine, G.W., et al., Predictive value of proximal femoral bone densitometry in determining local orthogonal material properties, *J. Biomech.*, 29, 753, 1996.
19. Goulet, R.W., Goldstein, S.A., Ciarelli, M.J., et al., The relationship between the structural and orthogonal compressive properties of trabecular bone, *J. Biomech.*, 27, 375, 1994.
20. Wong, M., Lawton, T., Goetinck, P.F., et al., Aggrecan core protein is expressed in membranous bone of the chick embryo. Molecular and biomechanical studies of normal and nanomelia embryos, *J. Biol. Chem.*, 267, 5592, 1992.
21. Choi, K. and Goldstein, S.A., A comparison of the fatigue behavior of human trabecular and cortical bone tissue, *J. Biomech.*, 25, 1371, 1992.
22. Jepsen, K.J., Schaffler, M.B., Kuhn, J.L., et al., Type I collagen mutation alters the strength and fatigue behavior of Mov13 cortical tissue, *J. Biomech.*, 30, 1141, 1997.
23. Tseng, K.F. and Goldstein, S.A., Systemic over-secretion of growth hormone in transgenic mice results in a specific pattern of skeletal modeling and adaptation, *J. Bone Miner. Res.*, 13, 706, 1998.

24. Riemer, B.A., Eadie, J.S., Weissman, D.E., et al., Characterization of the architecture, tissue properties, and continuum behavior of aging trabecular bone, *Trans. Orthop. Res. Soc.*, 19, 189, 1994.

25. Riemer, B.A., Eadie, J.S., Wenzel, T.E., et al., Microstructure and material property variations in compact and trabecular vertebral bone tissue, *Trans. Orthop. Res. Soc.*, 20, 529, 1995.

26. Townsend, P.R., Rose, R.M., and Radin, E.L., Buckling studies of single human trabeculae, *J. Biomech.*, 8, 199, 1975.

27. Rho, J.Y., Ashman, R.B., and Turner, C.H., Young's modulus of trabecular and cortical bone material: ultrasonic and microtensile measurements, *J. Biomech.*, 26, 111, 1993.

28. Mente, P.L. and Lewis, J.L., Experimental method for the measurement of the elastic modulus of trabecular bone tissue, *J. Orthop. Res.*, 7, 456, 1989.

29. Ascenzi, A. and Bonucci, E., The tensile properties of single osteons, *Anat. Rec.*, 158, 375, 1967.

30. Ascenzi, A., Baschieri, P., and Benvenuti, A., The bending properties of single osteons, *J. Biomech.*, 23, 763, 1990.

31. Hoffler, C.E., Guo, X.E., Zysset, P.K., et al., Evaluation of bone microstructural properties: effect of testing conditions, depth, repetition, time delay and displacement rate, in *Proceedings of the 1997 Bioengineering Conference*, Chandran, K.B., et al., Eds., ASME, New York, 1997, 567.

32. Zysset, P.K., Guo, X.E., Hoffler, C.E., and Goldstein, S.A., Elastic modulus of human cortical and trabecular tissue lamellae, *Trans. Orthop. Res. Soc.*, 22, 798, 1997.

33. Moore, K.E., Hoffler, C.E., Zysset, P.K., and Goldstein, S.A., Effect of anatomical location on elastic modulus of human bone tissue lamellae, *Trans. Orthop. Res. Soc.*, 23, 560, 1998.

34. Hoffler, C.E., Moore, K.E., Kozloff, K.M., et al., Femoral neck bone lamellae elastic properties are independent of age and gender, *Trans. Orthop. Res. Soc.*, 24, 753, 1999.

35. Lips, P., Epidemiology and predictors of fractures associated with osteoporosis, *Am. J. Med.*, 103, 3S, 1997.

36. Ko, C.C., Douglas, W.H., and Cheng, Y.S., Intrinsic mechanical competence of cortical and trabecular bone measured by nanoindentation and microindentation probes, in *Proceedings of the 1995 Bioengineering Conference,* Hochmuth, R.M., et al., Eds., ASME, New York, 1995, 415.

37. Roy, M., Rho, J.Y., Tsui, T.Y., and Pharr, G.M., Variations of Young's modulus and hardness in human lumbar vertebrae measured by nanoindentation, in *Advances in Bioengineering*, Rastegar, S., Ed., ASME, New York, 385, 1996.

38. Rho, J.Y., Tsui, T.Y., and Pharr, G.M., Elastic properties of human cortical and trabecular lamellar bone measured by nanoindentation, *Biomaterials*, 18, 1325, 1997.

39. Su, X.W., Feng, Q.L., Cui, F.Z., and Zhu, X.D., Microstructure and micromechanical properties of the mid-diaphyses of human fetal femurs, *Connect. Tissue Res.*, 36, 271, 1997.

40. Amprino, R., Investigations on some physical properties of bone tissue, *Acta Anat.*, 34, 161, 1958.

41. Weaver, J.K., The microscopic hardness of bone, *J. Bone Joint Surg.*, 48A, 273, 1966.

42. Katz, J.L. and Meunier, A., Scanning acoustic microscope studies of the elastic properties of osteons and osteon lamellae, *J. Biomech. Eng.*, 115, 543, 1993.

43. Hoffler, C.E., Zhang, N., Kozloff, K.M., et al., Comparison of scanning acoustic microscopy and nanoindentation measures of the elastic properties of human bone lamellae, in *Proceedings of the 1999 Bioengineering Conference,* Goel, V.K., et al., Eds., ASME, New York, 1999, 315.

44. Ascenzi, A., Benvenuti, A., and Bonucci, E., The tensile properties of single osteonic lamellae: technical problems and preliminary results, *J. Biomech.*, 15, 29, 1982.

45. Ascenzi, A. and Bonucci, E., The compressive properties of single osteons, *Anat. Rec.*, 161, 377, 1968.

46. Oxlund, H., Barckman, M., Ortoft, G., and Andreassen, T.T., Reduced concentrations of collagen cross-links are associated with reduced strength of bone, *Bone*, 17, 365S, 1995.

47. Burstein, A.H., Zika, J.M., Heiple, K.G., and Klein, L., Contribution of collagen and mineral to the elastic-plastic properties of bone, *J. Bone Joint Surg.*, 57A, 956, 1975.

48. Hasegawa, K., Turner, C.H., and Burr, D.B., Contribution of collagen and mineral to the elastic anisotropy of bone, *Calcif. Tissue Int.*, 55, 381, 1994.

49. Turner, C.H., Chandran, A., and Pidaparti, R.M., The anisotropy of osteonal bone and its ultrastructural implications, *Bone*, 17, 85, 1995.

50. Luo, Z.P., Bolander, M.E., and An, K.N., A method for determination of stiffness of collagen molecules, *Biochem. Biophys. Res. Commun.*, 232, 251, 1997.

51. Bonadio, J., Saunders, T.L., Tsai, E., et al., Transgenic mouse model of the mild dominant form of osteogenesis imperfecta, *Proc. Natl. Acad. Sci. U.S.A.*, 87, 7145, 1990.

52. Bonadio, J., Jepsen, K.J., Mansoura, M.K., et al., A murine skeletal adaptation that significantly increases cortical bone mechanical properties. Implications for human skeletal fragility, *J. Clin. Invest.*, 92, 1697, 1993.

53. Jepsen, K.J., Goldstein, S.A., Kuhn, J.L., et al., Type-I collagen mutation compromises the post-yield behavior of Mov13 long bone, *J. Orthop. Res.*, 14, 493, 1996.

54. Guldberg, R.E., Caldwell, N.J., Goulet, R.W., et al., Mechanical stimulation of bone repair: an evaluation of *in vivo* tissue strains in hydraulic bone chamber model, *Trans. Orthop. Res. Soc.*, 22, 114, 1997.

55. Ladd, A.J., Kinney, J.H., Haupt, D.L., and Goldstein, S.A., Finite-element modeling of trabecular bone: comparison with mechanical testing and determination of tissue modulus, *J. Orthop. Res.*, 16, 622, 1998.

56. Zysset, P.K., Goulet, R.W., and Hollister, S.J., Prediction of the elastic behavior of human trabecular bone from morphology and tissue properties, *Trans. Orthop. Res. Soc.*, 22, 64, 1997.

57. Gibson, L.J., The mechanical behavior of cancellous bone, *J. Biomech.*, 18, 317, 1985.

58. Hollister, S.J., Fyhrie, D.P., Jepsen, K.J., and Goldstein, S.A., Application of homogenization theory to the study of trabecular bone mechanics, *J. Biomech.*, 24, 825, 1991.

59. Guo, X.E., Zysset, P.K., and Goldstein, S.A., Study of post-yield behavior of trabecular bone using a 3-D microstructural model, in *Advances in Bioengineering*, Hull, M.L., Ed., ASME, New York, 1995, 165.

60. Guo, X.E., McMahon, T.A., Keaveny, T.M., et al., Finite element modeling of damage accumulation in trabecular bone under cyclic loading, *J. Biomech.*, 27, 145, 1994.

9 Nondestructive Mechanical Testing of Cancellous Bone

Frank Linde and Ivan Hvid

CONTENTS

I. INTRODUCTION

Cancellous bone is a tricky material to test mechanically. First of all it is not homogeneous. There can be an enormous variation of the strength in an anatomical site.[1] Second, cancellous bone is anisotropic, exhibiting differences up to tenfold in the stiffness of different directions within the same anatomical location.[2-4] Third, it is a structure, which becomes apparent when it is cut into test specimens since the surface of this structure behaves differently from the rest of the test specimen.[5-7] Furthermore, cancellous bone is viscoelastic.

A standard geometry of a test specimen in order to obtain even stress distribution is a specimen with a reduced diameter of the central part and a length to diameter ratio of 2:1. Furthermore, the axial deformation has to be measured at the part of the specimen with reduced diameter. Most cancellous bone is too fragile and too inhomogeneous to machine into such a specimen geometry. Therefore, the most popular type of testing has become a compression test using test specimens with cylindrical or cubic geometry, and with a strain measurement device attached to the test columns close to the test specimen (Figure 9.1).

This deviation from the standard engineering setup introduces systematic errors which tend to underestimate the stiffness of the test specimen (as the testing axis is noncoincident with a major structural axis[8] and the structural surface phenomena),[6-7] while other systematic errors tend to overestimate the stiffness (uneven stress distribution due to friction at the surface)[9] and viscoelasticity. The net results of these errors have been estimated to be an underestimation of the stiffness between 20 and 40%.[10]

0-8493-0266-9/00/$0.00+$.50

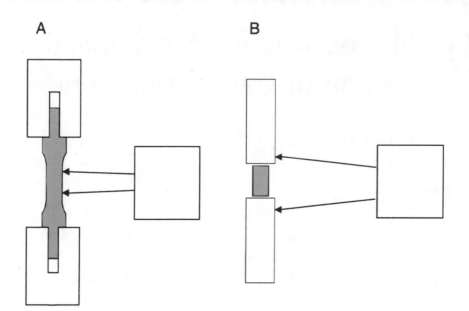

FIGURE 9.1 (A) The standard test setup for a mechanical test with an extensometer attached directly to the reduced section of the test sample. (B) The test setup used for compression testing of a cancellous bone specimen with the extensometer attached to the testing columns.

Why should one perform such an inaccurate test? It is obvious, when accurate data are imperative such as for providing bone data to put into finite-element models analyzing the relationship between implants and bone, that the data should be produced more accurately.[11] The trouble is that this is extremely difficult and maybe even impossible using weak bone. The advantages of a nondestructive test such as that described below are related to assessment of precision, the ability to determine mechanical properties in different directions, and the ability to determine viscoelastic properties.

This technique will be superior in studies where a test specimen can be its own control, such as in studies of the effect of different preservation methods,[12] temperature, water saturation, and extraction of different connective tissue elements (collagen, elastin) on the mechanical properties. By using cubic geometry the test specimen can also be its own control in analyzing anisotropy by nondestructive testing in different directions.[3] Since the precision can be determined, the technique also has a great advantage in studies where it is important to calculate the number of patients/samples which have to be included in a specific study in order to be able to detect a predetermined possible difference.

II. GUIDELINES FOR NONDESTRUCTIVE TESTING IN COMPRESSION

A. TYPE OF TEST MACHINE AND STRAIN MEASUREMENT DEVICES

The change in length during nondestructive testing of cancellous bone is so small that the quality of the test machine and deformation measurement device becomes critical for the outcome of the test.

It has been observed that machines driven by two screws occasionally produce an extra loop on the top of the hysteresis loop during nondestructive testing. The reason for this extra loop is probably a small tilting of the crosshead of the testing machine when it turns from loading to unloading. This can occur because the two screws are driven by one motor. In order to avoid this phenomenon a hydraulic machine is superior.

Sometimes a machine runs a little farther than the actual set limits. This overshoot is related to the speed of transmission and transformation of data. It is therefore obligatory for the research worker to be familiar with the specific test machine and data-collecting system, so that adjustments can be made.

Because of the small deformations involved in cancellous bone testing, the deformation of the machine and testing column are not insignificant, and the built-in deformation measurement device is not sufficient. It is imperative to use an extensometer or a similar accurate device placed on the test columns close to the test specimen or directly on the specimen in order to measure changes in the length accurately.

The following description of nondestructive testing implies the use of a strain measurement device attached to the test columns close to the test sample.

B. Handling the Test Specimens

A test specimen that has been stored frozen should be kept in saline at room temperature for a few hours before testing. The authors put a droplet of mineral oil on the ends of the testing column in order to reduce friction. Drying of a specimen is not a problem during the short time of nondestructive testing including the mechanical conditioning procedure. If the specimen is going to be retested later the same day, it should be kept in saline. It can be stored frozen for later retesting without damage.[12]

C. Preload

When the test is started it is necessary to have contact between the specimen and test columns in order to avoid artifacts from fluid on the surfaces and in order to define zero strain. This is best done by defining the zero strain to be at a specific loading stress. The authors usually use a stress of 0.1 MPa. This stress corresponds to a load of a few newtons (preload) when the diameter/side length of the testing specimen is between 5 and 7 mm (cylindrical/cubic geometry).

D. Upper Strain Limit

The options for setting the upper test limit in nondestructive testing are a fixed load, a percentage of the ultimate load determined from the density of the test specimen (obtained by quantitative computed tomography or photon absorptiometry) or a fixed strain. Whereas ultimate stress (the strength) varies considerably, ultimate strain is nearly constant. Accordingly, a strain limit has been found to be best in producing a stiffness which correlates strongly with the stiffness of a test to failure.[13]

The test is conducted between a lower stress limit (preload) and an upper strain limit. This upper strain limit should be chosen so that the test runs into the linear part of the load–displacement curve, but not so far that the slope of the curve is decreasing. By using the cutting/sawing technique (EXAKT Apparaturbau, Hamburg, Germany) for specimen preparation, it was found that for test specimens between 5 and 7.5 mm, the maximum strain limit in order to avoid beginning failure during testing was 0.8%; 0.6% strain was found to be the optimum safe upper strain limit. However, if the machining technique is more precise in producing parallel end plates, or less traumatizing to the trabecular struts at the surface, or if specimens longer than 7.5 mm are chosen, then the upper strain limit should be smaller.

It is advisable to run a pilot study by testing a number of specimens to failure. The average strain corresponding to the "middle" of the linear part of the load–displacement curve should be determined. The "middle" of the linear part can be determined by fitting a third-order (or higher order) polynomial to the stress–strain data set from zero strain to a point between yield strain and ultimate strain. The middle of the linear part can be defined and found as the strain corresponding to the point where the tangent changes from increasing to decreasing. A simpler method, and fairly accurate for that purpose, would be to draw the tangent to the point with maximum slope on a printout and determine the strain corresponding to the middle of that segment where the testing curve does not differ significantly from a straight line. The upper strain limit should be selected as 75% of that strain.

If the pilot study reveals an average strain corresponding to the middle of the linear part of the load–displacement curve larger than 1%, one should seriously consider if the technique of machining test specimens is sufficiently good or if there is a major error in displacement measurement.

E. Strain Rate and Testing Frequency

Since cancellous bone has viscoelastic properties, the results of testing are time dependent. As a consequence, the strain rate and testing frequency have to be fixed. A sequence of test cycles can be made by loading and unloading using the same strain rate without a pause between cycles, or a predetermined pause between cycles can be used. The authors find a strain rate of 0.01 s^{-1} and a testing frequency of 0.2 Hz to be suitable. This method provides a pause of about 4 s between cycles, which is sufficient time for resetting the strain channel during conditioning (see below).

F. Mechanical Conditioning

The reproducibility of the first test cycle is not particularly good. The end point of the testing curve will not coincide with the starting point. This is partly due to the viscoelastic properties of cancellous bone and probably partly due to smoothing of small surface irregularities during the first cycle. The end point of each cycle moves a little to the right (a small residual strain) during repetitive testing, but the difference between the starting point and the end point of a cycle becomes smaller and smaller by continued testing. A steady state (the end point of the curve coincides with the starting point) is usually reached by 5 to 15 cycles. The real test can be performed immediately after conditioning either as a single nondestructive test or as the average of a number of nondestructive tests.

Since the starting point of a new cycle moves to the right until a steady state has been reached, the strain at start is not zero and the strain interval will be smaller than selected (Figure 9.2). The magnitude of this shift to the right of the stating point may vary considerably between specimens. The authors found that the reproducibility of the final test was best, when the strain channel was reset to zero at the end of each test cycle, so that the final test was conducted within the zero strain limit and the selected upper strain limit for that particular cycle. The authors' laboratory uses a fixed number of conditioning cycles (15 or 20) or defines the steady state to be reached when the starting point was reproduced ±2 μm within three consecutive conditioning cycles.

G. Determination of Normalized Stiffness

The stiffness is defined as the steepest part of the loading curve. Since data are collected and stored by a computer, the maximum slope of the loading curve is easily calculated by fitting a third-order polynomial to the data set of the loading curve (Figure 9.3).

H. Determination of Energy Absorption

The area underneath the loading curve represents energy stored or absorbed by the specimen and the interface between specimen and test machine (loading energy). The area underneath the unloading curve represents energy regained during unloading (elastic energy). The area between the loading and the unloading curve represents energy lost during a cycle (hysteresis). This energy loss is the sum of viscoelastic energy absorbed by the test specimen and energy lost by friction at the interface between test specimen and test the columns (see Figure 9.3).

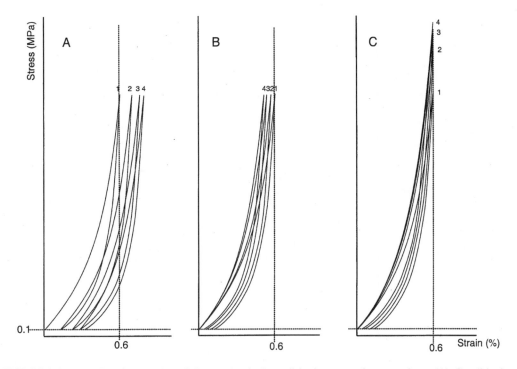

FIGURE 9.2   The first four cycles of the mechanical conditioning procedure are show. (A) Conditioning performed to a fixed load. Note that the cycles move to the right. The strain at the end of the loading curve is comparable to the changes in strain in a creep test. (B) The four cycles from (A) are put on top of each other with the same starting point. Note that the stiffness is increasing from test to test and the area of the hysteresis loop is decreasing. (C) Conditioning to a fixed strain by resetting the strain channel between each cycle. Note that the stiffness and the stress at the end of the loading curve increase from test to test.

III. VARIATION IN TEST TECHNIQUE

If cancellous bone from large mammals and from anatomical sites with strong bone is the subject of study, it may be possible to machine specimens with a 2 : 1 length-to-diameter ratio strong enough to attach a miniextensometer directly to the specimen without causing damage to it.[11] In that case a great part of the systematic error arising from the interface between specimen and test column will be eliminated. The upper strain limit should in that case be selected considerably smaller. An upper strain limit as small as 0.2% should be selected[14] in order to avoid signs of beginning failure (decreasing stiffness on repeated testing).

The technique described including the above-mentioned variation works with physiological strains. Nondestructive testing by small strain amplitudes (ultrasound) has been used for determination of both elastic and viscoelastic properties. Strong correlations have been found between properties obtained by ultrasound techniques and properties obtained by large strain mechanical testing technique. Since the stiffness obtained by the ultrasound technique usually is high, it may look less affected by those systematic errors listed in the beginning of this chapter. The ultrasound technique is also useful for determination of properties in different directions, and it is even possible to obtain the shear stiffness.[15,16]

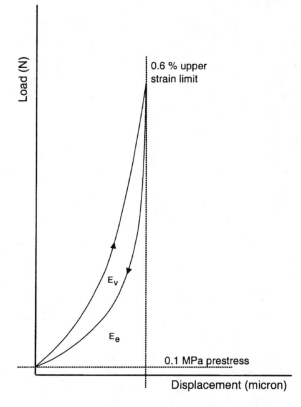

FIGURE 9.3 A typical load–displacement curve. The stiffness is the slope of the steepest part of the loading curve. The stiffness is normalized using the cross-sectional area and the original length of the specimen. Elastic energy is the area underneath the unloading curve. The energy loss (viscoelastic energy) is the area enclosed by the loading/unloading cycle.

REFERENCES

1. Hvid, I., Mechanical strength of trabecular bone at the knee, *Dan. Med. Bull.*, 35, 345, 1988.
2. Evans, F.G. and King, A.I., Regional differences in some physical properties of human spongy bone, in *Biomechanical Studies of the Musculo-Skeletal System*, Evans, F.G., Ed., Charles C Thomas, Springfield, 1961, 19.
3. Linde, F., Pongsoipetch, B., Frich, L.H., and Hvid, I., Three-axial strain controlled testing applied to bone specimens from the proximal tibial epiphysis, *J. Biomech.*, 23, 1167, 1990.
4. Martens, M., Van Audekercke, R., Delport, P., et al., The mechanical characteristics of cancellous bone at the upper femoral region, *J. Biomech.*, 16, 971, 1983.
5. Allard, R.N. and Ashman, R.B., A comparison between cancellous bone compressive moduli determined from surface strain and total specimen deflection, *Trans. Orthop. Res. Soc.*, 16, 151, 1991.
6. Linde, F. and Hvid, I., The effect of constraint on the mechanical behavior of trabecular bone specimens, *J. Biomech.*, 22, 485, 1989.
7. Odgaard, A. and Linde, F., The underestimation of Young's modulus in compression testing of cancellous bone specimens, *J. Biomech.* 24, 691, 1991.
8. Turner, C.H. and Cowin, S.C., Errors induced by off-axis measurement of the elastic properties of bone, *J. Biomech. Eng.*, 110, 213, 1988.
9. Dieter, G.E., *Mechanical Metallurgy.* McGraw-Hill, New York, 1961, 479.
10. Linde, F., Elastic and viscoelastic properties of trabecular bone by a compression testing approach, *Dan. Med. Bull.*, 41, 119, 1994

11. Keaveny, T.M., Guo, X.E., Wachtel, E.F., et al., Trabecular bone exhibits fully linear elastic behavior and yields at low strains, *J. Biomech.*, 27, 1127, 1994.

12. Linde, F. and Sørensen, H.C., The effect of different storage methods on the mechanical properties of trabecular bone, *J. Biomech.*, 26, 1249, 1993.

13. Linde, F., Gøthgen, C.B., Hvid, I., et al., Mechanical properties of trabecular bone by a nondestructive compression testing approach, *Eng. Med.*, 17, 23, 1988.

14. Røhl, L., Larsen, E., Linde, F., et al., Tensile and compressive properties of cancellous bone, *J. Biomech.*, 24, 1143, 1991.

15. Ashman, R.B., Experimental techniques, in *Bone Mechanics*, Cowin, S.C., Ed., CRC Press, Boca Raton, FL, 1989, 75.

16. Ashman, R.B., Rho, J.Y., and Turner, C.H., Anatomical variation of orthotropic elastic moduli of the proximal human tibia, *J. Biomech.*, 22, 895, 1989.

10 Synthetic Materials and Structures Used as Models for Bone

John A. Szivek

CONTENTS

I. CORTICAL BONE SUBSTITUTES

A. INTRODUCTION

Cadaver bones have routinely been used as support structures during bench-top testing to evaluate biomechanical changes caused by artificial joints,[1-3] orthopaedic fracture fixation devices,[4-6] and new orthopaedic procedures. Obtaining fresh disease-free cadaver bones to be used during mechanical testing of orthopaedic implants and fixation systems is becoming difficult and extremely expensive. Large interbone shape and materials property variations with standard deviations in excess of 100% have been noted.[1,7,8] Variations of this size imply that several hundred bones are required to approach statistical significance. Sample sizes reported in the literature are typically less than 50 specimens and are often as few as three specimens. Interbone variations have prompted investigations to carry out comparative testing within the same bone to assess biomechanical parameters prior to and following implant placement. This approach, in which the bone is used as its own control, limits experimental design considerably. Moreover, the handling and storing of human cadaver specimens prior to and during testing can also cause problems leading to changes in properties during the course of the test.

    These factors have prompted the development of synthetic support structures for use during mechanical testing. In general, accurately simulating the stiffness of bone is most important when "stress shielding" near artificial joints or fracture fixation devices are being evaluated, while accurately simulating the strength of bone is most important when screws or other orthopaedic attachment devices are being evaluated. Early studies that simulated the properties of bone as a support structure used tubular metal,[9] wood, and constructs such as laminated linen.[10-12] Although these constructs demonstrated consistent materials properties, they did not accurately simulate the strength, stiffness, and time-dependent properties of bone. In addition, the shape of these constructs did not allow accurate modeling of physiological loads. One of the earliest reports of the preparation and use of a fiber-reinforced proximal femur[13] described a structure which simulated bone strength and stiffness properties better and attempted to model the shape of the proximal femur. Fiber-reinforced femora of this kind were further developed and used to compare fracture fixation techniques[14] and evaluate stability of artificial hip designs.[15] Uta[16] suggested the use of polyurethane model bones to standardize testing of fracture fixation devices.

Fiber-reinforced epoxy bones became commercially available in the late 1980s (Pacific Research Labs, Inc., Vashon Island, WA). The first generation (F-type) amber-colored left femora were carbon fiber–reinforced epoxy. The geometric measurements of these bones fell within the spectrum of sizes corresponding to cadaver femora.[17,18] There were mixed reports on the usefulness of this type of bone. Beals[19] reported favorable results but Szivek et al.[20] concluded, from torsional and anatomical bending tests, that smaller variations in materials properties were needed for these to serve as valuable bone models and support structures for mechanical testing. Neither investigator had carried out a quantitative comparison with cadaver specimens of the same size. However, both authors agreed that the consistency in size of these "bones" facilitated the reuse of fixtures to run multiple comparisons using the synthetic bones. This offered advantages over the use of cadaver materials.

More recently, a second-generation glass fiber–reinforced bone was introduced by the same manufacturer. Examination of the mechanical properties[21] indicated that the "cortical" component of these synthetic bones demonstrated consistent mechanical properties and a similar deformation response to that of a size-matched cadaver bone. This study suggested that the polyurethane foam used to model the trabecular bone was weak,[21] although a recent report[22] indicated that the stiffness of this foam specified at 69 MPa falls within the range of properties reported for trabecular bone.[23] Other investigators have noted that these bones have a similar deformation response to cadaver bone in four-point bending,[22] axial loading,[22] and during simulated physiological loading,[21] but not during torsion testing.[20,22]

Otani et al.[25] have observed that these models are not reliable for circumferential strain measurement under axial load or for any type of strain measurement under torsion load. They indicated that differences in comparison to bone were likely a result of the cross-ply fiber orientation in the synthetic bones. They did not observe these discrepancies when micromotion measurements were collected for implant stability studies. Examination of femoral head deflection and strain distributions across proximal bone sections during axial testing[22] have also shown that while overall mechanical properties are quite consistent from one synthetic bone to another, local strains can vary. This suggests that testing a bone intact and then with an implant will provide the best understanding of the effect of the implant. It has been noted that while time constants on the viscoelastic response of these bones are short, it is beneficial to leave loads in place during static testing for up to 4 min.[22]

In addition to two sizes of composite femora, a synthetic tibia is now also available. There are no published comparisons of the deformation response of the synthetic tibia with that of the cadaver bone. These tibia models do offer the advantage of providing consistency in size, allowing the reuse of fixtures and making it easy to run multiple comparisons. The lack of mechanical properties information on these bones suggest that studies in which these are used should be carefully planned to allow adequate characterization of intact properties before using them to evaluate the performance of implants.

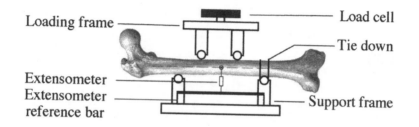

FIGURE 10.1 Diagram showing a four-point bend testing configuration which can be used to characterize overall bending stiffness of a synthetic bone with or without an implant.

B. PREPARATION OF SYNTHETIC BONES FOR TESTING AND TEST SELECTION

Variations in the fabrication process occasionally lead to some anomalies in the location of the fiberglass-reinforcing sleeve within the bones which can locally affect mechanical properties. X-raying the bones prior to testing provides a means of detecting gross differences, although it cannot be used as a predictive tool to assess the way in which mechanical properties are affected. The author has used a high-resolution Faxitron cabinet X-ray system (Hewlett-Packard, McMinniville, OR) with X-OMAT AR scientific imaging film (Eastman Kodak Co., Rochester, NY) as a screening tool. In order to reduce interbone variability during testing several specimens can be purchased and bones which pass radiographic scrutiny should be compared intact. Selection of a subgroup from this larger group provides test bones with very similar deformation responses. In preparation for testing, which requires accurate cortical and trabecular support, removal of the foam is recommended. It can be replaced with a polyurethane foam called Daro foam (see Section II on trabecular bone models for details) which can be produced with a range of stiffness from 63 to 104 MPa,[24] simulating the properties of the trabecular bone from a range of patient populations.

Test and measurement system selection should be based on the fact that synthetic femora have a similar deformation response to cadaver femora in four-point bending, axial loading, and during simulated physiological loading but not torsional loading. Deflection of components of the femur such as the head have also been noted to be consistent. Test design should include testing the femur intact and then with an implant in place to provide the best understanding of the effect of the implant. The viscoelastic response of these bones dictate that tests be separated by several minutes to allow viscoelastic effects to dissipate. Although these synthetic bones are more consistent during retesting than cadaver bones, retesting of the same construct at least three times is mandatory to assess reproducibility.[21,22]

C. EVALUATION OF MECHANICAL PROPERTIES PRIOR TO USE

The simplest testing procedure that allows comparison of whole-bone properties is four-point bending (Figure 10.1). It has been used to assess stiffness characteristics of fracture fixation systems. Four-point bending is preferable to three-point bending since it assures a uniform bending moment between the inner two supports and potentially more accurate deflection measurements from this region of the specimen. The separation of the roller supports is dependent on the size of the specimen being tested. Ideally, the supports should be as far apart as possible and located within the diaphysis so that the metaphyseal flares do not affect testing. A displacement transducer (commonly an extensometer) attached to the centerline of the middiaphysis of the bone and to a reference bar is used to evaluate deflection accurately. A small pin or K wire placed in the bone can facilitate attachment of the extensometer to the bone.

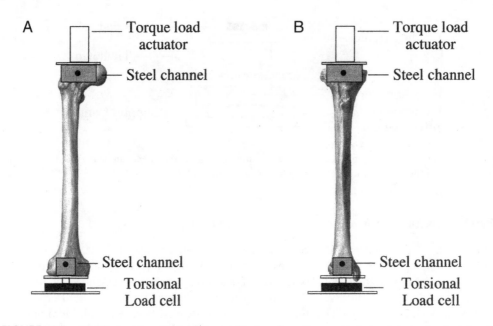

FIGURE 10.2   (A) Diagram showing the fixture and test configuration used to test an intact or implanted synthetic femur. (B) Diagram showing the fixture and test configuration used to test an intact or implanted synthetic tibia.

Alternatively, strain gauges can be attached to the lateral, medial, anterior, and posterior bone surfaces. Ideally, gauges used on the surface of these composite bones should have a self-temperature compensation factor eliminating errors due to thermal expansion of the gauge. They should also have a relatively large surface area and high resistance to minimize the amount of heating. For greatest accuracy a Micro-Measurements EA-00-250BK-10C uniaxial gauge (Measurements Group, Raleigh, NC) can be used. Since measurements are often taken over relatively short periods of time thermal factors generally have a small effect on accuracy, and it is common to use more readily available CEA-06-125UW-120 (Measurements Group, Raleigh, NC) uniaxial-type gauges. For biaxial and rosette strain measurements CEA-06-062WT-120 and WA-06-060WR-120, respectively, are satisfactory. These gauges can be attached using a suitable cyanoacrylate adhesive such as M-Bond 200 (Measurements Group, Raleigh, NC). Additional choices are available in the M-Line strain gauge accessories catalog (A-110-6, Measurements Group, Raleigh, NC). European investigators[22,26] have successfully used H.B.M. 6/120 LY 11 supplied by Hottinger Baldwin Messtechnik, Stuttgart, Germany.

Bones should be tested in ML (medial to lateral) and AP (anterior to posterior) bending. It is valuable to clamp or in some way fix one end of the femur to prevent rotation during the loading procedure. The triangular shape of the tibia may preclude the need to do this. Three to six repetitions of a test will provide an indication of the variation in response to a particular test setup. No conditioning effects should be observed; i.e., no progressive change in properties should be noted over the course of the repeated testing.

In cases where synthetic bones are to be used to evaluate implants which must support torsion loading, a simple whole-bone torque test can be used to characterize the response of the model bone prior to testing with an implant in place. The bone should be gripped securely at the ends and positioned with the center of the diaphysis aligned along the center of the torsion axis.

For testing of the femur, this alignment will place the intercondylar space and the neck of the femur on this centerline (Figure 10.2A). The fixture holding the proximal femur should be a stiff, channel-shaped part with a deep section so that the surface of the head, neck, and greater trochanter are all rotated simultaneously by the test machine actuator. The distal femur should be placed in

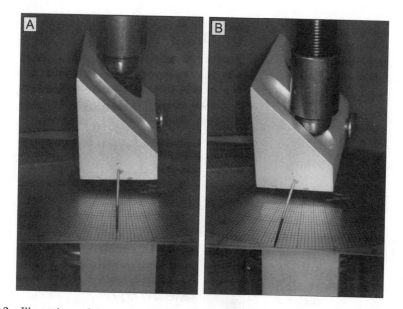

FIGURE 10.3 Illustrations of the way in which a loading ramp can be used to generate a torsion load on a bone if only an axial-loading fixture is available. (From Szivek, J.A., and Yapp, R.A., *J. Biomed. Mater. Res. Appl. Biomater.*, 23 (A1 Suppl.), 105, 1989. With permission.)

a rectangular steel channel the height of the condyles or, alternatively, can be embedded to a level above the condyles in a low-melting-point compound such as Cerrobend (Scottsdale Tool, Phoenix, AZ) or a polymethylmethacrylate (PMMA) such as a dental repair resin (Hygienic Repair Resin, Hygienic Corp., Akron, OH). The fixture ends should be observed closely during loading to ensure solid gripping so that torsional displacements measured by the actuator will be accurate. The direction of rotation will affect the response and should be chosen carefully to simulate the response of the bone accurately, e.g., internal rotation of the femoral head can be used to simulate the physiological loading during rising from a chair. A slight amount of initial torque load (up to 5 N·m) can be applied to ensure the system is tight. Specimens should not be tested beyond 30 N·m unless nonlinear responses are of interest in the study.

Torsion testing of a tibia is slightly more complex. A transcortical pin or screw embedded in a potting compound such as PMMA can be used to hold the distal tibia (Figure 10.2B). The proximal tibia can be fixtured in a similar way. This setup will work if testing of plates or external fixation devices is to be undertaken, although it may interfere with the ability to place intramedullary devices. In general, this type of setup will also allow the use of combined loading such as combined axial and torsion loading. This is best accomplished with a test machine that can independently apply torsion and axial loads, but for situations in which only an axial actuator is available a fixture with a loading ramp (Figure 10.3) can provide combined loading.[27]

Axial loading has also been used to characterize the axial deformation response of femora but is not commonly used to evaluate implants. For axial compression or tension testing, the same fixture design used for torsion testing can be employed. However, the deformations will be small and the most sensitive deformation measurement approach available is recommended. Strain gauges placed around the circumference of the bone are sufficiently sensitive for this task, but the ram excursion measurement from a servohydraulic test machine is generally not.

D. TESTING IMPLANTS WITH SYNTHETIC BONE MODELS

Using synthetic femurs for studies in which artificial joints or fracture fixation devices are tested is best done by simulating physiological loading. At the very least, body weight and the effects of

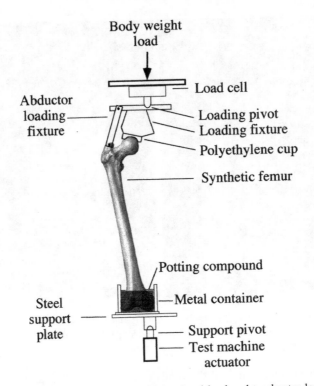

FIGURE 10.4   Diagram illustrating the way in which a head load and trochanter load can be applied to a femur.

the abductors should be modeled. Head and abductor loading angle can be altered to simulate several stance positions.[28] Prior to testing a model femur with implants in place, a control test of the intact femur alone is imperative. Figure 10.4 shows one design of a head and abductor loading arrangement used to apply a simulated stance load to a model femur. In this arrangement the abductor loading fixture can be strain-gauged and calibrated with a load cell or weights. The gauge circuit arrangement uses four gauges to provide uniform uniaxial strain measurements.[29] Alternatively, a small load cell can be purchased and incorporated into the fixture to measure load.

Testing using this arrangement can be carried out while monitoring strain gauges attached to the bone surface or while monitoring linear variable differential transformers placed near locations of interest on the bone or implant. It can also be used in conjunction with motion analysis systems to monitor motion or gross deformation of the bone. Markers such as K wires or pins allow monitoring of the motion of selected surface locations of interest.

Recently, there has been an interest in modeling additional muscle loads on this type of model, and Figure 10.5 shows one configuration of this test setup in which the addition of lateral muscle loads has been incorporated into the loading procedure. There is no consensus on the ideal loading arrangement for this type of testing, and a detailed discussion of the advantages of various loading arrangements is beyond the scope of this chapter but can be found in reviews of this topic such as Colgan et al.[30]

II. TRABECULAR BONE MODELING

A. INTRODUCTION

The reproducibility of biomechanical test results for orthopaedic implants tested in cadaver trabecular bone has often been hampered by the wide variation in the mechanical properties of the

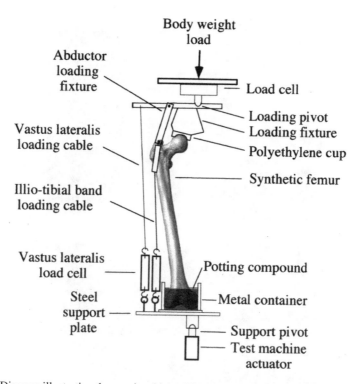

FIGURE 10.5   Diagram illustrating the way in which additional lateral muscle loads can be applied to a femur.

substrate material.[31-39] Differences between samples have been attributed to variations in specimen selection site,[32,34,40] and the age, sex, and metabolic conditions[35,36,39] of the donor. Materials with consistent and controllable mechanical properties similar to those of human cancellous bone would provide a valuable alternative to cadaver bone as a test substrate. In addition, the ability to produce unlimited numbers of these substrates in a variety of shapes offers a major advantage over cadaver specimens whose shapes are defined by the tissue bed from which they were harvested.

The structure of trabecular bone is a network of connecting rods and plates which form columns and struts.[41] This results in an interconnected pore structure within the bone. There have been no reports of synthetic porous structures with interconnecting pores having the same stiffness and strength characteristics of human trabecular bone. Implantable coralline hydroxyapatite (Interpore International Irvine, CA) or porous filters made of metals or ceramics (Astromet, Cincinnati, OH) could be used if interconnecting porosity is of primary importance and strength characteristics are of secondary consideration. If strength or stiffness need to be more accurately modeled, porous polymers are better candidates even though they have a closed pore structure.

One popular synthetic closed-cell polyurethane foam (Daro, Butler, WI) first used as a test bed for fracture fixation devices[42] and evaluation of the stability of artificial joint components[43,44] has been noted to have a structure with some similarities to human trabecular bone[24,45] (Figure 10.6). The two parts provided to form Daro foam are an isocyanate (methylene diisocyanate) and a resin (polyol). The foam is formed during a process when liquid polymer–coated gas bubbles impinge and solidify.[24,45] Varying the density (and bubble size) affects the mechanical properties of the foam, allowing some tailoring of the properties to model bone from a range of types of patients.

The stress–strain curve of this closed-cell foam is similar to that of trabecular bone when compression-loaded.[24,31,36,37] In both cases, the first phase of loading these materials leads to a linear elastic response as the components of the material are subjected to compression or tension loads. At higher loads, they yield as the cell walls begin to collapse. The resistance to load increases, causing a final increasingly steep slope to the stress–strain curve.[31,33]

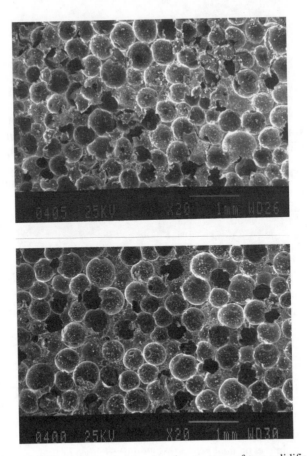

FIGURE 10.6   Scanning electron micrographs showing the structure of two solidified foams with different bubble densities.

Initial characterization of the mechanical properties of this foam were reported for a formulation representing "normal" trabecular bone.[24] Recent studies[45] have shown that by varying the ratio of resin to isocyanate the mechanical properties of the foam can be altered so that it can model the trabecular bone in a range of patient populations. This allows its use for the evaluation of implants or procedures specific to a particular patient group. Some examples include young healthy trauma patients, patients with osteoporosis, or those with rheumatoid arthritis.

B.   FOAM PREPARATION

Although the properties of Daro foam can be very consistent, factors that cause variations in its properties are the ratio of isocyanate and resin, temperature, humidity, mixing protocol, pouring protocol, container shape, container size, and thermal conductivity and whether the container is open or sealed during setting. Since the foam can form with different properties, care should be taken to control as many of these parameters as possible and to test small samples separately from each fabrication procedure to characterize property variations.

The first step in the preparation of the foam for evaluating orthopaedic devices requires the selection of a container to provide an appropriate shape or test bed. Although the implant to be tested will to some extent dictate a preferred shape, cube-shaped containers provide relatively more uniform properties compared with nonsymmetric or oddly shaped containers. To avoid edge effects (unless one is intentionally attempting to model bone property variations near surfaces) the foam blocks should be relatively large compared with the implant being tested. Analytical modeling of screw pullout has shown that the damage area is equivalent to two screw diameters.[46] Blocks with a width greater than twice the diameter of the screws should be made, and if multiple screws are pulled out of the same block they should be separated by this distance.

A skin of relatively denser material will form at all surfaces when foam is made. It can be used to simulate a cortical shell formed around trabecular surfaces of some bones, or this skin can be removed in order to model the trabecular bed only. In either case, it is imperative that a sample of material (in the form of a small cube or cylinder if possible) from the interior of the foam be tested in either uniaxial tension, compression, or shear to confirm its mechanical properties and to ensure interbatch consistency. If the skin is to be used to evaluate implants, the mechanical properties of samples of the skin (possibly in the form of a thin sheet) should also be characterized.

Ideally, the loading of the cubes, cylinders, or the skin samples should be similar to the way in which the implants inserted into the foam blocks will load the foam during implant evaluation. While the results of recent studies[27,45] were obtained using samples compressed without constraining specimen ends or sides, studies on trabecular bone have suggested that unconstrained testing procedures produce failure strength values that are low in comparison with those predicted by finite-element models which are constrained by surrounding bone.[47,48] However, most literature values for trabecular bone reported to date have been measured using unconstrained experimental testing. As such, it has been possible to compare synthetic material properties with these values. When contemplating the use of these foams, future characterization will benefit from testing with end and side constraints. Specimen ends can be constrained by using PMMA or epoxy to attach specimens to the platens of the test machine. Accurate side constraint is harder to achieve. A close-fitting sleeve around a loading piston with the exact cross-sectional area of the face of the test specimen is one option. Pushout testing through a block larger than the sample being compressed may provide more accurate side constraint modeling. Few test results from trabecular bone evaluated using these approaches are currently available.

Daro foam properties vary depending on the molding parameters. Figure 10.7 provides an example of the range of strength and stiffness properties noted when the ratio of resin to isocyanate is altered from 10.0 : 10.0 to 10 : 7.9 and 10.0 : 5.0.[24,45] Over this range of ratios, the bubble diameters increase by approximately 13%. The foam density changes by approximately the same percentage, decreasing from 269 g/cc to 235 g/cc. Although this is a fairly narrow range of foam density, published evidence over a wider range for other foams suggests a linear relationship between density and strength or stiffness.[49]

To ensure uniform properties throughout each foam, resin should be mixed prior to use and added to the isocyanate and then mixed with a blender or paint mixer at 1500 rpm for at least 20 s. Although properties as a function of mixing time have not been evaluated quantitatively, shorter mixing times do not allow thorough mixing and result in uneven bubble sizes and properties through the section of the foam. Some bubble size variation is to be expected and cannot be avoided even with much longer mixing times (Figure 10.8).

Mixtures must immediately be poured into a container and allowed to cure for 24 h. In cases in which a flat, dense skin is desirable to model a flat, cortical shell, the container should be enclosed. Properties of foams made using this procedure are slightly different and warrant examination since they could be used to study mandibular ridge or skull modeling applications.

In cases in which specimens are intended to simulate a trabecular bed only, a band saw should be used to remove the surface of the foam. It is advisable to mark the specimen orientation and to mark the orientation of any samples cut from it. Some variation in properties within specimens resulting from the foaming process and direction of bubble migration during solidification have been observed. Variations across specimens smaller than 5 cm in thickness are minor. When measuring sample shapes prior to testing, several measurements along each edge are recommended since cut tolerances for this material even when prepared by machining are not tight. However, since large specimens are easily prepared, this material characteristic will not adversely affect the ability to calculate failure stresses and stiffness values accurately.

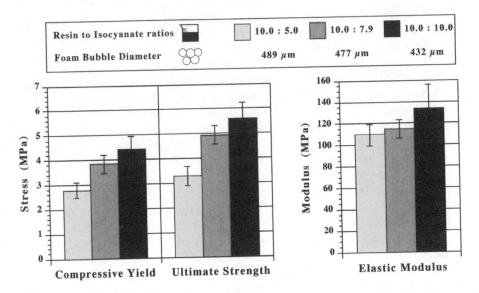

FIGURE 10.7 A graph summarizing the strength and stiffness of the foams as a function of isocyanate to resin mixtures. Values were drawn from published information.[24,45]

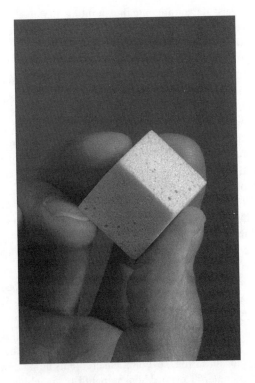

FIGURE 10.8 An example of a block taken from a foam prepared using a resin-to-isocyanate ratio of 10.0 : 5.0.

C. Foam Testing

The most facile specimen characterization technique is compressive loading. A load rate comparable to that to be used when testing the orthopaedic implant in the model material should be used in this test. Implants to be used in older, total-joint patients should be tested relatively slowly in comparison with tests of devices used in young athletes. A rate of 0.5 mm/s on a servohydraulic test frame provides a moderate test speed to evaluate the foam for tests involving study of implants during the postoperative period when patients are expected to have activities with moderate load rates. Each sample must be conditioned by axial loading three times to approximately 70% of the compressive yield strength, since surface damage caused by cutting will initially produce inaccurate stiffness readings. After conditioning, each sample should be compressed axially in the same direction until permanent damage is apparent. Deformation of test specimens can most easily be measured with the LVDT in the test frame. An extensometer can also be used for greater accuracy or if deformation in other than the loading direction is of interest. For greatest accuracy optical extensometry of the middle portion of a sample is ideal.[47] Load–deformation values should be plotted to establish the stiffness of the material and its failure strength. Failure stresses should be calculated using stress = force/area, and failure strain using strain = (change in height from failure load – original height)/original height. Stiffness is calculated using stiffness = stress/strain.

Shear testing of this material is more difficult and has not been described in the literature. While a rectangular specimen that is attached to the surfaces of a lap shear fixture with a high-strength epoxy could be used, a pushout-type test may be more appropriate for the type of specimen that can easily be created from these foams. Similarly, tensile testing would require epoxying specimens to platens which could be used to pull the specimens apart. Calculation of cross-sectional area and consequently failure strength values from this type of test are expected to be difficult. Since few implant interfaces are loaded in pure tension, this test may offer information of limited usefulness.

III. SUMMARY

The cortical and trabecular bone models developed to date offer the advantages of consistency in shape, strength, and stiffness. These advantages alone make them a better choice than cadaver bone as support materials for testing orthopaedic and dental implants in almost all applications. Continued development of fiber-reinforced epoxy to create a model with more similar torsional deformation to cortical bone would be valuable. Testing of a range of types of trabecular bone from patients with various diseases and additional development of polyurethane foams with an even greater range of properties would provide foams simulating the properties of trabecular bone in a wider range of patients. Recently developed standards[50] for polyurethane foam materials for use during mechanical testing should also be considered as a guide during the development of new trabecular bone substitutes.

REFERENCES

1. Diegel, P.D., Daniels, A.U., and Dunn, H.K., Initial effect of collarless stem stiffness on femoral bone strain, *J. Arthroplasty*, 4, 173, 1989.
2. Englehardt, J.A. and Saha, S., Effects of femoral component section modulus on the stress distribution in the proximal human femur, *Med. Biol. Eng. Comput.*, 26, 38, 1988.
3. Finlay, J.B., Chess, D.G., Hardie, W.R., et al., An evaluation of three loading configurations for the *in vitro* testing of femoral strains in total hip arthroplasty, *J. Orthop. Res.*, 9, 749, 1991.
4. Anderson, J.T., Erickson, J.M., Thompson, R.C., and Chao, E.Y., Pathologic femoral shaft fractures comparing fixation techniques using cement, *Clin. Orthop.*, 131, 273, 1978.

5. Laurence, M., Freeman, M.A., and Swanson, S.A.V., Engineering consideration in the internal fixation of fractures of the tibial shaft, *J. Bone Joint Surg.*, 51B, 754, 1969.

6. Cordey, J. and Perren, S.M., Stress protection in femora plated by carbon fiber and metallic plates; mathematical analysis and experimental verification, in *Biomaterials and Biomechanics*, Ducheyne, P., Van der Perre, G., and Aubert, A. E., Eds., Elsevier, Amsterdam, the Netherlands, 1984.

7. Crowninshield, R.D., Pederson, D.R., and Brand, R.A., A physiologically based criterion of muscle force prediction in locomotion, *J. Biomech. Eng.*, 102, 230, 1990.

8. Shybutt, G.T., Askew, M.J., Hori, R.Y., and Stulberg, S.D., Theoretical and experimental studies on femoral stresses following surface replacement hip arthroplasty, in Hip, *Proceedings of the 8th Open Scientific Meeting of the the Hip Society,* Frank Stinchfield Award Paper 192, The Hip Society, C. V. Mosby Co., St. Louis, MO, 1980.

9. Simon, B.R., Woo, S.L.-Y., Stanley, G.M., et al., Evaluation of one, two, and three dimensional finite element and experimental models of internal fixation plates, *J. Biomech.*, 10, 79, 1977.

10. Briggs, B.T. and Chao, E.Y.S., The mechanical performance of the standard Hoffman–Vidal external fixation apparatus, *J. Bone Joint Surg.*, 64A(4), 566, 1982.

11. Chao, E.Y. and An, K.N., Biomechanical analysis of external fixation devices for the treatment of open bone fractures in finite elements, in *Biomechanics*, Gallagher, R.H., Simon, B.R., Johnson, P.C., and Gross, J.F., Eds., John Wiley & Sons, New York, 1982.

12. Behrens, F., Johnson, W.D., Koch, T.W., and Kovacevic, N., Bending stiffness of unilateral and bilateral fixator frames, *Clin. Orthop.*, 178, 103, 1983.

13. Niederer, P.G. and Chiquet, C., Artificial proximal femur of fiber reinforced polyester for the study of load transmission of cemented hip prostheses: the prosthesis cement interface, *Trans. Annu. Soc. Biomater.*, 2, 88, 1978.

14. McKellop, H., Ebramzadeh, E., Matta, J., et al., Stability of femoral fractures with interlocking intramedullary rods, *Trans. Annu. Orthop. Res. Soc.,* 319, 1986.

15. McKellop, H., Ebramzadeh, E., Niederer, P.O., and Sarmiento, A., Comparison of the stability of press-fit prosthesis femoral stems using a synthetic femur model, *J. Orthop. Res.*, 9, 297, 1991.

16. Uta, S., Development of synthetic bone models for the evaluation of fracture fixation devices, *Nippon Seikegeka Gakai Zasshi,* 66, 1156, 1992.

17. Noble, P.C., Alexander, J.W., Lindahl, L.J., et al., The anatomical basis of femoral component design, *Clin. Orthop.*, 235, 148, 1988.

18. Rubin, P.J., Leyvraz, P.F., Aubaniac J.M., et al., The morphology of the proximal femur, *J. Bone Joint Surg.*, 74B, 28, 1992.

19. Beals, N., Evaluation of a Composite Sawbones Femur Model, Research Report ML-87-25, Richards Medical Company, Memphis, TN, 1987.

20. Szivek, J.A., Weng, M., and Karpman, R., Variability in the torsional and bending response of a commercially available composite femur, *J. Appl. Biomater.*, 1, 183, 1990.

21. Szivek, J.A. and Gealer, R.L., Comparison of the deformation response of synthetic and cadaveric femora during simulated one-legged stance, *J. Appl. Biomater.*, 2, 277, 1991.

22. Cristofolini, L., Viceconti, M., Cappello, A., and Toni, A., Mechanical validation of whole bone composite femur models, *J. Biomech.*, 29, 525, 1996.

23. Martens, M., Van Audekercke, R., Delport, P., et al., The mechanical characteristics of cancellous bone at the upper femoral region, *J. Biomech.*, 16, 971, 1983.

24. Szivek, J.A., Thomas, M., and Benjamin, J.B., Characterization of a synthetic foam as a model for human cancellous bone, *J. Appl. Biomater.*, 4, 269, 1993.

25. Otani, T., Whiteside, L.A., and White, S.E., Strain distribution in the proximal femur with flexible composite and metallic femoral components under axial and torsional loads, *J. Biomed. Mater. Res.*, 27, 575, 1993.

26. McNamara, B.P., Cristofolini, L., Toni, A., and Taylor, D., Evaluation of experimental and finite-element models of synthetic and cadaveric femora for pre-clinical design-analysis, *J. Clin. Mater.*, 17, 131, 1995.

27. Szivek, J.A. and Yapp, R.A., A testing technique allowing cyclic application of axial, bending, and torque loads to fracture plates to examine screw loosening, *J. Biomed. Mater. Res. Appl. Biomater.*, 23-A1, 105, 1989.

28. McLeish, R.D. and Charnley, J., Abduction forces in the one legged stance, *J. Biomech.*, 3, 191, 1970.

29. Measurements Group, Publication No. TN-514, 5, Raleigh, NC, 1988.
30. Colgan, D., Trench, P., Slemon, D., et al., A review of joint and muscle load simulation relevant to *in vitro* stress analysis of the hip, *Strain*, 30, 47, 1994.
31. Carter, D.R. and Hayes, W.C., The compressive behavior of bone as a two-phase porous structure, *J. Bone Joint Surg.*, 7, 954, 1977.
32. Galante, J., Rostoker, W., and Ray, R.D., Physical properties of trabecular bone, *Calcif. Tissue Res.*, 5, 236, 1970.
33. Gibson, L.J., The mechanical behavior of cancellous bone, *J. Biomech.*, 18, 317, 1985.
34. Goldstein, S.A., Wilson, D.L., Sonstigard, D.A., and Mathews, L., The mechanical properties of human tibial trabecular bone as a function of metaphyseal location, *J. Biomech.*, 16, 965, 1985.
35. Koeneman, J.B., Norman, J.P., and Szivek, J.A., The mechanical properties of cancellous bone in the femoral head: correlation with CT measurements, Trans. 20th International Society for Biomaterials, Kyoto, Japan, 11, 267, 1988.
36. Lindahl, O., Mechanical properties of dried defatted spongy bone, *Acta Orthop. Scand.*, 47, 19, 1976.
37. Linde, F., Hvid, I., and Pongsoipetch, B., Energy absorptive properties of human trabecular bone specimens during axial compression, *J. Orthop. Res.*, 7, 432, 1989.
38. Ashman, R.B., Rho, J.Y., and Turner, C.H., Anatomical variation of orthotropic elastic moduli of the proximal human tibia, *J. Biomech.*, 22, 895, 1989.
39. Wixson, R.L., Elasky, N., and Lewis, J., Cancellous bone material properties in osteoarthritic and rheumatoid total knee patients, *J. Orthop. Res.*, 7, 885, 1989.
40. Brown, T.D. and Ferguson, A.B., Mechanical property distributions in the cancellous bone of the human proximal femur, *Acta Orthop. Scand.*, 51, 429, 1980.
41. Mosekilde, L., Consequences of the remodeling process for vertebral trabecular structure: a scanning electron microscopy study (uncoupling of unloaded structures), *Bone Miner.*, 10, 13, 1990.
42. Hein, T.J., Hotchkiss, R., Perissinotto, A., and Chao, E.Y., Analysis of bone model material for external fracture fixation experiments, *J. Biomech. Instr.*, 22, 43, 1987.
43. Volz, R.G. and Lee, R.W., The effect of the stem and stem length on the mechanical stability of tibial knee components, *Trans. Orthop. Res. Soc.*, 13, 1988.
44. Lee, R.W., Volz, R.G., and Schroder, D.Q., Laboratory analysis of threaded acetabular cup stability, *Trans. Am. Acad. Orthop. Surg.*, New Orleans, LA, 1990.
45. Szivek, J.A., Thompson, J., and Benjamin, J.B., Three synthetic foams used to model a range of properties of human cancellous bone, *J. Appl. Biomater.*, 6, 125, 1995.
46. Thompson, J., Benjamin, J.B., and Szivek, J.A., Pullout strengths of cannulated and non-cannulated cancellous bone screws: a comparative study, *Clin. Orthop.*, 341, 241, 1997.
47. Odgaard, A., Hvid, I., and Linde, F., Compressive axial strain distributions in cancellous bone specimens, *J. Biomech.*, 22, 829, 1989.
48. Linde, F. and Hvid, I., The effect of constraint on the mechanical behavior of trabecular bone specimens, *J. Biomech.*, 22, 485, 1989.
49. Gibson, L.J. and Ashby, M.F., Material properties of cellular solids, in *Cellular Solids: Structure and Properties*, Cambridge University Press, Cambridge, U.K., 1997.
50. ASTM Subcommittee F04.21 of committee F-04 on Medical and Surgical Materials and Devices, *Standard Specification for Rigid Polyurethane Foam for Use as a Standard Material for Testing Orthopaedic Devices and Instruments*, Designation F 1839-97, American Society for Testing and Materials, West Conshohocken, PA, 1998.

Section II

Methods of Mechanical Testing of Bone

11 Tensile and Compression Testing of Bone

Tony S. Keller and Michael A. K. Liebschner

CONTENTS

I. INTRODUCTION

Mechanical testing studies of bone have been directed at determining the mechanical properties of whole bone and bone tissue under different loading conditions. In general, determination of mechanical properties of bone is done by the same methods used to study similar properties in metal, woods, and other structural materials and composites. These methods are based on fundamental principles of mechanics.[1-4] Consequently, some basic knowledge of mechanics and the terminology employed is essential in order to apply these principles.

Bone is a viscoelastic, composite material. The organization of the composite varies from animal to animal and is strongly influenced by aging, activity, and disease. Unlike engineering composite materials, however, bone has a fibrous structural component (collagen) as its matrix and exhibits a composite behavior microscopically as well as macroscopically. The main constituents

0-8493-0266-9/00/$0.00+$.50
© 2000 by CRC Press LLC

of bone are mineral (hydroxyapatite, $\approx\frac{2}{3}$ dry weight, $\approx\frac{1}{2}$ volume), collagen ($\approx\frac{1}{3}$ dry weight, $\approx\frac{1}{2}$ volume), and water. At the whole bone or organ level, bone consists of a dense tissue (cortical bone) which forms a stiff, hollow shaft coupled to a porous, less dense tissue (trabecular bone) that is located adjacent to joint articulations and which acts to dissipate loads and absorb energy. Thus, from a histological point of view, bone can be considered a composite material at both the tissue and organ levels. Furthermore, since bone tissue is a living composite material, methods of preservation, sectioning, and mechanical fixation must also be considered in order to ensure that reliable test results are obtained.

In this chapter, basic specimen preparation, standard materials testing, and stress–strain measurement procedures are reviewed.

II. PRACTICAL CONSIDERATIONS

Bone tissue is part of a biological structure and its mechanical properties can only be fully appreciated if one understands how the structure functions as a whole. The "functional behavior" of bone is one of the most practical aspects that the investigator must consider prior to testing. When one starts to investigate the mechanical properties of bone, therefore, it is first necessary to determine what structural level or levels of organization should be investigated. Starting at the highest level of organization, forces acting on the whole body can be considered. At lower levels, whole-bone, macromechanical specimens machined from whole-bone, micromechanical test specimens, or single bone cells can be investigated.[5-11] To some extent, the specific interests of the investigator may determine the level of organization to be studied. Some investigations may require examination of the bone structure at several levels of organization.

Aging and disease processes produce significant changes in the composition, geometry, and architecture of bone, each of which is associated with alterations in the mechanical properties of bone and consequently the response of bone to loading. If the goal is to study the fracture risk of "old" bones compared with "young" bones, one could begin by testing the whole bone. Subsequently, one may find that the load required to break old bones is less than that required to fracture young bones, but at this stage of the investigation intrinsic differences in the geometry, material quality, and/or structural organization of the young vs. old bone tissue is unknown. Quantification of geometry (histomorphometry) such as cortex thickness and cortical area are easily performed on the bone specimens at this point, and subsequent statistical analyses may reveal a significant correlation, for example, between bone cortex thickness and age. Whole-bone structural properties, however, are dependent upon both geometric and material properties. Thus, consideration of geometry alone may not account for all the observed differences in the whole bone or structural strength of the bone samples. Additional tests on machined bone samples may become necessary to determine how aging and changing composition influence bone mechanical properties. Tests conducted on machined bone specimens reveal bone material properties (at least at the macrostructural level). On the other hand, if the objective of the study is to determine how bone tissue histology influences bone mechanical behavior, one could begin by preparing machined specimens from whole bones, and then quantify how the material properties of the specimens change with histology. At this point one may find a clear relationship between bone material properties and histology, but it may be difficult to predict how bone material comprised of different histological types behaves as a composite. An investigator studying bone must therefore consider the possibility that the answer to a specific research question might be found only by investigating the properties of bone at several organization levels.

In principle, mechanical testing of bone is straightforward. Experimental results, however, can be affected by specimen preparation and test methods used and by environmental conditions. In particular, loading rate, deformation rate, specimen size, specimen shape, mode of loading, and the method of gripping test specimens can influence the mechanical response of bone and engineering materials. Recognizing this, strict standards for testing engineering materials have been well established. In the case of bone, however, standardized engineering materials testing methods cannot always be utilized due to restrictions imposed by the finite size of the bone specimens, difficulties in gripping the specimens, and/or relatively low loads that can be applied to bone. Nevertheless, it is important to implement standards developed for testing engineering materials whenever possible. American Society for Testing and Materials (ASTM) designations for compressive testing (ASTM C469, D1621), tensile testing (ASTM C565, D1623, D3039, D3044, E8, and E132), and shear testing (ASTM D143) provide a source of mechanical testing techniques.[12-15] These can generally be applied to bone, although modifications to specimen size and method of gripping the test specimens may be necessary.

Of the ASTM mechanical test methods available, the tension test is the easiest to apply accurately both to cortical and to trabecular bone specimens. Trabecular bone specimens, with dimensions implemented by Linde,[16] Keller et al.,[17] Keaveny et al.,[18] have become standard. Trabecular bone specimens are more difficult to grip in tensile testing. Two methods that have been used successfully to grip dry trabecular bone tensile test specimens involve bonding the trabecular bone specimen to flat plates or inside brass tubing using epoxy or cyanoacrylate adhesive.[18,19] Stresses up to 500 kPa can be applied using cyanoacrylate.

The relationship between load applied to a structure and deformation in response to the load is called a load–deformation curve. The load–deformation curve can be divided into two regions: the elastic deformation region and the plastic deformation region. Within the elastic deformation region the structure imitates a spring — the geometric deformation in the structure increases linearly with increasing load and, after the load is released, the structure returns to its original shape. The slope of the elastic region of the load–deformation curve represents the extrinsic stiffness or rigidity of the structure. Larger structures will have greater rigidity than smaller structures of similar composition. Load and deformation can be converted to stress and strain by engineering formulae. The slope of the resulting stress–strain curve within the elastic region is called the modulus of elasticity or Young's modulus. Young's modulus is independent of specimen size and is therefore a measure of the intrinsic stiffness of the material.

$$\text{stiffness} = \text{force/deformation} \tag{11.1}$$

$$\text{elastic modulus} = \text{stress/strain} \tag{11.2}$$

The definition of stiffness for trabecular bone is more difficult. Trabecular bone is a two-phase, porous, composite structure consisting of individual trabeculae organized in a lattice structure and marrow made up of cells, fat, and vessels. Whereas individual trabeculae are relatively uniform, the lattice structure may exhibit a large degree of variability in terms of porosity, structural orientation, and connectivity.[20-24] Indeed, the bony elements of trabecular bone can be organized as open- and closed-cell rodlike or platelike lattice structures. Thus, trabecular bone forms a complex structure that has its own unique stiffness. Consequently, trabecular bone exhibits both an intrinsic or "material stiffness," which is the stiffness of an individual trabeculae and an extrinsic or "structural stiffness," which is the stiffness of the trabecular structure.[25-27] Most biomechanical studies of trabecular bone concentrate on structural properties because material properties of individual trabeculae are difficult to measure. Structural properties, however, can vary appreciably (several orders of magnitude) for different anatomical regions, and are closely dependent upon the density, distribution, and orientation of the trabeculae.

Analysis of load–deformation and stress–strain behavior in bone is further complicated by the fact that bones and other biological materials do not behave as a perfect spring. Rather, most biological materials exhibit nonlinear load–deformation and stress–strain behavior, which are further influenced by loading rate and temperature. Such behavior is termed *viscoelastic* and is the result of internal energy losses due to friction in the structure (intrinsic viscoelasticity) or fluid flow (fluid-dependent viscoelasticity) during deformation. Bone exhibits only a slight degree of viscoelasticity, and it is therefore reasonable to treat bone as a linear-elastic or springlike (Hookean) material. Alternatively, nonlinear stress analyses may be implemented and the stress–strain dependency on the applied stress can be quantified.

These simple examples and basic mechanical testing definitions are intended to point out that neither testing the whole bone nor testing of standardized bone specimens alone may prove a complete or practical answer to questions of how aging affects bone fracture risk. Summarizing these points, practical evaluation of whole or machined bone mechanical functionality should include considerations of the following:

- Specimen geometry;
- Effect of loading type;
- Effect of test conditions (hydration) and preparation;
- Directional properties of the bone tissue;
- Composite nature of bone tissue;
- Composition of bone tissue;
- Lattice structure of trabecular bone;
- Viscoelastic properties of bone tissue;
- Nonlinear load–deformation and stress–strain behavior.

These variables influence and govern the overall mechanical properties of bone.

III. SPECIMEN PREPARATION

A. PRESERVATION

Water (matrix) accounts for approximately 6% of the weight and 11% of the volume of hydrated bone. Thus, changes in water content have a significant effect on mechanical properties. Mechanical properties have been shown to vary significantly depending upon the storage and handling procedures used following removal of the tissue from the body. Changes on the order of 10% are not uncommon.[28-31] Any treatment of bone, which changes the nature or relative composition of these components, can influence mechanical behavior. Thus, drying, freezing, storage in saline or alcohol solutions, and embalming affect the properties of bone.[32,33] The properties of fresh tissue can vary in a short period of time if bone is allowed to dry. For example, bone specimens maintained at room temperature for 24 h without preservation will demonstrate about a 3% decline in Young's modulus.[34]

For optimal preservation of bone physical and mechanical properties, the following storage methods are recommended. For long-term storage, bone should be frozen and kept as moist and hydrated as possible. In order to minimize freeze-drying of the bone tissue, the surrounding musculature should be left intact, and a plastic wrap and bag should cover the musculature to further minimize freeze-drying and freezer burn. If the musculature and surrounding soft tissues must be removed before freezing, the bone tissue should be wrapped in gauze, soaked in normal saline, wrapped with plastic wrap, and placed in sealed, airtight plastic bags. The bone tissue should be placed in the freezer within 1 h after it has been harvested and stored at –20°C. Upon removal from the freezer and during all stages of tissue preparation, the bone should be kept hydrated in saline.

For time periods of up to 3 months, small specimens (including machined bone) may be preserved at room temperature in a solution of 50% saline and 50% alcohol, or in biostatic saline. Preservation of bone in an ethanol/saline solution results in minimal changes in the mechanical properties of bone. Ashman[35] found that keeping samples in 50% ethanol and 50% saline solutions for up to 90 days resulted in less than a 2% decline in Young's modulus. Sedlin and Hirsch[34] found ethanol to be somewhat less effective as a preservative. Bone samples stored in 40% ethanol for 5 to 10 days had a 2.5 to 4% decrease in Young's modulus. Bone specimens preserved in ethanol solution will lose some residual water, so it is important to soak them in an isotonic saline solution for several hours prior to testing, during which time the specimens should be refrigerated.

Bone test specimens can also be fixed in formalin or glutaraldehyde. Fixation in this manner increases collagen cross-linking and will, therefore, alter the properties of the bone tissue more significantly than alcohol preservation.[34,36] Sedlin and Hirsch[34] reported that embalmed bone exhibits different values of strength and elasticity compared with fresh tissue. Evans[37] reported a 68% increase in Young's modulus and ultimate tensile strength. McElhaney et al.[36] found a 1 to 9% decrease in tensile strength and a 12 to 18% decrease in the compressive strength of bovine bone. Although the results of these two studies are equivocal, both indicate that embalming dramatically alters the mechanical behavior of bone. Mechanical testing of formalin-fixed samples only provides data relative to other fixed samples, and results from individual samples will not provide an accurate measure of the true properties of bone. Whenever possible, therefore, bone tissue should be tested in an unembalmed state. Unquestionably, the best method of long-term preservation is to store saline-soaked, gauze-wrapped specimens in airtight bags or containers at −20°C. Embalmed tissue should be stored in a manner similar to unembalmed tissue.

B. Cutting and Machining of Bone

Cutting and machining of bone samples can be one of the most time-consuming steps in preparation of bone specimens for mechanical testing (Figure 11.1). Rough cuts can be made through bone with a band saw, hacksaw, or a jigsaw, but it can be difficult to keep the bone moist while cutting and when using a band saw it is easy to overheat and even burn the bone tissue. Damage due to overheating during rough-cutting procedures generally affects an area of bone only 1 to 2 mm from the cut. The affected area can be removed using wet sandpaper. Alternatively, finer cuts can be made using a diamond-impregnated wire saw or a low-speed diamond-impregnated wafering saw. Diamond wafering saws produce smooth parallel cuts and are particularly well suited for preparing rectangular test specimens or for creating coplanar surfaces in cylindrical specimens. Cylindrical specimens can be cored using a diamond-coring tool. When using a coring tool, the specimen and tool should be completely immersed in a water or saline bath. For more intricate machining a vertical end mill or lathe can be used. When milling or lathing cortical or trabecular bone, cutting rates similar to those suggested for aluminum should be used. Irrigation with water or saline is necessary to prevent overheating of the bone samples during the machining process. Specimen surfaces should be examined microscopically for cracks and other defects caused by machining, cutting, or sawing. Radiographs of machined and sectioned bone specimens can also be used to identify cracks and voids within the specimens.

C. Specimen Geometry

A key factor that needs to be considered when preparing bone samples for mechanical testing is specimen geometry. The most common specimen geometries are cubes with a side length between 6 and 8 mm or cylinders with a length-to-diameter (L/D) ratio between 1 and 2 and a diameter between 6 and 8 mm (Figure 11.2). The extremes of dimensions for cubic specimens reported in the literature are 4.5 mm[38] and 10 mm.[39] Cylindrical specimens with a L/D ratio between 2[40] and ¼[41] have been used with diameters ranging from 5 mm[42] to 20 mm,[41] and lengths ranging from 2.75 mm[40] to 12 mm.[43] Considerations of specimen geometry are particularly important for tests conducted on trabecular bone, which has been shown to be very susceptible to experimental artifacts during compression testing.[40,44-48]

In a recent study, Keaveny et al.[46] performed a theoretical analysis of the effect of friction (between the bone specimen and compression platen) and the damage artifact (structural end phenomenon associated with cut surfaces) on the experimental determination of Young's modulus. These investigators found that Young's modulus determinations were significantly underestimated for certain bone specimen geometries. They noted that a specimen with an aspect ratio of 2:1 was least sensitive to the combined effects of friction and the damage artifact on modulus underestimation.

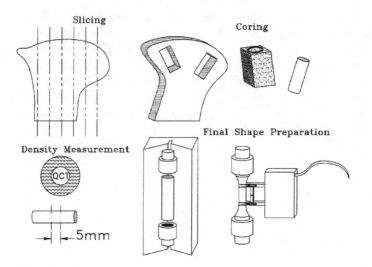

FIGURE 11.1 Trabecular bone specimen preparation for tensile or compressive mechanical testing. Steps include slicing of the bone section, X-raying of slices to avoid voids and precracks of specimens, cutting of cubic specimens with band saw and coring cylindrical specimens, density analysis using QCT, alignment of specimen in sockets, and final preparation of reduced diameter gauge section using a low-speed lathe.

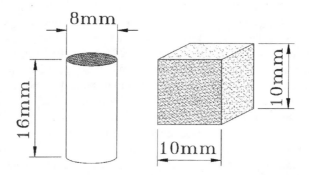

FIGURE 11.2 Geometric properties of test specimens commonly used in biomechanical testing.

They also argued against the use of cubic specimen geometry as a standard in biomechanical testing because cylinders can be made more easily and accurately than cubes, and because the surface-to-volume ratio is lower for cylinders than for cubes with the same aspect ratio (equal width). Both of these factors permit more accurate density measurements to be performed when using cylinders with a 2 : 1 aspect ratio. Furthermore, they found evidence that the correlation coefficient in the modulus–density regression increases as the aspect ratio increases, and noted that the 2 : 1 aspect ratio cylinder was superior to a cube in that respect. They also found more accurate (lower standard error of the estimate) predictions of modulus and strength could be made using 2 : 1 aspect ratio cylinders than with cubes of the same width. Experimental support for the theoretical analysis performed by Keaveny et al.[46] was provided from a study by Choi et al.[49] Zhu and associates[48] performed a comprehensive series of experiments on open-cell foams and human trabecular bone specimens and developed a surface damage theory to explain the modulus underestimation associated with the cut surface structural end phenomenon in porous materials such as trabecular bone. They recommended that the overall height of trabecular bone compression test specimens should be at least 10 mm. Linde et al.[40] also pointed out that the diameter of trabecular bone specimens should be large enough to satisfy continuum scale assumptions,[45,50,51] but at the same time should be small enough to ensure that specimen homogeneity was preserved.[52-54] Based on these and the aforementioned finding by

Keaveny and associates, a 5-mm-diameter, 2 : 1 aspect ratio cylindrical specimen with a specimen height of at least 10 mm would appear to be optimal for compression testing of human and bovine trabecular bone.

D. POTTING OF SPECIMENS IN BONE CEMENT

Bone specimens are often potted in cement (polymethylmethacrylate or PMMA) in order to obtain a reliable grip interface for the testing apparatus. However, some precautions should be taken when using potting procedures. First, removal of bone marrow and fat is essential for adequate bonding of PMMA to bone surfaces. Bone marrow and fat can be removed mechanically using a water jet or air jet or the fat can be removed chemically using a fat-dissolving detergent or alcohol or trichloroethylene. Usually, a combination of a mechanical and a chemical method provides the best results. The following is the suggested method for preparing bone specimens for potting:

- Clean the specimen mechanically with a high pressure water jet at the region to be cast.
- Defat the specimen at that particular region in trichlorethylene or 10% bleach + 90% water solution in an ultrasound bath for about 10 min.
- Air-dry the region to be cast using an air jet.

For small specimens and for low-force mechanical tests (e.g., nondestructive testing) the specimen can be potted immediately. For high-force mechanical tests (e.g., destructive testing) or testing of cortical bone samples with smooth surfaces, several layers of cyanoacrylate cement should be applied on the bone surface. Cyanoacrylate cement provides a stronger bond between the bone and the PMMA potting material. Specimens should be rehydrated immediately following the surface preparation and potting procedures in order to prevent any strength loss associated with preparation-related specimen dehydration.[55-57] In addition, the potting mold volume should not exceed three times the volume of the bone region that is embedded in bone cement. By using this rule of thumb, overheating of the specimen during the heat curing process of the PMMA ($\approx 60°C$) will be minimized. This also minimizes shrinkage of the potting mold. For bone tissue tests that include a bone–PMMA interface it may also be necessary to account for the material properties of PMMA. However, the authors are aware of only one study specifically conducted on bone–PMMA composite properties[58] and a similar study on planar reinforced plastic resin.[59]

IV. STANDARD MATERIALS TESTING METHODS

The strength of human cortical bone varies depending upon the kind of stress applied to the bone.[60] The ultimate tensile strength of femoral bone in the longitudinal direction is 135 MPa, the ultimate compressive strength is 205 MPa, and the shear strength is 67 MPa.[61] Like the Young's modulus, the strength of cortical bone also varies with direction. The tensile strength of the femur in the transverse direction is only 53 MPa, compared with 135 MPa in the longitudinal direction.[61] Tensile strength in trabecular bone can vary from 1 to over 20 MPa, and is strongly dependent upon apparent density and trabecular orientation.[39,48,62,63] The mechanical behavior of bone is also loading-rate and strain-rate dependent.[64-70]

A. GENERAL CONSIDERATIONS

In bone, like wood and many other biological structures, there is a "grain" or preferred direction associated with the structure. Consequently, the mechanical behavior of bone and other directional composites is dependent upon the direction of the applied load. Materials that have different properties in different directions are termed *anisotropic*, and as many as 21 independent elastic constants are required to characterize their mechanical behavior completely. Most materials have planes of symmetry that reduce the number of material constants. For example, materials having properties that differ in each of three mutually perpendicular directions are termed *orthotropic*, and nine elastic constants are required to characterize their mechanical behavior fully. Plexiform bone (e.g., bovine femur) is an example of a tissue with orthotropic material symmetry. Materials that have properties that are constant within a given plane are termed *transversely isotropic*. Human osteonal bone is an example of a transversely isotropic material because it has the same Young's modulus in all transverse directions, but has a higher Young's modulus in the longitudinal direction.[61,71-76] Materials that have the same elastic properties in all directions have the highest order of symmetry and are termed *isotropic*.

Complete characterization of the mechanical behavior of anisotropic material properties requires mechanical testing to be performed in several different orientations. For example, to determine the nine independent elastic coefficients of an orthotropic material the following mechanical tests are required:[73,77-79]

1. Tensile or compressive tests in each of three mutually perpendicular material directions;
2. Three lateral deflection tests to obtain Poisson's ratios; and
3. Three torsion tests to obtain shear moduli.

Ideally, mechanical test specimens should be oriented relative to the axes of material symmetry. In the case of cortical bone, the mutually perpendicular axes of material symmetry are generally one axis oriented parallel to the long axis of the bone, another oriented radially outward from the center, and the third oriented in a circumferential direction. In order to assure that specimens are cut in the proper orientation, the axes of material symmetry must be determined prior to testing, and are typically defined based upon histology. Loads applied in tension, compression, torsion, shear, and in combined modes on specimens cut in many different orientations are necessary to describe the anisotropic failure surface completely.[80-82] Table 11.1 summarizes the orthotropic and transversely isotropic material properties that have been reported for the human femur and tibia, respectively.

TABLE 11.1
Engineering Elastic Constants for Human Bone

	Femur[a]	Tibia[b]
E_1 (GPa)	11.5	6.91
E_2 (GPa)	11.5	8.51
E_3 (GPa)	17.0	18.4
G_{12} (GPa)	3.6	2.41
G_{31} (GPa)	3.28	3.56
G_{23} (GPa)	3.28	4.91
$?_{12}$	0.58	0.49
$?_{13}$	0.31	0.12
$?_{23}$	0.31	0.14
$?_{21}$	0.58	0.62
$?_{31}$	0.46	0.32
$?_{32}$	0.46	0.31

[a] Reilly, S.B., Burstein, A.H., Frankel, V.H., The elastic modulus of bone, *J. Biomech.*, 7, 271, 1974.

[b] Obrazcov, I., Adamovich, I., Burer, A., Knets, I. et al., *The Problems of Strength in Biomechanics*, Vishaya Shkola Publ. House, Moscow, 1988 (in Russian).

Several standards from the ASTM have been adapted for mechanical testing procedures on biological tissue.[84-90] The specimen shape most widely used in testing bone tissue is the so-called dog bone specimen, and the end portions of these specimens are enlarged diameter regions where the specimen will be attached to the testing apparatus. The test region or gauge section consists of a turned-down section of decreased cross-sectional area, and ideally it is in this region that the specimen should fail. If the specimen fails outside of the gauge region or near the edge of the gauge region, this is an indication that alignment errors or other interface artifacts caused premature failure of the specimen. The ultimate strength of the material being tested is underestimated when this occurs.

During mechanical testing of biological tissues, the test specimen should be saturated with saline, particularly during long-term fatigue tests.

B. Tensile Testing

Tensile testing can be one of the most accurate methods for measuring bone properties, but bone specimens must be relatively large and should be carefully machined. Tensile test specimens for cortical bone and cancellous bone are illustrated in Figures 11.3 and 11.4.

Dimensions are derived from ASTM standards. In Figure 11.3, the ratio d/D should be around ½ and the parallel length of the narrow section should be at least three times the size of the gauge diameter d. The radius of curvature R should be very large to avoid stress concentrations and should have the same dimensions as the parallel length A. The grip length M is one quarter of the whole specimen length L. Because of the relatively homogeneous microstructure of cortical bone, cortical bone specimens can be made comparatively small in size (gauge diameter = $d \approx 3$ mm).

In principle, the same geometry used for cortical bone tensile test specimens applies to trabecular bone.[91] However, because of the intrinsic lattice and inhomogeneous structure of trabecular bone, a minimum gauge diameter of 5 mm is required to ensure that continuum scale criteria are met.

Tensile test specimens are designed so that the highest strains will occur in the central portion or gauge region of the specimen. Strain measurements can be obtained by attaching a clip-on extensometer to the gauge section of the specimen (refer to Figure 11.1). Stress is calculated as the applied force divided by the bone cross-sectional area measured in the specimen midsection. Assuming that

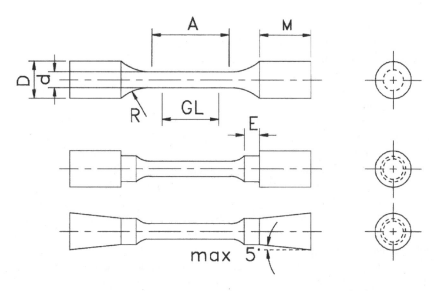

FIGURE 11.3 Tensile test specimen geometry for cortical bone tests. A = parallel length, GL = gauge length, M = grip length, E = neck length, R = curvature radius, D = specimen outer diameter, d = specimen gauge diameter.

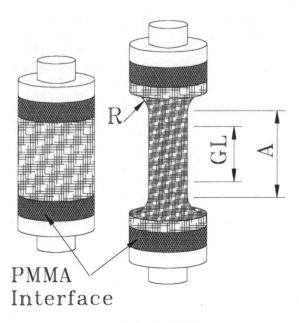

FIGURE 11.4   Tensile test specimen geometry for trabecular bone tests.

the force is applied without inducing a coupled bending moment, a tensile test will provide a very accurate measurement of the bone mechanical properties. A technical concern associated with tension testing is bending imposed on the specimen. Incorporating pivoting elements in the loading chain typically reduces bending. Attaching universal joints onto the sockets or self-aligning socket holders can accommodate eccentricities that may be present during specimen mounting and will therefore minimize bending artifacts. To correct for residual bending, four stress–strain tests should be run with the extensometer placed on each of the four sides of the specimen. The four moduli are then averaged. If strain is only measured in a single plane, bending can significantly affect the measured modulus.[92]

The elastic portion of the stress–strain curve is characterized by a straight line (Hooke's law) and the slope of this line, or the ratio of stress–strain within the elastic range, is defined as the modulus of elasticity E (Young's modulus). As the stress is increased, a point is reached where a further increase in stress will show a departure of the curve from the straight line. The greatest stress intensity for which stress is still proportional to strain is called the *proportional-elastic limit* (indicated by PEL in Figure 11.5). This is not strictly the same as the elastic limit. The *elastic limit* is defined as the greatest stress that can be applied without leaving a permanent deformation upon complete release of the load. To determine the elastic limit, it is necessary to load and unload the specimen with increasing values of the load until a permanent set is found after complete unloading. Since this procedure is time-consuming and since the elastic limit differs little from the proportional limit, the true elastic limit is seldom obtained in actual practice.

If the stress is increased further from the proportional limit, the stress–strain curve departs more and more from the straight line. Unloading the specimen at point A (Figure 11.5), the portion AB is linear and is essentially parallel to the original line OC. The horizontal distance OB is the plastic deformation corresponding to the stress at A. This is the basis for the construction of the arbitrary (offset) yield strength. To determine the offset yield strength, a straight line AB is drawn parallel to the initial elastic line OC but is displaced from it by an arbitrary value of permanent strain. The permanent strain most commonly used is 0.2% of the original gauge length. When reporting the yield strength, the permanent strain value should be specified. The arbitrary yield strength is typically used for those materials that do not exhibit a natural yield point, but is not necessarily limited to such materials. For analysis of brittle materials like cortical bone, one may need to choose a permanent strain value lower than 0.2%, since cortical bone typically has a relatively low failure strain (<3%).

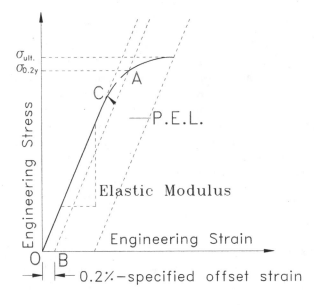

FIGURE 11.5 Typical stress–strain curve for tensile test.

The actual yield point in a stress–strain curve has been defined as the stress for which a marked increase in strain occurs without a corresponding increase in stress. In such materials both an upper and a lower yield point are usually identified. Following initial yielding, the stress drops and the curve remains approximately horizontal for a period of deformation before it begins to rise again. The upper yield point (σ_{ypH}) is the stress level at which the initial drop occurs. The lower yield point (σ_{ypL}) is taken as the lowest value of stress after the initial drop-off and before the load begins to rise continuously or, more properly, as the average stress during this interval (Figure 11.6). ASTM standards E6-36 specify that the term *yield point* should not be used in connection with

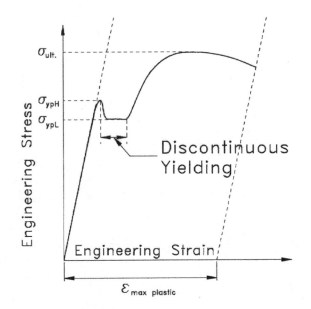

FIGURE 11.6 Typical stress–strain curve with visible yielding.

materials where the stress–strain diagram does not become horizontal or does not show an actual drop of stress with increasing strain in the yield region.

Upon further deformation, the load reaches a maximum value and then drops somewhat before fracture occurs. The tensile strength (ultimate tensile stress) is obtained by dividing the maximum load during the test by the original cross-sectional area. A measure of the ductility of a material after fracture is given by the percent elongation and also by the reduction of cross-sectional area. Percent elongation after fracture is determined by dividing the change in the original gauge length by the original gauge length (multiplied by 100%). The original gauge length should always be stated in reporting the percent elongation values. The percent reduction of area after fracture is the ratio of the change in the original area determined at the smallest cross section divided by the original area of cross section (multiplied by 100%).

As discussed earlier, there is a difference between intrinsic stiffness and extrinsic stiffness (rigidity). For a tensile test of bone the intrinsic stiffness is equal to the Young's modulus (E), while the extrinsic stiffness is equal to EAL, where A is the cross-sectional area of the specimen and L is the gauge length of the specimen. The extrinsic stiffness is dependent not only upon elasticity, but also on specimen size. In the case of trabecular bone the specimen must be large enough that the trabecular structure can be treated as a continuum. A specimen width of at least 4 to 8 mm is recommended for trabecular bone specimens.[51,93-96]

C. COMPRESSION TESTING

Compression testing of bone specimens is a popular technique, especially for cortical bone because relatively small specimens can be used. Compressive tests, however, tend to be less accurate than tensile tests due to friction and compression-platen end effects imposed on the bone specimen during the test. Friction at the load platen–bone surface interface can be minimized using polished stainless steel platens lubricated with a coating of lightweight machine oil. A surface roughness of 2 μm cm^{-1} is recommended.[48] If the load faces of the bone specimen are slightly misaligned with respect to the compression loading platen, then large stress concentrations can occur, resulting in 18618an underestimation of both Young's modulus and compressive strength. Placement of a pivoting platen in the load train reduces misalignment error (Figure 11.7). By using a micrometer, the parallelism of the load-contacting surfaces of each specimen can be assessed by measuring the height differences between each of the four sides and a central point of the load-contacting surfaces. Four height differences, recorded by assigning a value of zero to the lowest point among the five points, can be utilized to determine the parallelism index.[48]

$$I = G \left(D_{max} + D_{max} - D_1 + D_{max} - D_2 + D_{max} - D_3 \right)$$

$$I = D_{max} - G \left(D_1 + D_2 + D_3 \right) \tag{11.3}$$

where D_{max} is the maximum height difference, D_1, D_2, and D_3 are the other height differences ranging from 0 to D_{max}, and the factor ¼ is used to obtain an averaged nominal height difference. This index considers both the absolute differences between each point and zero reference point, and the relative difference between individual points. The higher the index, the greater the irregularity of the surface plane. This index may be normalized by the linear dimension of a cross-sectional area of a sample (width or diameter) to indicate a nominal flatness of a contacting surface.

Another problem associated with compressive testing of trabecular bone is the previously noted end effect created by cutting or machining the faces of trabecular bone test specimens.[53] At the boundary where the specimen contacts the loading platen, the cut surfaces of the trabeculae lattice are unsupported, and the strain tends to be much greater in the boundary region than in the middle of the specimen.[48] Elevated strains at the ends of the specimen result in an overestimation of the average specimen strain and concomitant underestimation of modulus. Thus, simple strain calcu-

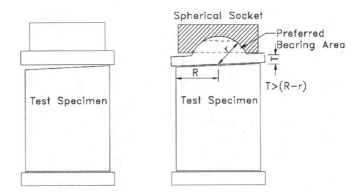

FIGURE 11.7   Spherical socket used to compensation for nonparallel load-bearing surfaces during compression testing.

lations tend to be inaccurate. More accurate specimen strain measurements can be obtained by directly measuring the local strain at the midsection of the specimen. Mechanical or optical extensometers can be used for local strain measurements in trabecular bone.

Although it is considerably more difficult to achieve accurate results using a compressive test compared with a tensile test, the compressive test has several advantages. First, compression test specimens need not be as large as tensile specimens, which is a major advantage when testing trabecular bone. Second, fabrication of compressive specimens is not as difficult as fabrication of tensile test specimens. Finally, in some regions of the skeleton (e.g., the vertebrae) compressive tests may more closely mimic the *in vivo* loading conditions to which the bone is exposed. Even with measurement error, compression tests are often very precise, particularly if one is simply interested in comparing data from experimental and control groups (assuming the measurement error did not change as a result of the treatment).

In a compression test, most ductile materials have stress–strain responses that are very similar to tensile stress–strain responses during the initial phases of testing. As the area of cross section increases (due to the Poisson effect), however, the stress–strain curve usually shows a gradual increase in slope, and does not exhibit the plastic deformation which is characteristic of the tension test. In addition, the compressive stress–strain curve does not necessarily reach an analytic maximum as in the case of tension, and unless shearing, splitting, or crumbling occurs there may not be any overt fracture.

Consequently, no definite compressive strength may be noted and compressive strength has no real meaning in such cases. Rather, porous composites and porous bone specimens will exhibit a crushing phenomenon associated with progressive pore collapse and stabilization (Figure 11.8). In this case failure is generally defined as the point at which pore collapse is first observed (typically the point at which the initial drop in load is observed). Fracture under compression does not occur in ductile materials since the material merely flows laterally as the height is decreasing. Thus, the definition of compressive strength depends upon the degree of distortion that is regarded as indicating failure of the material. In fact, many plastic materials will continue to deform in compression until a flat disk is produced. In such cases, the compressive stress (nominal) rises steadily without any well-defined fracture occurring. Fracture is usually of the shear type with sliding along inclined planes starting at the surface on which the pressure is applied. Low ductility or brittle materials may not necessarily have well-defined yield points, but do exhibit definite fail points, since they fail in compression by a shattering type of fracture. Fracture of brittle material depends upon

1. the ratio of height to lateral dimension (aspect ratio),
2. friction between the compression platens and the specimen, and
3. the shape of the specimen.

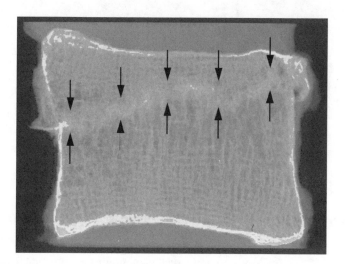

FIGURE 11.8   Fracture line on a 10-mm thick vertebral body section.

D. Fatigue Testing

Fatigue refers to the failure of materials under the action of repeated stresses. Fatigue is the result of slip occurring along certain crystallographic directions accompanied by local crystal fragmentation rupturing the atomic bonds, culminating in the formation of submicroscopic cracks, which soon become visible cracks.[98-104]

Standard testing methods are important since fatigue susceptibility of a material is dependent on specimen shape, size, and cyclic rate. Standard fatigue testing techniques have been established for engineering materials (ASTM C394, D671, D3166, and E206), but because of the size limitations, standard fatigue testing methods must be modified for bone material. In fatigue testing, the test specimen is subjected to periodically varying stresses by means of mechanical devices. The applied stresses may alternate between equal positive and negative values (fully reversed cyclic fatigue tests), from zero to maximum positive or negative values, or between unequal positive and negative values. Cyclic fatigue testing has been applied to both cortical and trabecular bone in fluctuating axial tension (0 to Tension), completely reversed axial loading (Compression to Tension), fluctuating bending (0 to Moment), and completely reversed bending (–Moment to +Moment).[41,62,101,105,106]

A series of fatigue tests is usually made on a number of specimens of the material at different stress levels.[107] The stress level endured is then plotted against the number of cycles sustained, and the resulting diagram is called the stress-cycle diagram or S–N diagram (Figure 11.9). From S–N curves, it is possible to predict fatigue failure at a particular stress level. By choosing lower and lower stresses, a value may be found which will not produce failure, regardless of the number of applied cycles. This stress value is called the endurance limit. The endurance limit may be established for most materials between 2 and 10 million cycles. Surface defects such as scratches or notches as well as surface roughness will reduce the fatigue strength of a specimen. In general, fatigue specimens are prepared with a turned-down or gauge section to ensure fracture will occur in the gauge region. Fatigue testing, more so than static mechanical testing, is dependent on specimen shape. The radius of curvature of the neck portion of the specimen and surface finish are critical factors influencing the fatigue life of the specimen.

As in single cycle, uniaxial, tensile, and compression mechanical testing, fatigue test results are strain-rate dependent. Cyclic loading frequencies from 2 to 125 Hz have been used to characterize the fatigue behavior of cortical bone.[41,62,101,106,108] Lafferty and Raju[106] presented corrections for the effects of cyclic rates on fatigue life. Load or deflections can be applied to the fatigue specimens, although the preferred method is to apply constant loads. Failure under load-control

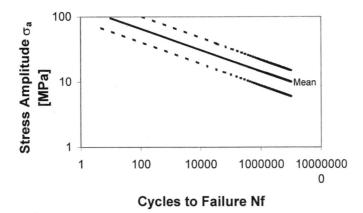

FIGURE 11.9 Comparison of stress amplitude vs. cycles to failure in fatigue study. Both axes are logarithmic scale.

fatigue testing occurs as a distinct fracture. Specimens subjected to controlled deflection fail in a more gradual manner due to relief of stress (stress relaxation) and decreased stiffness. Failure under controlled deflection or strain is often defined as the point at which stress has been reduced to 70% of its original value.[64,101]

E. TESTING WHOLE-BONE SPECIMENS

Performing tensile, compressive, or torsion tests on whole-bone specimens has the added difficulty of attaching the specimen to the testing machine. Whole-bone mechanical test specimens do not have a nice prismatic or symmetrical shape like the machined test specimens used for the standardized tensile, compression, and shear tests discussed in the previous section. Thus, special fixtures and casting procedures are required (Figure 11.10).[109] The cast should be symmetrical to allow easy attachment to the testing apparatus. Bone cement or epoxy resin is generally preferred as the casting material, and commonly used materials include methylmethacrylate and plastic padding (Figure 11.11).

In some cases an intact bone structure such as the vertebral motion segment (two vertebral bodies and the intervertebral disk) are placed between two compression platens and no casting material is used.[112-117] In such cases, a rough surface finish on the platens is used to prevent slipping during the compression test. However, such procedures may lead to asymmetrical loading of the specimen and can contribute to measurement error, typically seen as underestimation of the stiffness of the vertebral body.

For whole-bone mechanical test specimens the most common method of strain determination is measurement of the crosshead displacement. However, it is also possible to attach strain-measuring devices (strain gauges or extensometers) directly to the specimen,[111] or one can perform noncontact strain measurements using an optical motion analysis system.[118-120] Optical systems, based on measuring the translation of points on the surface by image analysis, have shown increasing success in accurately determining the mechanical properties of bone. By using CCD-cameras, the resolution of the optical system can be better than 0.01% of the field of view (FOV) provided that there is good contrast between the specimen and targets. The targets captured by the camera can be passive reflective markers, active markers (light emitting diodes or LEDs), or ink lines drawn by the test specimen. By using reflective markers it is possible to create an array of targets, which can be used to measure surface deflections in the direction of loading as well as in directions normal to the loading axis. With two cameras, laser tracking systems or magnetic field-based devices, three-dimensional data of an area of interest can be recorded and analyzed. Bonded strain gauges and acoustic measurement devices can also be used to quantify whole-bone deformation,[121,122] and are described later in this chapter.

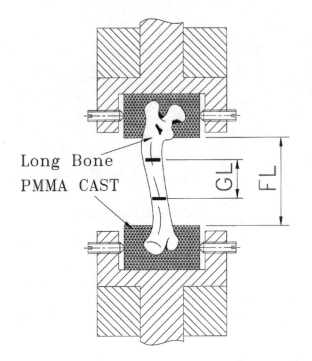

FIGURE 11.10   Mounted rodent whole-bone test specimen.[110,111] FL = free length, GL = arbitrary chosen gauge length.

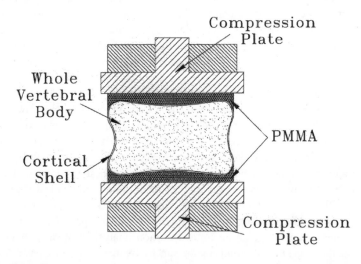

FIGURE 11.11   Whole vertebral body prepared for compression testing.

V. EQUIPMENT

Machines and apparatus for the mechanical testing of materials usually contain the following elements: (1) specimen gripping mechanism; (2) specimen loading mechanism; and (3) load measurement transducer. Some machines include an integrated apparatus for measurement of both load and deformation, while others may rely on an auxiliary apparatus to record the specimen deformation (e.g., extensometer, strain gauge). Testing machines can be screw driven, pneumatic, or hydraulic. More sophisticated testing apparatus tends to be servo-controlled. Servo-based testing machines can apply loads or deflections to bone specimens at a variety of different rates and magnitudes under feedback control. In most general-purpose mechanical testing systems, deformation can be controlled as the independent variable and the resulting load measured. In other systems, particularly those intended for use with low loads, the load is controlled and the resulting deformation is measured. Special features of general-purpose test systems are capabilities for constant rate of loading, constant strain rate, constant load, constant deformation, and cyclical loading (fatigue).

One of the simplest ways to control loading during mechanical testing is by crosshead position or stroke-control feedback. In stroke-control feedback, the crosshead motion is controlled at a fixed speed or constant displacement (strain) rate. For high-stiffness test specimens, however, motion of the crosshead is very small and it is very easy to break the specimen prematurely. Use of load-control feedback from a load cell attached in the load chain provides more precise control. In the load-control method, a load time history profile is programmed into the load-feedback loop and crosshead position is adjusted to provide the programmed load profile. Stress rate (Pa/s), rather than strain rate (ε/s), is controlled in a load-feedback test setup, and the actual strain rate is dependent on the modulus (Pa) of the test material:

$$\text{strain rate} = \text{stress rate/modulus} \tag{11.4}$$

The choice of strain rate depends on the nature of the investigation, but for studies of normal bone activity the strain rate should be selected to lie in the physiological range, i.e., 0.002 to 0.01/s (0.2 to 1% ε/s).[106] To simulate trauma and impact failure, strain rates of 0.1 to 1.0/s (10 to 100% ε/s) can be employed,[41,62] but higher strain rates may be limited by the functional capacity of the mechanical test apparatus. For most materials, an increased strain rate will result in an increase in the stress necessary to produce a given strain. Ordinarily, variations in strain rate of 10 to 1 or lower produce quite small changes in the measured stress. However, very large changes in the measured stress may occur when testing at impact-level strain rates of 100% or higher. This effect is known as hydraulic strengthening (HS) and is a fluid-flow phenomenon associated with viscoelastic materials such as bone tissue.[69] Strain rate effects on the apparent elastic modulus E_{app} can be accounted for by multiplying the true or specific modulus E_s by the apparent density/specific density ratio expressed as a power function of strain rate $f(\dot{\varepsilon})$:[69]

$$E_{app} = E_s \left(\frac{\rho_{app}}{\rho_s} \right)^{f(\dot{\varepsilon})} \tag{11.5}$$

For small ranges of strain rate, the strain rate power function exponent, $f(\dot{\varepsilon}) = 0.06$, obtained by Carter and Hayes[41,62] can be used to predict the apparent modulus:

$$E_{app} \propto \dot{\varepsilon}^{0.06} \tag{11.6}$$

Most mechanical testing machines are equipped with a load cell for detecting the applied load and a transducer for measuring the displacement of the crosshead. The crosshead displacement provides a measurement from which strain in the specimen can be calculated. Crosshead displacement measurements, however, are often inaccurate because inhomogeneous strains may be present within the specimen. In addition, crosshead displacement measurements include the deformation associated with the crosshead fixture, load cell fixture, and specimen grip fixtures. Consequently, more accurate strain measurement methods are obtained by attaching resistance strain gauges or extensometers directly to the specimen. Extensometers and strain gauges change electrical resistance when deformed. A Wheatstone bridge type of amplifier is generally used with these transducers to provide a precise voltage output for very small displacement and strain changes. Stress and strain can be recorded by connecting the readout channel from the testing machine, load cell, or strain measurement device to an *x–y* plotter, strip chart recorder, or a data acquisition system attached to a computer. Load and displacement output must be converted to stress and strain using

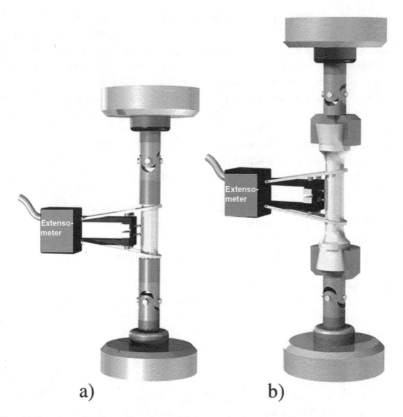

Figure 11.12   (a) Specimen holder with universal joints on both ends; (b) same as (a), however, with tapered specimen in a conic holder. The conic holder is made out of two halves connected with screws or clamps perpendicular to the loading direction.

appropriate formulae. Once the data are stored on computer, data analysis software is used to determine mechanical properties (Young's modulus, strength, yield stress, toughness, etc.).

Machine test grips are used to hold the specimen. Ideally, the test grips should not only hold the test specimen without slipping, but should also apply the load in the desired manner (pure tension, compression, and shear). In compression, centering of the load is important, and should not be neglected in tension testing if the material is brittle. Errors of up to 25% in strength prediction can result from misalignment during compression testing.[79] Swiveling (ball-and-socket, or pivoting) holders or compression blocks should be used for compression testing of all but very ductile materials, and rough surfaces should be smoothed or capped. In tensile tests, serrated wedge-type grips may be used to hold the shanks of ductile materials. A tapered specimen in a conical holder provides good protection against slipping and protects the specimen from grip damage. A taper of 1 in 6 on the wedge faces gives a self-tightening action without excessive jamming (Figure 11.12).

As noted previously, environmental testing conditions play a significant role during mechanical testing. Differences of up to 10% in material properties can result from changes in temperature and humidity alone (see previous section and References 123 and 124).

VI. MEASUREMENT PROCEDURES

A. COMPLIANCE AND VALIDATION

If a direct measurement of strain is too difficult (e.g., the specimens are too short for the application of extensometers or unsuitable for strain gauges), then the strain must be determined from the crosshead position measurements. When crosshead position measurements are used to determine strain, the compliance (1/stiffness) of the load frame, including the load cell and loading platens, must be considered. Standard specimens of steel, aluminum, and acrylic can be used to calibrate the stiffness of the system. Load frame stiffness can also be determined directly by loading the system without a specimen. The compliance-corrected (deflection/load) stiffness response of the bone test specimen, k_{bone}, is obtained from

$$1/k_{bone} = 1/k_{total} - 1/k_{machine} \qquad (11.7)$$

where k_{total} is the measured stiffness of the bone and machine, and $1/k_{machine}$ is the compliance of the machine (load cell, loading platens, load frame). Note that Equation 11.7 assumes that the load frame and bone specimen are a system of serially connected springs. With small testing machines, however, the stiffness of the bone specimen may be greater than that of the load frame, whereas for large testing machines the opposite is the usual case. In general, the compliance of the ideal testing apparatus should be 10^{-5} mm/N or better.

Standard materials should be used whenever possible to ensure experimental measurements are reliable and accurate. After a particular test procedure has been selected, the procedure should be verified using several standardized specimens. Plastics (e.g., Plexiglas) have a similar modulus to that of cortical bone and therefore make good materials standards for cortical bone. By using materials standards, the measurements derived from a given experimental method can be easily checked since the mechanical properties of a specific plastic are readily available from the manufacturer. Plastic standards are not only useful for machined bone specimens, but can also be used to calibrate whole-bone tests. In the case of whole bone, specimens that approximate the bone dimensions are useful to verify that there are no potential errors associated with the test apparatus or data reduction procedures. For example, when validating a simple compression test experiment on Plexiglas, Turner and Burr[125] found that the test procedure resulted in an underestimation of the Young's modulus of Plexiglas by 30% compared with the manufacturer's data sheet. They found that the addition of a pivoting platen to the load train corrected this error.

B. PRECISION AND ACCURACY

Precision (or reproducibility) and accuracy are two very different terms. *Precision* describes the variation in the determination of a property associated with a specific method, whereas *accuracy* describes the ability of the method to estimate the true value of a measurement procedure. Precision and accuracy are not necessarily related. For example, the precision of a method can be very good, but the accuracy of the same method may be very poor, or vice versa. Increasing the number of repeated measurements generally increases the precision, and is a simple addendum to nondestructive testing techniques.[126]

Precision derived from the yield point and the failure point during mechanical testing to failure cannot be assessed due to the singular nature of such test. Precision measurements derived from nondestructive tests, however, can easily be assessed by repeated measurements. For example, the precision of the stiffness and nondestructive energy absorption properties of bone have been determined in a number of studies.[40,127-131] These studies found that the precision of a series of repeated measurements was best when the specimens were not removed from the test machine between measurements. In addition, the precision of stiffness measurements was improved (smaller standard deviation) when the stiffness measurements were determined as the average stiffness of five consecutive test cycles as opposed to a single test. Furthermore, the stiffness precision was improved when measurements were performed after a number of conditioning cycles in comparison with tests conducted without conditioning.[73,132] Moreover, precision of stiffness and elastic energy storage was also better for larger specimens than for smaller bone specimens, whereas energy dissipation did not exhibit such a dependency. Viscoelastic energy dissipation measurements, however, are generally less precise than the stiffness and elastic energy storage.[133] A number of investigators have also examined the effects of the testing order in orthogonal tests on the precision of mechanical property measurements. Test order was not found to affect the precision.[40,127,129,131]

The measurement precision of load cell and deformation measurement devices is usually very good (0.3% of full scale). However, there are a number of factors that may reduce the precision of load and displacement measurements, including

- Misalignment of test columns;
- Placement of the specimen away from the centroidal axis;
- Nonparallel specimen ends;
- Nonhomogeneity of the specimen.

These factors tend to push the test columns farther away from the central axis of the test specimen. A compliant (sensitive) load cell and/or long testing column will amplify such a tendency. Other factors that can reduce measurement precision include changes in specimen hydration and temperature, the state of mechanical conditioning, or structural changes produced during a previous testing session.[123]

Factors affecting the accuracy of mechanical property measurements are usually related to the test machine, the bone specimen, and/or the interface between the grip or platen and the specimen. Although the stiffness of commercial test machines ($>10^5$ N/mm) is usually much larger than the stiffness of the bone sample, some deformation occurs in the load cell. Consequently, when using crosshead displacement measurements, it is easy to overestimate both the axial deformation of the bone specimen as well as the strain rate of the test. If necessary, mechanical properties (strength, stiffness) can be adjusted using power function relationships established between mechanical properties and strain rate.[41,62,134] Errors in mechanical property measurements that are due to an overestimation of strain rate, however, are generally very small in comparison to errors caused by over-estimation of axial deformation. As noted previously, specimen preparation can have a significant effect on the accuracy in determining the mechanical properties of bone. In particular, embalming is known to significantly and variably effect bone mechanical properties and should be avoided if possible.

Another problem that occurs primarily in screw driven test machines is a variable tendency to produce small "loops" at the bottom and top of the load–deformation curve during cyclic loading. This phenomenon would seem to indicate that the system is producing energy rather than dissipating energy. However, these small load–deformation loops are most likely caused by a slight tilting of the crosshead produced by asynchronous activation of the screw drives responsible for moving the crosshead. This generally occurs because the up/down (tension/compression) screw mechanism is from a single belt attached to the motor of the test machine. This phenomenon is often a major factor affecting the reproducibility of the test data, because repositioning of specimens that are not absolutely homogeneous or that have slightly nonparallel end plates may create slight changes in the mechanical test axis.

Retaining marrow *in situ* may be important in preventing water loss from the trabecular tissue lattice during storage and testing.[28,62,77,135] If marrow must be extracted, the specimens should be rehydrated prior to mechanical testing. Nevertheless, the properties of rehydrated trabecular bone may differ from trabecular bone tested with marrow *in situ*. Carter and Hayes[62] analyzed the dependence of mechanical properties on apparent density and strain rate using specimens allocated to either testing with marrow or testing without marrow. They found a variable effect of marrow on the strength and stiffness of the trabecular bone samples depending on the strain rate used to test the specimens. Trabecular bone strength and stiffness were higher in specimens tested with marrow in comparison with specimens tested without marrow at strain rates of 10 s^{-1}, but not at strain rates of 1 s^{-1} and lower. Experimental differences associated with the high strain rate tests may be due to the hydraulic strengthening effect.[68,69,136-138]

In uniaxial compression tests it is generally assumed that grip stresses are constant and that there is no friction between the surface of the test grip and the specimen. This is only true if the specimen is homogeneous and if the test column grips produce a constant stress on the specimen during loading. Ordinarily, however, the grip stresses will vary as the specimen dimensions change. When this occurs, the general effect is an uneven stress distribution at the specimen–platen interface, which in turn causes a triaxial stress field in the specimen.[139] The effect of a triaxial stress field was studied by Filon,[140] who analyzed the stress distribution in a cylindrical homogeneous specimen subjected to compression, tension, and shear. This investigator found that the central regions of the specimen were subjected to lower strains in comparison with regions near the specimen end. Such axial strain nonhomogeneity leads to an overestimation of Young's modulus. To investigate this phenomenon, Brown and Ferguson[141] performed a finite-element analysis of a cubic specimen, and found that Young's modulus was overestimated by about 5%. Odgaard and Linde[142] performed a similar finite-element analysis on a homogeneous, isotropic cube where the interface was held rigid, and no deformation in the test column was allowed. Using a Poisson's ratio of 0.22, which was considered realistic for trabecular bone, these authors found a 3% overestimation of Young's modulus. A recent study by Keaveny et al.[46] indicates that such modulus overestimations are highly dependent on the Poisson's ratio of the specimen.

The effect of friction at the interface between specimen and test column was investigated experimentally by Linde and Hvid.[130] These authors compared compressive mechanical properties derived from nondestructive testing of trabecular bone specimens between ordinary steel columns, steel columns with polished ends, and steel columns with polished ends lubricated with mineral oil. The compressive stiffness was reduced by 5% when polished steel columns were used in comparison with unpolished columns. When polished steel columns lubricated with mineral oil were used, the compressive stiffness was reduced 7% compared with the stiffness obtained using ordinary steel columns without oil as lubricant. Corresponding reductions were also found for viscoelastic energy dissipation. Their differences are of the same order of magnitude as the results obtained by finite-element analysis.[141,142] Thus, frictional effects on the mechanical behavior of bone can be appreciable. Indeed, if the bone surface is fully constrained from sliding by gluing the specimen with PMMA, then there is a 40% increase in stiffness compared with testing between ordinary steel columns without oil.[130] Differences in stiffness obtained between a system with a rigid interface and a system with minimal interface friction is even greater (nearly 50%)!

In another recent study, Allard and Ashman[143] made simultaneous compressive strain measurement using both crosshead deflection and extensometer measurements at the central region of cubic bone specimens. They found that the compressive stiffness derived from the central region of the bone specimen was considerably larger than that derived from the total deflection. This finding is well explained by the cut surface or structural end phenomenon of the specimen as described by Zhu et al.[48] As a result of the structural end phenomenon, axial compressive strain measurements based upon crosshead deflection measurements will always be overestimated to a certain extent, and the magnitude of this overestimation is inversely related to the specimen length.[40,48] Specimens with embedded ends for tensile testing, however, are not expected to be affected by the structural end phenomenon and will accordingly be expected to have a larger stiffness and smaller ultimate strain than specimens that are not so constrained at the grip interface.[144-146]

One of the most important factors influencing mechanical test measurement accuracy is related to errors in the strain measurement. The net underestimation of stiffness resulting from interface phenomena (including overestimation caused by friction and structural end effects) has been estimated to be 20 to 40% in specimens with a length of 7 to 7.5 mm,[131,142] and about 40% in 15-mm-long specimens with a 3:1 aspect ratio.[46] Stiffness overestimation is expected to be larger in shorter specimens and smaller in longer specimens.[40,48] In addition, since the axial stress distribution is heterogeneous in bone specimens with or without embedded ends, tests based upon local strain measurements (extensometers, strain gauges, and optical targets) may be the only reliable way to obtain accurate results. For local strain measurements, it is advisable to obtain specimen strain measurements from several sides of the specimen in order to take into account any bending that is imposed on the specimen.[35] Ignoring structural end phenomena, it should also be noted that the stiffness determined is not necessarily the true or intrinsic material stiffness, since testing is generally not performed at an infinitely low strain rate.

The accuracy of strength measurements is generally better than that of stiffness measurements and measurements of energy absorptive properties, since no strain measurement is involved. In the case of ultimate strain determinations, the accuracy is only affected by the general inaccuracy of the strain measurements. Ultimate strain is generally slightly overestimated, and the most accurate values are obtained from testing embedded specimens as is the case for stiffness and energy absorptive properties.

C. DATA ACQUISITION AND ANALYSIS

Whether tension or compression loads are used, it is advisable to apply the load to the specimen several times before recording the load and deflection, since some "settling" occurs between the specimen and grips during the first cycles. When presenting results, bone density, mineral content, age, sex, and health of the bone source should be included since such information serves as a benchmark for comparison with other studies. The following sections describe key stress–strain measurements and methods for compensating for artifacts in stress–strain measurements.

1. Determination of Mechanical and Structural Properties

Yield point

In a mechanical sense, the yield point is the point where structural changes begin. For bone specimens this point is presumed to be near the point where the slope of the stress–strain curve is seen to decrease. Such a definition, however, is not very precise, and methods for determination of the yield point vary accordingly. In analyzing a stress–strain curve wherein there is no distinct yield point the ASTM Committee on Mechanical Testing suggests that the 0.2% offset criteria for engineering material be used to determine the yield stress. The yield point by the offset criterion is defined as the intersection between the compression curve and a line parallel with the maximum slope and displaced 0.2% strain (ASTM E8). Although this definition is precise, it has some disadvantages. Significant structural changes have probably occurred before that point, and due to the slightly different shape of stress–strain curves of weak specimens compared with stronger specimens, a yield strain close to and even larger than the ultimate strain is sometimes found in weak specimens. A smaller strain offset will eliminate this problem, and for biomechanical testing a strain offset of 0.1% is preferred and may become standardized for future testing.[63]

A more physiological definition of the yield point would be the point where the slope has reached maximum in its mathematical sense. This point is easily determined whenever test data are stored directly on computers, and can be derived from the second-order differential equation of a third-order (or higher) polynomial fit to the stress–strain data. This point has been found to be about 0.8% strain in unconfined compression testing of trabecular bone specimens.[128]

Ultimate strength

The maximum stress the bone can sustain is called the ultimate strength, and the breaking strength is the stress at which the bone actually breaks. In bone the ultimate strength and the breaking strength usually have the same value, but this is not necessarily true for all materials. For example, a specimen of ductile steel will stretch considerably before it breaks, and due to this stretching, the stress sustained at fracture (breaking strength) may actually be less than the maximum stress attained (ultimate strength). It should be noted that strength, as it is defined above (e.g., stress), is an intrinsic property of bone. That is, strength values are independent of the size and shape of the bone. The force required to break the bone differs from the intrinsic strength, because the breaking load or fracture load will vary with bone or specimen size. One must keep this distinction in mind because intrinsic strength and breaking load can show very different trends between control and experimental groups in studies wherein the treatment affects the size of the bone. For example, fluoride treatment decreases the intrinsic strength of bone in young rats, but it also increases the bone size such that breaking load remains unchanged.

Tensile strength

The tensile strength is calculated by dividing the maximum load recorded (from the tensile test to failure) in newtons by the original minimum cross-sectional area of the specimen in square meters. This result is generally expressed in pascals (N/m^2) and should be reported to three significant figures as tensile strength at yield or as the tensile strength at break, whichever term is applicable. When a nominal yield or breaking load is less than the maximum, it may be desirable to calculate the corresponding tensile stress at yield or tensile stress at break and report these using at least three significant figures.

Percent elongation

If the test results in a yield load that is larger than the load at break, one should calculate the percent elongation at yield. Otherwise, the percent elongation at break should be calculated. Percent elongation is determined by reading the deformation (change in gauge length) at the moment the applicable load is reached, and dividing that value by the original gauge length (multiply by 100). Report percent elongation at yield or percent elongation at break to two significant figures. When a yield or breaking load is less than the maximum, both percent elongation at yield and percent elongation at break should be reported.

Modulus of elasticity

Calculate the modulus of elasticity by extending the initial linear portion of the load–deformation curve and dividing the difference in stress corresponding to any segment of the section on this straight line by the corresponding difference in strain. Compute all elastic modulus values using the average initial cross-sectional area of the test specimens in the calculations. Express the result in pascals and report to three significant figures.

The stress–strain relations of many biological tissues do not conform to Hooke's law throughout the elastic range but may deviate from this idealized linear stress–strain behavior at stresses well below the elastic limit. For such materials the slope of the tangent to the stress–strain curve at a low stress is usually taken as the modulus of elasticity. Since the existence of a true proportional limit in biological tissue is debatable, the appropriateness of applying the term *modulus of elasticity* to describe the stiffness of rigidity of a biological specimen has been seriously questioned. The exact stress–strain characteristics of biological materials are dependent on such factors as strain rate, temperature, previous specimen stress history, etc. Thus, when applied to biological tissue, the precise meaning of mechanical property is most useful if this dependency is understood.

Energy absorption

The area under the compression or tension curve represents the work put into the material by compression/tension (loading energy or strain energy). Unloading the specimen prior to reaching the elastic limit of an ideal elastic material results in the same amount of energy being released (unloading energy). In other words, the unloading curve coincides with the loading curve. However, since bone is a viscoelastic material, it dissipates energy. The loading energy within the elastic range is composed of elastic energy that is released during unloading and viscoelastic energy that is absorbed by the material and converted to other energy forms such as frictional heat. The unloading curve of a viscoelastic material will follow a lower course than the loading curve, and the two types of energy can be determined from such a loading–unloading cycle (the so-called hysteresis loop). The area underneath the unloading curve represents the energy released during unloading (elastic energy), and the area enclosed by the hysteresis loop represents energy dissipation during the loading cycle (viscoelastic energy). For each series of tests, calculate the arithmetic mean of all values obtained and report it as the average values for the particular property in question.

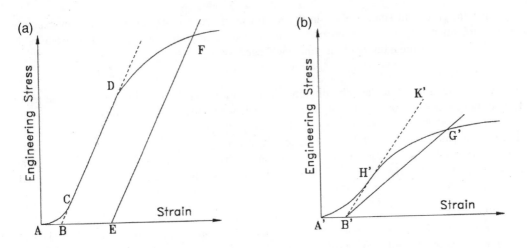

FIGURE 11.13 Typical stress–strain curve obtained from tensile testing: (a) with linear region; (b) without linear region.

2. Toe Region Compensation

In a typical stress–strain curve (Figure 11.13) there is a toe region, AC, that does not represent a property of the material.[147] The toe region is an artifact caused by a take-up of slack, alignment and/or seating of the test specimen. In order to obtain correct values of mechanical parameters such as modulus, yield, and ultimate strain, the corrected zero point on the strain or extension axis must be determined. In case of a material exhibiting a linear or Hookean stress–strain behavior, a continuation of the linear (CD) region of the curve is constructed through the zero-stress axis. This intersection (B) is the corrected zero-strain point from which all displacements or strains must be measured, including the yield offset point (BE), if applicable. The elastic modulus can be determined by dividing the stress at any point along the line CD (or its extension) by the strain at the same point (measured from point B, defined as zero strain).

In the case of a material that does not exhibit any linear region (refer to Figure 11.13), the same kind of toe correction for the zero-strain point can be made by constructing a tangent to the maximum slope at the inflection point (H′). This is extended to intersect the strain axis at point B′, which is the corrected zero-strain point. By using point B′ as the zero strain reference, the stress at any point (G′) on the curve can be divided by the strain at that point to obtain a secant modulus (slope of line B′G′). For those materials with no linear region, any attempt to use the tangent through the inflection point as a basis for determination of an offset yield point may result in unacceptable error.

VII. ANIMAL MODELS

The animal model chosen determines, to a large extent, the specific biomechanical tests that can be performed. Any of the aforementioned tests can be performed for bones from larger animals, but the test choice is more restrictive for smaller animals. With rats, for instance, tests are usually limited to bending or torsion of long bones and compression of vertebral bodies. It is difficult, but not impossible, to accurately measure the mechanical properties of trabecular bone in rodents. Trabecular bone cores can be prepared from rat vertebral bodies for purposes of compression testing, but more commonly compression tests of intact vertebral bodies are conducted since core preparations can be exceedingly difficult. When testing intact structures, such as an entire vertebral body, the contributions of both the cortical shell and trabecular bone core will have a significant influence on the mechanical test results. Another important consideration is the type of bone being studied. Many larger species (e.g., sheep and cows) have predominantly plexiform cortical bone, which differs mechanically from osteonal cortical bone, especially in fatigue.[148] Canine trabecular bone also differs appreciably from human trabecular bone.[149]

Because many mechanical tests are prone to experimental bias, a good experimental design should always include a control group. Fortunately, most biomechanical tests (e.g., compression, tension, bending, and torsion) are very precise and reasonably accurate, so that comparison between treatment groups and controls can be done very effectively.

VIII. SUMMARY

Knowledge of the mechanical properties of bone is of significant importance for understanding diseases such as osteoporosis and osteoarthritis. Bone loss associated with osteoporosis reduces the mechanical strength of trabecular bone, increases the risk of fracture, and produces painful and spontaneous collapse of bones, especially vertebral bodies. During the slow and progressive development of osteoarthritis, subchondral trabecular bone undergoes characteristic changes, and it has been hypothesized that the initial changes in osteoarthritis are the result of changes in the shock-absorptive properties of trabecular bone.

Knowledge of mechanical properties of bone is also of major importance for the design of fracture fixation devices, as well as the design, fixation, and survival of artificial joints. Artificial joints, such as the acetabular component in hip arthroplasty and the femoral and tibial components in knee arthroplasty are intimately associated with cortical and trabecular bone. An understanding of the mechanical properties of the bone is thus very important for the design of joint prostheses. A precise and accurate knowledge of bone mechanical properties is also a prerequisite for numerical design and optimization (finite-element analysis) of implants and for simulation of load-induced stress-morphology processes (remodeling) that take place in bone. The validity of such numerical analyses draws upon the accuracy of the mechanical property data used to describe bone, implant, and bone–implant interface.

Because of the wide variety of bone shapes and sizes, and the fact that there are no established standards for bone biomechanical testing, there are a large number of variables to consider when establishing testing procedures. Unfortunately, there are no well-established "industry standards" for biomechanical testing of bone. Consequently, a lot of published biomechanical test data are inaccurate because of poor testing techniques or inattention to confounding variables. This chapter was not intended to provide an exhaustive review of experimental techniques used by researchers; rather, the chapter focused on several common test protocols, which are currently used in biomechanical testing of bone tissue.

The following summarizes several important factors and guidelines that should be considered when performing mechanical tests of bone:

1. Specimen geometry has a highly significant influence on mechanical properties such as stiffness, ultimate strain, and energy absorption. A cube with a side length of 8 mm and a cylindrical specimen with a length of 16 mm and a diameter of 8 mm are suggested as standard geometries providing comparable results.
2. Standard testing of small trabecular bone specimens is associated with systematic errors. The most significant of these errors are believed to be related to the integrity of trabeculae at the cut or machined surfaces of the test specimen and friction at the specimen–platen interface.
3. The best method of long-term preservation prior to testing is to freeze the specimens at −20°C in saline-soaked gauze. Small specimens can be preserved up to 90 days if kept in a solution of 50% ethanol and 50% saline. During testing, care should be taken to ensure that the test specimens are kept hydrated.

4. Reproducibility can be improved by "preconditioning" the test specimens using a number of conditioning cycles to achieve a viscoelastic steady state.
5. The stiffness derived from nondestructive tests will generally be lower than that obtained from a destructive test because of inherent nonlinearity in the load–deformation curve.
6. For each experiment, a series of tests should be conducted so that calculations of the arithmetic mean of all values can be obtained.

REFERENCES

1. American Society for Metals International, Mechanical testing, in *Metals Handbook*, 8, ASM, Materials Park, OH, 1989, 589.
2. Evans, F.G. and Lebow, M., The strength of human bone as revealed by engineering techniques, *Am. J. Surg.*, 83, 326, 1952.
3. Gerard, G., *Introduction to Structural Stability Theory*, McGraw-Hill, New York, 1962, 19.
4. Roak, R.J. and Young, W.C., *Formulas for Stress and Strain*, McGraw-Hill, New York, 1975.
5. Banse, X., Delloye, C., Cornu, O., and Bourgois, R., Comparative left-right mechanical testing of cancellous bone from normal femoral heads, *J. Biomech.*, 29, 1249, 1996.
6. Bartley, M.H., Arnold, J.S., Haslam, R.K., and Jee, W.S., The relationship of bone strength and bone quantity in health, disease and aging, *J. Gerontol.*, 21, 517, 1966.
7. Evans, F.G. and Band, S., Differences and relationships between the physical properties and the relationships between the physical properties and the microscopic structure of human femoral, tibial and fibular cortical bone, *Am. J. Anat.*, 120, 79, 1967.
8. Gibson, L.J., The mechanical behavior of cancellous bone, *J. Biomech.*, 18, 317, 1985.
9. Goldstein, S.A., The mechanical properties of trabecular bone: dependence on anatomic location and function, *J. Biomech.*, 20, 1055, 1987.
10. Martin, R.B. and Atkinson, P.J., Age and sex-related changes in the structure and strength of the human femoral shaft, *J. Biomech.*, 10, 223, 1977.
11. Welch, D.O., The composite structure of bone and its response to mechanical stress, *Recent Adv. Eng. Sci.*, 5, 245, 1970.
12. ASTM, Standard: Standard test methods of compression testing of metallic materials at room temperature, *Annual Book of ASTM Standards,* ASTM, Philadelphia, E9-89a, 1983.
13. ASTM, Standard: Standard test method for compressive properties of rigid cellular plastics, D1621, ASTM, Philadelphia, 1991, 11.
14. ASTM, Standard: Standard test method for compressive properties of rigid plastics, D695, ASTM, Philadelphia, 1991, 276.
15. ASTM, Standard: Standard testing for compressive strength of cylindrical concrete specimens, C39, ASTM, Philadelphia, 1991, 86.
16. Linde, F., Elastic and viscoelastic properties of trabecular bone by a compression testing approach, *Dan. Med. Bull.*, 41, 119, 1994.
17. Keller, T.S., Hansson, T.H., Abram, A.C., et al., Regional variations in the compressive properties of lumbar vertebral trabeculae. Effects of disc degeneration, *Spine*, 14, 1012, 1989.
18. Keaveny, T.M., Borchers, R.D., Gibson, L.J., and Hayes, W.C., Trabecular bone modulus and strength can depend on specimen geometry, *J. Biomech.*, 26, 991, 1993.
19. Carter, D.R. and Spengler, D.M., Mechanical properties and composition of cortical bone, *Clin. Orthop.*, 135, 192, 1978.
20. Cowin, S.C., Mechanics of materials, in *Bone Mechanics*, Cowin, S.C., Ed., CRC Press, Boca Raton, FL, 1989, 15.
21. Currey, J.D., The mechanical properties of bone, *Clin. Orthop.*, 73, 210, 1970.
22. Hollister, S.J., Fyhrie, D.P., Jepsen, K.J., and Goldstein, S.A., Application of homogenization theory to the study of trabecular bone mechanics, *J. Biomech.*, 24, 825, 1991.
23. Mosekilde, Li., Viidik, A., and Mosekilde, Le., Correlation between the compressive strength of iliac and vertebral trabecular bone in normal individuals, *Bone*, 6, 291, 1985.
24. Mosekilde, Li., Mosekilde, Le., and Danielsen, C.C., Biomechanical competence of vertebral trabecular bone in relation to ash density and age in normal individuals, *Bone*, 8, 79, 1987.

25. Behrens, J.C., Walker, P.S., and Shoje, H., Variations in strength and structure of cancellous bone at the knee, *J. Biomech.*, 7, 201, 1974.

26. Cowin, S.C., The mechanical properties of cancellous bone, in *Bone Mechanics*, Cowin, S.C., Ed., CRC Press, Boca Raton, FL, 1989, 129.

27. Goldstein, S.A., Wilson, D.L., Sonstegard, D.A., and Matthews, L.S., The mechanical properties of human tibial trabecular bone as a function of metaphyseal location, *J. Biomech.*, 16, 965, 1983.

28. Lindahl, O., Mechanical properties of dried defatted spongy bone, *Acta Orthop. Scand.*, 47, 11, 1976.

29. Panjabi, M.M., Krag, M.K., Summers, M.K., and Videman, T., Biomechanical time-tolerance of fresh cadaveric human tissue specimens, *J. Orthop. Res.*, 3, 292, 1985.

30. Pelker, R.R., Friedlaender, G.E., Markham, T.C., et al., Effects of freezing and freeze-drying on the biomechanical properties of rat bone, *J. Orthop. Res.*, 1, 405, 1984.

31. Sonstegard, D.A. and Matthews, L.S., Mechanical property dependence on storage technique and local of knee joint trabecular bone, *Trans. Orthop. Res. Soc.*, 2, 283, 1977.

32. Komender, A., Influences of preservation on some mechanical properties of human Haversian bone, *Mater. Med. Pol.*, 8, 13, 1976.

33. Linde, F. and Sørensen, H.C., The effect of different storage methods on mechanical properties of trabecular bone, *J. Biomech.*, 26, 1249, 1993.

34. Sedlin, E.D. and Hirsch, C., Factors affecting the determination of the physical properties of femoral cortical bone, *Acta Orthop. Scand.*, 37, 29, 1966.

35. Ashman, R.B., Experimental techniques, in *Bone Mechanics*, Cowin, S.C., CRC Press, Boca Raton, FL, 1989, 75.

36. McElhaney, J.H., Fogle, J., Byars, E., and Weaver, G., Effect of embalming on the mechanical properties of beef bone, *J. Appl. Physiol.*, 19, 12334, 1964.

37. Evans, F.G., *Mechanical Properties of Bone,* Charles C Thomas, Springfield, IL, 1973.

38. Hvid, I. and Hansen, S.L., Trabecular bone strength patterns at the proximal tibial epiphysis, *J. Orthop. Res.*, 3, 464, 1985.

39. Keller, T.S., Predicting the mechanical behavior of bone, *J. Biomech.*, 27, 1159, 1994.

40. Linde, F., Hvid, I., and Madsen, F., The effect of specimen size and geometry on the mechanical behavior of trabecular bone, *J. Biomech.*, 25, 359, 1992.

41. Carter, D.R. and Hayes, W.C., Compact bone fatigue damage, *Clin. Orthop.*, 127, 265, 1977.

42. Odgaard, A., Hvid, I., and Linde, F., Compressive axial strain distribution in cancellous bone specimen, *J. Biomech.*, 22, 829, 1989.

43. Rohlmann, A., Zilch, H., Bergmann, G., and Koebel, R., Material properties of femoral cancellous bone in axial loading. Part I: Time independent properties, *Arch. Orthop. Trauma Surg.*, 97, 95, 1980.

44. Hansson, T.H., Keller, T.S., and Panjabi, M.M., A study of the compressive properties of lumbar vertebral trabeculae: effects of tissue characteristics, *Spine*, 12, 56, 1987.

45. Hvid, I., Mechanical strength of trabecular bone at the knee, *Dan. Med. Bull.*, 35, 345, 1988.

46. Keaveny, T.M., Borchers, R.E., Gibson, L.J., and Hayes, W.C., Theoretical analysis of the experimental artifact in trabecular bone compressive modulus, *J. Biomech.*, 26, 599, 1993.

47. Tanner, K.E., Sharp, D.J., Turner, S., and Bonfield, W., Specimen length and the measured mechanical properties of trabecular bone, *Trans. World Congr. Biomech.*, 1, 131, 1990.

48. Zhu, M., Keller, T.S., and Spengler, D.M., Effects of specimen load-bearing and free surface layers on the compressive mechanical properties of cellular materials, *J. Biomech.*, 27, 57, 1994.

49. Choi, K., Kuhn, J.L., Ciarelli, M.J., and Goldstein, S.A., The elastic moduli of subchondral, trabecular, and cortical bone tissue and the size-dependency of cortical bone modulus, *J. Biomech.*, 23, 1103, 1990.

50. Cowin, S.C. and Mehrabidi, M.M., Identification of the elastic symmetry of bone and other materials, *J. Biomech.*, 22, 503, 1989.

51. Harrigan, T.P., Jasty, M., Mann, R.W., and Harris, W.H., Limitations of the continuum assumptions in cancellous bone, *J. Biomech.*, 21, 269, 1988.

52. Bachus, K.N., Bloebaum, R.D., and Hofmann, A.A., Minimum trabecular width: the biomechanical limit of load bearing cancellous bone, *Trans. Orthop. Res. Soc.*, 15, 54, 1990.

53. Sumner, D.R., Turner, T.M., and Galante, J.O., Symmetry of the canine femur: implications for experimental sample size requirements, *J. Orthop. Res.*, 6, 758, 1988.

54. Tanner, K.E., Harris, J.R., Evans, G.P., and Bonfield, W., Assessment of parameters which affect the measured mechanical properties of human cancellous bone, *Proc. Meet. Eur. Soc. Biomech.*, 8, 66, 1992.

55. Currey, J.D., The effects of drying and re-wetting on some mechanical properties of cortical bone, *J. Biomech.*, 21, 439, 1988.
56. Currey, J.D., Physical characteristics affecting the tensile failure properties of cortical bone, *J. Biomech.*, 23, 837, 1990.
57. Jameson, M.W., Hood, J.A., and Tidmarsh, B.G., The effects of dehydration and rehydration on some mechanical properties of human dentine, *J. Biomech.*, 26, 1055, 1993.
58. Williams, J.L. and Johnson, W.J., Elastic constants of composites formed from PMMA bone cement and anisotropic bovine tibial cancellous bone, *J. Biomech.*, 22, 673, 1989.
59. Padawer, G.E. and Beecher, N., On the strength and stiffness of planar reinforced plastic resins, *Polym. Eng. Sci.*, 10, 185, 1994.
60. Gray, R.J. and Korbacher, G.K., Compressive fatigue behavior of bovine compact bone, *J. Biomech.*, 7, 287, 292.
61. Reilly, S.B. and Burstein, A.H., The elastic and ultimate properties of compact bone tissue, *J. Biomech.*, 8, 393, 1975.
62. Carter, D.R. and Hayes, W.C., The compressive behavior of bone as a two phase porous structure, *J. Bone Joint Surg.*, 59A, 954, 1977.
63. Turner, C.H., Yield behavior of bovine cancellous bone, *J. Biomech. Eng.*, 111, 256, 1989.
64. Carter, D.R., Caler, W.E., Spengler, D.M., and Frankel, V.H., Fatigue behavior of adult cortical bone: the influence of mean strain and strain range, *Acta Orthop. Scand.*, 52, 481, 1981.
65. Crowninshield, R.D. and Pope, M.H., The response of compact bone in tension at various strain rate, *Ann. Biomed. Eng.*, 2, 217, 1974.
66. Currey, J.D., The effects of strain rate, reconstruction, and mineral content on some mechanical properties of bovine bone, *J. Biomech.*, 8, 81, 1975.
67. Ducheyne, P., Heymans, L., Martens, M., et al., The mechanical behavior of intracondylar cancellous bone of the femur at different loading rates, *J. Biomech.*, 10, 747, 1977.
68. Kafka, V., On hydraulic strengthening of bones, *Biorheology*, 20, 789, 1983.
69. Liebschner, M.A.K. and Keller, T.S., Cortical Bone Exhibits Hydraulic Strengthening, *44th Annual Meeting of the Orthopaedic Research Society*, New Orleans, LA, 23, 559, 1998.
70. Panjabi, M.M., White, A.A., III, and Southwick, W.O., Mechanical properties of bone as a function of rate of deformation, *J. Bone Joint Surg.*, 55A, 322, 1973.
71. Ciarelli, M.J., Goldstein, S.A., Kuhn, J.L., et al., Evaluation of the orthogonal mechanical properties and density of human trabecular bone from the major metaphyseal regions with materials testing and computed tomography, *J. Orthop. Res.*, 9, 674, 1991.
72. Dempster, W.T. and Liddicoat, R., Compact bone as a non-isotropic material, *Am. J. Anat.*, 91, 331, 1952.
73. Fondrik, M., Bahniuk, E., Davy, D.T., and Michaels, C., Some viscoelastic characteristics of bovine and human cortical bone, *J. Biomech.*, 21, 623, 1988.
74. Rice, J.C., Cowin, S.C., and Bowman, J.A., On the dependence of the elastic and strength of cancellous bone on apparent density, *J. Biomech.*, 21, 155, 1988.
75. Røhl, L., Larsen, E., Linde, F., et al., Tensile and compressive properties of cancellous bone, *J. Biomech.*, 24, 1143, 1991.
76. Stone, J.L., Beaupre, G.S., and Hayes, W.C., Multiaxial strength characteristics of trabecular bone, *J. Biomech.*, 16, 743, 1983.
77. Ashman, R.B. and Rho, J.Y., Elastic moduli of trabecular bone material, *J. Biomech.*, 21, 177, 1988.
78. Bird, F., Becker, H., Healer, J., and Messer, M., Experimental determination of the mechanical properties of bone, *Aerospace Med.*, 39, 44, 1968.
79. Reilly, S.B., Burstein, A.H., and Frankel, V.H., The elastic modulus of bone, *J. Biomech.*, 7, 271, 1974.
80. Katz, J.L., Anisotropy of Young's modulus of bone, *Nature* (London), 283, 106, 1980.
81. Klever, F.J., Klumpert, R., Horenberg, J., et al., Global mechanical properties of trabecular bone: experimental determination and prediction from a structural model, in *Biomechanics: Current Interdisciplinary Research*, Perren, S.M. and Schneider, E., Eds., Martinus Nijhoff, Dordrecht, the Netherlands, 1985, 167.
82. Tsai, S.W. and Wu, E.M., A general theory of strength for anisotropic material, *J. Compos. Mater.*, 5, 58, 1971.

83. Burstein, A.H., Currey, J.D., Frankel, V.H., and Reilly, D.T., The ultimate properties of bone tissue: the effects of yielding, *J. Biomech.*, 5, 35, 1973.

84. Jonas, J., Burns, J., Able E.W., et al., A technique for the tensile testing of demineralized bone, *J. Biomech.*, 26, 271, 1993.

85. Katsamanis, F. and Raftopoulos, D.D., Determination of mechanical properties of human femoral cortical bone by the Hopkinson bar stress technique, *J. Biomech.*, 23, 1173, 1990.

86. Knauss, P., Material properties and strength behavior of spongy bone tissue at the proximal human femur (Part I), *Biomed. Tech.*, 26, 200, 1981 [translated from German].

87. Lewis, J.L. and Goldsmith, W., The dynamic fracture and prefracture response of compact bone by split Hopkinson bar methods, *J. Biomech.*, 8, 27, 1975.

88. Mente, P.L. and Lewis, J.L., Experimental method for measurement of the elastic modulus of trabecular bone tissue, *J. Orthop. Res.*, 7, 456, 1989.

89. Tarnopol'skii, I.M. and Kincis, T., Static Test Method for Composites, Van Nostrand Reinhold, New York, 1985.

90. Yahia, L.H., Drouin, G., and Duval, P., A methodology for mechanical measurements of technical constants of trabecular bone, *Eng. Med.*, 17, 169, 1988.

91. Carter, D.R., Schwab, G.H., and Spengler, D.M., Tensile fracture of cancellous bone, *Acta Orthop. Scand.*, 51, 733, 1980.

92. Turner, C.H. and Cowin, S.C., Errors induced by off-axis measurement of the elastic properties of bone, *J. Biomech. Eng.*, 110, 213, 1988.

93. Hayes, W.C. and Black, D., Post-yield energy absorption characteristics of trabecular bone. In *1979 Biomechanics Symposium,* Van Buskirk, W.C., Ed., ASME, New York, 1979, 177.

94. Hodgkinson, R. and Currey, J.D., The effect of variation in structure on the Young's modulus of cancellous bone: a comparison of human and non-human material, *Proc. Inst. Mech. Eng. H: J. Eng. Med.,* 204, 115, 1990.

95. Inoue, N., Sakakida, K., Yamashita, F., et al., The elasto-plastic behavior of bovine cancellous bone under tensile loading, *Proc. Meet. Eur. Soc. Biomech.*, 6, 8A, 1988.

96. Keaveny, T.M., Guo, X.E., Wachtel, E.F., et al., Trabecular bone exhibits fully linear elastic behavior and yields at low strain, *J. Biomech.*, 27, 1127, 1994.

97. Kopperdahl, D.L. and Keaveny, T.M., Damage behavior of vertebral sections is dependent on applied strains and dominated by trabecular bone, in *Trans. Orthop. Res. Soc.*, 34, 1033, 1999.

98. Caler, W.E. and Carter, D.R., Bone creep-fatigue damage accumulation, *J. Biomech.*, 22, 625, 1989.

99. Carter, D.R. and Hayes, W.C., Fatigue life of compact bone — I. Effects of stress amplitude, temperature and density, *J. Biomech*, 9, 27, 1976.

100. Chamay, A., Mechanical and morphological aspects of experimental overload and fatigue in bone, *J. Biomech.*, 3, 263, 1970.

101. Keller, T.S., Lovin, J.D., Spengler, D.M., and, Carter, D.R., Fatigue of immature baboon cortical bone, *J. Biomech.*, 18, 297, 1985.

102. Michel, M.C., Xiang-Dong, E.G., Gibson, L.J., et al., Compressive fatigue behavior of bovine trabecular bone, *J. Biomech.*, 26, 453, 1993.

103. Wachtel, E.F. and Keaveny, T.M., The effects of unloading conditions and strain-rate on the residual properties of damaged trabecular bone, *ASME Adv. Bioeng.*, BED, 31, 159, 1995.

104. Wagner, H.D. and Weiner, S., On the relationship between the microstructure of bone and its mechanical stiffness, *J. Biomech.*, 25, 1311, 1992.

105. Carter, D.R. and Caler, W.E., Cycle dependent and time dependent bone fracture with repeated loading, *J. Biomech. Eng.*, 105, 166, 1983.

106. Lafferty, J.F. and Raju, P.V., The influence of stress frequency on the fatigue strength of cortical bone, *J. Biomech Eng.*, 101, 112, 1979.

107. Choi, K. and Goldstein, S.A., A comparison of the fatigue behavior of human trabecular and cortical bone tissue, *J. Biomech.*, 25, 1371, 1992.

108. Schaffler, M.B., Radin, E.L., and Burr, D.B., Long-term fatigue behavior of compact bone at low strain magnitude and rate, *Bone*, 11, 321, 1990.

109. McBroom, R.J., Hayes, W.C., Edwards, W.T., et al., Prediction of the vertebral body compressive fracture using quantitative computed tomography, *J. Bone Joint Surg.*, 67A, 1206, 1985.

110. Keller, T.S., Spengler, D.M., and Carter, D.R., The influence of exercise on maturing rat long bone structural and material properties, *Trans. Orthop. Res. Soc.*, 29, 60, 1983.

111. Keller, T.S., Spengler, D.M., and Carter, D.R., Geometric, elastic, and structural properties of maturing rat femora, *J. Orthop. Res.*, 4, 57, 1986.

112. Bell, G.H., Dunbar, O., Beck, J.S., and Gibb, A., Variations in strength of vertebrae with age and their relations to osteoporosis, *Calcif. Tissue Res.*, 1, 75, 1967.

113. Hansson, T.H., Keller, T.S., and Spengler, D.M., Mechanical behavior of the human lumbar spine. II. Fatigue strength during dynamic compressive loading, *J. Orthop. Res.*, 5, 479, 1987.

114. Hansson, T., Roos, B., and Nachemson, A., The bone mineral content and ultimate compressive strength of lumbar vertebrae, *Spine*, 5, 46, 1980.

115. Hardy, W.G., Lissner, H.R., Webster, J.E., and Gurdijian, E.S., Repeated loading tests of the lumbar, *Spine Surg. Forum*, 9, 690, 1958.

116. Keller, T.S., Spengler, D.M., and Hansson, T.H., Mechanical behavior of the human lumbar spine. I. Creep analysis during static compressive loading, *J. Orthop. Res.*, 5, 467, 1987.

117. McCubbrey, D.A., Cody, D.D., Kuhn, J.L., et al., Static and fatigue failure properties of thoracic and lumbar vertebral bodies and their regional density, *Trans. Orthop. Res. Soc.*, 15, 178, 1990.

118. Derwin, K.A., Soslowsky, L.J., Green, W.D., and Elder, S.H., A new optical system for the determination of deformations and strains: calibration characteristics and experimental results, *J. Biomech.*, 27, 1277, 1994.

119. Woo, S.L., Gomez, M.A., Seguchi, Y., et al., Measurement of mechanical properties of ligament substance from a bone-ligament-bone preparation, *J. Orthop. Res.*, 1, 22, 1983.

120. Woo, S.L., Danto, M.I., and Ohland, K.J., The use of a laser micrometer system to determine the cross-sectional shape and area of ligaments: a comparative study with two existing methods, *J. Biomech. Eng.*, 112, 426, 1990.

121. Wright, T.M. and Hayes, W.C., Strain gauge application on compact bone, *J. Biomech.*, 12, 471, 1979.

122. Wright, T.M., Vosburgh, F., and Burstein, A.H., Permanent deformation of compact bone monitored by acoustic emission, *J. Biomech.*, 14, 405, 1981.

123. Bonfield, W., and Li, C.H., The temperature dependence of the deformation of bone, *J. Biomech.*, 1, 323, 1968.

124. Brear, K., Currey, J.D., Rainers, S., and Smith, K.J., Density and temperature effects on some mechanical properties of cancellous bone, *Eng. Med.*, 17, 163, 1988.

125. Turner, C.H. and Burr, D.B., Basic biomechanical measurements of bone: a tutorial, *Bone*, 14, 595, 1993.

126. Wall, J.C., Chatterji, S., and Jeffery, J.W., On the origin of scatter in results of human bone strength tests, *Med. Biol. Eng.*, 8, 171, 1970.

127. Linde, F., Hvid, I., and Jensen, N.C., Material properties of cancellous bone in repetitive axial loading, *Eng. Med.*, 14, 173, 1985.

128. Linde, F. and Hvid, I., Stiffness behavior of trabecular bone specimens, *J. Biomech.*, 20, 82, 1987.

129. Linde, F., Gøthgen, C.B., Hvid, I., et al., Mechanical properties of trabecular bone by a nondestructive compression testing approach, *Eng. Med.*, 17, 23, 1988.

130. Linde, F. and Hvid, I., The effect of constraint on the mechanical behavior of trabecular bone specimens, *J. Biomech.*, 22, 485, 1989.

131. Linde, F., Hvid, I., and Pongsoipetch, B., Energy absorptive properties of human trabecular bone specimens during axial compression, *J. Orthop. Res.*, 7, 432, 1989.

132. Burstein, A.H. and Frankel, V.H., The visco-elastic properties of some biological materials, *Ann. N.Y. Acad. Sci.*, 146, 158, 1968.

133. Madsen, F., Odgaard, A., and Linde, F., The consequences of compression strain level on energy absorption in trabecular bone specimens, *Proc. Meet. Eur. Soc. Biomech.*, 6, 7A, 1988.

134. Lakes, R.S., Katz, J.L., and Sternstein, S.S., Viscoelastic properties of wet cortical bone — I. Torsional and biaxial studies, *J. Biomech.*, 12, 657, 1979.

135. Kaplan, S.J., Hayes, W.C., Stone, J.L., and Beaupre, G.S., Tensile strength of bovine trabecular bone, *J. Biomech.*, 18, 732, 1985.

136. Linde, F., Nørgaard, P., Hvid, I., et al., Mechanical properties of trabecular bone. Dependency on stain rate, *J. Biomech.*, 24, 803, 1991.

137. Saha, S. and Hayes, W.C., Tensile impact properties of human compact bone, *J. Biomech.*, 9, 243, 1976.

138. Schaffler, M.B., Radin, E.L., and Burr, D.B., Mechanical and morphological effects of strain-rate on fatigue of compact bone, *Bone*, 10, 207, 1989.

139. Vrijhoef, M.M. and Driessens, F.C., On the interaction between specimen and testing machine in the mechanical testing procedures, *J. Biomech.*, 4, 233, 1971.

140. Filon, L.N., On the elastic equilibrium of circular cylinders under certain practical systems of load, *Philos. Trans. R. Soc. London A,* 198, 147, 1992.

141. Brown, T.D. and Ferguson, A.B., Mechanical property distributions in the cancellous bone of the human proximal femur, *Acta Orthop. Scand.*, 51, 429, 1980.

142. Odgaard, A., and Linde, F., The underestimation of Young's modulus in compression testing of cancellous bone specimens, *J. Biomech.*, 24, 691, 1991.

143. Allard, R.N. and Ashman, R.B., A comparison between cancellous bone compressive moduli determined from surface strain and total specimen deflection, *Trans. Orthop. Res. Soc.*, 16, 151, 1991.

144. Aspden, R.M., Constraining the lateral dimensions of uniaxially loaded materials increases the calculated strength and stiffness: application to muscle and bone, *J. Mater. Sci. Mater. Med.*, 1, 100, 1990.

145. Guo, X.E., Gibson, L.J., and McMahon, T.A., Fatigue of trabecular bone: avoiding end-crushing artifacts, *Trans. Orthop. Res. Soc.*, 18, 584, 1993.

146. Keaveny, T.M., Pinilla, T.P., Crawford, R.P., et al., Systematic and random errors in compression testing of trabecular bone, *J. Orthop. Res.*, 15, 101, 1997.

147. Keaveny, T.M., Wachtel, E.F., Ford, C.M., and Hayes, W.C., Differences between the tensile and compressive strength of bovine tibial trabecular bone depend on modulus, *J. Biomech.*, 27, 1137, 1994.

148. Carter, D.R. and Hayes, W.C., Bone compressive strength: the influence of density and strain-rate, *Science*, 194, 1174, 1976.

149. Kuhn, J.L., Goldstein, S.A., Ciarelli, M.J., and Matthews, L.S., The limitation of canine trabecular bone as a model for human: a biomechanical study, *J. Biomech.*, 22, 95, 1989.

12 Bending Tests of Bone

Mandi J. Lopez and Mark D. Markel

CONTENTS

I. INTRODUCTION

The purpose of bending tests of bone is to establish the relative strength of the bone when loads are applied in a manner that causes it to bend about an axis. The tests may be applied to bone alone or with fixation devices such as interlocking nails, plates and screws, and external fixators. The bone may be intact, ostectomized, osteotomized, or otherwise modified. For most experimental models, the contralateral limb is used as the control condition. Regardless of the bone or alterations made to its structure, the same basic principles for bending tests apply.

A bone is subjected to a combination of tension and compression when it is loaded in bending. Compressive stresses and strains act on one side of the neutral axis while tensile stresses and strains act on the other.[1,2] There are no normal stresses or strains acting along the neutral axis (Figure 12.1). The magnitude of the stresses is proportional to their distance from the neutral axis. The farther the stresses are from the neutral axis, the higher their magnitude. Due to asymmetry of the bone, the tensile and compressive stresses may not be equal. Since bone is weakest in tension, fractures propagate from the tensile surface of the bone to the compressive surface transversely until shear forces acting on a 45° plane become high enough to result in a butterfly component on the compressive side of the bone (Figure 12.2).[3,4]

During a bending test, the load applied can be controlled by load control with feedback from the load cell, or through displacement control with feedback from the crosshead. Both methods have been employed in bending testing of bone.[5-7] Load is typically applied over a single-cycle

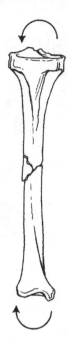

FIGURE 12.1   Typical fracture morphology in bending. Initially the bone fails in tension and the fracture propagates toward the compression surface of the bone, resulting in a large butterfly fragment.

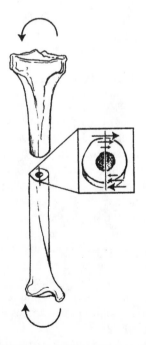

FIGURE 12.2   Illustration of a cross section of a tibia subjected to bending, showing the distribution of stresses around the neutral axis (solid line). Tensile stresses act on the anterior surface of the bone and compressive stresses act on the posterior surface. The stresses are highest on the periosteal surface of the bone and lower near the neutral axis. The tensile and compressive stresses are unequal because the bone is asymmetrical.

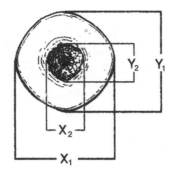

FIGURE 12.3 Diagram of cross-sectional distances measured to calculate the area moment of inertia: X_1 = lateral-to-medial total width (minimum outside radius), X_2 = lateral-to-medial medullary canal width (minimum inside radius), Y_1 = dorsal-to-palmar total width (major outside radius), and Y_2 = dorsal-to-palmar medullary canal width (major inside radius) for the anterior-to-posterior axis.

ramp function. The rate of load application depends on the nature of the investigation, but should be in the physiological range for studies of normal bone activity, and higher for trauma fracture studies.[5] For nondestructive testing, preliminary trials may be required to determine the maximum load or deformation the bone can withstand without sustaining plastic deformation.[6,8] Similarly, if specific loading rate values are not available for fracture studies, trials may be needed to determine a loading rate that consistently fractures the bone in a predetermined time period.[7] The specifics of load and displacement control are covered in depth elsewhere in this text.

II. THREE-POINT BENDING

Three-point bending occurs when three forces acting on a bone produce two equal moments. Each moment is the product of one of the two peripheral forces and its perpendicular distance from the axis of rotation, the point of application of the middle force (Figure 12.3). If loading continues to the yield point, the structure should break at the application point of the middle force, assuming that the structure is homogeneous and symmetrical. Typical three-point bending fractures include "boot top" tibial fractures sustained by snow skiers.[1]

A. WHOLE BONE

1. Sample Preparation

Bone specimens to be tested should be harvested as soon as possible postmortem. They are disarticulated from surrounding joints, wrapped in saline-soaked towels, and sealed in plastic bags with soft tissues left intact.[9] They are then frozen at −20°C until testing. Bones are allowed to thaw and reach 20 to 22°C (room temperature) before testing. After removal from the freezer, specimens should be maintained wet, in saline, during all further stages of tissue preparation. For ease of application, soft tissues are usually removed prior to application of fixation devices, but for all cases of bone testing in bending the soft tissues should be removed so that a soft tissue component is not included in testing values. The time between thawing and testing should be kept to a minimum. One author recommends that no more than 12 h occur between removal from the freezer and completion of a test so that the conditions of fresh bone are as closely simulated as possible.[10]

2. Testing Methods

Typically, the support span for bending testing of an entire bone extends from metaphysis to metaphysis (Figure 12.4).[11,12] Segments of bone such as the diaphysis can be tested as well.[6] In

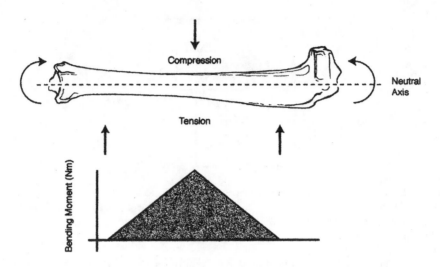

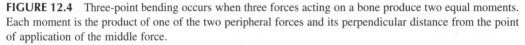

FIGURE 12.4 Three-point bending occurs when three forces acting on a bone produce two equal moments. Each moment is the product of one of the two peripheral forces and its perpendicular distance from the point of application of the middle force.

such cases, the support span typically extends from each end of the segment with just enough bone extending over the end supports to ensure good contact. The support should be strong enough to withstand the forces necessary to test the bone in bending, wide enough to support the bone width, and of sufficient length for the area of interest to be contained within the support span. The end supports should be smooth, flat, and perpendicular to the horizontal axis. Typically, the samples tested are close enough in size such that a single support designed for the average bone can be used, although adjustable end supports have been used as well.[10,12]

Three-point bending requires the use of an actuator with a single point of application. The application point of the actuator should be located on the midline between the two end supports (Figure 12.3). The actuator is applied according to the desired direction of bending. For example, posterior to anterior bending is performed with the anterior surface of the bone facing downward on the support and the load applied on the posterior aspect of the bone. Lateromedial bending is performed with the load applied on the lateral surface.

The testing loading rate depends on the experimental study as discussed above and data obtained from preliminary trials. These authors prefer to test bone nondestructively by applying load over a single-cycle ramp function at a constant displacement rate of 10 mm/min until a maximum displacement of 0.8 mm is obtained. To test specimens to failure, the same displacement rate is used but with no displacement end limit.

3. Data Collection and Calculation

Force and crosshead displacements are recorded from the materials testing system during testing. The authors collect data at 0.1-s intervals and record it on a personal computer directly linked to the materials testing system. One of the most important points relevant to data collection is that the frequency of collection should be high enough to reflect continuous data collection as closely as possible. Load–deformation curves are generated for all tests. For bending tests, load is represented as the bending moment (N·m). Stiffness values are calculated as the slope of the linear regression fit from the straight portion of the curve. Failure is generally defined as the point at which the bone fractures or the central load applicator visibly crushes the underlying cortex.

Most equations to calculate the structural and material properties of bone in bending are based on long prismatic beams where the beam is initially straight, the cross section of the beam does not vary along its length, and the beam is made of an isotropic, homogeneous, linearly elastic material. Bone does not conform to many of these assumptions, but calculations based on these equations provide a means for comparison between studies. Three properties of bones commonly calculated for three-point bending include area moment of inertia, breaking strength, and modulus of elasticity.[6,7,10,13-16]

Bending moment is determined by the formula:

$$M = FL/4 \qquad (12.1)$$

where M = bending moment (N·m), F = applied force, L = distance between two end supports.[17] Bending moment allows comparisons of force to be made between bones of different lengths.

Stress is defined as force per unit area. The area moment of inertia accounts not only for differences in area, but also for differences in shape of the bone cross section through which the force is applied. Bending stress can be calculated from the flexure formula:

$$S = Mc/I \qquad (12.2)$$

where S = stress (N/m²), M = bending moment on the cross section, c = distance from the farthest point in the cross section to the neutral axis, and I = area moment of inertia.

Again, assuming prismatic beam theories, the area moment of inertia can be calculated for a whole bone in posterior-to-anterior bending with the formula:

$$I = \pi/64(X_1 Y_1^3 - X_2 Y_2^3) \qquad (12.3)$$

where I = area moment of inertia, X_1 = lateral-to-medial total width (minimum outside radius), X_2 = lateral-to-medial medullary canal width (minimum inside radius), Y_1 = anterior-to-posterior total width (major outside radius), and Y_2 = anterior-to-posterior medullary canal width (major inside radius) for the anterior-to-posterior axis (Figure 12.4).[6,8,10,12,16]

When bending is performed about the opposite axis, x and y values should be interchanged. For the most applicable results, specimens should be measured where the fracture originates through the cortex.[16]

Stress allows comparisons to be made between strengths of bones that differ in length, size, and shape. For three-point bending, breaking stress is calculated with the formula:

$$BS_{max} = M_{max}\, C/I = (FLC/4I) \qquad (12.4)$$

where BS = breaking stress (N/m²), F = load at failure, L = distance between end supports, and $C = y_1/2$ = distance from the centroid to the surface (see Figure 12.4), and I = area moment of inertia.[16]

Bending stress is calculated using Equation 12.4 at a point prior to the failure point.

The modulus of elasticity for a bone in three-point bending is calculated with the formula:

$$E = (BS_{max}\, L^3)/(48\, I d_a) \qquad (12.5)$$

where E = modulus of elasticity, BS_{max} = breaking strength, d_a = the deformation at the point of load application measured as actuator displacement, and L = distance between end supports.[8,12,15,18]

Strain takes into account the amount of bending or deformation that occurs in the bone as it is being tested. Strain is unitless since it is the change in length per unit length. The formula for calculation of strain in three-point bending is

$$\varepsilon = (12d_a C)/L^2 \qquad (12.6)$$

where d_a = the deformation at the point of load application measured as actuator displacement, C = $y_1/2$ = distance from the centroid to the surface, and L = distance between end supports.[18]

B. Cancellous Bone

The same principles of harvesting and preservation for whole bone apply to cancellous bone. Samples of cancellous bone may be prepared at the same time as collection or after thawing.[19,20] The shape of the samples is generally cylindrical, but other shapes are used, and the area moment of inertia is calculated accordingly. Depending on the directional strength of interest, the samples may be cut longitudinally, transversely, or in any trabecular orientation.[19-22] Often, samples from different areas within the bone are collected.[20,21] Cancellous bone samples are usually cored from the appropriate bone while using a physiological solution lavage.[19,20] In a typical longitudinal section preparation, a stainless-steel coring bit is used to extract cylindrical dowels of cancellous bone beginning at the articular surface and continuing proximally in a plane perpendicular to the ground, usually with the bone in a normal standing weight-bearing orientation. A physiological solution is used during drilling to moisten and cool the specimen. Ideally, it is forced through the drill bit while drilling. The cylinders are then cut to the appropriate length using a low-speed saw with parallel cutting blades again while using a physiological lavage solution. Care is taken to exclude the subchondral bone. Cylinder length and diameter are normally measured using a caliper. Testing methods are similar to those described for whole-bone three-point bending. The size and specifications of the testing support correspond to the size of the specimens. Loading rates are again dependent upon the chosen model (i.e., fracture vs. physiological loading). A sample loading rate for cancellous bone is 0.05 mm/sec.[20]

Data collection for cancellous bone is similar to that of whole bone. Once again, the frequency of data collection should reflect continuous collection as closely as possible. Calculation of data for a solid cylinder or rectangle generally requires fewer manipulations than that of whole bone. Bending moment, bending and breaking stresses, and modulus of elasticity can be calculated from Equations 12.1, 12.4, and 12.5, respectively. The formula for area moment of inertia for a solid cylinder is:

$$I_{cylinder} = \pi r^4/4 \qquad\qquad (12.7)$$

where r = radius of the sample.[4] The formula for area moment of inertia of a solid rectangle is

$$I_{rectangle} = bh^3/12 \qquad\qquad (12.8)$$

where b = base and h = height.[4]

C. Cortical Bone

Collection and preservation of bones for cortical sample collection are the same as for whole bones. Long bones are usually sectioned with a band saw prior to removal of cortical samples.[23,24] The cortex can then be divided into regions and the samples subsequently lathed into right cylinders, or cylinders can be cored from diaphyseal sections using a diamond-tipped hole saw.[23,24] As before, physiological solution is applied to the bone during all trimming to provide moisture and cooling. Cortical samples are often collected from different areas of the bone for comparative purposes.[24] Samples are typically oriented with the long axis of the bone, although any direction is possible. The same methods of testing whole and cancellous bone samples in three-point bending described in Sections II.A and II.B, respectively, apply to cortical bone samples. The same methods and formulas as for cancellous bone described in Section II.B accomplish data collection and calculation.

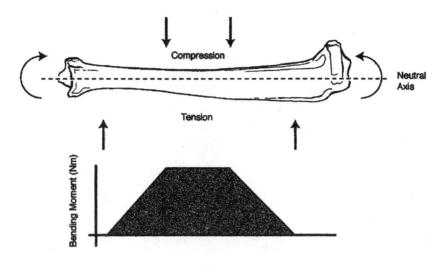

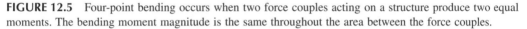

FIGURE 12.5 Four-point bending occurs when two force couples acting on a structure produce two equal moments. The bending moment magnitude is the same throughout the area between the force couples.

III. FOUR-POINT BENDING

Four-point bending occurs when two force couples acting on a structure produce two equal moments. A force couple refers to a pair of parallel forces of equal magnitude but opposite direction applied to a structure (Figure 12.5). The bending moment magnitude is the same throughout the area between the force couples; hence, the structure being tested should fracture at its weakest point. This arrangement is advantageous for testing where one might be uncertain about the strongest or weakest point and does not wish to influence the test by locating the maximum bending moment at a specific place. A clinical example of a four-point bending fracture is a femoral fracture through a previous fracture site resulting from one force couple formed by the posterior knee joint capsule and tibia and the other by the femoral head and hip joint capsule.

A. WHOLE BONE

Whole bone sample preparation is described in Section II.A.

The testing methods described in Section II.A for loading rates, application direction, and support span construction are essentially the same for three- and four-point bending. The major difference between three- and four-point bending is the construction of the actuator. The arms of the actuator are usually spaced such that the area of interest is located between them (see Figure 12.5). This ensures that the bending moment is uniform throughout that area. The size and material structure of the support span and actuator are again dictated by the specimen to be tested. For accurate results, the two central points of load application must contact the bone at the same time. Due to the irregular surface shape of some bones, the span between the actuator arms and hence the span tested may be limited. All points in contact with bone should be smooth and rounded to prevent stress concentration.

Data collection is the same as described for three-point bending in Section II.A. Calculations for some of the biomechanical parameters of interest are different due to differences in load application. Equations 12.2 and 12.3 can be used to calculate bending stress and area moment of inertia, respectively. For four-point bending, bending moment is calculated with the formula:

$$M = FL/6 \qquad\qquad (12.9)$$

where M = bending moment (N·m), F = applied force, and L = distance between two end supports. Breaking stress is calculated with the formula:

$$BS_{max} = M_{max}\, C/I = (F/2a)C/I \tag{12.10}$$

where BS = breaking stress (N/m^2), F = load at failure, a = distance from the end support to the nearest point of load application, $C = y_1/2$ = distance from the centroid to the surface (see Figure 12.4), and I = area moment of inertia.[6] Bending stress is calculated using Equation 12.10 at a point prior to the failure point. The modulus of elasticity is calculated with the formula:

$$E = [BS_{max}/2a^2(3L - 4a)]/(6Id_a) \tag{12.11}$$

where E = modulus of elasticity, BS_{max} = breaking stress, a = distance from the end support to the nearest point of load application, L = distance between end supports, I = area moment of inertia, and d_a = the deformation at the point of load application measured as actuator displacement.[6]

B. CANCELLOUS BONE

Cancellous bone sample preparation is described in Section II.B for three-point bending.[29] Testing methods are the same as described in Section II.B for three-point bending with the exception of the actuator, which must be modified for four-point bending as described previously for whole-bone four-point bending. Data collection is the same as described for three-point bending in Section II.A. The same basic formulas are used for biomechanical parameter calculation as in whole bone four-point bending with differences owing to the shape. Equation 12.9 is used to calculate bending moment. Equation 12.7 or 12.8 is used to calculate area moment of inertia of the sample depending on its shape. Equations 12.10 and 12.11 are used to calculate breaking and bending stresses and modulus of elasticity, respectively.

C. CORTICAL BONE

Cortical bone sample preparation is described in Section II.C for three-point bending. Testing methods are the same as described in Section II.C for three-point bending with actuator modifications as described previously. Data collection and calculation is accomplished by the same methods and formulas for cancellous bone described in Section III.B.[25]

IV. CANTILEVER TEST

Cantilever bending refers to a loading arrangement in which one end of the specimen is rigidly fixed while the other end is completely free. The bending moment varies from a maximum at the fixed end to zero at the force application point (Figure 12.6). This particular bending test may be applied to a whole bone or to part of a whole bone as well as to cancellous and cortical specimens.

A. WHOLE BONE

Whole bone sample collection and preservation is described in Section II.A. For cantilever testing, one end of the bone must be fixed with the area of interest free. This may be accomplished in a number of ways, the most common of which is to pot one end of the bone into a container. Potting materials include such substances as polyester resins and low-melting alloys.[26,27] Care must be taken to ensure that the material used to pot the bone does not affect the bone substance during the polymerization phase. The container may be made from anything ranging from PVC tubing to stainless steel, depending on the size of the specimen and the forces to be applied.[26-29] It is important

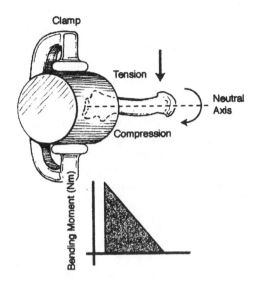

FIGURE 12.6   Cantilever bending refers to a loading arrangement in which one specimen end is rigidly fixed while the other end is completely free. The bending moment varies from a maximum at the fixed end to zero at the force application point.

to pot the bone centrally and to direct it parallel to the longitudinal axis of the potting container so that the orientation of applied forces does not vary between specimens when the sample is clamped in the mechanical testing system. A part of a whole bone may be prepared for cantilever bending as well. A specific example is application of vertical force to the femoral head of an intact proximal femur. The distal aspect of the femur is potted with the same principles of potting materials and orientation as for a whole-bone sample.[28]

The majority of cantilever bending testing is performed with the force applied at the point on the free end most distant from the fixed end of the bone so that the highest bending moment is obtained and the majority of the sample is included in the testing. The forces can be applied at different levels on the sample, however, with care taken to ensure that they are not applied directly on the area of interest. The side of the bone to which the load is applied depends on which surfaces are to be under tensile or compressive loads and thus which bending direction is desired. Specimens can also be oriented at different angles within the materials testing system to simulate various anatomical positions.[27] Cantilever bending requires an actuator with a single load application point. The actuator size and shape is dependent on the bone being tested. As described previously for other testing structures, the actuator should be smooth and of adequate material properties to withstand applied loads. Loading rates depend on the desired model and the bone being testing as described before. Examples of loading rates include 5 mm/min displacement for cantilever testing of human phalangeal specimens and 16 N/s loading for cantilever testing of intact rat femora.[26,27]

Data collection is the same as described for three-point bending in Section II.A. Area moment of inertia is calculated using Equation 12.3. The formula for bending moment for cantilever bending is:

$$M = FL \tag{12.12}$$

where M = bending moment (N·m), F = applied force, and L = distance between fixed end and applied load.[4] Breaking stress is provided by the formula:

$$BS_{max} = (F)(d)(C/2I) = F \sin \alpha / A + [(F \cos \alpha)d]C/I \tag{12.13}$$

where BS_{max} = breaking stress (N/m^2), F = load at failure, α = angle between fracture surface and the vertical, A = total cross-sectional area, d = distance between the fixed end and the applied load, C = distance from the centroid to the surface, and I = area moment of inertia.[28] Bending stress is calculated using Equation 12.13 at a point prior to the failure point.

B. CANCELLOUS BONE

Cancellous bone sample preparation is described in Section II.B for three-point bending. Potting procedures are the same as for cantilever testing of whole-bone specimens in Section IV.A. Cantilever testing methods for cancellous bone are the same as those for whole bone described in Section IV.A. with considerations made for size and shape of the samples. Data collection is the same as described for three-point bending in Section II.A. Area moment of inertia, bending moment, and bending and breaking stresses are calculated using Equations 12.7 or 12.8, 12.12, and 12.13, respectively.

C. CORTICAL BONE

Cortical bone sample preparation is described in Section II.C. for three-point bending. Potting procedures are the same as for cantilever testing of whole-bone specimens in Section IV.A. Cantilever testing methods for cancellous bone are the same as those for whole bone described in Section IV.A. with considerations made for size and shape of the samples. Data collection and calculation for cantilever bending of cortical bone are the same as for cancellous bone described in Section IV.B.

REFERENCES

1. Nordin, M. and Frankel, V.H., Biomechanics of bone, in *Basic Biomechanics of the Musculoskeletal System*, Nordin, R.W. and Frankel, V.H., Eds., Lea & Febiger, Philadelphia, 1989, 3.
2. Trostle, S.S. and Markel, M.D., Fracture biology, biomechanics, and internal fixation, *Vet. Clin. North Am. Food Anim. Pract.*, 12, 19, 1996.
3. Markel, M.D., Fracture biomechanics, in *Equine Fracture Repair*, Nixon, Ed., W.B. Saunders, Philadelphia, 1996, 10.
4. Tencer, A.F., Johnson, K.D., Kyle, R.F., and Fu, F.H., Biomechanics of fractures and fracture fixation, in *Instructional Course Lectures, American Academy of Orthopaedic Surgeons*, Heckman, J.D., Ed., Rand McNally, Taunton, MA, 1993, 19.
5. Ashman, R.B., Experimental techniques, in *Bone Mechanics*, Cowin, S.C., Ed., CRC Press, Boca Raton, FL, 1989, 75.
6. Hanson, P., Markel, M., and Vanderby, R., Jr., Diaphyseal structural properties of equine long bones, *Am. J. Vet. Res.*, 56, 233, 1995.
7. McDuffee, L.A., Stover, S.M., Taylor, K.T., and Les, C.M., An *in vitro* biomechanical investigation of an interlocking nail for fixation of diaphyseal tibial fractures in adult horses, *Vet. Surg.*, 23, 219, 1994.
8. Kasra, M., Vanin, C.M., MacLusky, N.J., et al., Effects of different estrogen and progestin regimens on the mechanical properties of rat femur, *J. Orthop. Res.*, 15, 118, 1997.
9. Walter, M.C., Smith, G.K., and Newton, C.D., Canine lumbar spinal internal fixation techniques, *Vet. Surg.*, 15, 191, 1986.
10. Bynum, D., Ledbetter, W.B., Boyd, C.L., and Ray, D.R., Flexural properties of equine metacarpus, *J. Biomed. Mater. Res.*, 5, 63, 1971.
11. Combs, N.R., Kornegay, E.T., Lindemann, M.D., et al., Calcium and phosphorus requirement of swine from weaning to market weight: II. Development of response curves for bone criteria and comparison of bending and shear bone testing, *J. Anim. Sci.*, 69, 682, 1991.
12. Jarvinen, T.L., Sievanen, H., Kannus, P., and Jarvinen M., Dual-energy X-ray absorptiometry in predicting mechanical characteristics of rat femur, *Bone*, 22, 551, 1998.

13. Currey, J.D., The mechanical consequences of variation in the mineral content of bone, *J. Biomech.*, 2, 1, 1969.
14. Pope, M.H. and Outwater, J.O, Mechanical properties of bone as a function of position and orientation, *J. Biomech.*, 7, 61, 1974.
15. Simkin, A. and Robin, G., The mechanical testing of bone in bending, *J. Biomech.*, 6, 31, 1973.
16. Specht, T.E., Miller, G.J., and Colahan, P.T., Effects of clustered drill holes on the breaking strength of the equine third metacarpal bone, *Am. J. Vet. Res.*, 51, 1242, 1990.
17. Brennan, J.J. and Aherne, F.X., The effect of dietary calcium and phosphorus levels on performance, bone bending moment and the severity of osteochondrosis and lameness in boars and gilts slaughtered at 100 or 130 kg body weight, *Can. J. Anim. Sci.*, 66, 777, 1986.
18. Crenshaw, T.D., Peo, E.R., Jr., Lewis, A.J., et al., Influence of age, sex and calcium and phosphorus levels on the mechanical properties of various bones in swine, *J. Anim. Sci.*, 52, 1319, 1981.
19. Kaneps, A.J., Stover, S.M., and Lane, N.E., Changes in canine cortical and cancellous bone mechanical properties following immobilization and remobilization with exercise, *Bone*, 21, 419, 1997.
20. Oden, Z.M., Selvitelli, D.M., Hayes, W.C., and Meyers, E.R., The effect of trabecular structure on DXA-based predictions of bovine bone failure, *Calcif. Tissue Int.*, 63, 67, 1998.
21. Banse, X., Delloye, C., Cornu, O., and Bourgois, R., Comparative left-right mechanical testing of cancellous bone from normal femoral heads, *J. Biomech.*, 29, 1247, 1996.
22. Wohl, G.R., Loehrke, L., Watkins, B.A., and Zernicke, R.F., Effects of high-fat diet on mature bone mineral content, structure, and mechanical properties, *Calcif. Tissue Int.*, 63, 74, 1998.
23. Courtney, A.C., Hayes, W.C., and Gibson, L.J., Age-related differences in post-yield damage in human cortical bone. Experiment and model, *J. Biomech.*, 29, 1463, 1996.
24. Les, C.M., Stover, S.M., Keyak, J.H., et al., The distribution of material properties in the equine third metacarpal bone serves to enhance saggital bending, *J. Biomech.*, 30, 355, 1997.
25. Bigot, G., Bouzidi, A., Rumelhart, C., and Martin-Rosset, W., Evolution during growth of the mechanical properties of the cortical bone in equine cannon-bones, *Med. Eng. Phys.*, 18, 79, 1996.
26. Battraw, G.A., Miera, V., and Anderson, P.L., et al., *J. Biomed. Mater. Res.*, 32, 285, 1996.
27. Campbell, J.T., Schon, L.C., Parks, B.G., et al., Mechanical comparison of biplanar proximal closing wedge osteotomy with plantar plate fixation vs. crescentic fixation for the correction of metatarsus primus varus, *Foot Ankle Int.*, 19, 293, 1998.
28. Hou, J.C., Salem, G.J., Zernicke, R.F., and Barnard, R.J., Structural and mechanical adaptations of immature trabecular bone to strenuous exercise, *J. Appl. Physiol.*, 69, 1309, 1990.
29. Salem, G.J., Zernicke, R.F., Martinez, D.A., and Vailas, A.C., Adaptations of immature trabecular bone to moderate exercise: geometrical, biochemical, and biomechanical correlates, *Bone*, 14, 647, 1993.

13 Torsional Testing of Bone

Benjamin R. Furman and Subrata Saha

CONTENTS

I. INTRODUCTION

During normal daily activities, the skeletal system is subjected to a complex system of loading exerted by the forces of gravity and the muscles attached to the bones. Such loading modes include tensile, compressive, bending, and torsional forces applied to the bones of the skeletal system. Therefore, in evaluating the tolerance limits of bones, it is important to determine the failure behavior of bones under all of these loading conditions. This chapter will discuss the testing of bones in torsion. This is important as many of the long bones as well as the spine are often subjected to a significant amount of torsional load. However, only limited information is available in the literature on the mechanical behavior of bones under torsion.[1-3] This is true for the torsional testing of whole bones as well as for testing machined compact and cancellous bone samples.[3,4] This is partly because most mechanical testing machines (both screw driven and servohydraulic) available in engineering schools in this country and abroad are suitable for tension, compression, or bending tests. One needs to use a specially designed test setup or a biaxial servohydraulic mechanical testing system for torsional testing of bones. Although screw-driven torsional testing machines exist, they are very rare. On the other hand, a pendulum type of torsional impact tester was popularized by Frankel and Burstein[5] in the 1960s and is a common mechanical testing machine in many biomechanics

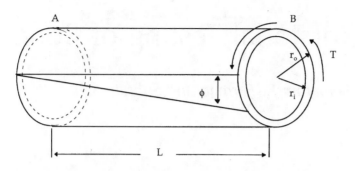

FIGURE 13.1   Simple torsional rotation of the free end of a hollow cylinder.

laboratories in this country, particularly in medical schools.[5-7] However, unless instrumented, such an impact tester only provides the information on the total energy to failure. When instrumented with a dynamic load cell and a suitable rotational measurement device, a pendulum-type torsional tester can provide information regarding the rotational stiffness, maximum torque, and the maximum rotational angle before failure.

It should be pointed out that for testing torsional properties of metallic implants, certain standards have been adopted by the American Society for Testing and Materials (ASTM).[8] However, no such standards exist for the mechanical testing of bones. Thus, when mechanical testing of bones is being planned, one should consider using the loading rate which would approximate the loading situation simulating the *in vivo* condition being examined.[9] Moreover, one should also remember that as bone is a viscoelastic material, mechanical property data generated from different experiments can only be compared if the loading rates employed are similar. It should also be noted that torsional testing is important in the evaluation of many surgical constructs using orthopaedic implants.[10-12]

II. THEORY OF TORSION FOR CYLINDERS

A diaphyseal segment from a long bone might be grossly approximated as a hollow cylindrical shaft made from a homogeneous, linear elastic material. Such a shaft might have a certain inner radius, r_i, an outer radius, r_o, and a length, L. If one end, A, of the shaft is fixed, and a torsional force, T, is applied to the opposite end, B, then end B will rotate in its own plane through some angle ϕ with respect to end A, as illustrated in Figure 13.1.

In order to find the shear stress, τ, in the material at any radius within the cross section of the shaft, the following simple formula is used as a guide[13]:

$$\tau = \frac{T\rho}{J} \qquad (13.1)$$

where J is the polar moment of inertia, which for a hollow cylinder is equal to $\pi(r_o^4 - r_i^4)/2$, and ρ is a specified radius, bounded by r_o and r_i. Thus, the maximum shear stress, τ_{max} is given by

$$\tau_{max} = \frac{Tr_o}{J} \qquad (13.2)$$

The relative angle between ends A and B is similarly given by

$$\phi = \frac{TL}{JG} \qquad (13.3)$$

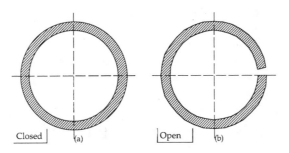

FIGURE 13.2   Cross-sectional view of a closed (a) and an open (b) cylinder.

where G is the elastic modulus of the bone in shear.

Since a cylindrical shaft is perfectly round in its perpendicular cross section, all cross sections along the entire length of the shaft will remain planar and parallel to one another. Any deviation in form away from this idealized cylindrical form will cause out-of-plane deformation to occur as torsional load is applied. Realizing that bones are not normally perfectly cylindrical in form, the authors emphasize that Equations 13.1 and 13.2 can only give rough approximations of the behavior observed in real bones. A closer approximation can be obtained from computed mechanical models using actual mechanical test data, especially when examining localized behaviors within a complex formation. An example of such a detailed analysis can be found in the work of Levenston et al.[14]

III. EFFECT OF STRUCTURAL DEFECTS

The theories described by Equations 13.1 and 13.2 are only valid for closed-section structures such as *intact* cortical bone. However, it is important to bear in mind two important structural deviations from the norm: so-called open structures, and closed structures containing small defects or holes.

First, consider that the torsional rigidity of *any* cylindrical structure, no matter how irregular, will be considerably reduced by a longitudinal cut or slit that continues along the entire or part of the length of the shaft. Such a slit is usually referred to as an "opening" in the structure.

To return again to an idealized case where there are ideal hollow cylinders, one open and one closed, which are otherwise identical in cross section (Figure 13.2), the open structure will have a torsional load-carrying capacity that is reduced (multiplied) by a factor of $t/3r$, where t is the wall thickness of the cylinder and r is its mean radius, with respect to the closed structure. One should always account for this difference, using the theoretical value as a rough guideline wherever a complete opening exists in the test specimen. This is especially important, for example, when comparing device designs for intramedullary nails. Exaggerated cases of open structure include devices having C-, U-, V-, and I-shaped cross sections.

Also of concern are holes, or incomplete openings, in the wall of a cylindrical material structure. Examples include pinholes in cortical bone or screw holes in prosthetic devices. Such defects will considerably reduce torsional strength as a matter of principle.[7,15,16] It is frequently useful in bio-mechanical testing to evaluate the effects of round holes placed in cortical bone to predict the relative likelihood of *in vivo* injury due to pin and/or screw placement. Most often, the effect of holes on the strength of the material is referred to as a *stress concentration* effect, whereby the localized stress in the material immediately surrounding the defect is higher than that predicted for the bulk of the material structure.[17-19] Perfectly round holes will increase the localized stress in the material by a certain *factor*, $\tau_{max}/\tau_{nominal}$, which is equal to 3 for an idealized structure loaded in simple torsion.[20] Other holes will have different stress concentration factors, depending on their size, shape, and orientation in combination with the loading mode for the structure. The intuitive conclusion is that peak failure loads should be expected to be considerably reduced, and this must always be planned for when setting up the expected ranges for load and deformation during a mechanical test.

Wherever it is desirable to predict the behavior of whole bones, which have complex geometries and orthotropic material properties, it is most convenient for the surgeon to investigate empirical results from mechanical testing. Mechanical testing, and torsional testing in particular, may be performed with a wide variety of equipment on a wide variety of bones — even those with unusual geometries — using a wide variety of loading modes. Please see the Further Reading list at the end of this chapter for a few examples.

IV. FIXATION TO THE TEST SYSTEM

For *in vitro* torsional testing, it is usually helpful to embed, or "pot," a portion of the bone into a moldable material such that intimate fixation can be achieved. This embedding material may, in turn, be held within a metal sleeve, cap, or other similar device in order to mate appropriately with the test machine.

The ideal embedding material should be easily formed, adhere well to the bony surface, become perfectly rigid once set, and be easily removable. While it is unrealistic to expect all of these characteristics from one material, there are a few materials available which may approximate to the ideal properties.

Epoxies and other self-curing, thermosetting polymers are perhaps the best embedding materials. They are available in liquid, paste, and dough forms that can all be suitably formed into close apposition with the bony surface. They undergo a low degree of shrinkage during curing and are also adhesive, thereby forming a strong bond with both the bone and any supporting metal devices once it is fully cured. The resulting construct is rigid enough for all practical purposes. If additional stiffness is required, reinforcing glass particles or short fibers may be added to the epoxy. Epoxies have the additional advantage of resistance to moisture. Once the epoxy has set, it can be completely submerged in saline without fear of loosening.

Many previous investigators have used polymethylmethacrylate (PMMA) bone cement as a embedding material because it is perceived to be "compatible" with bone. While it does have excellent working properties and sets up to be reasonably rigid in a short period of time, it may not be cost effective to use when compared with the "hardware store" epoxies. Moreover, the exotherm generated by curing PMMA is much higher than that of the epoxies.

Beyond the polymers, another choice of embedding material is Wood's metal. This alloy has a melting temperature of 70°C, which is accessible with a small warming plate. Unfortunately, the temperature is also high enough to cause protein denaturation; however, the metal quenches quite rapidly. Wood's metal offers the advantage of higher elastic modulus, as compared with the thermosetting polymers, while still conforming readily to irregular bony structures and being easy to use.[21]

In addition to or in place of embedding materials, pins and clamps may be used to hold the epiphyses of long bones. If used alone, they have the advantage of being easily removed. The fixtures will necessarily cause pinhole and clamping stresses at the attachment points; however, this should not cause any great difficulty if the test length of the specimen is far away from the attachment points and is expected to fail more readily than the fixed ends. Figure 13.3 shows an example of such fixation of a spine segment in a clamp, and Figure 13.4 shows the results of such torsional testing of a thoracolumbar spine segment using such a clamp.[22] If combined with an embedding material, pins can provide an additional mechanical interlock with the fixture.

V. AUTOMATED MECHANICAL TESTING SYSTEMS

A. SERVOHYDRAULIC SYSTEMS

The most flexible and commonly used mechanical testing systems for examining the torsional properties of materials under a wide variety of loading conditions are modern servohydraulic

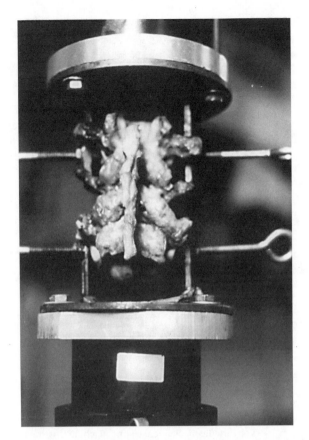

FIGURE 13.3 A thoracolumbar spine segment held by clamps for torsional testing in a servohydraulic mechanical testing system.

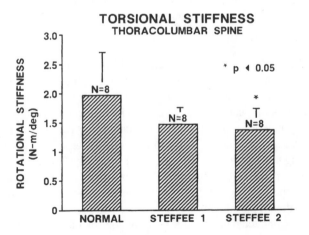

FIGURE 13.4 A comparison of the torsional stiffnesses of spine segments as evaluated by torsional testing. (Data from Reference 22.)

machines. All servohydraulic testing machines have a large load frame, a substantial hydraulic pump, a valve-controlled actuator piston, a linear variable differential transducer (LVDT) to measure the axial motion, and a load transducer or load "cell" to measure the axial thrust.[23]

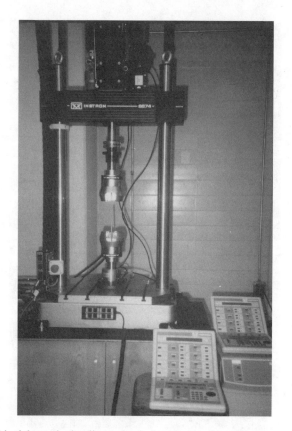

FIGURE 13.5   A new biaxial servohydraulic mechanical testing machine (Instron model 8874) with hydraulic grips. The electronic control panels are shown in the bottom right corner.

Biaxial testing systems are a special class of servohydraulic machines which can exert and respond to the torsional loads in addition to the axial loads (Figure 13.5).[23] In addition to the components mentioned above, these machines require a torsional actuation mechanism, a rotational variable differential transducer (RVDT) to measure the angular rotation, and a torque cell to measure the applied torque.

The LVDT, RVDT, load cell, and torque cell are all electromechanical transducers that yield to mechanical deformation and produce an electrical signal output which can be used as the *feedback* signal. Other transducers that generate useful feedback signals include resistive strain gauges and extensometers that can be applied externally to the specimen. In exactly the opposite way, the *actuator* responds to an electrical signal, called the *command* signal, by producing a mechanical motion. All servohydraulic control systems operate by carefully balancing the command and feedback signals to produce motion when necessary and generate information about the load–deformation response of the specimen. The machines cannot operate without the presence of a specimen because the specimen serves as a link between the command and feedback systems, as shown in the simplified diagram (Figure 13.6).

Testing is generally conducted under three types of control, or control mode: *load*, *deformation*, and *strain*. Most testing is conducted under displacement control; however, there are situations where the other two control modes are quite useful.

In load control mode, the system controller allows a specified command signal (voltage) to be applied to the actuator, which responds immediately by moving. The system controller oversees the test by continually monitoring the load/torque cell feedback. After some time, when a specified

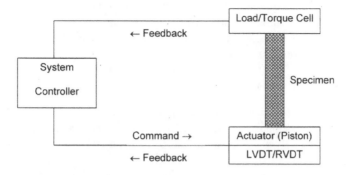

FIGURE 13.6 Control/feedback linkage including specimen.

feedback from the load/torque cell is detected by the system controller, the controller will no longer signal the actuator to move, and the loading cycle is completed. The difference between the starting load and the total expected load is called the *load range* for the test. The rate at which voltage is applied to the actuator by the system controller is determined by the machine operator and is called the *loading rate*. The voltage may vary linearly, sinusoidally, or according to some other continuous function. This type of control mode is quite useful for fatigue testing, where load is varied cyclically over a specified range.

In deformation control mode, the machine operator again determines the rate at which voltage is applied to the controller, but in this case the controller input is a signal from the LVDT/RVDT. The total expected actuator motion is called the *displacement range*, and the controller voltage is based on the *displacement rate*. For biological materials, which are generally much more compliant than the machine itself, the machine displacement may be considered approximately equal to the overall specimen deformation. Once a test has begun, feedback from the LVDT/RVDT is recorded and measured vs. either (1) the displacement feedback from the LVDT/RVDT or (2) the specimen strain feedback from an external transducer. The resulting plot indicates how well the specimen has withstood a given loading. Most tests performed in this way are run slowly, or *quasi-statically*. After the specimen has failed, the actuator continues to move until a displacement limit has been reached. It is usually convenient to stop the test manually.

In strain control mode, the controller will apply a command signal until a specified level of feedback from an external strain gauge or extensometer is detected. Fatigue testing can be performed over a specified *strain range*, and some machine operators prefer this control method to load control.

The feedback signals from the electromechanical transducers are usually amplified by circuitry in the controller, and the amplified signals can be used to drive a host of plotters to generate curves of applied load vs. linear displacement, torque vs. angular rotation, etc. The most sophisticated systems read the output signals by computer, and the associated software packages are usually quite convenient for calculating the work of fracture and the elastic moduli for a given test.

Biaxial servohydraulic testing systems (see Figure 13.5) often require a significant amount of floor space and other resources to operate but can give a wealth of information in return. More recently, system manufacturers have been introducing smaller, more specialized machines to handle small-scale testing. It is important to match machine size with the expected range of specimens to be tested.

Another point of significance is that servohydraulic machines are very quick to respond to controller input and are capable of generating extremely high or extremely low loading rates. This can be useful for simulating impact in one test and creep in the next. It should be noted here, however, that no mechanical testing system may be able to match perfectly the desired loading profile with respect to time, whether it be linear, sinusoidal, or some other profile. The most sophisticated servohydraulic systems offer digital control and very fine sensitivity; however, simpler systems can often be used with good success depending upon the desired accuracy. These include the manually operated pendulum machines described in the introduction as well as electromechanical systems made from inexpensive equipment. Electromechanical systems make up the second most versatile class of automated testing equipment.

B. ELECTROMECHANICAL SYSTEMS

For the purpose of testing long bones, some researchers have devised cost-effective, purpose-built torsional machines from existing motor-driven equipment (such as a lathe). It has been demonstrated that these systems can reliably and consistently perform torque-to-failure tests when using angular testing rates in the range of 3 to 12°/second.[24]

One group of Finnish researchers used a particularly cost-effective approach.[25] They replaced the original motor of an existing lathe with an overscaled asynchronous motor capable of producing continuous torque up to 250 N·m. Generally, electric motors operate best at a nearly fixed rotational speed, and so the group was careful to select a motor rated for maximal torque at a desirable speed. They chose an angular rate of 6°/s. (It is to be understood that no electric motor has a perfectly linear response, and yet the results can be reliable if the average speed of the motor falls within the range described above and has minimal deviation.) The lathe was equipped with a torque cell at the fixed end. The total machine inaccuracy, including the linearity error of the motor, strain gauge sensitivity, repeatability error, sensor asymmetry, and output baseline instability, was determined to be less than 1.0%. The whole-method error for torsional testing of sheep tibiae was reported to be 3.0%. This is sufficiently accurate for the routine testing of long bones.

It should be noted here that very high loading rates can increase the apparent torque required to fracture long bones since less time is allowed for microcracks to develop and to dissipate fracture energy.[6] While it can be useful to test bones at a high rate to simulate transient loading conditions *in vivo*, it would be unwise to try to simulate slow fracture with an abbreviated test.

C. SYSTEM SELECTION

Custom-built equipment is naturally less flexible but can be less expensive than a complex servohydraulic system. The researcher must therefore determine the type of tests necessary to fulfill both the short- and long-term goals. When selecting a test machine, one should first consider the geometric needs and constraints: (1) What are the longest and shortest bones to be tested? (2) Will there ever be any bulky augmentation, such as external fixators, applied to the bone? Second, determine precisely what loading modes are most important: (1) Will the testing be limited to simple torsion? (2) Will biaxial loading be necessary in future studies? (3) Will there be a need for transient loads, such as impact, to be applied at any point during any of the tests?

VI. *IN VITRO* TESTING METHODOLOGY FOR SERVOHYDRAULIC SYSTEMS

A. ADJUSTING THE CROSSHEAD POSITION

The crosshead of the machine may be lowered or raised in order to bring the actuator and load cell closer together or farther apart, respectively. It is the relative position of the crosshead that lends versatility to servohydraulic machines in terms of the range of specimen sizes that can be tested. The actual testing ranges are generally much smaller.

Lowering of the crosshead is performed by the action of gravity alone, and the hydraulic pump should not be turned on during this operation. Lowering is achieved by releasing the hydraulic clamp and lowering valve in succession. Alternatively, the crosshead may be raised only when the hydraulic pump is *on*. Again, the hydraulic clamp is released, followed by the raising valve. The rate of crosshead motion is controlled by the degree to which the valves are opened and is stopped by closing the valves and the clamp. It is important to close but not to overtighten the valves.

B. Internal Controller Calibration

Many recent control systems are self-calibrating, but older units will occasionally require that the internal feedback and command signals be brought into alignment as a taring operation whenever fixtures and/or specimens are changed. Follow the manufacturer's instructions carefully to determine whether and how an adjustment should be made. For most tests, it is desirable for the load, torque, and displacements to begin at zero.

C. External Load Calibration

Another important calibration determines whether the output device (plotter, computer, etc.) registers a known load correctly. All load/torque cells will have a range over which they should respond linearly to applied forces, and that range should not be exceeded. The use of three or more different dead loads will allow the checking of the accuracy of the readout as well as the linearity of the load/torque cell. If the readout is not accurate, then the output device must be adjusted. If the readout is not linear to within a specified error, then the load/torque cell should be checked before testing.

D. Test Preparation: The Ramp Test

A number of settings can be made before the machine is actually turned on. These are detailed as follows. For a linear ramp test, the system controller function generator output must be set to increase linearly with time. This is true whether the test is to be controlled by load or by displacement. Make sure that the function selector of the function generator is switched to the ramp function. Afterward, select the mode of the test as being positive or negative, depending on which direction of actuator motion is desired.

Destructive tensile, compressive, torsional, and combined tests are often performed to determine the load under which yielding or ultimate failure takes place. In order to conduct this type of test, the test is often run in the displacement control mode. This type of control results in a continuous change in the position of the actuator with respect to time, and the displacement rate is predetermined before testing begins. The displacement rate is given as a measure of the displacement per unit time and is determined by reverse-calculation from the available controller settings.

The full displacement range of many actuators is less than 4 in. axially and $\pm 45°$ rotationally. If torsional testing is to be combined with tension or compression, the percentage of the total axial displacement range to be used is sometimes manually selected. This is important when the displacement range of the test to be conducted is much less than the overall range of the device. The reason is that the feedback signal from the LVDT will be relatively weak at small fractions of its total range, and the controller must therefore be set to amplify the signal. Generally, it is important to match the axial displacement capabilities of the machine with the type of tests to be done, but reliable data can be obtained using as little as 10% of the available displacement. Finally, the plotter resolution can be adjusted for the desired output scale over the expected range of the test.

E. General Ramp Testing Procedure

The hydraulic pump should be turned on and allowed to build pressure for a few minutes. While the pump is building pressure, the specimen may be fixed appropriately to the load/torque cell of the machine. Afterward, it is desirable to re-zero the load and displacement feedback signals at the controller. Next, the actuator may be turned on. It may "jump" slightly upon being turned on; however, the operator should also be certain that the function generator of the controller is not running. Once the hydraulic actuator is on, the actuator piston can be lowered or raised until the upper fixture is in the appropriate position for mounting the remaining free end of the specimen. If careful preparation has been made, the piston should not have to move very far.

Note: Safety glasses **must** be worn any time the actuator is on. This is of extreme importance for the safety of all personnel working directly with or in the close vicinity of the machine. Prescription glasses are acceptable for this purpose only if they have polycarbonate lenses with side shields.

Once the actuator is turned on under active displacement control, any change in the command signal from the controller will cause the actuator to move. Engaging the function generator of the controller begins the test. Before operating the function generator, be sure that the load feedback at the start of the test is at the desired level. If the test is to be performed after some preload, make sure to apply it manually prior to starting the function generator. Likewise, if the test fixtures have generated any unwanted preload, it may be manually relaxed.

Note: In some cases it is appropriate to "condition" the specimen by applying a small fraction of the expected load and then releasing it. This is especially important for any specimen that is difficult to seat in the testing fixtures.

Again, ensure that the ramp function of the function generator is selected and that the test will occur in the appropriate direction ("+" or "−"). Double check all controller settings, paying special attention to the function generator ramp rate. Finally, prepare the recording device and begin the test. Be ready to use any available emergency stop switches in case of difficulty. At the completion of the test, stop the function generator and wait for it to reset to its original position.

F. TEST PREPARATION: THE FATIGUE TEST

Fatigue testing is almost always performed with a sinusoidally varying command signal, and the function generator of the controller should be set to operate in that capacity with the desired frequency and load/strain ranges. Many controllers operate based on the half-cycle amplitude of the function. Be sure to check the manufacturer's instructions for calculating the function parameters correctly. Fatigue tests can be conducted in either load or strain control mode. However, it may be easier to start it in displacement control mode and then transfer to load or strain control after the preloading conditions have been achieved.

Rotational and axial fatigue can both be performed in five different capacities: positive-positive, negative-negative, zero-positive, zero-negative, and positive-negative. As an example, take the case of positive-positive torsional fatigue under load control. The specimen will experience positive torsional loading at all times. A positive torsional preload, or *mean level*, is placed on the specimen, and subsequent loading cycles are superimposed over that level. For example, the preload may be equal to 5 N·m while the half-cycle amplitude is 1 N·m. The test will then cycle between 4 and 6 N·m. Negative-negative tests behave the same way, but in the reverse direction. Zero-positive and zero-negative tests have no preload. Positive-negative tests may use any type of preload (or none at all) as long as the torsional direction reverses at some point in each cycle.

Load-controlled tests will obtain their feedback from the load/torque cell, while strain-controlled tests require the use of external gauges. The latter must be calibrated to work properly with the system controller and its function generator. As with the ramp test, the displacement ranges should also be set to provide the appropriate amplification of the LVDT/RVDT feedback signal if the displacement is to be monitored.

G. GENERAL FATIGUE TESTING PROCEDURE

Begin the test in displacement control mode, as with the ramp test. Preload the specimen to the desired level, and adjust the mean level of the load/strain controller to match the preload. Once the preload has been applied, the control modes may be switched. After changing control modes, the function generator of the controller may be started. This begins the test. After the test specimen has failed, the machine will continue to run unless axial and rotational displacement limits have been applied. These should be available and apparent on the controller. Refer to the manufacturer's instructions for setting the limits. Once a limit has been exceeded, the actuator will turn itself off. Cycle counters and oscilloscopes can be easily used to monitor the load/torque cell feedback instantaneously. Alternatively, computer software acquisition will allow a more complete feedback history to be recorded.

H. THE CREEP TEST

The creep test is the simplest test to operate from a machine perspective, yet it can be the most difficult test to instrument. It will always be performed under load control. As with the fatigue test, however, the servohydraulic machine may be difficult to start in the load control mode. Rather, the test may be started under stroke control, and the operator may manually adjust the controller to obtain a desired static preload. Once the preload is achieved, the machine may be switched to load control, at which point the machine will maintain the set preload for as long as is desired. Over time, the bone will begin to creep, and the resulting machine displacement or strain feedback signals can be monitored. Since creep is a very slow and small-scale phenomenon, the displacement feedback will most likely be of little use. Resistive strain gauges, on the other hand, can provide more detailed information about what changes have taken place over a small region of the bone. These gauges must be carefully placed over the region of interest with cyanoacrylate adhesives. They are delicate instruments, and it is most useful to monitor the small feedback signals with a computerized acquisition system.

Some authors have used a specially designed apparatus to study the torsional creep behavior of compact bone.[26] Such equipment can be built inexpensively by applying the torque by means of dead loads with pulleys and lever arms.

VII. SUMMARY

Torsional testing is a uniquely capable technique for examining the *in vitro* mechanical properties of a wide variety of bones. Servohydraulic testing equipment can be a straightforward means to obtain a large amount of torsional data using different loading modes. Electromechanical and manually operated machines can be produced economically for purpose-specific torsional studies. Gross approximations of torsional stress in diaphyseal bone may be calculated using simple linear elastic mechanic theories; however, more accurate and detailed theoretical treatments may require the use of computational mathematics. Empirical torsional testing is often the most efficient means for the surgeon to obtain useful mechanical data. Torsional data may correlate well with many common injury scenarios.

REFERENCES

1. Evans, F.G., *Mechanical Properties of Bone*, Charles C Thomas, Springfield, IL, 1973.
2. Evans, F.G., *Stress and Strain in Bones*, Charles C Thomas, Springfield, IL, 1957.
3. Hayes, W.C. and Carter, D.R., Biomechanics of bone, in *Skeletal Research: An Experimental Approach*, Simmons, D.J. and Kunin, A.S., Eds., Academic Press, New York, 1979, 263.

4. Saha, S., Dynamic strength of bone and its relevance, in *Osteoarthromechanics,* Ghista, D.N., Ed., McGraw-Hill, New York, 1982, 1.
5. Burstein, A.H. and Frankel, V.H., A standard test for laboratory animal bone, *J. Biomech.,* 4, 155, 1971.
6. Sammarco, G.J., Burstein, A.H., Davis, W.L., and Frankel, V.H., The biomechanics of torsional fractures: the effect of loading on ultimate properties, *J. Biomech.,* 4, 113, 1971.
7. Medige, J., Mindell, E.R., and Doolittle, T., Remodeling of large, persistent bone defects, *Clin. Orthop.,* 69, 275, 1982.
8. ASTM, Standard test method for measuring the torsional properties of metallic bone screws, in *1997 Book of ASTM Standards,* 13.01, ASTM, West Conshohocken, PA, 1997, 958.
9. Archdeacon, M.T., Davy, K.J., and Jepsen, K.J., Time dependent damage accumulation in bovine cortical bone loaded in torsion, *Orthop. Trans.,* 21, 731, 1997–98.
10. Bankston, A.B., Keating, M., and Saha, S., The biomechanical evaluation of intramedullary nails in distal femoral shaft fractures, *Clin. Orthop.,* 276, 272, 1992.
11. Hajek, P.D., Bicknell, H.R., Bronson, W.E., et al., Clinical and biomechanical analysis of one vs. two distal screws in the treatment of femoral shaft fractures with locked intramedullary nails, *J. Bone Joint Surg.,* 75A, 519, 1993.
12. Albright, J.A., Thompson, T., and Saha, S., The principles of internal fixation, in *Orthopaedic Mechanics: Procedures and Devices,* Ghista, D.N. and Roaf, R., Eds., Academic Press, New York, 1978, 124.
13. Beer, F.P. and Johnston, E.R., Jr., *Mechanics of Materials,* McGraw-Hill, New York, 1992, 114.
14. Levenston, M.E., Beaupré, G.S., and Van der Meulen, M.C.H., Improved method for analysis of whole bone torsion tests, *J. Bone Miner. Res.,* 9, 1459, 1994.
15. Brooks, D.B., Burstein, A.H., and Frankel, V.H., The biomechanics of torsional fractures — the stress concentration effect of a screw hole, *J. Bone Joint Surg.,* 52A, 507, 1970.
16. Clark, C.R., Morgan, C., Sonstegard, D.A., and Mathews, L.S., The effect of biopsy-hole shape and size on bone strength, *J. Bone Joint Surg.,* 59A, 213, 1977.
17. Currey J., Stress concentration in bone, *Q. J. Microsc. Sci.,* 103, 111, 1962.
18. Nowinski, J.L., Effects of holes and perforations on the strength and stress distribution in bone elements, in *Osteoarthromechanics,* Ghista, D.N., Ed., Hemisphere Publishing, Washington, D.C., 1982, 180.
19. Saha, S., Stress concentration in bone: an experimental and theoretical investigation, in *Biomedical Engineering II: Recent Developments,* Hall, C.W., Ed., Pergamon Press, New York, 1983, 367.
20. Ugural, A.C. and Fenster, S.K., *Advanced Strength and Applied Elasticity,* Prentice-Hall, Upper Saddle River, NJ, 1995.
21. Won, H.Y., Lounci, S., Chen, D., et al., Influence of bounding conditions on torsional structural testing of canine tibial diaphysis, in *Proceedings of the Combined Orthopaedic Research Societies Meeting,* September 28–30, Hamamatsu, Japan, 1998.
22. Lipka, J.M., Saha, S., Keating, E.M., and Albright, J.A., The biomechanical analysis of a simulated spondylolysis fracture and its contribution to lumbar spine rigidity, in *Biomedical Engineering V: Recent Developments,* Saha, S., Ed., Pergamon Press, New York, 1986, 521.
23. Instron, *Guide to Advanced Materials Testing,* Instron Corporation, Canton, MA, 1997.
24. Strömberg, L. and Dálen, N., Experimental measurement of maximum torque capacity of long bones, *Acta Orthop. Scand.,* 47, 257, 1976.
25. Jämsä, T. and Jalovaara, P., A cost-effective, accurate machine for testing the torsional strength of sheep long bones, *Med. Eng. Phys.,* 18, 433, 1996.
26. Lakes, R. and Saha, S., Long term torsional creep in compact bone, *J. Biomech. Eng.,* 102, 178, 1980.

FURTHER READING

Brånemark, R., Öhrnell, L.-O., Nilsson, P., and Thomsen, P., Biomechanical characterization of osseointegration during healing: an experimental *in vivo* study in the rat, *Biomaterials,* 18, 969, 1997.
Cervantes, C., Badison, J. B., Miller, G.J., and Casar, R.S., An *in vitro* biomechanical study of a multiplanar circular external fixator applied to equine third metacarpal bones, *Vet. Surg.,* 25, 1, 1996.
Dueland, R.T., Berglund, L., Venderby, R., and Chao, E.Y., Structural properties of interlocking nails, canine femora, and femur-interlocking nail constructs, *Vet. Surg.,* 25, 386, 1996.

Farfan, H.F., Cossette, J.W., Wells, R.V., and Kraus, H., The effects of torsion on the lumbar intervertebral joints: the role of torsion in the production of disc degeneration, *J. Bone Joint Surg.*, 52A, 468, 1970.

Hopper, S.A., Schneider, R.K., Ratzlaff, M.H., et al., Effect of pin hole size and number on *in vitro* bone strength in the equine radius loaded in torsion, *Am. J. Vet. Res.*, 59, 201, 1998.

Malkani, A.L., Voor, M.J., Fee, K.A., and Bates, C.S., Femoral component revision using impacted morsellised cancellous graft: a biomechanical study of implant stability, *J. Bone Joint Surg.*, 78B, 973, 1996.

Netz, P., Eriksson, K., and Strömberg, L., Material reaction of diaphyseal bone under torsion: an experimental study on dogs, *Acta Orthop. Scand.*, 51, 223, 1980.

Seltzer, K.L., Stover, S.M., Taylor, K.T., and Willits, N.H., The effect of hole diameter on the torsional mechanical properties of the equine third metacarpal bone, *Vet. Surg.*, 25, 371, 1996.

14 Indentation Testing of Bone

Brodie E. McKoy, Qian Kang, and Yuehuei H. An

CONTENTS

I. INTRODUCTION

Hardness of a solid material is defined as its resistance to penetration by another solid body. Hardness or indentation tests measure hardness by driving an indenter with a specified geometry into a sectional surface of the material. The tests can be categorized based on the geometry and/or the size of the indenter employed. With different geometries there are Brinell, Rockwell, Vickers, and Knoop indenters (Figure 14.1). Based on the size of the indenter, macroindentation, micro-hardness, and nanoindentation are defined. All of these tests are used for biomechanical studies of bone. Each of these methods assesses bone structures at different scales based on the sizes of the specimens and the indenters.

    Bone is a hierarchical structure.[1] In order to understand its mechanical properties as a whole, one must understand the mechanical properties of its constituent parts. The various levels of organization of bone can be tested by the different categories of indentation tests. Based on the work by Rho et al.[1] and Hoffler et al. (Chapter 8), the hierarchical structure of bone can be simplified into four levels: (1) macrostructure: cancellous or cortical bone; (2) microstructure (1 to 500 μm): Haversian systems, osteons; (3) submicrostructure/nanostructure (200 nm to 1 μm): fibrillar collagen and lamella; and (4) subnanostructure (less than 200 nm): molecular structure of constituent elements. Macroindentation, microhardness, and nanoindentation tests can be used to study the macro-structure, microstructure, and submicrostructure of bone, respectively. Hardness values differ according to the bone structure being indented. Since it is not possible to extrapolate the mechanical properties of the bone from a single indentation test, it is ideal to perform different tests at various levels of the bone structure.

II. MAJOR INDENTATION TESTS

A. MACROINDENTATION TESTS

Macroindentation testing evaluates bone mechanical properties at the macrostructural level. Bone at this level is considered either cortical or cancellous. These types of bone are distinguished most readily by their amount of porosity.[2,3] Definitive differentiation is achieved only by microscopic

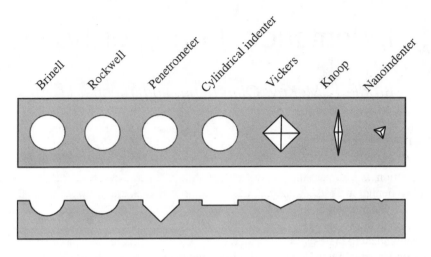

FIGURE 14.1   The typical indentations of common indentation tests.

evaluation of the tissue microstructure. The mechanical properties of bone at this level, including hardness, are important for bone-related research as well as clinical purposes. Numerous investigators have studied the mechanical properties of bone using this type of indentation testing. Several different tests are of historical as well as functional interest.

The first indentation test was reported in 1900 by Brinell and co-workers using a spherical indenter (a steel ball).[4] The Brinell hardness value can be obtained by the following equations:

$$\text{Brinell Hardness (BH)} = P/A \quad (\text{N/mm}^2) \tag{14.1}$$

where P is the applied load and A is indentation area measured after withdrawing the ball. Following the pioneering work of Brinell, Lexer in 1929 evaluated the hardness of bone macroscopically.[5] Using a 3-mm steel ball and a large load, this investigator produced indentations in bone to assess its hardness. He found no variation of hardness with illness or age. The design of these original tests have persisted throughout the twentieth century with only minor modifications.

The Brinell method has been used to measure the hardness of cancellous bone of human patella[4] and fracture callus material.[6,7] Equation 14.1 was used by Björkstrom and Goldie.[4] For the method used by Markel et al.,[6,7] only a simple value of indentation (N/mm) was drawn from the test when the indentation depth was maintained the same for all of the specimens. A modified Brinell's hardness test was reported by Aro et al.[8] using the following equation for calculation of hardness value:

$$\text{Modified Brinell Hardness (MBH)} = 2P/\pi dD \quad (\text{N/mm}^2) \tag{14.2}$$

where P is the applied load, d is the diameter of the indenter, and D is the depth of the indentation.

The Rockwell superficial hardness test is another indentation test which measures hardness of materials at the macrostructural level.[9] Originally, this test was used to test metals with a rough surface finish. Doppler modified this test to allow the testing of cancellous bone samples by decreasing the major load.[10] A minor load (3 kg) is first applied and the resulting indenter position is used as the zero point. Next, the major load (5 kg) is applied and then removed. The permanent indentation depth produced by the major load is measured.[11,12] Recently, several investigators have used this technique to measure the hardness of bovine and human bone.[9,13] As in the Brinell hardness test, a spherical indenter is used. However, the incremental depth is used as hardness number without considering the indentation area.

The osteopenetrometer reported by Sneppen and Hvid et al.[14-16] also measures the hardness of bone at the macrostructural level. The osteopenetrometer was originally developed as purely a mechanical construction which measured the force of penetration of a needle into bone by means of strain gauges, and depth of penetration by means of a differential transformer. The current systems contain a hydraulic system between the recording unit and the needle.[17] The osteo-penetrometer operates by recording the force necessary to penetrate the cancellous bone with a 2.5-mm-diameter pointed needle, with the shaft milled to 2.3 mm to avoid friction, as a function of the depth of penetration. This test is an indentation test with a small indenter (a 90° conical profile) which travels into the bone up to 6 to 12 mm. The evaluation program disregards the initial 1.5 mm depth interval, which "represents increasing contact with the measuring profile"; the average force per unit area of the measuring needle of the following consecutive 2 mm depth intervals (2 to 5 mm) is used to represent the penetration strength of that interval. Agreement has been found between the penetration test and conventional compression test on the same bony structure. Hvid et al.[18] found correlation coefficients of close to 0.90 when ultimate stress data was compared between the osteopenetrometer and conventional compression tests. The advantage of this method is that it can be used during surgery. Intraoperative recording of bone strength may be beneficial in individualizing the choice of prosthetic design and postoperative rehabilitation programs. The authors used this method for measuring the bone strength of human upper tibia and calcaneous.

The most popular macroindentation test uses flat-ended cylindrical indenters.[19-21] It has been used for examining the mechanical properties of cancellous bone from different subjects. In this indentation test, an indenter is driven into a sectional bone surface. Although the failure mechanisms are more complicated and less clear than the conventional compression test, it is useful for examining the mechanical properties of small cancellous bones of different species. Because of the ease of specimen fabrication, the use of the indentation test has increased in recent years.[22] The test is simpler than the compression test which uses cubed or cylindrical samples. Only a flat sample surface of minimal thickness is needed for indentation tests. Recent reports describe the use of the indentation test for measuring the mechanical properties of rat,[23] rabbit,[22] canine,[24] and bovine[25] cancellous bone.

B. MICROHARDNESS TESTS

The microhardness test is an indentation test using a specially designed testing device with a very small indentor.[26] Microhardness indentations range from 20 to 150 mm in length. At this range, this test evaluates materials at the microstructural level of bone such as individual osteons or Haversian systems. In 1936, Lips and Sack[27] introduced the first metallurgical microscope and with this microhardness testers became available.

Vickers and Knoop are the two main types of microhardness indenters used today. The Vickers has a pyramidal diamond indenter with an apical angle of 136° between the faces. Vickers can also be used as a macrohardness test. The Knoop indenter has a rhombic-shaped pyramidal diamond, with a longitudinal angle of 172° 30′ and a transverse angle of 130°. Both methods are mainly used to examine the hardness of metals, plastics, composites,[27] or polymers. Several investigators have reported on the application of microhardness tests to bone samples[5,28-30] including cortical bone,[31,32] trabecular bone,[33] woven callus bone,[34,35] and bone adjacent to endosseous implants.[36,37]

Using the Vickers and Knoop indenters, the hardness values have units of kg/mm². The Vickers microhardness number (VHN or HV) is calculated using the following equation:[38,39]

$$VHN = HV = 1.8544P/D^2$$

(14.3)

where P is the applied load in kg and D is the mean of the length of d_1 and d_2 (the two diagonals of the indentation) in mm. The Knoop microhardness number (HK) is calculated using the following equation:[31,40]

$$HK = \frac{P}{A} = \frac{P}{CL^2} \qquad (14.4)$$

where P is the applied load in kg, A is the unrecovered projected area of indentation (mm^2), L is the measured length (mm) of the long diagonal, and C (0.07028) is a constant for the indenter relating the projected area of the indentation to the square of the length of the long diagonal.

C. Nanoindentation Tests

Nanoindentation tests allow very small microstructural features to be studied. This method can evaluate bone at the submicrostructural level which includes individual lamella of an osteon and trabeculae.[41,42] The development of nanoindentation over the past several years has allowed the evaluation of component properties (*in situ*). This technique allows the intrinsic properties of individual submicrostructural components to be studied without the influences of inhomogeneities in the macro- and microstructure.

Recently, nanoindentation has been used to study individual trabeculae of human vertebrae and tibia.[41,42] Elastic moduli and the hardness of individual lamella within an osteon have been evaluated. Investigators have used this technique to show differences in hardness in both transverse and longitudinal directions of bone. Even though this test is currently performed predominately with dry bone, nanoindentation has greatly increased knowledge of bone mechanical properties.

III. MACROINDENTATION TESTS USING A CYLINDRICAL INDENTER

Numerous investigators have used this method to assess the hardness of bone. In humans, the indentation stiffness of the patella,[5] distal femur,[20] tibial plateau,[21] distal tibia,[43] and head and neck of the femur[44] has been evaluated. Several animal models have been studied with the flat-ended indenter. This method of indentation is accepted by many researchers.

The indentation test using a flat-ended cylindrical indenter has been applied to different animal bones in the authors' laboratory, including epiphysometaphyseal cancellous bones of rats, rabbits, dogs, and goats.[22,23,45] The methods of performing the indentation tests in these various animals are similar. In the authors' laboratory, the selected bones (rat, rabbit, dogs, and cows) are rough-cut using a band saw. They are then ground on a rotating wheel grinder to a proscribed level in the cancellous bone at the epiphysis or metaphysis to create a surface for testing.

After the first surface is created, two different methods can be used to position the specimen on the testing platform. In the first method, a parallel cut is made next to the first ground surface to create a second surface to be set against the specimen-holding platform. The second method involves potting the specimen. Instead of performing the second cut, the specimen can be potted in dental stone or plaster of paris for positioning on the platform. Both of these methods have been used successfully in the authors' laboratory. The latter is especially suitable for small specimens.

In the authors' laboratory, a mechanical testing system (MTS, Minneapolis, MN) is used for the indentation test. It is operated in displacement control, and is calibrated using an extensometer. After the specimen to be tested is prepared, the platform holding the specimen is leveled to ensure that the loading is perpendicular to the specimen surface to be tested. A cylindrical stainless-steel indenter with a flat-ended surface, ranging from 1.3 to 5.0 mm in diameter, is used. After the specimen is positioned on the platform and the indenter adjusted close to the specimen surface, the indenter is driven into the bone at a constant slow rate (1 mm/min in the authors' laboratory).

The loading is stopped manually when the load–displacement curve passes the ultimate load (the highest point of the curve).

Using this indentation test, the ultimate load, stiffness, ultimate strength (ultimate stress), and elastic modulus of the bone can be obtained directly or calculated from the load–deformation curve. The ultimate indentation strength is calculated using the following equation:

$$\sigma = 4\ P/\pi d^2 \qquad\qquad (14.5)$$

where P is the ultimate indentation load and d is the diameter of the indenter. By utilizing the formula developed by Timoshenko and Goodier[46] and validated recently by Sumner et al.,[24] the local modulus of elasticity (E) for each test site is calculated with the following formula:

$$E = S(1 - v^2)/d \qquad\qquad (14.6)$$

where S is the indentation stiffness (N/mm) and d (mm) is the diameter of the indenter. As used by Sumner et al.[24] and Aitken et al.,[43] the Poisson's ratio (v) is assumed to be 0.2 according to Vasu et al.[47]

Recent reports describe the use of the indentation test for measuring the mechanical properties of rat,[23] rabbit,[22] canine, and bovine[48] cancellous bones. Differences in mechanical properties were found between epiphyseal cancellous bones at different locations. The reason for this phenomenon is the functional difference between the different locations.[49] For example, the humeral head bears less load compared with the femoral head, so the ultimate strength of the cancellous bones of humeral head is less than that of the femoral head. Correlation has been obtained between indentation depth (at 50 N load) and ultimate strength ($R = -0.937$, $p < 0.05$), meaning that with the increase of ultimate strength the indentation depth or deformation decreased proportionally.

Sumner et al.[24] have verified that the data obtained from the indentation tests correlate well with that from conventional compressive tests. Kang et al.[25] showed that ultimate load, stiffness, and ultimate strength, measured by the indentation test were higher than those measured by the compression test. This group also found a significant correlation between compression testing and indentation testing with correlation values of 0.823 to 0.952. Although the ultimate strength and elastic modulus of different cancellous bones from different subjects are not the same, they generally fall into a certain range, like that of compression tests. According to the data pooled from the literature[21,24,25,43,50] and the data generated from this study, the ultimate strength of cancellous bones obtained by the indentation test ranges from 38 to 71 MPa. The wide range of these values is not surprising and is due to different subjects and different locations. Even with the conventional compressive test, the range of elastic modulus was much larger, ranging from several to 3000 MPa.[48] Trabecular bone modulus can vary 100-fold from one location to another even within the same metaphysis.

Indentation testing with a flat-ended cylindrical indenter has been used often due to its several advantages. Indentation testing may be more representative of the *in vivo* condition, which can be considered as a constrained compression test. The mechanical properties (mostly obtained from compression testing) of a cube or cylinder bone sample separated from the bone such as the femur or tibia are not the same as that when the cube or cylinder were in the bone tissue. The preparation of bone required with compression testing introduces errors. With indentation testing, the bone can be tested as a whole and numerous areas of the same bone may be tested. The indentation test is a simple procedure. Only a flat surface of the sample is needed for testing, and it is less invasive than the conventional compression test. The indentation test makes mechanical testing on smaller bones feasible. There have been no reports to the authors' knowledge of attempts to study rat bones using compression tests, possibly because the bone size is too small. Because the structure of cancellous bone is anisotropic and heterogeneous, which is more apparent for smaller bones, indentation testing may be more appropriate. Also, fewer variables are involved with indentation testing compared with conventional compression testing. When the conditions of the test machine are the same, indentation tests only require the specimen deformation and the surface area of the indenter and the load to be known. When using a compression test with cylindrical samples, the length (which cannot be easily controlled), end surface area, and the deformation have to be known. Finally, macroindentation using a cylindrical indenter requires only a conventional material testing machine available in most material testing laboratories.

REFERENCES

1. Rho, J.Y., Kuhn-Spearing, L., and Zioupos, P., Mechanical properties and the hierarchical structure of bone, *Med. Eng. Phys.,* 20, 92, 1998.
2. Carter, D.R. and Hayes, W.C., The compressive behavior of bone as a two-phase porous structure, *J. Bone Joint Surg.,* 59A, 954, 1977.
3. Gibson, L.J., The mechanical behavior of cancellous bone, *J. Biomech.,* 18, 317, 1985.
4. Björkstrom, S. and Goldie, I.F., Hardness of the subchondral bone of the patella in the normal state, in chondromalacia, and in osteoarthrosis, *Acta Orthop. Scand.,* 53, 451, 1982.
5. Weaver, J.K., The microscopic hardness of bone, *J. Bone Joint Surg.,* 48A, 273, 1966.
6. Markel, M.D., Wikenheiser, M.A., and Chao, E.Y., A study of fracture callus material properties: relationship to the torsional strength of bone, *J. Orthop. Res.,* 8, 843, 1990.
7. Markel, M.D., Wikenheiser, M.A., and Chao, E.Y., Formation of bone in tibial defects in a canine model. Histomorphometric and biomechanical studies, *J. Bone Joint Surg.,* 73A, 914, 1991.
8. Aro, H.T., Wippermann, B.W., Hodgson, S.F., et al., Prediction of properties of fracture callus by measurement of mineral density using micro-bone densitometry, *J. Bone Joint Surg.,* 71A, 1020, 1989.
9. Houde, J., Marchetti, M., Duquette, J., et al., Correlation of bone mineral density and femoral neck hardness in bovine and human samples, *Calcif. Tissue Int.,* 57, 201, 1995.
10. Doppler, R.A., Bone Mechanical Property Determination through Superficial Rockwell Hardness Testing, M.S. thesis, Worcester Polytechnic Institute, Worcester, MA, 1993.
11. Standards, A., Standard test methods for Rockwell hardness and Rockwell superficial hardness of metallic materials, *ASTM Standards — Specifications,* E18, ASTM, Philadelphia, 1989, 176.
12. Evans, F.G. and Lebow, M., Regional differences in some of the physical properties of the human femur, *J. Appl. Physiol.,* 3, 563, 1951.
13. Duquette, J., Lin, J., Hoffman, A., et al., Correlations among bone mineral density, broadband ultrasound attenuation, mechanical indentation testing, and bone orientation in bovine femoral neck samples, *Calcif. Tissue Int.,* 60, 181, 1997.
14. Sneppen, O., Christensen, P., Larsen, H., and Vang, P.S., Mechanical testing of trabecular bone in knee replacement, *Int. Orthop.,* 5, 251, 1981.
15. Hvid, I., Trabecular bone strength at the knee, *Clin. Orthop.,* 227, 210, 1988.
16. Jensen, N.C., Madsen, L.P., and Linde, F., Topographical distribution of trabecular bone strength in the human os calcanei, *J. Biomech.,* 24, 49, 1991.
17. Hvid, I., Andersen, K., and Olesen, S., Cancellous bone strength measurements with the osteopenetrometer, *Eng. Med.,* 13, 73, 1984.
18. Hvid, I., Jensen, J., and Nielsen, S., Bone strength measurements at the proximal tibia. Penetration tests and epiphyseal compressive strength, *Int. Orthop.,* 10, 271, 1986.
19. Josechak, R.G., Finlay, J.B., Bourne, R.B., and Rorabeck, C.H., Cancellous bone support for patellar resurfacing, *Clin. Orthop.,* 192, 1987.
20. Nakabayashi, Y., Wevers, H.W., Cooke, T.D., and Griffin, M., Bone strength and histomorphometry of the distal femur, *J. Arthroplasty,* 9, 307, 1994.
21. Behrens, J.C., Walker, P.S., and Shoji, H., Variations in strength and structure of cancellous bone at the knee, *J. Biomech.,* 7, 201, 1974.
22. An, Y.H., Kang, Q., and Friedman, R.J., Mechanical symmetry of rabbit bones studied by bending and indentation testing, *Am. J. Vet. Res.,* 57, 1786, 1996.
23. An, Y.H., Zhang, J.H., Kang, Q., and Friedman, R.J., Mechanical properties of rat epiphyseal cancellous bones studied by indentation test, *J. Mater. Sci. Mater. Med.,* 8, 493, 1997.

24. Sumner, D.R., Willke, T.L., Berzins, A., and Turner, T.M., Distribution of Young's modulus in the cancellous bone of the proximal canine tibia, *J. Biomech.,* 27, 1095, 1994.

25. Kang, Q., An, Y.H., and Friedman, R.J., The mechanical properties and bone densities of canine cancellous bones, *J. Mater. Sci. Mater. Med.,* 9, 1998.

26. Wassell, R.W., McCabe, J.F., and Walls, A.W., Subsurface deformation associated with hardness measurements of composites, *Dent. Mater.,* 8, 218, 1992.

27. Lips, E.M. and Sack, J., A hardness tester for microscopical objects, *Nature,* 138, 328, 1936.

28. Ramrakhiani, M., Pal, D., and Murty, T.S., Micro-indentation hardness studies on human bones, *Acta Anat.,* 103, 358, 1979.

29. Ramrakhiani, M., Pal, D., and Datta, S.C., Effect of heating on the hardness of human bone, *Acta Anat.,* 108, 316, 1980.

30. Amprino, R., Investigations on some physical properties of bone tissue, *Acta Anat.,* 34, 161, 1958.

31. Riches, P.E., Everitt, N.M., Heggie, A.R., and McNally, D.S., Microhardness anisotropy of lamellar bone, *J. Biomech.,* 30, 1059, 1997.

32. Ziv, V., Wagner, H.D., and Weiner, S., Microstructure–microhardness relations in parallel-fibered and lamellar bone, *Bone,* 18, 417, 1996.

33. Lenart, G., Toth, I., and Piner, J., Experiments on the hardness of bone by Vickers microhardness measurements, *Acta Biochem. Biophys. Acad. Sci. Hung.,* 3, 1968.

34. Huja, S.S., Qian, H., Roberts, W.E., and Katona, T.R., Effects of callus and bonding on strains in bone surrounding an implant under bending, *Int. J. Oral Maxillofac. Implants,* 13, 630, 1998.

35. Blackburn, J., Hodgskinson, R., Currey, J.D., and Mason, J.E., Mechanical properties of microcallus in human cancellous bone, *J. Orthop. Res.,* 10, 237, 1992.

36. Stea, S., Savarino, L., Toni, A., et al., Microradiographic and histochemical evaluation of mineralization inhibition at the bone-alumina interface, *Biomaterials,* 13, 664, 1992.

37. Stea, S., Visentin, M., Savarino, L., et al., Microhardness of bone at the interface with ceramic-coated metal implants, *J. Biomed. Mater. Res.,* 29, 695, 1995.

38. Simske, S.J. and Sachdeva, R., Cranial bone apposition and ingrowth in a porous nickel-titanium implant, *J. Biomed. Mater. Res.,* 29, 527, 1995.

39. Evans, G.P., Behiri, J.C., Currey, J.D., and Bonfield, W., Microhardness and Young's modulus in cortical bone exhibiting a wide range of mineral voume fractions, and in a bone analogue, *J. Mater. Sci. Mater. Med.,* 1, 38, 1990.

40. Huja, S.S., Katona, T.R., Moore, B.K., and Roberts, W.E., Microhardness and anisotropy of the vital osseous interface and endosseous implant supporting bone, *J. Orthop. Res.,* 16, 54, 1998.

41. Rho, J.Y., Tsui, T.Y., and Pharr, G.M., Elastic properties of human cortical and trabecular lamellar bone measured by nanoindentation, *Biomaterials,* 18, 1325, 1997.

42. Lee, F.Y., Rho, J.Y., Harten, R., Jr., et al., Micromechanical properties of epiphyseal trabecular bone and primary spongiosa around the physis: an *in situ* nanoindentation study, *J. Pediatr. Orthop.,* 18, 582, 1998.

43. Aitken, G.K., Bourne, R.B., Finlay, J.B., et al., Indentation stiffness of the cancellous bone in the distal human tibia, *Clin. Orthop.,* 264, 1985.

44. Hardinge, M.G., Determination of the strength of the cancellous bone in the head and neck of the femur, *Surg. Gynecol. Obstetr.,* 89, 439, 1949.

45. An, Y.H., Kang, Q., and Friedman, R.J., et al., Do mechanical properties of epiphyseal cancellous bones vary? *J. Invest. Surg.,* 10, 221, 1997.

46. Timoshenko, S.P. and Goodier, J.N. Axisymmetric stress and deformation in a solid of revolution. Load distributed over a part of a boundary of an infinite solid, in *Theory of Elasticity,* Clark, B.J. and Maisel, J.W., Eds., McGraw-Hill, New York, 1970, 380.

47. Vasu, R., Carter, D.R., and Harris, W.H., Stress distributions in the acetabular region — I. Before and after total joint replacement, *J. Biomech.,* 15, 155, 1982.

48. Kang, Q., An, Y.H., and Friedman, R.J., Effects of multiple freezing–thawing cycles on ultimate indentation load and stiffness of bovine cancellous bone, *Am. J. Vet. Res.,* 58, 1171, 1997.

49. Goldstein, S.A., The mechanical properties of trabecular bone: dependence on anatomic location and function, *J. Biomech.,* 20, 1055, 1987.

50. Saitoh, S., Nakatsuchi, Y., Latta, L., and Milne, E., An absence of structural changes in the proximal femur with osteoporosis, *Skeletal Radiol.,* 22, 425, 1993.

15 Penetration Testing of Bone Using an Osteopenetrometer

Ivan Hvid and Frank Linde

CONTENTS

I. INTRODUCTION

Penetration testing was originally developed to characterize the quality of soil. A measuring profile is driven from the surface into the structure or material under investigation, while the force necessary to advance the probe is recorded as a function of the depth of penetration.

The motivation to develop and use this particular method of mechanical testing was a desire to characterize trabecular bone mechanically at the knee joint during total knee arthroplasty. This work was initiated in the 1970s, when mechanical loosening was still a significant problem in the emerging semi- and nonconstrained total knee designs, the long-term function of which were dependent upon the mechanical quality of tibial and femoral condylar trabecular bone.[1] As it turned out, the problem of mechanical loosening was minimized by a combination of improved implant design and development of instrumentation to assure proper implant alignment. Even with these refinements, however, the strength of condylar trabecular bone remains an important factor for the risk of mechanical loosening.[2] Reduced physical activity, low body weight, and rheumatoid arthritis were shown to be related to reduced trabecular bone strength around the knee.[2,3] Trabecular bone strength was universally (normal knees, osteoarthrosis, rheumatoid arthritis) shown to diminish quite significantly with the distance from the subchondral bone plate,[2-4] indicating that bone resection during total knee replacement should be minimized.

In the laboratory, the method was used to obtain closely spaced bone strength measurements to describe accurately the variation of bone strength across the surface of joints.[3-6] The findings correlated qualitatively to findings of gait analysis,[7,8] tending to justify the simplifying assumptions inherent in the model solutions in these kinds of studies.

II. GUIDELINES FOR PENETRATION TESTING OF TRABECULAR BONE

A. THE OSTEOPENETROMETER: DESIGNED FOR *IN VIVO* TESTING

Since the idea was to develop a tool to measure bone strength intraoperatively, the device had to be quite small to facilitate handheld operation. It should be able to endure repeated exposure to high pressure and high temperature for sterilization purposes.

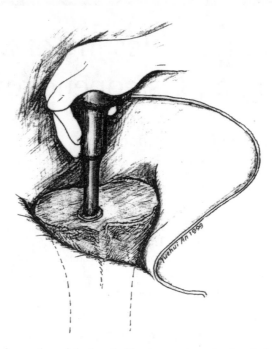

FIGURE 15.1   Sketch of operation of the handheld osteopenetrometer for clinical, intraoperative use. The operator must resist the reaction force used to drive the measuring probe into the trabecular bone.

A number of mechanical restraints were necessary. Since counterpressure must be exerted by the operator (Figure 15.1), the maximal measurable force could not exceed 500 to 600 N. Accordingly, the penetration needle had to be relatively thin. This was also desirable from the point of view that minimal damage should be inflicted on the bone structure. A measuring profile diameter of 2.5 mm (4.9 mm^2 projected cross section, Figure 15.2) was finally chosen after some experimentation. The speed of penetration was to be kept constant since bone is a viscoelastic substance, so that mechanical properties are strain rate dependent. In fact, penetration strength was found to be penetration rate (speed) dependent in laboratory studies.[9] The penetration speed used routinely in the authors' clinical and laboratory studies was 1 mm s^{-1}.

The first prototype in clinical use was a mechanical device.[1] It was soon abandoned because it tolerated sterilization procedures poorly. A hydraulically powered penetrometer, using sterile demineralized water as hydraulic fluid, was then developed (Figure 15.3).[9] This osteopenetrometer needed hydraulic fluid refills between every few sterilizations, but was otherwise stable and relatively easy to use. It was indirectly powered by a computer-controlled electromotor, and the same custom-built computer was used to calibrate the device automatically and store a series of 12 measuring cycles.

The measurement obtained was the force of penetration as a function of the depth of penetration (Figure 15.4). Penetration strength (MPa) was reported as the force of penetration (N) averaged over an arbitrary depth interval, and normalized for the projected cross-sectional area of the needle (in mm^2). Penetration tests — as hardness tests — do not reflect any well-defined property of bone. They do, however, correlate quite closely to some important mechanical properties of bone.[5,9] A systematic series of tests was done relating the results of penetration tests to those of compression tests on unconfined machined specimens in a regular materials testing machine. Such a comparison presents a crucial inherent problem in that both types of tests are destructive. However, using two different approaches[5,9] yielding very similar results, it was possible to establish empirical relationships to yield strength, ultimate strength, Young's modulus, and energy absorption as determined from regular materials testing. These observations were later confirmed using bone

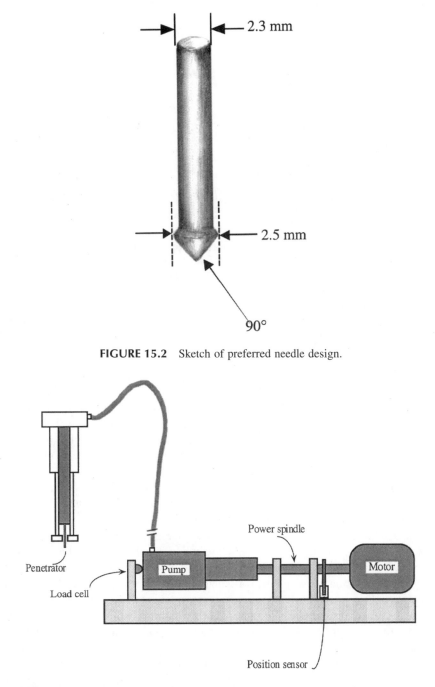

FIGURE 15.2   Sketch of preferred needle design.

FIGURE 15.3   Design diagram of osteopenetrometer developed for clinical measurement.

density measurements obtained by quantitative computed X-ray tomography scanning as a link between the two modes of mechanical testing.[10]

Obviously, the measurement obtained is dependent upon the design of the needle used to penetrate the trabecular bone. A systematic approach to find a suitable needle design was undertaken.[9] Blunt needles and needles with a stem diameter identical to that of the base of the measuring profile resulted in empirical relationships to ultimate strength and ultimate strain energy that were

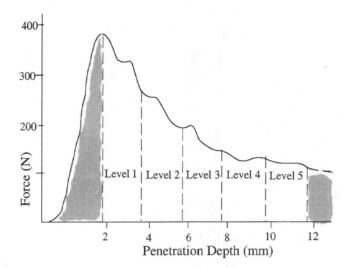

FIGURE 15.4 Typical measurement curve. An example of data extraction from the curve is shown. Initial 1.5 mm of penetration disregarded — this is needed to engage the leading profile of the needle fully with bone. The curve is then further subdivided in arbitrary intervals, depending upon the depth resolution desired. Finally, force is averaged over each depth interval, and the resulting force normalized with respect to the projected cross-sectional area of the measuring profile. When force is measured in N and the cross-sectional area expressed in mm^2, the strength expression will be in MPa.

functions of the depth of penetration (higher penetration strength values relative to ultimate properties were obtained from deep portions of the penetration path than from superficial portions). This was interpreted to be a result of impaction of bone beneath the blunt needle and frictional forces along the stem of the needle, respectively. The needle design finally chosen for future measurements (see Figure 15.2) featured a 90° conical measuring profile with a base diameter of 2.5 mm, and the needle shaft milled to 2.3 mm, since this needle produced indistinguishable regression lines from superficial and deep aspects of the bone.

In the laboratory, the osteopenetrometer could be mounted on a heavy metal frame. In this way, it was more or less comparable with a regular materials testing machine with the crosshead equipped with a needle. Early on, it was shown that the 2.5-mm needle resulted only in very localized damage to the trabecular bone structure, leaving trabeculae outside the actual measuring pathway of the needle virtually unharmed.[1] Therefore, the method would be suitable to obtain fairly closely spaced measurements which would be of considerable interest in establishing a deeper insight in the patterns of load transmission across joints, particularly the rather complex knee joint. It was found that 5 mm between the center of each measurement was sufficient to avoid measurable deterioration of the mechanical properties of trabecular bone located within the confines of four penetration tests in a squared pattern,[5] and "cross talk" between penetration tests using this minimal distance between individual measurements could not be demonstrated.[3]

Following transverse resection of the joint surface just below the subchondral bone plates of the condyles, measurements were taken across the proximal tibial epiphysis using penetration tests 5 mm apart in a squared pattern. This revealed a smooth topographical pattern of strength with a higher medial than lateral peak strength localized centrally and posteriorly, respectively. Toward the periphery of the condyles, bone strength diminished progressively to very low values near the edges, indirectly demonstrating the effectiveness of the menisci in distributing the forces at the normal knee joint and minimizing strength/stiffness gradients in joint cartilage and subchondral bone.[3] Viewed in concert with the marked reduction of strength away from the joint surface (about 50% over 10 mm at the stronger central parts of the condyles) certain proximal tibial fracture patterns can be explained.

One more problem related to this unique needle design needs to be addressed. As with other mechanical tests not performed on individual trabeculae, the strength of the trabecular structure rather than of the bone as such is measured. Therefore, the bone is assumed to be a continuum. To meet this assumption, a linear distance of ten intercept lengths (bone–marrow interfaces as seen microscopically), corresponding to five intertrabecular widths (approximately 5 mm in the human proximal tibia) must be engaged by the measuring device according to Harrigan et al.[11] Penetration tests on human trabecular bone using a 2.5-mm-diameter needle obviously violates the continuum assumption. However, when measuring human trabecular bone around the knee with this particular needle dimension, the estimated error is moderate, less than ±10%.[12] This error could be huge if measurements were done in other parts of the human skeleton: consider the aged human vertebra where trabeculae may be several millimeters apart.

The osteopenetrometer as described above is not commercially available. Modern imaging techniques offer the opportunity of assaying bone strength by measuring bone density very accurately.[10,13-15] With present-day technology, these methods of assaying bone strength are probably as accurate as *in vivo* osteopenetrometer testing, and, in addition, they are noninvasive. The doses of ionizing radiation necessary to obtain these measurements are decreasing, while the structural resolution is increasing, leading to even better noninvasive assays of the mechanical properties of bone. Accordingly, although the use of the osteopenetrometer has produced some interesting results in the past, it must be regarded as obsolete for clinical use.

B. LABORATORY PENETRATION TESTING

As mentioned above, penetration tests can be performed on a regular materials testing machine. The needle must be mounted on the crosshead of the machine. The needle can then be advanced into trabecular bone samples at a constant crosshead speed. The load cell is most conveniently mounted between the crosshead and the needle. The bony structure being studied must be rigidly supported.

Measurements should usually be obtained by advancing the needle at right angles to the bone surface. This will limit the usefulness of the method or call for elaborate adjustable fixation devices, e.g., in measuring the bone strength distribution under curved surfaces such as the femoral condyles and the femoral head. Failure to engage the surface of the bone specimen at right angles, especially when the bone is relatively strong, may lead to bending of the needle and invalidation of the measurement. When trying to measure extremely strong bone, e.g., the sclerotic subchondral bone in severe osteoarthrosis, the needle may buckle, again invalidating the measurement. To deal with such problems, one might consider the use of a needle of heavier design. However, it should be remembered that the penetration test has not been validated measuring very dense bone, and therefore the results obtained may not be readily interpretable. Other methods should be considered. Indentation testing, for instance, can be used to obtain a dense pattern of measurement, and a quasi-continuous measurement deep to the surface could be established by removing bone successively from the surface doing repeated measurements as needed.

The use of larger needles or penetrators has been reported,[16] but has not been validated. In the authors' opinion, large needle penetration tests are not useful for laboratory use, since better methods exist.

The authors believe that the penetration test has been very useful in describing topographical variations of trabecular bone strength in subchondral bone regions, i.e., close to joints, and has provided valuable (indirect) information on the mode of load transmission through various joints. For such purposes this method can be recommended, and is still being used.[17] The method does provide quasi-three-dimensional information on the mechanical strength of trabecular bone not readily obtainable by other methods. While the standard method of mechanically testing trabecular bone as a structure is likely to remain compression tests on machined specimens large enough to satisfy the continuum assumption, it is worth remembering that this method is blind to variations within the test volume. One significant accomplishment of the penetration test was to document the 50% decrease of bone strength within the first few millimeters of subchondral bone at the proximal tibia, which was not revealed by previous studies using standard testing of machined specimens.

REFERENCES

1. Sneppen, O., Christensen, P., Larsen, H., and Vang, P-S., Mechanical testing of trabecular bone in knee replacement, *Int. Orthop.*, 5, 251, 1981.
2. Hvid, I., Trabecular bone strength at the knee, *Clin. Orthop.*, 227, 210, 1988.
3. Hvid, I. and Hansen S.L., Trabecular bone strength patterns at the proximal tibial epiphysis, *J. Orthop. Res.*, 3, 464, 1985.
4. Hvid, I. and Hansen, S.L., Subchondral bone strength in arthrosis. Cadaver studies of tibial condyles, *Acta Orthop. Scand.*, 57, 47, 1986.
5. Hvid, I., Cancellous bone at the knee: a comparison of two methods of strength measurement, *Arch. Orthop. Trauma Surg.*, 104, 211, 1985.
6. Hvid, I., Rasmussen, O., Jensen, N.C., and Nielsen, S., Trabecular bone strength profiles at the ankle joint, *Clin. Orthop.*, 199, 306, 1985.
7. Morrison, J.B., The mechanics of the knee joint in relation to normal walking, *J. Biomech.*, 3, 51, 1970.
8. Harrington, I.J., Static and dynamic loading patterns in knee joints with deformities, *J. Bone Joint Surg.*, 65A, 247, 1983.
9. Hvid, I., Andersen, K., and Olesen, S., Cancellous bone strength measurements with the osteopenetrometer, *Eng. Med.*, 13, 73, 1984.
10. Bentzen, S.M., Hvid, I., and Jørgensen, J., Mechanical strength of tibial trabecular bone evaluated by X-ray computed tomography, *J. Biomech.*, 20, 743, 1987.
11. Harrigan, T.P., Jasty, M., Mann, R.W., and Harris, W.H., Limitations of the continuum assumption in cancellous bone, *J. Biomech.*, 21, 269, 1988.
12. Hvid, I., Mechanical Strength of Trabecular Bone at the Knee, thesis, University of Aarhus, Laegeforeningens Forlag, Aarhus, Denmark, 1988, 15.
13. Hvid, I., Bentzen, S.M., and Jørgensen, J., Bone density at the proximal tibia after total knee replacement. A two-year follow-up study using quantitative X-ray computed tomography, *Acta Orthop. Scand.*, 59, 567, 1988.
14. Petersen, M.M., Nielsen, P.T., Lauritzen, J.B., and Lund, B., Changes in bone mineral density of the proximal tibia after uncemented total knee arthoplasty. A 3-year follow-up of 25 knees, *Acta Orthop. Scand.*, 66, 513, 1995.
15. Petersen, M.M., Jensen, N.C., Gehrchen, P.M., and Nielsen, P.K., The relation between trabecular bone strength and bone mineral density assessed by dual photon and dual energy X-ray absorptiometry in the proximal tibia, *Calcif. Tissue Int.*, 59, 311, 1996.
16. Yuzuki, O., Study on the mechanical strength and the inner structure of the knee, *J. Jpn. Orthop. Assoc.*, 52, 537, 1978.
17. Müller-Gerbl, M., Dalstra, M., Ding, M., et al., Distribution of strength and mineralization in the subchondral bone plate of human tibial heads, *Trans. Eur. Orthop. Res. Soc.*, 8, 94, 1998.

16 Microhardness Testing of Bone

Sarandeep S. Huja, Thomas R. Katona, and W. Eugene Roberts

CONTENTS

I. INTRODUCTION

Hardness is a reflection of the resistance to penetration or indentation. Two types of hardness tests are recognized based on the magnitude of the indentation load. Macrohardness testing involves using loads greater than 1 kg, while microhardness tests use loads less than 1 kg.[1] Macrohardness testing was used in the past to gain information about the mechanical properties of bone.[2] However, microhardness testing is routine and preferred for testing small bone specimens. Others classify hardness testing into microhardness, low-load hardness, and standard hardness tests.[3] Recently, nanoindentation techniques have also been applied to bone.[4] For perspective, the size of an osteon is about 200 to 300 µm, and each lamella in bone is 3 to 7 µm wide.[5] Microhardness indentations range from 20 to 150 µm in length, while nanoindentations can be of the order of 1 µm. Bone is a hierarchal structure[6] and it is possible that hardness values will differ with the particular bone structure (e.g., collagen fiber, lamella, osteon) being indented.

The literature reports a number of studies detailing the experimental basis of microhardness testing,[1,3,7,8] the application of microhardness testing to bone,[9,10] and dental enamel.[11] Some studies attempt to relate microhardness to mechanical properties.[12-15] A review of the above-cited articles should provide the reader with a comprehensive understanding of the use and limitations of microhardness testing of biological tissues.

The intent of this chapter is to aid researchers in developing a suitable protocol for conducting bone microhardness tests. Factors that could influence results will be discussed. In addition, the reader will be referred throughout the chapter to articles that provide information about specific important factors.

The prototype for microhardness testers became available in 1936 with the introduction of a metallurgic microscope by Lips and Sack.[16] (See Lysaght[7] for a description of the evolution of hardness and microhardness testers.) At the outset, microhardness testing enabled metallurgists and engineers to test brittle materials and microconstituents of metals and alloys which could not be examined by macrohardness tests. Bone microhardness testing was first reported by Carlstrom.[17] He measured Vickers microhardness on a human femur section that contained three groups of Haversian systems with differences in mineralization of about 10%. Carlstrom concluded that there was a close relationship between mineralization, as measured by microradiographic density, and microhardness. His Vickers microhardness numbers ranged from 29.5 to 38.3 kg/mm^2. Similar observations about mineralization were made by Weaver.[9] While mineralization is an important determinant of microhardness, Amprino[10] suggests that other factors such as collagen fiber orientation may also influence microhardness. Subsequent to these early studies, the microhardnesses of cortical bone,[18,19] trabecular bone,[9,20] woven bone callus,[21,22] bone adjacent to endosseous implants,[21,23,24] bone with an Haversian system,[9] and dental enamel[11] have been measured. In addition, microhardness has been used to test in-plane anisotropy of cortical bone and parallel-fibered bone in different animal species.[10,18,19,21] In many of these studies, there would not have been other means of obtaining information about the mechanical properties of the bone structures. Constraints imposed by specimen size or shape would have precluded conventional mechanical testing (e.g., preparing dumbbell/coupon-shaped specimens). Therein lies the uniqueness and applicability of microhardness testing.

II. MICROHARDNESS INDENTERS

Vickers and Knoop are the two types of microhardness indenters that are commonly used. In 1920, the Vickers indenter was developed in England and was initially used for macrohardness testing.[25] In 1939, the Knoop indenter was introduced by the National Bureau of Standards in the United States.[26] The instrument of choice has partly been determined by the part of the world in which the studies have been conducted. Since most, but not all,[9] of the early bone microhardness studies were conducted in Europe,[10,17,20] the literature reports mostly Vickers microhardness results.

The Vickers indenter is a square-shaped diamond (Figure 16.1a) with face angles of 136°. The Knoop indenter (Figure 16.1b) is a rhombic-shaped pyramidal diamond, with a longitudinal angle of 172°30′ and a transverse angle of 130°. For both indenters, the microhardness number is the ratio of applied load to indented area, and they have the units of kg/mm^2.

The Vickers microhardness number (HV) is given by

$$2P \sin(\theta/2)/d^2 \tag{16.1}$$

where P is the applied load in kg, d is the mean of the length of d_1 and d_2 in mm, and θ is 136°.

The Knoop microhardness number (HK) is given by

$$P/A = P/C(d_1)^2 \tag{16.2}$$

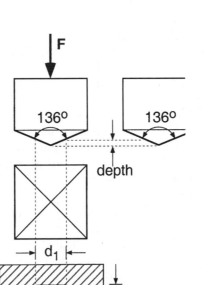

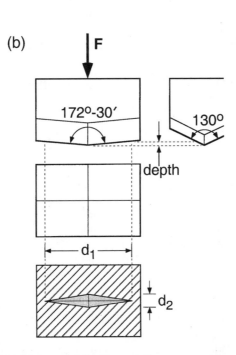

FIGURE 16.1 Schematics of (a) Vickers and (b) Knoop indenter geometries and their indentations in the cross-hatched surfaces. The angles between the faces of the indenters are indicated. The d_1/d_2 ratios are 1 : 1 and 1 : 7 for the Vickers and Knoop indenters, respectively. With the same load, the Vickers indenter penetrates approximately two times deeper than the Knoop indenter.

where P is the applied load in kg, and A is the unrecovered projected area (mm^2). The unrecovered area is calculated from the length of the long diagonal d_1 and a constant C (0.07028) which relates the length of the long diagonal to the projected area.

The depths of the Vickers and Knoop indentations are ⅐th and 1/30th of the respective lengths of their diagonals. For a given material, the Knoop diagonal is approximately three times as long as the Vickers, while the Vickers indenter penetrates nearly twice as deep as the Knoop indenter. Microhardness and macrohardness indentations can be made using the same Vickers indenter. This is not the case with the Knoop indenter, which is used primarily for microhardness tests.

The Knoop indenter is, in essence, a specialized case of the Vickers indenter. Knoop and his colleagues attempted to develop a universal indentation scale.[8] Knoop wanted a d_1/d_2 ratio between 5 and 10. After experimentation they chose a ratio of 7. A ratio of 5 may have allowed elastic recovery, and a ratio of 10 decreased sensitivity due to lack of ability to locate the ends of the indentations. With the Knoop indenter, the maximum strain (deformation) is along its width, the least is at the tips of its length.[8]

In making comparisons between the two indenters, it has been suggested that the Knoop indenter cuts, while the Vickers deforms.[1,10,27] It has also been stated that the Knoop indenter allows elastic recovery of the impression to occur primarily along the shorter diagonal. This is because the stresses are distributed in such a manner that only the minor axis dimensions are subject to recovery.[27] Since the long diagonal dimension is affected minimally by elastic recovery, it is used to calculate HK.[7,8] With lighter loads on the Knoop indenter, inflated microhardness numbers may result for two reasons. Lighter loads allow for greater elastic recovery of the long diagonal,[7] and, second, the recovery makes the actual ends of the diagonal more difficult to locate under the microscope.

Bückle[3] disputes that the change in indentation dimensions is related to the elastic properties of the material. He states that elastic recovery with a (Vickers) indenter is negligible along the diagonals, but it can occur along the depth of the indentation. He ascribes changes in the diagonal length to secondary causes such as "formation of pile-ups, the reflecting power of the specimen, the numerical aperture of the objective." Pileups are plastic flow of the material in the vicinity of the indentation. Thus, Bückle is of the opinion that operator and machine error are responsible for dimensional changes.

III. FACTORS AFFECTING MICROHARDNESS OF BONE

It is important to understand the effects of the following factors prior to conducting bone microhardness tests.

A. SPECIMEN PREPARATION

1. Storage Temperature

It is recommended that bone specimens be stored in saline-soaked gauze at –20°C prior to mechanical testing.[28] Effects of storage on microscopic hardness have been examined.[9] It was found that rapid freezing and storage of bone at –20°C in a sealed container had no appreciable effect on hardness, provided the surface is prepared within 1 h of testing.

2. Fixation

The effect fixation has on microhardness is unclear. It is thought that fixation causes cross-linking of collagen. Amprino,[10] citing Rössle[29] and Lexer,[30] suggested that brief (i.e., 24 h vs. weeks) fixation in formalin has no effect on hardness. However, Weaver[9] found that storage in 10% neutral formalin for 24 h caused a 20% increase in microhardness. Blackburn et al.[22] demonstrated that fixation in 4% formaldehyde for 24 h at room temperature had no effect on microhardness. As this is a variable which may affect microhardness, it is prudent to eliminate it by using unfixed specimens when possible.

3. Embedding in Resin and Infiltration

The literature does not make a clear distinction between *embedding* and *infiltration* of bone specimens in resin. While testing trabecular bone specimens or callus, it is beneficial to provide support by embedding the specimen. This, however, is different from infiltration, in which the objective is to allow the methyl methacrylate to occupy the smallest spaces (e.g., lacunae) within the substance of bone.

Embedding (in reality, infiltrating) bone in methyl methacrylate has been reported to increase microhardness by 30 to 40%.[9] When unfixed and noninfiltrated specimens were used in studies of different animal species[18,21] similar cortical bone Knoop values were obtained, suggesting the relative importance of these two variables. However, when specimens are infiltrated, the Knoop microhardness number does not increase.[31] It is therefore preferable to use noninfiltrated specimens for microhardness testing.

4. Degreasing/Defatting

Defatting allows for sharper indent outlines. Defatting with a chloroform/methanol mixture had no effect on microhardness.[22]

5. Drying vs. Testing Wet

There is a general consensus that drying bone specimens prior to testing will increase the microhardness values substantially. The chief reason to dry specimens is to provide clear indentation outlines, thereby allowing accurate measurements. Drying causes a significant increase in microhardness in primary and secondary bone — the higher the drying temperature (38°C, 60°C, 120°C for a few hours), the greater the increase.[10] This is in agreement with Blackburn et al.[22] who dried their specimens at 40°C prior to testing. This resulted in an increase in microhardness by approximately 20%. These findings are also in agreement with Evans and Lebow[2] who found that air drying (105°C) increased elastic modulus by 17.6% and macrohardness by 54.3%. While some investigators dry the specimens prior to testing, it would be preferable to use specimens that have not been subjected to heat. In addition, however, it has been found that microhardness of rehydrated bone is very close to that of wet fresh bone.[10]

B. ANATOMICAL VARIABLES

1. Type of Bone — Cortical, Trabecular, and Woven Bone Callus

When using a Vickers indenter, trabecular bone has lower microhardness than cortical bone.[9,20] Blackburn et al.[22] demonstrated that the microhardness of nodular-type microcallus and trabecular bone were similar. However, the mean microhardness values for the former are lower, but with more variability. Huja et al.[21] examined woven bone calluses that stabilize endosseous implants at 12 weeks postimplantation in dog midfemoral diaphysis. They found that periosteal and endosteal callus had significantly lower HK values than the layer of rapidly remodeling bone adjacent to the implant. Both the callus and implant adjacent bone, in turn, had lower HK than the cortical bone.

2. Anatomical Location of Bone and Site Within Bone

Ramarakhiani et al.[32] found HV to be different for different embalmed dry bones of the human skeleton. Riches et al.[18] and Weaver[9] found that HV was lower in the epiphyseal and metaphyseal regions than in the diaphysis. HV was also uniform throughout the diaphysis.

3. Age, Sex

Two studies[9,32] report no sex specific differences in microhardness of cortical bone. However, Weaver[9] was able to demonstrate an increase in microhardness with age.

4. Disease States

Amprino[10] examined the microhardness of bone specimens in patients with Paget's disease, renal rickets, and osteogenesis imperfecta. Others found no detectable change in the microhardness of osteoporotic bone.[9] In addition, hardness of subchondral bone in chondromalacia and osteoarthrosis has been examined.[33]

C. TESTING VARIABLES

The precision, bias, repeatability, and reproducibility of Vickers and Knoop microhardness indentations for metallic specimens of varying hardnesses have been determined.[34] Similarly, factors that determine the accuracy of indentation microhardness tests have been discussed.[35] With instruments available today, the rate of load application, duration of dwell, and removal of the load from the specimen are usually automated. Other factors that should be taken into consideration are discussed below.

1. Specimen Thickness

Generally, the thickness of the specimen should be at least ten times the depth of the anticipated impression.[7]

2. Indentation Spacing

When making multiple tests of the same specimen, it is important not to place additional indentations within the strain field of previous indentations. It has been suggested that additional Vickers indentations be made no closer than 1.5 to 2× the length of the original indentation.[7,10]

3. Load Dependency

By using a number of different materials, it has been shown that HK increases as the load decreases. In contrast, HV shows the opposite trend.[1] These effects are only seen at relatively low (below approximately 50 g) loads for both indenters. Amprino[10] addressed the question of whether similar HV values can be obtained from a given bone structure under different loads (15, 25, 50, 100, 200, 300 g). He found that with increasing load there was a slight tendency to a lowering of the microhardness value. Ramarakhiani et al.[32] measured HV using 5, 10, 20, 30, 50, 75, 100, 130, 150 g loads and found that HV increased with loads to 50 g, and then became independent of load in subsequent measurements. In another study,[21] loads of 25 and 50 g did not reveal statistically significant ($p = 0.74$) differences in HK values of cortical bone. Other studies have also rigorously addressed this issue.[8,34] For cortical bone, a 50-g load seems appropriate.

4. Duration of Dwell

Mott[25] stated that the reason for applying a load for a standard time is to ensure static conditions; i.e., there should be no flow/creep of a material leading to increase in the size of an indentation. This becomes more important for viscoelastic materials. It has been stated that consistent results were obtained on bone specimens by leaving the indenter in place for longer than 3 to 4 s.[9] A 10 to 15 s dwell on bone specimens seems to be adequate. Additional information is available on the effects of this factor.[3,8]

5. Dimension of Indentation and Magnification of the Optical System

When making pilot indentations in a test material, a balance between the size of the indentation and the microscope magnification must be struck. As a general rule, the larger the indentation, the greater the accuracy.[1] In bone specimens, the dimension of the structure may limit the size of the indentation. If an indentation is too large for a given magnification, the load must be decreased. For example, a 25-g load with a Knoop indenter on cortical bone may result in a small (e.g., 70 μm) indentation, necessitating a higher magnification (e.g., ×400). A 50-g load and ×200 magnification could then be chosen. To allow for comparisons between studies, it is imperative to specify the load.

IV. GUIDELINES FOR MICROHARDNESS TESTING

The following guidelines for testing bone specimens are recommended. Specimens, frozen during storage, must be thawed. Water lubrication during cutting is advisable, particularly if an implant–bone block is being sectioned. It is advisable to test bone specimens which have not been fixed in formalin or infiltrated with resin. Generally, the bone specimens must be mounted in a resin block to provide support for polishing and testing.

A good surface polish is essential. Procedures similar to those used to obtain a metallurgic finish are recommended. A method that has been used successfully to polish cortical bone specimens is described below.[21] A rotary wheel (Vari/Pol, VP-150, Leco, St. Joseph, MI) set at 150 rpm with successive 400-, 800-, and 1200-grit SiC papers and water lubrication is used. The 400-grit paper is used for a brief interval, with light pressure, as it can leave deep gouges in the bone. Frequently changing the orientation of the specimen ensures a good finish without scratches. The bone specimen is examined under a stage microscope to confirm a smooth surface. The bone is polished further using a napless Metcloth (Buehler polishing cloth, #40-7158, Lake Bluff, IL) with diluted water slurry of 1 μm aluminum oxide paste (Buehler Micropolish C alpha Alumina, Lake Bluff, IL). The specimen is sonicated in cleaning solution (Ultramet Sonic, Buehler, Lake Bluff, IL). Blotting with paper towels for 10 min to obtain a dry surface will remove excess moisture.

The specimen is then mounted in a leveling vise of the microhardness testing machine. The vise allows the indenter to penetrate the surface at right angles. The loading mechanism should be free of vibration and any effects of inertia. An accurate optical system for measuring the indentations should be available with most indenters. Under the microscope, the operator selects the area where the indentation is to be made. Automatic test cycle features ensure standardization of the test cycle. The rate of descent of the indenter, duration of dwell, and return of the indenter to its original position is uniform from one test to the next. Changing the direction of specimen illumination can make a difference in the clarity of the indentations and should be standardized to obtain the best view. With the Knoop and Vickers indenter, a difference of more than 20% between the two mirror halves of the indentation around the axes is usually an indication that the indenter is not entering perpendicular to the specimen surface. Asymmetric readings should be discarded.

A "weeping" problem has been observed with bone specimens that have been blotted dry without heat.[21,22] This is due to the exudate from the specimen. Weeping is recognized by the observation of indistinct indentation margins or the inability to focus on the surface. Reblotting the specimen for about 3 min with paper towels adequately resolves this problem. In most testers, the HV or HK is calculated automatically after the load and length of the indentation are provided.

Routine maintenance and calibration of the equipment by a qualified technician is important for consistent results. Intraobserver variability should be evaluated prior to starting the research project. Close to 5% error on bone and stainless steel indentations has been reported.[21,34]

V. MEASURING MICROHARDNESS ANISOTROPY

Measurement of anisotropy has been conducted with conventional mechanical tests,[36] acoustic techniques,[37] and microhardness indenters.[19] With the latter, anisotropy has been investigated using two methods. First, multiple indentations can be made on a single surface by orientating the indentor in specific directions[18,21] (e.g., relative to the lamellae.). Second, a cubic bone specimen[19] can be machined to coincide with the orthogonal directions of bone, and indentations made on the different surfaces can be compared.

Amprino[10] demonstrated that Vickers microhardness measurements on collagen fibers were independent of the Vickers pyramid face alignment. In his experiment, indentations were made so that collagen bundles from avian long bone (ethanol fixed and air dried) were cut either (1) with one diagonal of the Vickers parallel to the collagen bundle and the other perpendicular to it, or (2) both diagonals crossing at 45° to the long axis of the collagen fibers. Amprino ascribed his results partly to the "characteristic shape of the *Vickers* pyramid; which does not act as a wedge-shaped tip, and therefore pressures prevail over splitting components." This suggests that the Vickers indenter can only provide one hardness measurement per surface. Similarly, Weaver[9] made Vickers indentations along the transverse and longitudinal axes of the same Haversian system in a fibular cortex. He did not find microhardness differences in the two directions of his infiltrated sections. In contrast, the Knoop indentor has been successfully used to detect in-plane anisotropy.[18,21] Riches et al.[18] were able to detect a microhardness anisotropy ratio of approximately 1.3 in the transverse vs. the longitudinal direction on specimens of rat tibiae. Similarly, Huja et al.,[21] using a Knoop indenter, demonstrated microhardness anisotropy in lamellar bone near the endocortical surfaces of the femur. Riches et al.[18] suggest that the Knoop indenter is more sensitive than a Vickers indenter in detecting anisotropy of bone.

Amprino[10] also made measurements on two perpendicular surfaces. In these sections the collagen fibers were cut either perpendicular or along their long axes. Various animal species were tested and the HV microhardness reading was higher by approximately 20 to 25% on the surface where the collagen fibers were cut perpendicular to their long axes. Ziv et al.[19] used a Vickers indenter on cubic specimens and were able to demonstrate anisotropy in three orthogonal directions on parallel-fibered bone. Although these authors acknowledged that the building blocks of lamellar bone are anisotropic, they found lamellar bone to be isotropic. This was probably due to the large size of their indentations.

VI. CONCLUSION

Microhardness testing has been used to measure the resistance to indentation of various bone types. It is generally acknowledged that microhardness results are not easily interpreted[14] and that hardness represents a combination of several material properties.[25] What these microhardness measurements mean remains unclear. However, relative comparisons between two microhardness measurements using the same methodology are accurate.

However, there are at least three studies[11,12,15] which have found strong correlations between microhardness and variables such as volume fraction of mineral, Young's modulus, yield stress, and calcium content. Currey and Brear,[12] referring to the relationship between hardness and elastic modulus, state that "hardness will not, of course, actually determine the other mechanical properties; these mechanical relationships doubtless indicate a common relationship with another variable, almost certainly mineral content of the tissues." Equations to estimate elastic modulus and yield stress from microhardness are available.[12,13] These equations have been derived for a range of mineralization levels. However, these formulae can only be used if identical methodology to that used in the original study is utilized. No such equations are available for the Knoop indenter.

These limitations do not detract from the usefulness of microhardness testing. Instead, information gained from microhardness tests could be corroborated by other methods to study the mechanical properties of bone and could serve to develop newer methods of investigating micro-structural properties of bone. One hopes the methods will lead to a better understanding of the complicated structure of bone and the mechanical properties of various subunits of bone, including the level of interaction between the collagen and hydroxyapatite crystals. Microhardness tests can be valuable tools in bone biomechanics, once the limitations of the tests are fully understood.

ACKNOWLEDGMENTS

The authors are extremely grateful to Dr. David B. Burr and Dr. B. Keith Moore for their invaluable assistance. This work was supported by National Institutes of Dental Research Grant PHS R55 DE09822.

REFERENCES

1. Fee, A.R., Segabache, R., and Tobolski, E.L., Hardness testing, in *Metals Handbook,* Vol. 8, American Society for Metals Mechanical Testing, Metals Park, OH, 1985, 87.
2. Evans, F.G. and Lebow, M., Regional differences in some of the physical properties of the human femur, *J. Appl. Physiol.*, 3, 563, 1951.
3. Bückle, I., Progress in micro-indentation hardness testing, *Metall. Rev.*, 4, 49, 1959.
4. Rho, J-Y., Tsui, T.Y., and Pharr, G.M., Elastic properties of human cortical and trabecular lamellar bone measured by nanoindentation, *Biomaterials*, 18, 1325, 1997.
5. Martin, R.B. and Burr, D.B., *Structure, Function and Adaptation of Compact Bone*, Raven Press, New York, 1989, 186.
6. Katz, J.L., Hierarchical modeling of compact Haversian bone as a fiber reinforced material, in *Advances in Bioengineering*, Mates, R.E and Smith, C.R., Eds., ASME, New York, 1976, 18.
7. Lysaght, V.E., *Indentation Hardness Testing*, Reinhold, New York, 1949, 234.
8. Knoop, P., Peters, C.G., and Emerson, W.B., A sensitive pyramidal-diamond tool for indentation measurements, *J. Res. Natl. Bur. Stand.*, 23, 39, 1939.
9. Weaver, J.K., The microscopic hardness of bone, *J. Bone Joint Surg.*, 48A, 273, 1966.
10. Amprino, R., Investigations on some physical properties of bone tissue, *Acta Anat.*, 34, 161, 1958.
11. Featherstone, J.D., ten Cate, J.M., Shariati, M., and Arends, J., Comparison of artificial caries-like lesions by quantitative microradiography and microhardness profiles, *Caries Res.*, 17, 385, 1983.
12. Currey, J.D. and Brear, K., Hardness, Young's modulus and yield stress in mammalian mineralized tissue, *J. Mater. Sci. Mater. Med.*, 1, 14, 1990.
13. Evans, G.P., Behiri, J.C., Currey, J.D., and Bonfield, W., Microhardness and Young's modulus in cortical bone exhibiting a wide range of mineral volume fractions, and in a bone analogue, *J. Mater. Sci. Mater. Med.*, 1, 38, 1990.
14. Hodgskinson, R., Currey, J.D., and Evans, F.G., Hardness, an indicator of the mechanical competence of cancellous bone, *J. Orthop. Res.*, 7, 754, 1989.
15. Evans, G.P., Behiri, J.C., and Bonfield, W., Microhardness, Young's modulus and mineral content in bone and bone analogue, in *Implant Materials in Biofunction; Advances in Biomaterials,* Vol. 8, de Putter, C., de Lange, G.L., de Groot, K., and Lee, A.J., Eds., Elsevier Science, Amsterdam, 1988, 311.
16. Lips, E.M. and Sack, J., A hardness tester for microscopical objects, *Nature*, 138, 328, 1936.
17. Carlstrom, D., Micro-hardness measurements on single Haversian systems in bone, *Acta Anat.*, 15, 171, 1952.
18. Riches, P.E., Everitt, N.M., Heggie, A.R., and McNally, D.S., Microhardness anisotropy of lamellar bone, *J. Biomech.*, 30, 1059, 1997.
19. Ziv, V., Wagner, H.D., and Weiner, S., Microstructure-microhardness relations in parallel-fibered and lamellar bone, *Bone*, 18, 417, 1996.
20. Lenart, G., Toth, I., and Pinter, J., Experiments on the hardness of bone by Vickers microhardness measurements, *Acta Biochim. Biophys. Acad. Sci. Hung.*, 3, 205, 1968.
21. Huja, S.S., Katona, T.R., Moore, B.K., and Roberts, W.E., Microhardness and anisotropy of the vital osseous interface and endosseous implant supporting bone, *J. Orthop. Res.*, 16, 54, 1998.
22. Blackburn, J., Hodgskinson, R., Currey, J.D., and Mason, J.E., Mechanical properties of microcallus in human cancellous bone, *J. Orthop. Res.*, 10, 237, 1992.
23. Stea, S., Tarabusi, C., Ciapetti, G., et al., Microhardness evaluation of the bone growing into porous implants, *J. Mater. Sci. Mater. Med.*, 3, 252, 1992.
24. Stea, S., Visentin, M., Savarino, L., et al., Microhardness of bone at the interface with ceramic-coated metal implants, *J. Biomed. Mater. Res.*, 29, 695, 1995.
25. Mott, B.W., Measuring "hardness," *New Sci.*, 9, 103, 1964.

26. Lysaght, V.E., *Indentation hardness testing*, Reinhold Publishing, New York, 1949, 188.
27. Anusavice, K.J., *Phillips' Science of Dental Materials*, 10th ed., W.B. Saunders, Philadelphia, 1996, 69.
28. Turner, C.H. and Burr, D.B., Basic biomechanical measurement of bone: a tutorial, *Bone*, 14, 595, 1993.
29. Rössle, R., Untersuchungen über Knochenhärte, *Beitr. Pathol. Anat.*, 77, 174, 1927.
30. Lexer, E.W., Untersuchungen über die Knochenhärte des Humerus, *Z. KonstLehre*, 14, 227, 1929.
31. Chachra, D., Turner, C.H., Dunipace, A.J., and Grynpas, M.D., The effect of fluoride treatment on bone mineral in rabbits, *Calcif. Tissue Int.*, 64, 345, 1999.
32. Ramarakhiani, M., Pal, D., and Murty, T.S., Micro-indentation hardness studies on human bones, *Acta Anat.*, 103, 358, 1979.
33. Björkström, J. and Goldie, I.F., Hardness of the subchondral bone of the patella in the normal state, in chondromalacia, and in osteoarthrosis, *Acta Orthop. Scand.*, 55, 453, 1982.
34. Vander Voort, G.F., Results of an ASTM E-4 Round-Robin on the precision and bias of measurements of microindentation hardness impressions, in *Factors That Affect the Precision of Mechanical Tests*, Papirno, R. and Weiss, H. C., Eds., ASTM, Baltimore, 1989, 3.
35. Tobolski, E.L., Factors that affect the accuracy of indentation hardness tests, in *Factors That Affect the Precision of Mechanical Tests*, Papirno, R. and Weiss, H.C., Eds., ASTM, Baltimore, 1989, 46.
36. Reilly, D.T., Burstein, A.H., and Frankel, V.H., The elastic modulus for bone, *J. Biomech.*, 7, 271, 1974.
37. Ashman, R.B., Cowin, S.C., Van Buskirk, W.C. and Rice, J.C., A continuous wave technique for the measurement of the elastic properties of cortical bone, *J. Biomech.*, 17, 349, 1984.

17 Nanoindentation Testing of Bone

Jae-Young Rho and George M. Pharr

CONTENTS

I. INTRODUCTION

Nanoindentation, developed over the last 10 years, is now used widely in the materials science community for probing the mechanical properties of thin films, small volumes, and small microstructural features.[1,2] The availability of depth-sensing nanoindentation instruments with capabilities for measuring displacements on the order of nanometers makes it possible to study the mechanical properties of thin films and other finely structured materials where small volumes need to be probed.[3] From analysis of nanoindentation load–displacement data, it is possible to derive values of the elastic modulus,[1,2] hardness,[1,2] and properties associated with time-dependent deformation such as strain rate sensitivity and the stress exponent for creep.[4] Since nanoindentation can be used to probe a surface and map its properties on a spatially resolved basis, often with a resolution of better than 1 mm, it can be used to measure the properties of small microstructural features such as individual osteons and trabeculae.[5-8]

The mechanical properties of bone have been extensively studied at the macrostructural and microstructural level. Conventional mechanical testing has a lower limit of a few hundreds of microns at best. Microindentation measures a dimension of a few tenths to hundreds of microns,[9,10] while nanoindentation can study on a 1 μm or smaller length scale. Since many important microstructural components of bone have dimensions of only a few microns or less, the nanoindentation technique can be used to investigate the mechanical properties of osteonal, interstitial, and trabecular lamellar bone at the largely unexplored micron and submicron level. As an example, the nanoindentation method has been used to examine variations in the individual lamellar properties within osteons, as a function of distance from the osteonal center. To the best of the authors' knowledge, in only one previous study has mechanical property measurement of individual lamellae within osteons been attempted,[11] and it met with little success due to technical difficulties. The nanoindentation method also potentially allows one to examine the properties in different directions and therefore explore elastic anisotropy, even in very small specimens such as individual trabeculae.

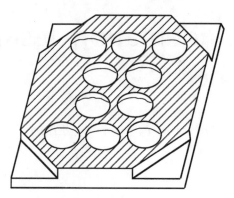

FIGURE 17.1   Schematic diagram of a typical specimen holder.

At present, microstructurally based theories of bone behavior are difficult to test due to a lack of microscopic mechanical property data.[12] Characterization of lamellar bone properties by nano-indentation methods would thus aid in further theoretical developments of the mechanisms of fracture in bone.

Because of experimental complications associated with testing in liquid environments and keeping specimens wet during testing, most nanoindentation work has focused on dried bone.[5] It is well documented, however, that the mechanical properties of bone show notable changes after dehydration.[13-16] In general, drying increases the Young's modulus of bone, decreases its toughness, and reduces the strain to fracture. An important question thus arises of the degree to which nanoindentation mechanical property measurements are affected by drying. To this end, a series of tests was recently conducted on wet and dry bovine femur using a special testing fixture in which specimens could be tested fully immersed in a liquid.[17] Drying was found to increase the elastic modulus by 9.7% for interstitial lamellae and 15.4% for osteons. The hardness was found to increase by 12.2% for interstitial lamellae and 17.6% for osteons.

The nanoindentation techniques elucidated in this chapter can be used to study mechanical properties at bone–implant interfaces, pathological metabolic bone diseases, the properties of woven bone and calcified cartilage in fracture callus, the properties of the growth plate, and biological aspects of implant loosening. Such results would fill a gap in the present knowledge by providing a better understanding of the mechanical function of bone at the microstructural and submicro-structural level.

II. SAMPLE PREPARATION

Nanoindentation specimens are normally in the form of polished, metallographic samples mounted in plastic mounts or glued to metal disks. The specimen holder is a metal plate into which holes have been drilled (Figure 17.1). Sample mounts are fitted into the holes and are held in place with set screws.

To test dried bone, bone sections can be dehydrated in a series of alcohol baths and embedded without vacuum in epoxy resin at room temperature. In the case of trabecular bone, a low-viscosity epoxy is preferred to infiltrate and provide support for the porous network. The embedded samples are metallographically polished to produce the smooth surfaces needed for nanoindentation testing. After being ground using silicon carbide abrasive papers of decreasing grit size (600, 800, and 1200 grit) under deionized water, the specimens are polished on micro-cloths with successively finer grades of alumina powder, the finest being 0.05 mm grit. The last polishing step is on plain microcloth under deionized water, and the specimens are cleaned ultrasonically to remove surface debris.

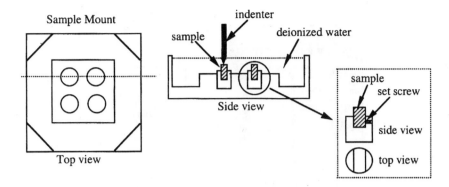

FIGURE 17.2   Mounting stage used for testing wet specimens. (From Rho, J. and Pharr, G., *J. Mater. Sci. Mater. Med.,* 1999. With permission.)

Wet specimens can be tested using a specially designed test fixture such as that shown in Figure 17.2, for which cortical bone specimens can be tested without embedding in plastic. The specimen is held securely in place by two set screws with the polished surface extending slightly above the aluminum mount. An appropriate solution is added to the test fixture until the specimen is completely immersed, but to avoid problems caused by water rising too far up the indenter shaft, the levels must be controlled carefully so that water extends only 50 to 100 mm above the specimen surface. At this level, the indenter tip is immersed during testing, but water does not rise high enough up the indenter shaft to damage the testing system. The proper water level can be determined by using an optical microscope to focus separately on the specimen surface and the water surface, noting when the two focal planes are separated by 50 to 100 mm. Reducing the surface tension of the water by adding a drop of liquid dishwashing detergent to the water aids in keeping water on the specimen surface and reduces the force needed for the indenter to penetrate the water surface at the beginning of a test. The latter effect helps in identifying the point of first surface contact during indenter approach to the specimen surface.

III. INDENTATION PROCEDURES

Experiments elucidated here were conducted using a commercially available nanoindenter, a schematic illustration of which is shown in Figure 17.3. This fully automated hardness testing system makes small indentations at precise positions on a specimen surface while continuously monitoring the loads and displacements of the indenter with resolutions of 75 nN and 0.04 nm, respectively. The specimens are held on an x–y–z table whose position relative to the microscope or the indenter is controlled with a joystick. The spatial resolution of the position of the table in the x–y plane is 400 nm. However, the optical microscope used for locating indentation sites may limit the positioning resolution to roughly 1 mm. The apparatus is enclosed in an insulated cabinet to provide thermal stability and suspended on a pneumatic antivibration table to isolate it from external vibrations.

A typical indent cycle is (1) approach to locate the specimen surface as accurately as possible; (2) load at a set rate to a set force or displacement limit; (3) hold a short time for the system to equilibrate fully before proceeding to an unloading; (4) unload at the same rate to typically 90% of maximum load; (5) hold for a relatively longer time to calculate the thermal drift; and (6) complete unload.

As an example, tests are typically conducted with a Berkovich diamond indenter (a three-sided pyramid) in load control using the load–time sequence such as that shown in Figure 17.4. As seen in the plot, it is useful to load and unload the indenter several times and include intervening periods

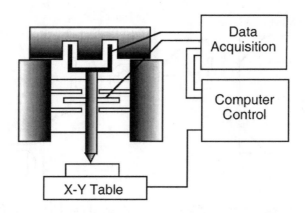

FIGURE 17.3   The mechanical properties microprobe.

during which the load is held constant. The multiple loading scheme is used to examine the extent to which the load–displacement data are influenced by viscoelastic deformation. Figure 17.5 presents a typical set of load–displacement data obtained from a test conducted in an osteon of dried human bone. After the initial loading, in which most of the plastic deformation occurs and the hardness impression is formed, there is a hysteresis in the data which indicates that a non-negligible portion of the indentation displacement is viscoelastic. Viscoelastic deformation is also apparent in the creep displacements observed during the constant load hold period at peak load. Viscoelastic deformation is important because analysis procedures used to obtain mechanical properties from the nanoindentation load–displacement data are premised on the notion that the upper portion of the unloading curve is dominated by elastic rather than viscoelastic recovery. Thus, to minimize the effects of viscoelasticity and creep on property measurements, a relatively long constant load hold period should be inserted prior to the final unloading, during which the viscoelastic deformation can diminish to a negligible rate. The second constant load hold period, near the end of the test at 90% of the peak load, is used to establish the rate of thermal expansion or contraction of the testing apparatus to correct the displacement data for thermal drift. Viscoelastic recovery is significant during the initial portion of the hold period, but after a period of time (about 200 s in the experiment shown in Figure 17.5) the viscoelastic effects become relatively small compared with the thermal effects. Data from the latter portion of the second hold period are used to establish the thermal drift rate and correct the displacement data. To minimize thermal drift effects, care must be taken to let the system thermally equilibrate for an extended period of time prior to testing. The indentation is then completely withdrawn. The upper half of the data obtained in the final unloading segment is used to determine the hardness and elastic modulus.[1] Fused silica, which exhibits elastic isotropy and has a relatively low modulus-to-hardness ratio, is used to calibrate the indenter shape function. The elastic modulus of fused silica is 72 GPa, and its Poisson's ratio is 0.17. Figure 17.6 shows a plot of elastic modulus of fused silica as a function of depth. The elastic modulus of fused silica is independent of indentation depth.

IV. ANALYZING NANOINDENTATION LOAD–DISPLACEMENT DATA

The most common method for analyzing nanoindentation load–displacement data is that of Oliver and Pharr[1] which expands on ideas developed by Doerner and Nix,[2] but is not constrained by the assumption of a flat punch indenter geometry. A typical load–displacement indentation curve is shown in Figure 17.7. During loading, both elastic and plastic deformation occur under the indenter as the contacts are changed with increasing depth. The unloading part of the curve is dominated by elastic displacements. The hardness is found by computing the mean pressure under the indenter

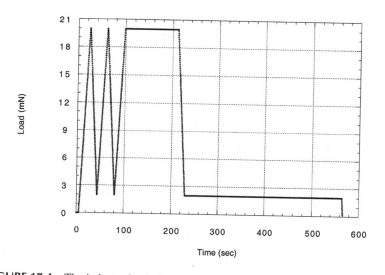

FIGURE 17.4 The indenter load–time sequence used for all nanoindentation testing.

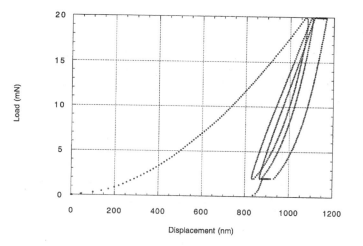

FIGURE 17.5 Typical load–displacement data (tested in an osteon).

at the point of maximum load. This requires a knowledge of the contact area at that point. Because the unloading curve is dominated by elastic displacement, it is possible to determine the elastic modulus of the material being indented from the slope of the unloading curve.[1,18]

Figure 17.8 shows a cross section of an indentation and identifies the parameters used in the analysis. At any time during loading, the total displacement h is written as

$$h = h_c + h_s,\qquad(17.1)$$

where h_c is the vertical distance along which contact is made (called contact depth) and h_s is the displacement of the surface at the perimeter of the contact. At peak load, the load and displacement are P_{max} and h_{max}, respectively. Upon unloading, the elastic displacements are recovered, and when the indenter is fully withdrawn, the final depth of the residual hardness impression is h_f.

The analysis begins by fitting the unloading curve to the power-law relation

$$P = b(h - h_f)^m,\qquad(17.2)$$

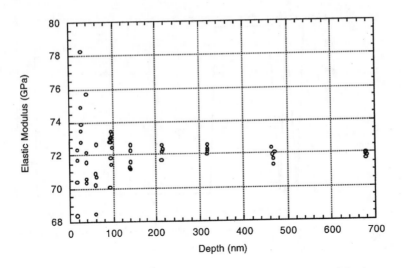

FIGURE 17.6 Elastic modulus of fused silica as a function of depth.

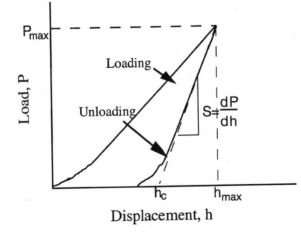

FIGURE 17.7 A schematic representation of load vs. indenter displacement showing quantities used in the analysis as well as a graphical interpretation of the contact depth.

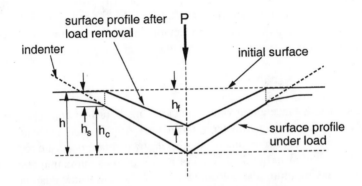

FIGURE 17.8 A schematic representation of a section through an indentation showing various quantities used in the analysis.

where P is the indentation load, h is the displacement, b and m are empirically determined fitting parameters, h_f is the final displacement after complete unloading determined by curve fitting. The unloading stiffness, S, that is, the slope of the unloading curve during the initial stages of unloading, is then established by differentiating Equation 17.2 at the maximum depth of penetration, $h = h_{max}$, giving

$$S = \frac{dP}{dh}\bigg|_{h=h_{max}} = mb(h_{max} - h_f)^{m-1}, \qquad (17.3)$$

The depth along which contact is made between the indenter and the specimen, h_c, can also be estimated from the load–displacement data using

$$h_c = h_{max} - \varepsilon\frac{P_{max}}{S}, \qquad (17.4)$$

where P_{max} is the peak indentation load and ε is a constant which depends on the geometry of the indenter — $\varepsilon = 1$ for the flat punch; $\varepsilon = 0.75$ for the paraboloid of revolution (Berkovich indenter); $\varepsilon = 0.72$ for the conical indenter. With these basic measurements, the projected contact area of the hardness impression, A, is derived by evaluating an empirically determined indenter shape function at the contact depth, h_c; that is, $A = f(h_c)$.

Finally, the hardness, H, and effective elastic modulus, E_{eff}, are derived from

$$H = \frac{P_{max}}{A} \qquad (17.5)$$

and

$$E_{eff} = \frac{1}{\beta}\frac{\sqrt{\pi}}{2}\frac{S}{\sqrt{A}}, \qquad (17.6)$$

where β is 1 for circular (flat punch), 1.034 for triangular (Berkovich indenter), and 1.012 for square (Vickers indenter). Note that the values of β for the triangular and square geometries deviate from the circular one by only 3.4 and 1.2%.[19]

An effective modulus is used in the analysis to account for the fact that elastic deformation occurs in both the specimen and the indenter. The effective modulus is related to the specimen modulus through

$$\frac{1}{E_{eff}} = \frac{1-v^2}{E} + \frac{1-v_i^2}{E_i}, \qquad (17.7)$$

where E and v are indentation modulus and Poisson's ratio for the specimen, and E_i and v_i are the same quantities for the indenter. The elastic properties of the diamond indenter, v_i and E_i, are 0.07 and 1140 GPa, respectively. We assume that Poisson's ratio for bone is $v = 0.3$. A sensitivity study showed that varying v in the range 0.2 to 0.4 changed the measured values of E by no more than 8%.

The attractiveness of this approach is that direct observation and measurement of the contact area is not needed for the evaluation of H and E, thus facilitating property measurement from very small indentations. Clearly, however, the accuracy with which H and E can be measured depends on how well Equations 17.3 through 17.6 describe the indentation deformation behavior. In this regard, it is important to note these equations were derived by Sneddon,[20] assuming elastic deformation only. One important way in which an elastic solution fails to describe properly the elastic/plastic behavior observed in indentation concerns the pileup or sink-in of material around the indenter. In the purely elastic contact solution, material always sinks in, while for elastic/plastic contact, material may either sink in or pile up. Since this has important effects on the indentation contact area, it is not entirely surprising that the Oliver–Pharr method has been found to work well for hard ceramics, in which sink-in predominates, but significant errors can be encountered when the method is applied to soft metals that exhibits extensive pileup.[21] Pileup leads to contact areas that are greater than the cross-sectional area of the indenter at a given depth. These effects lead to errors in the absolute measurement of mechanical properties by nanoindentation.[3] However, the elastic and plastic properties of bone are such that pileup is not an important issue, and can largely be ignored (see Figure 17.10).

V. DETERMINATION OF LOAD FRAME COMPLIANCE AND DIAMOND AREA FUNCTION

A method for calibrating the shape of the indenter tip and load frame compliance has been developed by Oliver and Pharr.[1] It is based on the measurement of contact stiffness and requires no imaging of the indentations. The area function for a perfect Berkovich indenter can be described by

$$A(h_c) = 24.5h_c^2. \tag{17.8}$$

However, all Berkovich indenters have some deviation from this geometry at the tip. Since the measured indentation displacement is the sum of the displacements in the specimen and the load frame, the load frame compliance must be known to determine specimen displacements accurately. To a good approximation, the load frame and the specimen can be modeled as two springs in series, for which case the total measured compliance is

$$C = C_s + C_m, \tag{17.9}$$

where C_s is the compliance of the specimen (the contact compliance), and C_m is the compliance of the testing machine. The contact compliance depends on the contact area at that point, A. Since the specimen compliance during elastic contact is given by the inverse of the contact stiffness, S, Equations 17.6 and 17.9 combine to yield

$$C = C_m + \frac{1}{\beta} \frac{\sqrt{\pi}}{2E_{eff}} \frac{1}{\sqrt{A}}. \tag{17.10}$$

Equation 17.10 shows that a plot of C vs. $A^{-1/2}$ is linear. The intercept of the plot is the load frame compliance, C_m, and the slope is proportional to $1/E_{eff}$. The best values of C_m are obtained when the second term on the right-hand side of Equation 17.10 is small, i.e., for large indentations. To implement the procedure, a series of indentations are made in aluminum, some of which can be quite large due to its low hardness. For the larger aluminum indentations, the area function is assumed to be that for a perfect Berkovich indenter (Equation 17.8), which provides a first estimate of the contact area. Initial estimates of C_m and E_{eff} are then obtained by plotting C vs. $A^{-1/2}$. By using these values, the contact area is computed by rewriting Equation 17.10 as

$$A = \frac{\pi}{4} \frac{1}{E_{eff}^2} \frac{1}{(C - C_m)^2}. \tag{17.11}$$

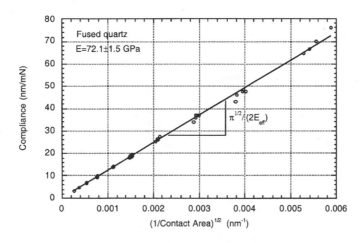

FIGURE 17.9   Unloading compliance vs. contact area for the indentation of fused quartz. Equation 17.10 is well obeyed. The effective elastic modulus can be found from the slope of the curve.

An initial guess at the area function is made by fitting the A vs. h_c data to a relationship such as

$$A(h_c) = 24.5h_c^2 + n_1 h_c^1 + n_2 h_c^{1/2} + n_3 h_c^{1/4} + \ldots n_8 h_c^{1/128} \qquad (17.12)$$

where n_1 through n_8 are constants.

The procedure is not complete at this stage because the exact form of the area function influences the values of C_m and E_{eff}, so using the new area function the procedure is applied again and iterated several times until convergence is achieved. To determine area function at shallower depths, a similar method involving indentations in fused quartz is used (fused quartz is much harder than aluminum, so it is easier to make small indenters), assuming the same machine compliance as measured in the aluminum experiments. This area function is assumed to describe the tip geometry completely, and thus it yields the contact area of any indentation made to a known depth. In this approach, the cross-sectional area of the tip and the contact area of the indenter and the specimen, at a given depth, are treated implicitly as if they are the same.[3] However, the tip-end geometry needs to be known precisely to determine the true contact area between the indenter and the material being tested when the contact area is small, or the machine compliance must be accurately determined where the specimen is stiff.[22]

Figure 17.9 shows a plot of the measured compliance vs. contact area for a sample of fused quartz. We noted that Equation 17.10 is very well obeyed and that the elastic modulus of quartz can be found from the slope of the curve.

VI. LIMITATIONS

The analytical methods outlined here are derived under the assumption that the material is homogeneous and isotropic in its elastic properties. When used to measure the elastic modulus of an anisotropic material such as bone, the modulus derived from the method is an average of the anisotropic elastic constants biased toward the modulus in the direction of testing.[5] The relationship between the elastic modulus measured by nanoindentation using the Oliver–Pharr method and the anisotropic elastic constants has been examined by Vlassak and Nix.[23,24] They showed that the elastic modulus obtained from nanoindentation techniques and the actual Young's modulus are the same only for elastically isotropic media. For materials with lower symmetry, elastic anisotropy affects the indentation measurements. The influence of anisotropy on experimental measurements has been studied by Hay et al.[25] who examined single crystals of β-silicon nitride with the long axis of the crystal oriented parallel to the c-direction of the hexagonal crystal structure. They found that the elastic modulus obtained from nanoindentation in the longitudinal direction underestimates the single-crystal Young's modulus while in the transverse direction, the nanoindentation elastic modulus overestimates the single-crystal Young's modulus. Hay et al.[25] also found that the elastic modulus obtained from nanoindentation is dominantly controlled by the elastic properties in the indentation direction, and is only weakly influenced by properties in the transverse directions. However, without some prior knowledge of the type of elastic anisotropy and an estimate of the associated anisotropic elastic constants, it is difficult to estimate how large the influences of anisotropy may be. This problem needs to be investigated further.

VII. RESULTS FOR MEASUREMENTS IN BONE

Recently, the elastic properties of several microstructural components of dry human vertebrae and tibiae have been investigated in the longitudinal and transverse directions using nanoindentation.[6] The bone sections were prepared in the same way as mentioned above. A total of 373 indentations were produced in this study. In the vertebrae, three to five indentations were made in 12 separate trabeculae in the longitudinal direction (i.e., perpendicular to the transverse section) and 29 separate trabeculae in the transverse direction. For the tibiae, three to five indentations were made in 15 osteons and 14 interstitial lamellae in the longitudinal direction. In the transverse direction (i.e., perpendicular to the longitudinal section), it was difficult to distinguish osteons microstructurally from interstitial lamellae (Figure 17.10), so individual measurements were not possible. Consequently, the transverse direction data represent an average over all the indentations in the longitudinal section without regard to their exact locations in the two microstructural components. Basic modulus and hardness results are summarized in Table 17.1. The elastic modulus was found to be highest for the interstitial lamellae, intermediate for osteonal lamellae, and lowest for trabecular bone. As regards direction, moduli determined in the longitudinal direction were always greater than those determined in the transverse direction for a given microstructural constituent. The ratio of elastic moduli in the longitudinal to transverse directions was found to be 1.35 for osteons and 1.29 for trabecular bone. The hardnesses follow in similar order. The ratio of hardness in the longitudinal to transverse direction is 1.10 for osteons and 1.19 for trabeculae. The mean values of elastic moduli for all of the bone components were found to be statistically different ($p < 0.05$). Therefore, for a given microstructural component, there is an anisotropy between the longitudinal and transverse directions. Similar conclusions hold for the hardnesses.

More recently, the nanoindentation method was used to examine variations in the individual lamellar properties within osteons, as a function of distance from the osteonal center (Haversian canal).[7] Elastic moduli and hardnesses of the individual lamellae within the osteon decrease monotonically as a function of increasing distance from the osteonal center. The mechanical properties of osteons are significantly lower than those of the interstitial bone ($p < 0.0001$). There were statistically significant differences ($p = 0.0005$ and 0.0004, respectively) between lamellar properties obtained from the two innermost osteonal lamellae ($E = 20.8 \pm 1.3$ GPa and $H = 0.65 \pm 0.06$ GPa) and those from the two outermost osteonal lamellae ($E = 18.8 \pm 1.0$ GPa and $H = 0.55 \pm 0.05$ GPa). The ratio (E_1/E_2) of the elastic moduli of the outermost osteonal lamella (E_1) (considered to be the soft part of the osteons) and that of interstitial bone (E_2) was approximately 0.7. These results contradict expectations based on the current understanding of the physiology and the mechanism of osteonal remodeling, but they may have important implications for the mechanical contribution of individual osteons for bone biomechanics.

TABLE 17.1

Mean Elastic Moduli and Hardnesses for the Microstructural Components of Cortical and Trabecular Bone as Measured in This Study

Bone Type	Direction to Be Tested	No. of Subjects	No. of Indentations	No. of Microstructural Components	Elastic Modulus, GPa (SD)	Hardness, GPa (SD)
Cortical bone	Longitudinal					
	Osteons	2	72	15	22.4 (1.2)	0.617 (0.039)
	Interstitial lamellae	2	58	14	25.7 (1.0)	0.736 (0.044)
	Transverse	2	58	13	16.6 (1.1)	0.564 (0.034)
Trabecular bone	Longitudinal	3	53	12	19.4 (2.3)	0.618 (0.061)
	Transverse	7	132	29	15.0 (2.5)	0.515 (0.082)

Note: Standard deviations are shown in parentheses (SD). The transverse cortical bone data represent an average over all the transverse section indentations without regard to their exact locations in the two microstructural components.

Source: Rho, J. et al., *J. Biomed. Mater. Res.,* 45, 48–54. © 1999 John Wiley & Sons, Inc. With permission.

(a)

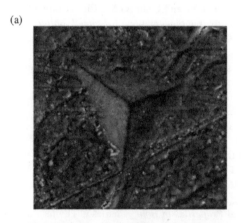

(b)

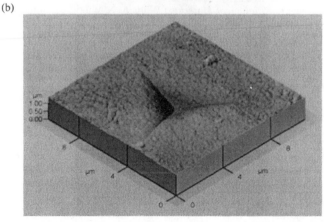

FIGURE 17.10 Typical nanoindentation of interstitial lamellar bone of tibia. (a) Scanning electron micrograph (×5000) and (b) atomic force microscopy.

ACKNOWLEDGMENTS

This research was sponsored by a faculty summer research fellowship from the Oak Ridge Institute for Science and Technology (ORISE) and the National Institutes of Health AR45297 (JY). Analytical instrumentation for the nanoindentation testing was provided by the Division of Materials Sciences, U.S. Department of Energy, under Contract DE-AC05-96OR22464 with Lockheed Martin Energy Research Corp. and through the SHaRE Program under Contract DE-AC05-76OR00033 between the U.S. Department of Energy and Oak Ridge Associated Universities.

REFERENCES

1. Oliver, W.C. and Pharr, G.M., An improved technique for determining hardness and elastic modulus using load and displacement sensing indentation experiments, *J. Mater. Res.*, 7, 1564, 1992.
2. Doerner, M.F. and Nix, W.D., A method for interpreting the data from depth-sensing indentation instruments, *J. Mater. Res.*, 601, 1986.
3. McElhaney, K.W., Vlassak, J.J., and Nix, W.D., Determination of indenter tip geometry and indentation contact area for depth-sensing indentation experiments, *J. Mater. Res.*, 13, 1300, 1998.
4. Mayo, M.J., Siegel, R.W., Liao, Y.X., and Nix, W.D., Nanoindentation of nanocrystalline ZnO, *J. Mater. Res.*, 7, 973, 1992.
5. Rho, J.Y., Tsui, T.Y., and Pharr, G.M., Elastic properties of human cortical and trabecular lamellar bone measured by nanoindentation, *Biomaterials*, 8, 1325, 1997.
6. Rho, J.Y., Roy, M.E., Tsui, T.Y., and Pharr, G.M., Elastic properties of microstructural components of human bone measured by nanoindentation, *J. Biomed. Mater. Res.*, 45, 48, 1999.
7. Rho, J.Y., Zioupos, P., Currey, J.D., and Pharr, G.M., Variations in the individual lamellar properties within osteons by nanoindentation, *Bone*, in press.
8. Roy, M.E., Rho, J.Y., Tsui, T.Y., et al., Mechanical and morphological variation of the human lumbar vertebral cortical and trabecular bone, *J. Biomed. Mater. Res.*, 44, 191, 1999.
9. Blackburn, J., Hodgskinson, R., Currey, J.D., and Mason, J.E., Mechanical properties of microcallus in human bone, *J. Orthop. Res.*, 10, 237, 1992.
10. Ziv, V., Wagner, H.D., and Weiner, S., Microstructure–microhardness relations in parallel-fibered and lamellar bone, *Bone*, 18, 417, 1996.
11. Ascenzi, A., Benvenuti, A., and Bonucci, E., The tensile properties of single osteonic lamellae: technical problems and preliminary results, *J. Biomech.*, 5, 29, 1982.
12. Prendergast, P.J. and Huiskes, R., Microdamage and osteocyte-lacuna strain in bone: a microstructural finite element analysis, *J. Biomech. Eng.*, 118, 240, 1996.
13. Evans F.G., *Mechanical Properties of Bone*, Charles C Thomas, Springfield, IL, 1973.
14. Yamada, H., *Strength of Biological Materials*, Williams & Wilkins, Baltimore, MD, 1970.
15. Townsend P.R. and Rose, R.M., Buckling studies of single human trabeculae, *J. Biomech.*, 8, 199, 1975.
16. Currey, J.D., The effects of drying and re-wetting on some mechanical properties of cortical bone, *J. Biomech.*, 21, 439, 1988.
17. Rho, J.Y. and Pharr, G.M., Effects of drying on the mechanical properties of bovine femur measured by nanoindentation, *J. Mater. Sci. Mater. Med.*, 10, 485, 1999.
18. Nix, W.D., Elastic and plastic properties of thin films on substrates: nanoindentation techniques, *Mater. Sci. Eng.*, A234, 37, 1997.
19. Pharr, G.M., Oliver, W.C., and Brotzen, F.R., On the generality of the relationship among contact stiffness, contact area, and elastic modulus during indentation, *J. Mater. Res.*, 7, 613, 1992.
20. Sneddon, I.N., The relation between load and penetration in the axisymmetric Boussinesq problem for a punch of arbitrary profile, *Int. J. Eng. Sci.*, 3, 47, 1965.
21. Bolshakov, A. and Pharr, G.M., Influences of pileup on the measurement of mechanical properties by load and depth sensing indentation techniques, *J. Mater. Res.*, 13, 1049, 1998.
22. Hainsworth, S.V., Chandler, H.W., and Page, T.F., Analysis of nanoindentation load–displacement loading curves, *J. Mater. Res.*, 11, 1987, 1996.
23. Vlassak, J.J. and Nix. W.D., Indentation modulus of elastically anisotropic half spaces, *Philos. Mag. A*, 67, 1045, 1993.

24. Vlassak, J.J. and Nix, W.D., Measuring the elastic properties of anisotropic materials by means of indentation experiments, *J. Mech. Phys. Solids*, 42, 1223, 1994.
25. Hay, J.C., Sun, E.Y., Pharr, G.M., et al., Elastic anisotropy of β-silicon nitride whiskers, *J. Am. Ceram. Soc.*, 81, 2661, 1998.

18 Single Osteon Micromechanical Testing

Maria-Grazia Ascenzi, Alessandro Benvenuti, and Antonio Ascenzi

CONTENTS

I. INTRODUCTION

Because sample dimensions may affect the mechanical behavior of a material, mechanics differentiates into micro- and macromechanics. The mechanics of biological materials, micro- and macrobiomechanics, can be viewed as a fundamental expression of skeleton physiology and pathology[1,2] and, hence, as complements of skeletal anatomy. This chapter treats the microbiomechanics of single secondary osteons.

While the observations of Galileo Galilei[3] in the 1600s can be considered to have initiated bone macromechanics, bone micromechanics began much later, between 1937 and 1942, with the studies conducted at the Anatomy School of Bologna, according to Evans.[4] Such studies did not, however, include techniques for isolation of single microscopic structural units.

The justification for studying bone micromechanics is found in bone morphology. The bone component of bone samples is not at all structured as a simple aggregation of molecular and supramolecular organic and inorganic units, which results in a homogeneous macroscopic entity. Petersen[5] first introduced the concept that bone structures can be viewed as a four-order hierarchy, arranged in decreasing size. The first order comprises the structures corresponding to gross shape and differentiation between compact and cancellous bone. The second order of compact bone includes Haversian systems, cylindrical lamellar systems, and additional related structures, e.g., bone marrow. The third order consists of collagen fibrils which lie in the ground substance; one of their roles, in association with osteocytes, is the constitution of lamellae. The fourth order consists of the molecular patterning between organic and inorganic substances. This four-order hierarchy forms through a slow, continuous process of replacement of primary or woven bone, which begins as woven bone is formed, in the fetus or soon after birth, and continues throughout life.

In view of the structural hierarchical orders described, the mechanical analysis of a first-order sample is possible only with knowledge of the properties of the three lower orders; conversely, from knowledge of properties of the three lower structural orders, mechanical behavior of the first-order sample can be derived. This is the case under both normal and pathological conditions so long as the pathology does not alter the structural configuration of the four orders.

An additional motivation to study the mechanics of osteons resides in the lack of knowledge about the structure of some of the microscopic entities which comprise them, such as lamellae in alternate osteons. Increased knowledge of osteon mechanics may shed light on the microstructural problems of such entities.

II. ELEMENTS OF MICROMECHANICAL TESTING

The methods for single osteon micromechanical testing share three well-established steps: (1) osteon selection; (2) sample isolation; (3) sample loading by an apparatus crafted in accordance with sample shape and dimensions, as well as load type and magnitude. Listed here are aspects of these steps, which apply to each of the micromechanical testing methods to be presented individually.

Any human or vertebrate secondary osteon may be selected and isolated. Ortner and Yong[6] and Frasca et al.[7] describe methods for isolating whole osteons. However, whole osteons display irregular shape, and such irregularity prevents accurate mechanical loading and comparison of mechanical loading results. Consideration of osteon samples of simple and same geometric shape, rather than whole osteons, allows comparison of mechanical loading results. Human osteons, the osteons considered in this chapter, have a somewhat cylindrical shape around a vascular canal. The osteon sample shape that suitably represents osteons and their mechanical properties is accordingly a cylindrical shape around a central vascular canal.

The selection of specific osteons for isolation depends on two factors: (1) sample dimensions, especially when the experimentation requires samples of approximately the same size; (2) sample type, described in terms of the two principal bone mechanical components which present three characteristics. The two components are collagen bundles and hydroxyapatite crystallites, and the three characteristics are distribution of collagen bundles, orientation of collagen bundles, and amount of hydroxyapatite crystallites.

Osteons are selected from one or more sections of fresh compact bone, not previously fixed. Sections are obtained by grinding on a glass plate while air cooling to prevent heating of material or by using a rotating-saw microtome equipped with a continuous waterspout to prevent heating of material. Sections of the same thickness are generally cut in parallel (longitudinal sections) or perpendicularly (transverse or cross sections) to the axes of the osteons.

The classic theory categorizes osteons structurally according to the types of coaxial lamellae which comprise them. Two lamellar types are evidenced in bone sections by the polarizing microscope. Classical theory supposes that lamellae which appear bright in longitudinal sections and dark or extinct in cross sections under the polarizing microscope consist of collagen bundles parallel to the osteon axis. They are called longitudinal lamellae. Classical theory supposes that lamellae which appear dark in longitudinal sections and bright in cross sections under the polarizing microscope consist of collagen bundles perpendicular to the osteon axis. They are called transverse or circularly fibered lamellae. In the last 20 years, Frasca et al.[8] A. Ascenzi and Benvenuti,[9,10] and Giraud-Guille[11] reported the additional presence of oblique bundles with discrete or continuous orientations relative to osteon axis. Pending definitive ascertainment, the terms *transverse* or *circularly fibered* lamella are used.

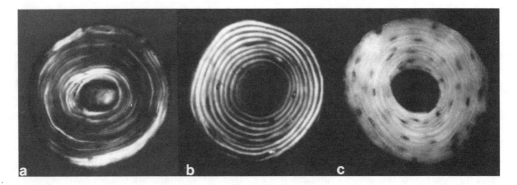

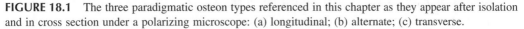

FIGURE 18.1   The three paradigmatic osteon types referenced in this chapter as they appear after isolation and in cross section under a polarizing microscope: (a) longitudinal; (b) alternate; (c) transverse.

Among the various arrangements of longitudinal and transverse lamellae, those characterizing two typical osteon types were chosen for the experiments that this chapter describes. In the first type, collagen bundles have a marked longitudinal spiral course, with the pitch of the spiral changing so slightly that the bundles in one lamella make an angle of approximately 0° with the bundles of the next lamella; under the polarizing microscope, such osteons appear homogeneously bright in longitudinal section and dark in cross section with few bright lamellae at the periphery and around the Haversian canal. A few, very thin, incomplete bright lamellae may also be present. Such osteons are called longitudinal osteons (Figure 18.1a). In the second type, bundles in one lamella make an angle of approximately 90° with the bundles of the next lamella; under the polarizing microscope, such osteons show an alternation of bright and dark lamellae in both longitudinal and cross section (Figure 18.1b), as reported by Gebhardt[12] and Amprino,[13] and they are called alternate osteons. In only a few studies was a third typical osteon type selected, that called transverse or circular. In the third type, collagen fibrils have a marked transverse spiral course in successive lamellae; under the polarizing microscope, such osteons appear homogeneously dark in longitudinal section and bright in cross section (Figure 18.1c).

The three mentioned osteon types are representative of osteons because they are outstanding appearances of a continuous distribution of osteon structures. The continuity of the distribution is due to the varying mesh of longitudinal and transverse lamellae.

The degree of calcification of single osteons is assessed by means of the microradiographic technique. On a micro-X-ray, the calcium amount in each unit is revealed by a shade ranging from light to dark gray. Since a micro-X-ray is a magnified negative film, the image of osteonic section at initial (final, respectively) stage of calcification is dark (light, respectively) gray. Osteons at an intermediate stage of calcification show an intermediate shade of gray. When osteons at either initial or final stage of calcification are desired, their recognition is straightforward. To assess exactly intermediate stages of calcification, a scale of comparison is necessary. In this case, a scale made of very thin, superimposed aluminum sheets is microradiographed together with the bone section on the same X-ray film.

After complete isolation of a cylindrical sample, the regularity of the sample is assessed in terms of the position and orientation of the canal. The distance between the vascular canal and external surface of the sample at various rotational angles and levels is required to be constant. The percent of discarded samples may reach 93 to 95% of prepared samples.

Skilled technicians designed and made the osteon loading apparatus which this chapter describes. Such apparatus proved useful and manageable to A. Ascenzi's research group. Apparatus based on other principles, but of similar sensitivity, could, of course, also be manufactured.

Osteon samples are loaded under physiological conditions, i.e., after rehydration by soaking in saline solution. Currey verified the validity of this method.[14]

The experiments are preferably performed at a temperature of 20 to 22°C.

III. TESTING METHODS

Methods for the study of mechanical properties of isolated osteon samples follow. Results are briefly reported after each mechanical test description to facilitate understanding of the method.

A. TENSION TEST

Design and preparation of osteon samples for axial tensional loading was a time-consuming process which involved diverse and repeated attempts.

Initially, it seemed unfeasible to obtain osteon samples of cylindrical shape around a vascular canal. Hence, hemidiametral osteon sections, 50 to 60 μm thick, were prepared. This type of sample at first presented some advantages: preparation by dissection and assessment of osteon type were straightforward. Tension testing showed that longitudinal osteons were stronger in tension than alternate osteons, as anticipated by structural considerations.[15,16] However, stress–strain curves of alternate osteon samples showed frequent abrupt changes in slope, so-called knees, at low stresses, similar to those recorded in some cross-ply laminates. Electron microscope examination revealed that such knees were due to failure of interfibrillar cementing substance in the lamellae whose collagen bundles were mainly perpendicularly oriented to the loading direction.[17] Hemidiametral sample preparation eliminated the longitudinal initial stress that ordinarily protects alternate osteons at low axial stresses.[18-21] Hence, this kind of sample was inadequately representative of osteon mechanical properties.

Studies were accordingly redirected toward development of a method for isolation of a cylindrical sample around the vascular canal which would also allow certain assessment of osteon type. This goal was achieved and the method follows.

A longitudinal section of thickness slightly larger than the osteon diameter, i.e., 300 to 350 μm, is cut from a bone shaft. It is difficult to locate longitudinal and alternate osteons on the section: the overlapping of concentric lamellae may mean that fewer or no dark lamellae are visible under a polarizing microscope; therefore, an alternate osteon might appear bright and be mistaken as a longitudinal one. Definite identification of osteon type is possible only after testing. It is accomplished by observing under a polarizing microscope a thin cross section cut with a microscopic drill. Longitudinal and alternate osteons, at initial and final stages of calcification, are tentatively chosen.

Isolation of osteon samples from sections occurs in two steps. In Step 1, a dental drill is inserted into the body of a microscope in place of the tube. The bone section is firmly secured on the microscope stage, perpendicularly oriented with respect to the drill. As the drill and microscope stage are operated simultaneously, the device allows longitudinal cuts so as to coarsely free an osteon sample around the vascular canal from the surrounding material. The shape of the sample is thinner in the middle portion, which is a parallelepiped, and larger at the rectangular cross-sectional ends (Figure 18.2a). Such lugs serve to secure the sample to the loading device when inserted into the loading device rectangular jaws. The total length of the sample measures 500 μm, the maximum osteonic stretch that does not contain Volkmann's canals, which would create discontinuities. Samples are air-cooled during coarse isolation to avoid overheating.

In Step 2, the middle portion of the sample is transformed from a parallelepiped to a cylindrical shape whose axis coincides with the axis of the vascular canal (Figure 18.2b) by means of a microgrinding lathe designed by A. Ascenzi's research group and manufactured by CECOM Company.

The microgrinding lathe features two jaws, powered by an electric motor and synchronously rotating around a common axis; they are used to secure the osteon sample. Once the shape of the sample has been corrected, the rotating axis of the system should coincide with the axis of the vascular canal. A small steel blade, whose edge measures nearly 500 μm in length, produces the grinding effect. The blade moves forward or backward and its movements are monitored by a

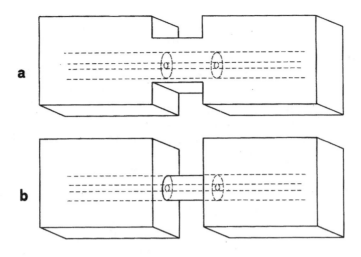

FIGURE 18.2   Diagram showing the preparation steps of a cylindrical osteon sample for tensional loading.
(a) Step 1. The sample has been isolated from the bone section by means of a dental drill. The sample is still
surrounded by bone material, is thinner in the middle portion, and has a rectangular cross section.
(b) Step 2. The material surrounding the middle portion of the sample has now been removed by means of a
special microgrinding lathe. The sample shows a middle cylindrical shape. (From Ascenzi, A., Baschieri, P.,
and Benvenuti, A., The torsional properties of single selected osteons, *J. Biomech.*, 27, 875, 1994. With
permission from Elsevier Science.)

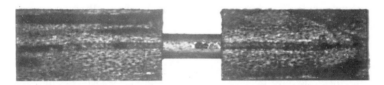

FIGURE 18.3   Osteon sample with its lugs. (From Ascenzi, A., Baschieri, P., and Benvenuti, A., The torsional
properties of single selected osteons, *J. Biomech.*, 27, 875, 1994. With permission from Elsevier Science.)

micrometer. The maximum penetration of the blade into the sample roughly corresponds to the
minimum osteon radius in order to eliminate significant residues of adjacent structures. Samples
are air-cooled during grinding to avoid overheating. At this point, complete isolation of a cylindrical
sample is achieved (Figure 18.3). The transverse area of the cylindrical portion of the sample is
used to calculate the ultimate tensile stress.

The loading apparatus consists of an extensometer furnished with a microwave micrometer
which allows loading of osteon samples and measurement of sample elongations. It was devised
by A. Gozzini, late holder of the chair of Solid State Physics at the Scuola Normale Superiore, Pisa.[22]

The informing principle of the apparatus follows. Let h and D be height and diameter, respectively, of a metallic cylinder whose cavity functions as a resonator for electromagnetic waves. The
resonance frequency, f_o, of this cavity will depend on h, D, and the electromagnetic field configuration inside its cavity, called mode. When the Te_{012} mode is the chosen configuration type, the
following relation holds:[23]

$$f_o^2 = (C/D)^2 (1.488 + (C/h)^2) \tag{18.1}$$

where C is the velocity of light in a vacuum.

Figure 18.4 shows a diagram of the apparatus used to measure the elongation of osteon samples under tensile load. Each of the two ends of the sample is secured into a jaw; one of the two jaws supports a Plexiglas disk whose lower metal-coated surface forms the upper plane of the cylindrical metal cavity. The disk, which may slide into the vertically oriented cavity, has a very thin nylon thread attached to its center. The thread runs along the longitudinal axis of the cavity and exits through a small hole at the center of the lower fixed end of the cylindrical metal cavity. To exert traction on the osteon sample, an increasing number of weights is attached to the free end of the thread. As the osteon sample elongates, the sample pulls the lug affixed to the upper disk of the cylindrical cavity; the upper disk slides into the cavity reducing the height of the cavity; such reduction produces a change in resonance frequency in the cavity. Therefore, as elongation of sample (Δl) takes place, the height of the cavity reduces by the same amount ($-\Delta l$) and resonance frequency changes by Δf_o in the cavity. In this apparatus, Δl and Δf_o are small with respect to h. Equation 18.1 gives, for small Δl's,

$$\Delta l = \Delta f_o \, (1+1.488(h/\Delta)^2)(h/f_o) \qquad\qquad (18.2)$$

A pulse technique[22] is used to measure Δf_o. An oscilloscope, based on Equation 18.2 and inserted in the apparatus, transforms Δf_o values into Δl values. The pulse technique has the advantages of being relatively simple to use, highly sensitive, and accurate. Accuracy in osteon sample elongation measurements is within 1%; accuracy partially depends on exact alignment of the osteon sample and apparatus.

In accordance with the results obtained on hemidiametral osteon samples, longitudinal osteon cylindrical samples resist tension better than alternate osteon cylindrical samples at both initial and final stages of calcification. A structural explanation may reside in the supposed diversity of the orientation of collagen bundles in alternate osteon samples, especially with regard to the presence of transverse bundles.

B. COMPRESSION TEST

Over the years, two methods have been developed to load and measure sample length changes in compression. In contrast with tension methods, both compressive methods are equally viable and the first one presented allows for recognition of osteon type before sample isolation.

Thickness of bone sections may measure at most 500 μm to be transparent enough to allow examination under the polarizing microscope. For thicker sections, bone transparency may be somewhat improved by soaking the section in bromoform, if necessary. A transverse section of long bone diaphysis 500 μm thick contains many straight, nonbranching portions of osteons which may be suitable for testing, once isolated.[24]

Longitudinal, alternate, and transverse osteons at both initial and final degree of calcification were selected on transverse sections 500 μm thick.

The specially designed device used for sample isolation consists of a very thin, carefully sharpened steel needle inserted off-center in a dental drill. As the drill turns, the tip of the needle describes a circle whose diameter may be adjusted to match the diameter of the sample. When the needle rotation axis is perpendicular to bone section surfaces, i.e., coincides with the osteon axis, the tip of the needle cuts an osteon sample of cylindrical shape with walls of uniform thickness just inside its limits. To ensure that the needle rotation axis is perpendicular to bone section surfaces, the drill handle is inserted in a microscope body in place of the tube and the section is firmly secured onto the microscope stage. Coarse microscope adjustment easily controls the needle movements into the bone section. Osteon cutting is controllable by watching the operation through a stereoscopic microscope. Figure 18.5 shows the shape of samples prepared with the above-described technique.

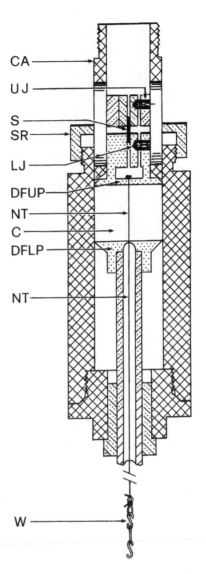

FIGURE 18.4 Diagram of cavity used as extensometer. From top to bottom: CA, cylindrical appendage; UJ, upper jaw with its screw; S, sample; SR, screw ring; LJ, lower jaw with its screw; DFUP, disk forming the upper plane of the cavity; NT, nylon thread; C, cavity; DFLP, disk forming the lower plane of the cavity; W, weights. (From Ascenzi, A., Bonucci, E., and Checcucci, A., *Studies on the Anatomy and Function of Bone and Joints*, F.G. Evans, Ed., Springer-Verlag, Berlin, 1966. With permission from Springer-Verlag, New York. From Ascenzi, A. and Bonucci, E., The tensile properties of single osteons, *Anat. Rec.*, 158, 375, 1967, The Wistar Institute. Reprinted by permission of Wiley-Liss, Inc., a division of John Wiley & Sons, Inc.)

Length and diameter of samples are accurately measured by means of an eyepiece micrometer. In experiments, the ratio of length to diameter ranged between 2.5 to 1 and 3 to 1.[24]

A microcompressor furnished with a microwave micrometer based on the cavity and pulse technique described in Section III.A above was used to load the specimens.

Figure 18.6 shows the apparatus diagram. The lower end of the sample is supported by the upper base of the fixed cylinder. The upper end is in contact with the push cylinder whose upper surface is the lower plane of the cylindrical cavity, which functions as a resonator for electromagnetic waves.

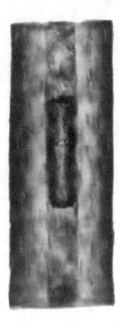

FIGURE 18.5 Isolated osteon sample to be loaded in compression, as seen in transmitted light. (From Ascenzi, A. and Bonucci, E., The compressive properties of single osteons, *Anat. Rec.*, 61, 377, 1968, The Wistar Institute. Reprinted by permission of Wiley-Liss, Inc., a division of John Wiley & Sons, Inc.)

The light (3.5 g) push cylinder can move freely inside the vertically oriented cavity. When weights are added to the thread attached to the push cylinder, the osteon sample undergoes a shortening which makes the cylindrical cavity lower plane slide, thus increasing the cavity height. Because sample shortening ($-\Delta l$) is equal in magnitude to cavity height elongation (Δl), sample shortenings are deduced from resonant frequency changes through Equation 18.2. Length change measurements are accurate up to 1%.

Longitudinal and alternate osteon samples show a compressive behavior opposite to tensional behavior. Modulus of elasticity and ultimate tensile strength values are maximum, intermediate, and minimum, respectively, for transverse, alternate, and longitudinal osteon types at the same degree of calcification. Modulus of elasticity and ultimate tensile strength values increase as calcification progresses.

The second compression test method differs from the previous one because the osteon sample shape is the sample shape used for tension loading, namely, a cylindrical central portion with rectangular cross-sectional ends. Consequently, the sample is secured to the loading apparatus by means of jaws as opposed to simply laying it in contact with the fixed cylinder surface and the push cylinder surface. The use of jaws allows loading under both tension and compression and, in particular, under tension–compression cyclic loading (see Section III.G). The disadvantage of the second method remains that definite identification of osteon type occurs only after loading.

C. Shearing Test

A. Ascenzi and Bonucci[25] have tested osteon samples loaded centrally and off-center with respect to their axes by means of a technique that may be viewed as a double-shearing strength test.

Longitudinal, alternate, and transverse osteons at both initial and final degree of calcification were selected on 300-μm-thick transverse sections. Each chosen osteon must pass through the section as shown by the appearance of its sectioned ends on both sides of the section.

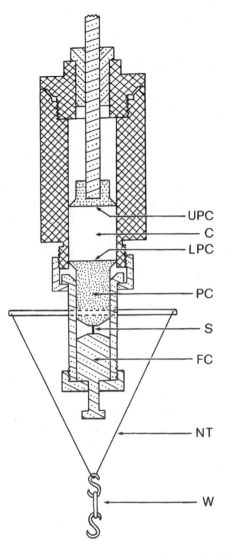

FIGURE 18.6   Diagram of cavity used as microwave micrometer and testing apparatus in compression. UPC, upper plane of cavity; C, cavity; LPC, lower plane cavity; PC, push cylinder; S, sample; FC, fixed cylinder; NT, nylon thread; W, weights. (From Ascenzi, A. and Bonucci, E., The compressive properties of single osteons, *Anat. Rec.*, 161, 377, 1968, The Wistar Institute. Reprinted by permission of Wiley-Liss, Inc., a division of John Wiley & Sons, Inc.)

Unlike previously described testing, sample isolation for a shearing test is part of sample loading. Hence, for shearing, isolation is examined in association with the apparatus description.

Figure 18.7 illustrates the method. It shows a compact bone transverse section with an osteon oriented perpendicularly to the upper and lower surface of the section itself. The section is supported by a rigid plane with a hole at its center. A steel cylinder, whose axis is aligned to the osteon axis of the sample, rests on the osteon upper end and acts as a punch when loaded with weights. In A. Ascenzi's group's investigation, the punch diameter was slightly smaller than the osteon diameter; although it may be smaller, according to the shearing surfaces to be studied. As the punch is loaded by adding small weights, the punch presses on the osteon; as soon as the punch displacement caused by an additional weight stopped, additional weights were added. At first, the punch induces

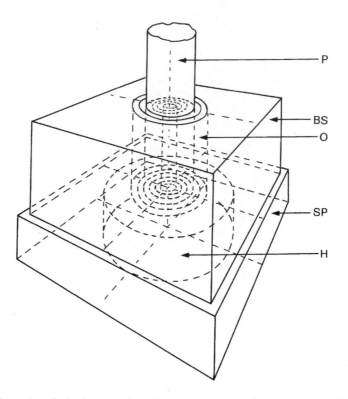

FIGURE 18.7   Illustration of criteria used to investigate osteon sample shearing strength. From top to bottom: P, punch; BS, bone section; O, osteon; SP, supporting plane; H, hole. (From Ascenzi, A. and Bonucci, E., The shearing properties of single osteons, *Anat. Rec.*, 172, 499, 1972, The Wistar Institute. Reprinted by permission of Wiley-Liss, Inc., a division of John Wiley & Sons, Inc.)

a deformation, then the connections between adjacent lamellae, at the immediate periphery of the punch, break. Consequently, as soon as ultimate shearing strength is reached and connections break, a cylindrical osteon sample begins to slip through the lower surface of the section and through the supporting plane hole (Figure 18.8). The diameter of the osteon sample coincides with the diameter of the punch.

A microwave micrometer based on cavity and pulse technique measures the progressive descent of the punch until ultimate strength is reached. The principle of the microwave micrometer is described in Section III.A.

Longitudinal osteons are the osteons least able to resist shearing stress. This suggests that bone compactness of the other osteon types is strengthened by circular collagen bundles. Ultimate strength and elasticity modulus in shear increases as calcification proceeds. Shearing properties of osteons loaded centrally with respect to their axes seem to be mainly related to lamellar structure as a whole. In fact, osteon samples loaded off-center are not cylindrical in shape and they fracture.

D. "PIN TEST"

This is a method for measuring the resistance of osteon walls to internal pressure. It was specially devised for micromechanical testing and is inspired by the standard "pin test" for copper and copper-alloy tubing expansion testing.[26] It consists of loading of an osteon sample by progressive penetration of a steel cone into the vascular canal until fracture occurs.[27]

Longitudinal, alternate, and transverse osteons at both initial and final degree of calcification were selected on 100-μm-thick transverse sections. Sections are cut by means of a rotating saw to ensure constant osteon sample height.

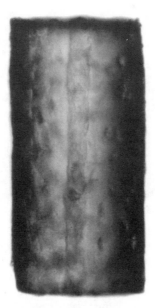

FIGURE 18.8 Fully calcified alternate osteon sample which has slipped out of an axially loaded bone section during shear testing. (From Ascenzi, A. and Bonucci, E., The shearing properties of single osteons, *Anat. Rec.*, 172, 499, 1972, The Wistar Institute. Reprinted by permission of Wiley-Liss, Inc., a division of John Wiley & Sons, Inc.)

Cylindrically shaped samples are obtained by using the first technique described in Section III.B. Uniform thickness of each osteon sample is checked with special care before the pin test: the outer and inner diameter measurements of each sample are checked at least eight times at 45° displacement.

Substitution of the punch in the apparatus for osteon testing in compression (Section III.B) with a steel cone yields an apparatus for the pin test. The angular width of the steel cone measures 35°. The choice of 35° allows the most accurate comparison between results, according to the A. Ascenzi group's experience. Progressive cone loading by means of weights causes the cone to press with increasing force on the upper circumferential end of the vascular canal. As soon as the cone displacement caused by an additional weight stopped, additional weights were added. At first, osteon deformation occurs and then lamellae increasingly fracture starting with lamellae closest to the vascular canal. A microwave micrometer based on cavity and pulse technique measures the progressive descent of the steel cone until ultimate strength is reached. The principle of the microwave micrometer is described in Section III.A. To allow comparison between load–deflection data of samples, dilating strength and strain are computed. Dilating strength equals $P/(r(R - r))$ and dilating strain equals $d/(R - r)$ where P is the load, r and R are inner and outer osteon radii, respectively, and d is the radius increase due to cone forward movement.

Transverse, alternate, and longitudinal osteon samples show, respectively, maximum, intermediate, and minimum ultimate dilating strength. This is further direct evidence that the presence of transverse lamellae increases osteon wall resistance.

E. Bending Test

Distribution of longitudinal and transverse lamellae in long bone sections is compatible with the force distribution usually acting on long bone under normal conditions.[28-33] Femoral lamellar distribution has been found to vary in accordance with a bending deformity consequent to severe rickets suffered in infancy.[34] Hence, a relationship exists in femur between modified microscopic

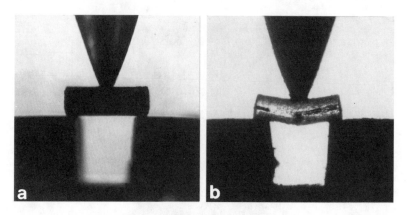

FIGURE 18.9   (a) Fully calcified alternate osteon sample ready to be loaded in bending. (b) Fully calcified alternate osteon sample at ultimate bending strength. (From Ascenzi, A., Baschieri, P., and Benvenuti, A., The bending properties of single osteons, *J. Biomech.*, 23, 763, 1990. With permission from Elsevier Science.)

structure and macroscopic features under bending. Such results motivated A. Ascenzi et al.[35] to explore micromechanical properties of a single osteon loaded in bending.

Longitudinal and alternate osteons at final degree of calcification were selected on 500-μm-thick transverse sections of a femoral diaphysis.

Cylindrically shaped samples are obtained by using the first technique described in Section III.B. Sample axis coinciding with the axis of the vascular canal is checked with particular care. The outer and inner diameter measurements of each sample need to be checked at least eight times at 45° displacement.

A 500-μm-long sample is laid on the edges of two small steel strips carefully placed on exactly the same horizontal plane. Since the distance between the edges measures 400 μm, an osteon sample is supported by each surface edge over a length of 50 μm. In this way, there are no constraints to angular rotation of the sample at the points of support, because both sample ends are free to move while the sample is loaded in bending (Figure 18.9a). The central part of the sample is loaded by means of a steel point which has linear contact with the sample (Figure 18.9b). Avoidance of longitudinal or rotational displacement of the sample relative to the point during loading is necessary for testing accuracy.

A microwave micrometer based on the cavity and pulse technique measures the advancement of the steel point. The principle of the microwave micrometer is described in Section III.A. Measurement of changes in bending is accurate within 1%.

Note that because the length of the sample is short with respect to the its external diameter, a large shearing stress is generated at the failure site. Such shearing stress makes for an improper bending test. However, this occurrence seems negligible because the aim of the present investigation is to provide comparative, as opposed to absolute, behavior in bending.

Ultimate bending load, ultimate bending deformation, elastic modulus, and rupture modulus are either obtained experimentally or computed from experimental data by means of beam theory. Longitudinal osteon samples are less able to withstand bending than alternate osteon samples. An interpretation resides in the very few transverse collagen bundles present in longitudinal osteons. In other words, alternate osteon samples are stiffer in bending because they are structurally more compact.

F. TORSION TEST

Frasca et al.[7,36] developed a method for torsional loading of whole osteons and A. Ascenzi et al.[37] developed a method for torsional loading of osteon samples.

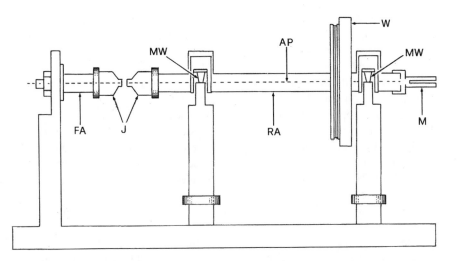

FIGURE 18.10 Simplified diagram of torsional device. Fixed axis (FA) and rotation axis (RA), each with its jaw (J) for securing sample to device; two hard metal wedges of pendulum loading system (MW); wheel (W) around which the tungsten thread with weights is attached; axis of pendulum (AP); mirror (M). (From Ascenzi, A., Baschieri, P., and Benvenuti, A., The torsional properties of single selected osteons, *J. Biomech.*, 27, 875, 1994. With permission from Elsevier Science.)

1. Frasca Method

Single osteons and osteon groups were chosen without regard to structural type and degree of calcification. Single osteons and osteon groups measuring approximately 5 to 8 mm in length are dissected from longitudinal and transverse bone sections by a method which separates each sample at its natural boundaries. Microfractures are produced and slowly propagated along the boundaries of each sample using scalpel and tweezers under a ×30 stereoscopic microscope. Samples are tested wet and dry. A laboratory-built microtorsional device is used for testing. In essence, it consists of an R-F coil immersed in a 5000 gauss magnetic field and connected to an oscillator. Angular amplitudes are measured by reflecting a laser light spot from a rotating mirror. Results indicate strain and frequency dependence of shear storage modulus of single osteons and osteon groups. They establish differences in wet and dry torsional behavior of both single osteons and osteon groups.

2. A. Ascenzi Method

A. Ascenzi et al.[35] have found that it is necessary to prepare the sample very accurately and to use a highly sensitive apparatus. Longitudinal and alternate osteons at final degree of calcification were tentatively selected on longitudinal sections 300 to 350 μm thick. Definitive identification of osteon type is possible only after loading. Osteon samples are isolated from sections by means of the second method described in Section III.B. In addition to usual sample regularity requirements, each sample needs to be carefully examined under an optical microscope to exclude the possibility of interference of small surface defects with experimental results. A special torsional device was manufactured according to researchers' specifications by the CECOM Company (Figure 18.10). This device consists of a fixed axis and a rotational axis horizontally aligned; each axis is furnished with a set of jaws that grips the osteon sample during testing. The center of each set of jaws lies on the associated axis. By means of a stereoscopic microscope, the rotational axis is verified to coincide with the osteon axis; i.e., the center of each jaw needs to correspond to one end of the axis of the osteon sample canal. The jaws are not free to move axially. This establishes an axial loading effect which could influence absolute measurements, but here such loading effect may be neglected because this investigation concerns comparative measurements.

One set of jaws is fixed, while the other turns in synchrony with a wheel measuring 61 mm in diameter. To reduce the rotating friction of the turning jaw to a negligible minimum, a pendulum loading system is adopted whose fulcrum is the tip of two hard metal wedges. The maximum oscillation of the pendulum is 55°. A tungsten thread, whose section measures 20 μm in diameter, winds around the rim of the wheel as 0.1 g weights are attached one after the other at one end of the tungsten thread until sample failure occurs. The interval between the application of two consecutive weights is kept constant at 4 s. The weight which produces an unchecked twisting of the sample; i.e., a sudden nonstop acceleration of the system, is considered to be the one responsible for osteon failure. The angles through which a specimen twists during a test are measured optically; such optical measure is based on the reflection of a laser beam from a small mirror inserted in the rotating set of jaws. The variations in the torsional angle are read on a graduated scale placed 160 cm from the device.

Precision and accuracy of the graduated scale and apparatus coincide, as checked by applying standard experimental procedures.

Ultimate torque, ultimate angular deflection, shear modulus, energy absorbed up to failure, and torsional shear stress are either obtained experimentally or computed from experimental data by means of beam theory. Ultimate torque and shear modulus values are higher for longitudinal osteon samples than alternate osteon samples. Moreover, osteon shear modulus resulting from such testing is as much as four times larger than shear modulus of macroscopic samples.[38,39] Lakes[40] explains that such moduli are actually in agreement through Cosserat elasticity theory. More precisely, slender specimens are stiffer than thick ones and the lower stiffness in thick specimens is attributed to localized slippage at the cement lines. Cosserat elasticity theory is a suitable model to represent presence (absence, respectively) of slippage under torsion in macrosamples (osteons, respectively) because it allows a moment per unit area in addition to the usual force per unit area of classic elasticity theory.

G. CYCLIC LOADING IN TENSION AND COMPRESSION

Availability of the technique which provides a cylindrical osteon sample with rectangular cross-sectional ends suggested to A. Ascenzi's research group to load osteon samples cyclically in tension and compression and to investigate their hysteresis loops.[41,42] Longitudinal and alternate osteons at final degree of calcification were tentatively selected on longitudinal sections 300 to 350 μm thick. Definitive identification of osteon type is possible only after loading. The technique of Section III.A is used here.

A. Gozzini, late holder of the chair of Solid State Physics at the Scuola Normale Superiore, Pisa, designed and assembled the apparatus. In essence, it comprises two parts: (1) a microwave micrometer based on cavity and pulse technique; (2) an electromechanical device functioning as a transducer to allow sample cyclic loading.

The microwave micrometer is an improved version of previously described apparatuses for loading in tension and in compression. The working frequency, f_o, was reduced from 24 GHz ($l = 1.25$ cm) to 14 GHz ($l = 2.2$ cm). A higher-quality klystron, which generates the microwaves, and crystal detectors had become available by 1985 in the latter frequency region; they ensure an increase in sensitivity and stability despite the increase in cylinder height from 1.78 to approximately 2 cm. The two hollow cylinders of the apparatus (one acting as a measuring cavity and the other used for comparison) were obtained from a single copper block to eliminate temperature differences between them and to minimize mechanical noises.

The transducer causing changes in cavity height ($-\Delta l$) was replaced by a more sophisticated electromechanical device whose description follows. Figure 18.11 shows a diagram of the electromechanical device. It consists of a measuring cavity (C_m) with two terminal walls: one terminal wall is mobile and can either penetrate into or withdraw from the cavity. The terminal wall is set in motion by an asynchronous motor (AM) whose rotating direction is reversible. The motor allows rotation of a metal bar (B) bearing both right and left screw threads connected to form a continuous

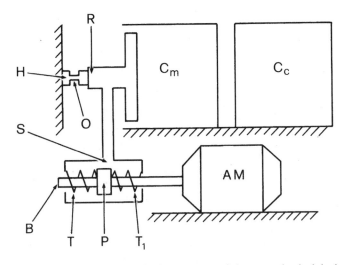

FIGURE 18.11 Simplified diagram of mechanical component of electromechanical device for osteon sample tension–compression cyclic loading and transformation of sample length changes into frequency variations of electromagnetic waves in resonator cavities. O, osteon sample with its lugs into securing jaws H and R; C_m, measuring cavity; C_c, comparing cavity; AM, asynchronous motor; B, bar; P, pin; T and T_1, coiled springs; S, slide. (From Ascenzi, A., Benvenuti, A., Mango, F., and Simili, R., Pinching in longitudinal and alternate osteons during cyclic loading, *J. Biomech.*, 18, 391, 1985. With permission from Elsevier Science.)

track. As result of bar rotations, a pin (P) inserted into the screw track undergoes alternating movements. The pin exerts alternating compression and decompression on each spring (T and T_1) coiled around the metal bar.

The coiled springs act on a slide (S) attached to the mobile terminal wall of the cavity C_m. The slide moves on two rectilinear rails of cemented steel through four ball bearings. One osteon sample lug is secured to the mobile part (R) and the other lug to the immobile part (H) of the device. Therefore, the moving slide exerts tension (compression, respectively) on the sample as the spring T (T_1, respectively) undergoes compression.

When tension (compression, respectively) is applied, the sample elongates (shortens, respectively), the mobile wall of the cavity advances (recedes, respectively), and cavity height decreases (increases, respectively). Since the length change of the sample is equal in magnitude to the cavity height change, the length change of the sample is deduced from the corresponding resonance frequency change of the cavity by means of Equation 18.2 of Section III.A.

Reduction of slide friction to a minimum and careful preparation of jaws to achieve perfect alignment between sample and jaws without sliding are crucial to accuracy.

Here the load limit is deduced from preliminary trials so that the stress limit, which varies from osteon to osteon because of the section variability, approximately corresponds to a middle value between the proportional stress limit and ultimate strength. An electronic system, which carries out the following operations, was devised: (1) recording of complete turns and fraction of turns; (2) recording of turns of the motor for each displacement in either direction; (3) memorization and comparison of computed data; (4) transmission of an electric signal to reverse motor rotation; and (5) provision to a recorder Y-axis of an electronic potential difference, proportional to the displacement and consequently to the load acting on the sample.

Sample deflection is registered by transformation of pulses coming from the two resonance cavities C_m and C_c into a difference of electric potential. Because the apparatus can detect fractional changes in resonance frequency on the order of 10^{-8}, sample length changes as small as a few Ångstroms can be measured. Since bone sample measurements require a sensitivity much lower than a few Ångstroms, high accuracy is assured.

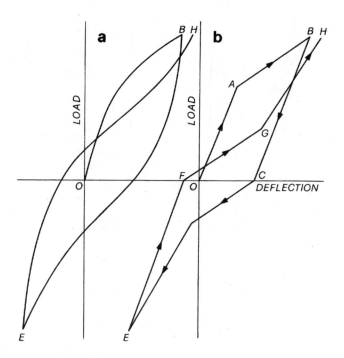

FIGURE 18.12   (a) Idealized curvilinear hysteresis model of curve prior to cycling and at the first cycle. Compressive half-cycle BE and tensional half-cycle EH are S-shaped or pinched as consequence of load reversal in both compression and tension. (b) Idealized bilinear hysteresis model of curve prior to cycling and at the first cycle used for structural interpretations. (From Ascenzi, A., Benvenuti, A., Bigi, A., et al., *Calcif. Tissue Int.*, 62, 266, 1998. With permission from Springer-Verlag, New York.)

A direct check for the apparatus is provided by loading of thin calibrated samples of a variety of material with predictable hysteresis loops, under the same experimental conditions as osteon samples. In addition, the conclusion is drawn that incidental variations in temperature do not appreciably affect test results.

The investigation of the A. Ascenzi group was performed with a mean loading–unloading cycle duration of 105 s, mean load rate of 0.05 N/s, and maximum load limit in both tension and compression of 1 N. The cycles applied to each sample varied in number; they were interrupted before spontaneous specimen rupture. Interruption is necessary because definitive identification of osteon type is possible only before rupture, but after testing.

A mathematical model of the hysteresis loops of osteon samples served to show that, as the number of cycles increases, strain limit increases, stiffness degrades, and energy absorption increases, all because of the increasing extent of lesions and possible increasing buckling. At equal degrees of calcification, the strain limit is greater in compression than in tension for longitudinal osteon samples because the high number of longitudinal fibers renders longitudinal osteon samples more resistant to tension than compression. The strain limit is smaller in compression than in tension for alternate osteon samples because the transverse and oblique collagen bundles minimize buckling and render alternate osteon samples more resistant to compression than tension.

In addition to stiffness degradation, another degradation effect occurs. Hysteresis loops are S-shaped or pinched (Figures 18.12 and 18.13) and such pinching degrades as the number of cycles increases. Pinching is due to temporary repair under compression and resolution under tension of lesions, and consequent abrupt changes in stiffness. Pinching degradation is less significant and energy absorption is more significant for longitudinal than alternate osteon samples. An interpretation is that, in longitudinal osteons, the simpler structure allows for easier repair and resolution of lesions while the lack of transverse collagen bundles increases the extent of the lesions.

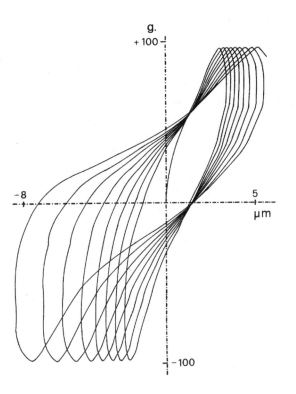

FIGURE 18.13 Stress–strain hysteresis loop of longitudinal osteon. Strain limit increases more rapidly and maximum curvature is smaller during compression than tension. (From Ascenzi, A., Benvenuti, A., Mango, F., and Simili, R., Pinching in longitudinal and alternate osteons during cyclic loading, *J. Biomech.*, 18, 391, 1985. With permission from Elsevier Science.)

IV. ACQUIRED KNOWLEDGE AND PENDING QUESTIONS

Analysis of secondary compact bone focused on the learning of osteon function through mechanical testing of osteonic lamellar structure is painstaking and time-consuming research which would be of limited value if not justified by a large breadth of useful results. Although this chapter's focus is mechanical testing of single osteons, a few words to summarize results to date and to list pending questions are included to stimulate researchers' interest.

1. The countless types of human osteons result from arrangements of longitudinal and transverse lamellae. Longitudinal (transverse, respectively) lamellae appear dark (bright, respectively) in cross section under a polarizing microscope. Longitudinal lamellae resist tension and torsion better than transverse lamellae. Under compression, shearing, and bending, transverse lamellae resist loading better than longitudinal lamellae.
2. The distribution of osteonic lamellae and interstitial bone in cross sections of long bone shafts is not random.
3. The distribution of osteonic lamellae in cross sections of long bone shafts shows a pattern compatible with the shaft shape and the distribution of forces usually operating on long bone under both normal and pathological condition. In general terms, there is indication of a high incidence of longitudinal (transverse, respectively) lamellae in bone sectors loaded in tension (compression, respectively).

4. Under normal conditions, the progressive increase of longitudinal lamellar concentration from the inner to the outer edge of a section is hypothesized as related to a condition of initial stress that would reduce the extent of the response of long bones to forces acting on them.

5. Variation in osteonic lamellar distribution of a long bone shaft is a sophisticated process, as proved by slight structural asymmetries found in shafts of subjects who had shown some simple asymmetric use of limbs during life.

6. The high concentration of transverse lamellae along the elongated sides of elliptical cross sections of a pathologically bowed shaft increases the bending stiffness of the deformed bone.

7. Pending questions are (a) the relation between osteonic lamellar distribution and geometry of the bone shaft loaded in bending and torsion, with respect to the mechanical properties of longitudinal and transverse lamellae; (b) the relation between osteonic lamellar distribution and geometry of the bone shape in determining fractures, especially in bending, with respect to the mechanical properties of longitudinal and transverse lamellae; and (c) the structural classification of osteons in diaphysis of vertebrates, whose lamellar structure somewhat differs from that of humans, to increase accuracy of interpretations.[43,44]

ACKNOWLEDGMENTS

Research Grant 97.03992.04 from the National Research Council of Italy supported this work. The authors thank Lucio Virgilii for figure preparation.

REFERENCES

1. Ascenzi, A., The micromechanics vs. the macromechanics of cortical bone — A comprehensive presentation, *J. Biomech. Eng.*, 110, 357, 1988.
2. Ascenzi, A., Boyde, A., Portigliatti-Barbos, M., and Carando, S., Micro-biomechanics vs. Macro-biomechanics in cortical bone. A micromechanical investigation of femurs deformed by bending, *J. Biomech.*, 20, 1045, 1987.
3. Ascenzi, A., Biomechanics and Galileo Galilei, *J. Biomech.*, 26, 95, 1993.
4. Evans, F.G., *Mechanical Properties of Bone*, Charles C Thomas, Springfield, IL, 1973.
5. Petersen, H., Die Organe des Skeletsystems, in *Handbuch der mikroskopischen Anatomie des Menschen*, Möllendorff (v.), W., Ed., Springer, Berlin, 1930.
6. Ortner, D.J. and Yong, D., A precision microdissection procedure for undecalcified bone thin sections, *Calcif. Tissue Res.*, 17, 169, 1975.
7. Frasca, P., Harper, R.A., and Katz, J.L., Isolation of single osteons and osteon lamellae, *Acta Anat.*, 95, 122, 1976.
8. Frasca, P., Harper, R.A., and Katz, J.L., Collagen fiber orientation in human secondary osteons, *Acta Anat.*, 98, 1, 1977.
9. Ascenzi, A. and Benvenuti, A., Orientation of collagen fibers at the boundary between two successive osteonic lamellae and its mechanical interpretation, *J. Biomech.*, 19, 455, 1986.
10. Ascenzi, A. and Benvenuti, A., The revisited osteon, in preparation.
11. Giraud-Guille, M.-M., Twisted plywood architecture of collagen fibrils in human compact bone osteons, *Calcif. Tissue Int.*, 42, 167, 1988.
12. Gebhardt, W., Über funktionell wichtige Anordnungsweisen der feineren und gröberen Bauelemente des Wirbeltierknochens. II. Spezieller Teil 1. Der Bau der Haversschen Lamellensysteme und seine funktionelle Bedeutung, *Arch. Entwmech. Org.*, 20, 187, 1906.
13. Amprino, R., Reported in *Trattato di Istologia*, Levi, G., Ed., Unione Tipografico-Editrice Torinese, Turin, 1946, 513.

14. Currey, J.D., The effect of drying and re-wetting on some mechanical properties of cortical bone, *J. Biomech.*, 21, 439, 1988.
15. Ascenzi, A., Bonucci, E., and Checcucci, A., The tensile properties of single osteons studied using a microwave extensometer, in *Studies on the Anatomy and Function of Bone and Joints*, Evans, F.G., Ed., Springer-Verlag, Berlin, 1966.
16. Ascenzi, A. and Bonucci, E., The tensile properties of single osteons, *Anat. Rec.*, 158, 375, 1967.
17. Ascenzi, A. and Bonucci, E., Mechanical similarities between alternate osteons and cross-ply laminates, *J. Biomech.*, 9, 65, 1976.
18. Ascenzi, A. and Benvenuti, A., Evidence of a state of initial stress in osteonic lamellae, *J. Biomech.*, 10, 447, 1977.
19. Ascenzi, A. and Benvenuti, A., Evidence of a state of initial stress in osteonic lamellae, *Acta Orthop. Belg.*, 46, 580, 1980.
20. Ascenzi, M.-G., A first estimation of prestress in so-called circularly fibered osteonic lamellae, *J. Biomech.*, 32, 935, 1999.
21. Ascenzi, M.-G., A first estimate of prestress in so-called circularly fibered osteonic lamellae, Abstracts of the 11th conference of the European Society of Biomechanics, *J. Biomech.*, 31 (Suppl. 1), 22, 1998.
22. Battaglia, A., Bruin, F., and Gozzini, A., Microwave apparatus for the measurement of the refraction dispersion and absorption of gases at relatively high pressure, *Nuovo Cimento*, 7, 1, 1958.
23. Montgomery, G., *Technique of Microwave Measurements*, McGraw-Hill, New York, 1947.
24. Ascenzi, A. and Bonucci, E., The compressive properties of single osteons, *Anat. Rec.*, 161, 377, 1968.
25. Ascenzi, A. and Bonucci, E., The shearing properties of single osteons, *Anat. Rec.*, 172, 499, 1972.
26. ASTM, Standards expansion (pin test) of copper and copper-alloy tubing, Designation: B 153–58, 3, 17, 1958.
27. Ascenzi, A. and Bonucci, E., Relationship between ultrastructure and "pin test" in osteons, *Clin. Orthop.*, 121, 275, 1976.
28. Portigliatti-Barbos, M., Bianco, P., and Ascenzi, A., Distribution of osteonic and interstitial components in the human femoral shaft with reference to structure, calcification, and mechanical properties, *Acta Anat.*, 15, 178, 1983.
29. Boyde, A., Bianco, P., Portigliatti-Barbos, M., and Ascenzi, A., Collagen orientation in compact bone: I. A new method for the determination of the proportion of collagen parallel to the plane of compact bone sections, *Metab. Bone Dis. Relat. Res.*, 5, 299, 1984.
30. Portigliatti-Barbos, M., Bianco, P., Ascenzi, A., and Boyde, A., Collagen orientation in compact bone: II. Distribution of lamellae in the whole of the human femoral shaft with reference to its mechanical properties, *Metab. Bone Dis. Relat. Res.*, 5, 309, 1984.
31. Carando, S., Portigliatti-Barbos, M., Ascenzi, A., and Boyde, A., Orientation of collagen in human tibial and fibular shaft and possible correlation with mechanical properties, *Bone*, 10, 139, 1989.
32. Carando, S., Portigliatti-Barbos, M., Ascenzi, A., et al., Macroscopic shape of, and lamellar distribution within, the upper limb shafts, allowing inferences about mechanical properties, *Bone*, 12, 265, 1991.
33. Portigliatti-Barbos, M., Carando, S., Ascenzi, A., and Boyde, A., On the structural symmetry of human femurs, *Bone*, 8, 165, 1987.
34. Ascenzi, A., Improta, S., Portigliatti-Barbos, M., et al., Distribution of lamellae in human femoral shafts deformed by bending with inferences on mechanical properties, *Bone*, 8, 319, 1987.
35. Ascenzi, A., Baschieri P., and Benvenuti, A., The bending properties of single osteons, *J. Biomech.*, 23, 763, 1990.
36. Frasca, P., Harper, R.A., and Katz, J. L., Strain and frequency dependence of shear storage modulus for human single osteons and cortical bone microsample-size and hydration effects, *J. Biomech.*, 14, 679, 1981.
37. Ascenzi, A., Baschieri P., and Benvenuti, A., The torsional properties of single selected osteons, *J. Biomech.*, 27, 875, 1994.
38. Pfafrod, G.O., Knets, I.V., Saulgozis,Y.Z, et al., Age-related changes in the strength of compact bone tissue under torsion, *Polym. Mech.*, 3, 493, 1975 [in Russian].
39. Evans, P.G., Relations between torsion properties and histology of adult human compact bone, *J. Biomech.*, 11, 157, 1978.
40. Lakes, R., On the torsional properties of single osteons, *J. Biomech.*, 28, 1409, 1995.

41. Ascenzi, A., Benvenuti, A., Mango, F., and Simili, R., Mechanical hysteresis loops from single osteons: technical devices and preliminary results, *J. Biomech.*, 18, 391, 1985.
42. Ascenzi, A., Ascenzi M.-G., Benvenuti, A., and Mango, F., Pinching in longitudinal and alternate osteons during cyclic loading, *J. Biomech.*, 30, 689, 1997.
43. Riggs, C.M., Lanyon, L.E., and Boyde, A., Functional associations between collagen fibre orientation and locomotor strain direction in cortical bone of the equine radius, *Anat. Embryol.*, 187, 231, 1993.
44. Riggs, C.M., Vaughan, L.C., Evans, G.P., et al., Mechanical implications of collagen fibre orientation in cortical bone of the equine radius, *Anat. Embryol.*, 187, 239, 1993.

19 Micromechanical Testing of Single Trabeculae

Peter L. Mente

CONTENTS

I. INTRODUCTION

Trabecular (or cancellous) bone is the relatively porous bony tissue found in the marrow cavities at the ends of the long bones and within the vertebrae and other small bones; the trabecular bone is encased by a denser and more highly structured cortical bone shell. The individual trabeculae that make up the trabecular tissue tend to have one of two basic shapes, either slender rods (or beamlike struts) or relatively thin, flat plates. These struts and plates form a three-dimensional scaffolding within the cortical shell. Structurally, trabecular bone helps to distribute loading from the articular surfaces to the cortical shell. Trabecular tissue is also very important for the stability and fixation of joint implants and other fixation devices placed into bone.

Because of its structural importance, many studies have focused on measuring the material properties of trabecular tissue. The majority of these studies have tested cubic or cylindrical specimens with dimensions on the order of 5 to 10 mm, and therefore have measured the bulk material properties of the tissue (see Chapter 11). The bulk material property combines the contributions of trabecular architecture (shape and spatial distribution of the trabecular scaffolding), porosity of the tissue, and the material properties of the bony tissue itself. It is important to make a distinction between the trabecular bone bulk modulus and the tissue modulus. Throughout this chapter, *tissue modulus* will be used to refer to the modulus of the bony material that makes up individual trabeculae and *bulk modulus* will refer to the modulus calculated from larger samples (including the effects of architecture and porosity). Originally, many models of trabecular bone assumed that the tissue modulus of trabecular bone was the same as the tissue modulus of cortical bone and that the bulk tissue stiffness of trabecular bone could thus be modeled by assuming that trabecular bone was simply a more porous cortical bone tissue. As models of trabecular bone become more refined and begin to include the internal trabecular architecture,[1-7] knowledge of the mechanical properties of the trabecular tissue has become more important. In order to determine if trabecular bone tissue is different from cortical bone tissue, and to understand how this might affect these models of the trabecular tissue, it is necessary to be able to perform mechanical testing on individual trabeculae and measure the modulus of the trabecular tissue itself.

The modulus of cortical bone tissue has been characterized extensively, in part because its size and relatively solid nature allow specimens to be machined into relatively standard test configurations for tensile and compressive testing (see Chapter 11). This, however, is not possible with trabecular bone tissue; the extremely small size and ill-defined shape of individual trabeculae make determining the modulus of trabecular tissue an extremely difficult task. Testing of these small, irregularly shaped specimens requires the use of nonstandard measurement techniques. In this chapter mechanical testing methods that have been employed to test individual trabeculae will be examined. These nonstandard techniques generally require specially built testing apparatus and special consideration of the specimen geometry. The first attempts to determine the modulus of individual trabeculae used a buckling analysis where the modulus was determined based on the critical buckling load during the controlled compression of individual trabecular specimens.[8,9] More recent testing methods which this chapter will cover have used more conventional engineering beam analysis to determine the modulus of this tissue. Three different mechanical testing techniques will be discussed: three-point bending, tensile testing, and cantilever beam testing. The three-point bending tests and tensile testing techniques use specimens of known or assumed geometry which allow the calculation of the tissue modulus using general engineering beam equations. The cantilever beam method uses a finite-element model of the test in order to determine the modulus of the specimen by matching model and experimental results.

II. TESTING METHODS

A. THREE-POINT BENDING TESTS

Kuhn et al.[10] and Choi et al.[11] tested rectangular beam specimens of trabecular bone in three-point bending to measure their tissue modulus. Their trabecular beam specimens were created by micromachining individual trabeculae down to a uniform rectangular cross section. To obtain trabecular specimens with uniform cross sections, blocks of bulk trabecular bone were first sectioned to a thickness of 75 to 100 µm using a Buehler Isomet and a low-speed diamond cutting blade (Buehler, Lake Bluff, IL), creating sections of tissue with two flat and parallel faces. Trabeculae that were continuous and homogeneous were dissected from the sections and placed in the holding fixture of a specially designed miniature milling machine using pressure plates lined with sandpaper. In the micromilling machine the two remaining uncut sides of the trabeculae were milled parallel to each other to a thickness of 50 to 200 µm. Specimens obtained in this manner had an overall length on the order of 1500 to 2000 µm. Cutting and machining was done under irrigation to prevent the specimens from drying out. Specimen dimensions were confirmed using digitized photographs of the trabecular beams taken at a magnification of 60×.

In a three-point bending test, a specimen is placed across two supports and a force is applied midway between the supports, causing the specimen to deflect (Figure 19.1). The modulus of beams tested in this manner can be calculated using the equation:

$$E = \frac{P}{\delta} \frac{L^3}{48I} \tag{19.1}$$

where E = Young's (tissue) modulus, P = applied load, δ = displacement at the point of application of the load (midpoint of the beam), L = distance between the supports, I = specimen moment of inertia (for a rectangular specimen this is equal to $\frac{1}{12}bh^3$, where b is the width of the specimen and h is its thickness).

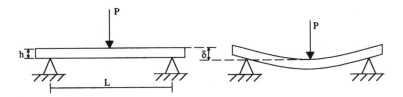

FIGURE 19.1   Schematic diagram of a three-point bending test geometry.

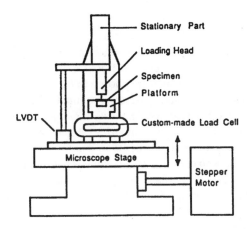

FIGURE 19.2   Schematic diagram of the three-point bending test apparatus used by Kuhn et al.[10] and Choi et al.[11] (From Choi, K., Kuhn, J.L., Ciarelli, M.J., and Goldstein, S.A., *J. Biomech.*, 23, 1103, 1990. With permission.)

Because relatively slender specimens were tested, Kuhn et al.[10] and Choi et al.[11] employed a modification of this general equation that includes terms that take into account the concentrated nature of the applied force.[12]

$$E = \frac{P}{\delta} \frac{L^3}{48I} \left[1 + 2.85 \left(\frac{h}{L} \right)^2 - 0.84 \left(\frac{h}{L} \right)^3 \right]$$ (19.2)

The testing apparatus used in these two studies was a modified microscope base (Figure 19.2). The two supports were fixed to the top of a load cell approximately 1 mm apart and the load cell in turn was attached to the specimen stage of the microscope. The loading head (positioned midway between the supports) was attached to the microscope stationary body tube. Specimens were deformed by moving the specimen stage up against the stationary loading head, using a stepper motor attached to the fine adjustment knob of the microscope. This allowed the specimens to be loaded at a controlled rate. Rates used in these tests were 0.081 mm/s[10] and 0.11 mm/s.[11] Vertical displacement of the stage relative to the loading head (which represents the specimen displacement at the point of application of the load) was measured using a linear variable differential transformer (LVDT) with a full-scale range of ±2.5 mm; the load cell that was used had a maximum compressive range of 0.6 N. The maximum load applied in the experiments was 0.2 to 0.3 N, and the maximum resulting specimen deflection at the point of application of the force was approximately 0.1 mm. The applied force (P) and specimen deflection at the point of application of the force (δ) were acquired by computer and the slope (P/δ) calculated by fitting a straight line to the experimental data. The experimentally measured slope, along with the measurements of the specimen geometry, allowed the trabecular tissue modulus to be determined from Equation 19.2.

B. TENSILE TESTING

Tensile tests on individual trabeculae have been performed by two groups, Ryan and Williams,[13] and Rho et al.[14] Standard tensile test specimens are normally machined or cut along the middle segment of their free length so that stress and strain measurements can be made on an area of reduced cross-sectional area. In this way, measurements are made well away from the fixed ends, where edge effects and stress concentrations due to the grips influence the general homogeneous stress state. The modulus for a standard specimen tested in tension is given by

$$E = \frac{P}{\delta} \frac{L}{A} \qquad (19.3)$$

where E = Young's (tissue) modulus, P = applied load, L = reference length, δ = elongation of the reference length L, and A = specimen cross-sectional area.

Both groups tested rodlike specimens excised from the bulk trabecular tissue using a scalpel under a dissecting microscope. Specimens were chosen to be as straight and uniform as possible. The specimens tested by Ryan and Williams[13] were approximately 0.3 mm in diameter with lengths on the order of 4 mm. Rho et al.[14] tested specimens with diameters and lengths of approximately 0.18 and 2.3 mm, respectively. The difference in size of tested specimens reflects the species and location from which specimens were obtained; Ryan and Williams[13] tested trabeculae from the distal end of bovine femurs and Rho et al.[14] tested specimens collected from a proximal human tibia.

Because individual trabeculae are so small, test specimens cannot be easily machined to create an area of reduced cross section, nor can specimens be obtained that are long enough for displacement changes to be measured away from the grips to avoid edge effects. Relative displacement measurements on trabeculae specimens tested in tension have therefore been made over the entire specimen length, using grip displacement as a measurement of specimen elongation. The cross-sectional area measurement used for these specimens represents the average cross-sectional area along the length. Although the cross-sectional area is generally elliptical with a major and minor radius, for modeling purposes the cross-sectional area was assumed to be circular with a constant radius over the entire free length between the grips. Ryan and Williams[13] noted that at a given cross section, the maximum and minimum radius could differ by as much as a factor of 2, although both studies indicated that measured specimen diameters varied by less than 10% along their test length.

Ryan and Williams[13] tested their specimens by clamping each end of their rodlike specimens between plates lined with 320-grit sandpaper (Figure 19.3). A set screw between the pair of grips set the free length at 1.524 mm for all specimens. The specimens were placed in the grips so that their longitudinal axes were aligned as closely as possible with the direction of loading. Two guide rods running between the grips maintained the orientation of the specimen and helped to prevent bending of the specimens during testing. Specimens were distracted at a strain rate of approximately 0.001 ε/s. A load cell (maximum load 6 N) and an extensometer (maximum displacement 2.5 mm) attached across the two grips were used to measure the force and specimen elongation, respectively. Specimen elongation ranged from 0.04 to 0.32 mm and the applied tensile force ranged from 2.2 to 5.5 N. The resulting force–displacement curves were plotted on an x–y plotter and the slope of the curves (P/δ) measured, using a straight line drawn on the graph, to determine specimen stiffness. The specimen stiffness along with the measured geometry (specimen free length and cross-sectional area) were then used in Equation 19.3 to calculate the tissue modulus.

The grips used in the tensile testing performed by Rho et al.[14] were rods with hollow ends into which the ends of the trabeculae were fixed using a cyanoacrylate glue (Figure 19.4). This attachment method required the specimens to be dry to ensure a good glue bond (specimens were not rewetted before testing). Specimens were aligned in the grips under a stereomicroscope to ensure they were straight and to minimize the bending moments that would develop from nonaxial loading. Specimens were loaded at a strain rate of 5.5 με/s using a motor geared to a slider that advanced the grip (see Figure 19.4). A purpose-built load cell was used to measure

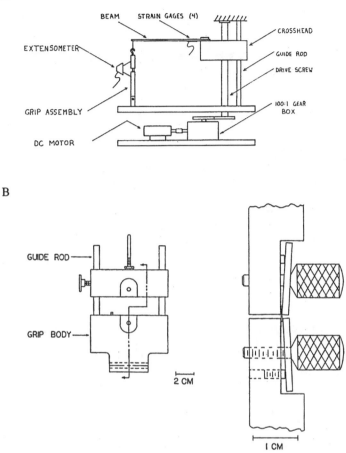

FIGURE 19.3   (A) Schematic diagram of the tensile testing apparatus used by Ryan and Williams.[13] (From Ryan, S.D., Tensile Testing of Individual Bovine Trabeculae, Master's thesis, Northeastern University, Boston, 1988. With permission). (B) A detail of the grip assembly used to hold specimens. (From Ryan, S.D. and Williams, J.L., Tensile testing of rodlike trabeculae excised from bovine femoral bone, *J. Biomech.*, 22, 351, 1989. With permission.)

load and an extensometer (maximum range 3 mm) attached to the two grip rods was used to measure specimen elongation. Load and elongation were recorded on an *x–y* plotter; maximum applied loads were on the order of 1 N and maximum specimen elongation was approximately 0.01 mm. As with Ryan and Williams,[13] the slope of the force–displacement curve (*P/δ*) along with the measured geometry (specimen free length and cross-sectional area) were used in Equation 19.3 to calculate the tissue modulus.

C. CANTILEVER BEAM TESTING

The third testing method that has been used to measure trabecular tissue modulus is cantilever beam testing.[15] A cantilever beam has one end fixed and the other end free, and loads are applied along the length of the specimen perpendicular to the long axis of the specimen, causing the specimen to bend. Trabecular bone specimens were tested in this configuration using a two-step procedure: first individual trabeculae were mechanically loaded and their bending response recorded, then a three-dimensional finite-element model of the trabeculae was created and subjected

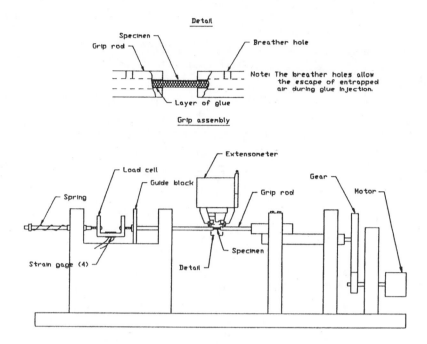

FIGURE 19.4 Schematic diagram of the tensile testing apparatus used by Rho et al.,[14] including a detail of the glue attachment of a specimen to the grip rods. (From Rho, J.Y., Ashman, R.B., and Turner, C.H., Young's modulus of trabecular and cortical bone material: ultrasonic and microtensile measurements, *J. Biomech.*, 26, 111, 1993. With permission.)

to simulated test conditions. The tissue modulus was determined by changing the modulus of the trabecular bone elements in the finite-element model until the displacement of the model matched the displacement of the specimen measured during experimental testing, for a given applied load.

Since finite-element models were created for each trabecular specimen tested, it was not necessary to select specimens with a uniform cross section; in fact, both flat, platelike specimens and rodlike specimens could be tested using this methodology. Specimens of trabecular bone were obtained by cutting open the end of a long bone to expose the internal trabecular scaffolding. Sections of the bulk trabecular tissue were cut from the bone using a scalpel and the marrow was removed using a water pick. When the marrow was removed, the trabecular scaffolding could be visualized and individual trabeculae excised using a scalpel. The main selection criteria for specimens was overall length. Side struts on the trabeculae that did not contribute to the bending stiffness were trimmed, to eliminate features that would add complexity to the finite-element model. For platelike trabeculae, the specimen width was trimmed to a maximum of 4.0 mm so that specimens would fit in the test apparatus. Trimming of the platelike specimens was also used to eliminate holes and other defects in the specimens to facilitate later modeling; specimen thickness was not altered, only specimen width.

Epoxy bases to hold the trabeculae were created using 8-mm-diameter electron microscopy specimen capsules. Epoxy (Shell Epon 828 and Hysol HD 3404 hardener in a 10 : 1 ratio) was poured into the capsules and allowed to set. Once the epoxy was hardened, the top surface was squared off and the top 3 mm turned down to a diameter of 5 mm. The remaining ledge on the base was used as a landmark from which geometry measurements could be referenced. A score along the length of the base served as an angular reference landmark to define the specimen orientation. A hole 4 mm in diameter by 3 mm deep was drilled into the top of the base to accept the specimens. The ends of the trabeculae were fixed by filling the hollowed out top of the epoxy

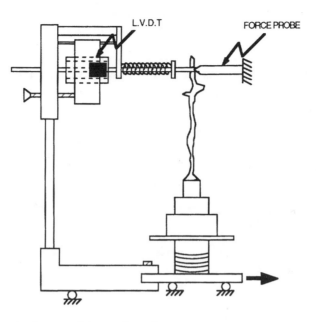

FIGURE 19.5 Schematic diagram of the cantilever beam test apparatus used by Mente and Lewis. (From Mente, P. L. and Lewis, J. L., Experimental method for the measurement of the elastic modulus of trabecular bone tissue, *J. Orthop. Res.*, 7, 456, 1989. With permission.)

base with fresh epoxy and pushing the trabecula specimens into the epoxy and holding them straight while the epoxy cured. This particular epoxy took 2 h to cure under a heat lamp. During the curing time the trabeculae dried out; to rewet the specimens they were soaked for a minimum of 1 h in saline before testing. When the epoxy set, it wicked up around the base of the specimen, creating a variably sized epoxy meniscus. The size and shape of the meniscus was found to have a significant effect on the specimen bending response and had to be included in the final models.

Specimens were tested by attaching the epoxy base to an *x–y* platform with the trabeculae standing vertically (Figure 19.5). The trabeculae were positioned against a horizontally oriented force probe with a full scale rating of 0.6 N (Model UC3; Statham Instruments Inc., Hato Rey, PR). The height of the force probe above the machined ledge on the epoxy base was measured and the specimen orientation about its vertical axis was adjusted to place the flattest contact area against the force probe. Since specimens were not symmetric and did not have a regular geometry, the direction of loading relative to the specimen had a significant effect on the specimen bending response. The reference line on the epoxy base allowed the rotational position of the specimen relative to the force probe to be recorded. The amount of contact between the specimen and the force probe was also recorded for use in the later modeling.

Specimen loading was produced by displacing the base relative to the fixed force probe (see Figure 19.5). As the base was displaced by hand, no consistent loading rate was used in these tests. The displacement of the base relative to the force probe was measured with an LVDT with a ±0.6 mm linear range (Model 025 MHR, Schaevitz, Pennsauken, NJ). The LVDT was held against the force probe by a calibrated compression spring (spring constant 0.019 N/mm). Each trial was run to a maximum displacement of 0.4 mm; the resulting applied force ranged from 0.01 to 0.09 N. The force–displacement response was recorded on an x-y plotter. A straight line was drawn to best approximate the experimental force–displacement plots and the slope of line calculated. The stiffness of the spring holding the LVDT against the force probe was subtracted from the experimentally measured slope to determine the specimen stiffness (P/δ). Specimens were loaded at several different heights to create several different load cases, and each test was repeated several times to obtain an average response. Specimens were rewetted periodically throughout the testing procedure to prevent them from drying over the course of the tests.

The finite-element models of the individual trabeculae were created after mechanical testing using photographs of the trabecular cross sections taken as the specimens were ground down. In order to prepare a specimen to be ground down it was bleached, encased in a hollow cylinder that was then filled with epoxy colored with carbon black, and subjected to a vacuum to remove any air bubbles from the epoxy. This procedure produced excellent contrast between the white bleached bone tissue, the black potting epoxy, and the lighter epoxy of the meniscus and base. The cylinders encasing the trabeculae were engraved internally with four longitudinal lines at 90° intervals to act as markers for a superimposed grid (1.27 mm Bausch and Lomb reticule); the lines on the cylinder were aligned with the reference line on the epoxy base of the specimen. The reticule provided a consistent local x–y coordinate system and length standard in each cross-sectional photograph so that successive levels could be properly aligned with each other. The specimens were ground down, by hand, with 600-grit silicon carbide paper under water irrigation at intervals of 0.25 mm until the meniscus was reached, at which point they were ground down at intervals of 0.125 mm. Parallel surfaces were obtained by advancing the epoxy-encased specimen up through the center of an aluminum annulus by means of a screw advance (accuracy = 0.025 mm) and then grinding the specimen down until the annulus was reached. Specimens were ground down until the machined ledge on the base was reached; this allowed the z-position of each section to be referenced relative to the landmarks used during testing. Knowing the z-position of the local coordinate system of each section, which was defined by the reticule in the photographs, a global coordinate system for the specimens could be defined with its origin at the center of the epoxy base on the plane created by the ledge of the base. This global coordinate system allowed the test geometry to be transferred to the finite-element model.

Tracings of the cross-sectional outline of the trabeculae were made and then sectioned into three to five quadrilaterals. The corner points of these quadrilaterals were digitized into the computer

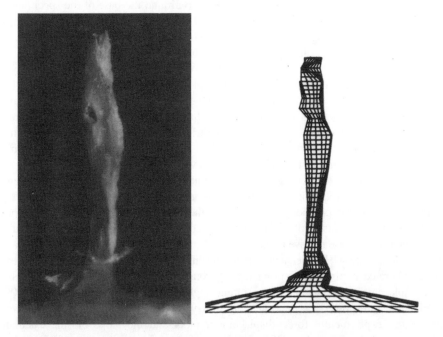

FIGURE 19.6 View of a cantilever beam trabecular specimen and its corresponding three-dimensional finite-element model. (From Mente, P.L. and Lewis, J.L., Experimental method for the measurement of the elastic modulus of trabecular bone tissue, *J. Orthop. Res.*, 7, 456, 1989. With permission.)

and connected together vertically to the corresponding quadrilaterals on neighboring levels to form three-dimensional brick elements (Figure 19.6). These elements were further subdivided into additional elements to ensure that there would be a minimum of four elements in the bending direction. Three different materials were defined in the finite-element models: epoxy, air (used to model holes in the specimens), and the bony tissue. The elastic modulus and Poisson's ratio used for epoxy elements were 3.1 GPa and 0.36, respectively, and for air elements 1 Pa and 0.30, respectively. The initial material properties used for the trabecular tissue was a tissue modulus of 15.0 GPa and a Poisson's ratio of 0.28. Fixation at the base of the specimen was simulated by constraining all of the nodes on the lowest cross section against displacements in all three directions. The trabecular model was rotated to match the specimen rotation during testing and a horizontal force was applied at the nodes that most closely approximated the contact area between the specimen and the force probe at the height recorded during testing. The magnitude of the force was divided equally among each of the nodes.

The nodal displacements at the point of application of the force, obtained from the finite-element solution (FEM displacement), were compared with the corresponding displacement calculated using the experimentally measured slope (F–δ displacement). A discrepancy in these displacements would indicate that the initial tissue modulus used was incorrect. Because of the approximate linearity of the finite-element nodal displacements with the elastic modulus that was used for the bone tissue elements (FEM modulus), the actual tissue modulus (the modulus that would make the two displacements equal) could be determined using the equation:

$$\text{Tissue modulus} = \left[\frac{\text{FEM displacement}}{\text{F–}\delta \text{ displacement}} \right] \text{FEM modulus} \tag{19.4}$$

In addition to testing trabecular bone, small cortical bone and aluminum rectangular cantilever beam specimens were also tested. These specimens were machined to a uniform rectangular cross section (approximate dimensions $0.5 \times 3.0 \times 10.0$ mm). This allowed the experimental procedure (mechanical testing and finite-element modeling) to be tested using specimens with a known geometry and modulus. For regular rectangular beam specimens tested as cantilever beams the modulus can be calculated using the equation:

$$E = \frac{P}{\delta} \frac{L^3}{3I} \tag{19.5}$$

where E = Young's modulus, P = applied load, δ = displacement at the point of application of the load, L = distance from the fixed end of the specimen to the applied load, and I = specimen moment of inertia (for a rectangular specimen this is equal to $\frac{1}{12}bh^3$, where b is the width of the specimen and h is its thickness)

Being able to calculate the modulus directly allowed the accuracy of the apparatus and the finite-element models to be determined. Tests of aluminum specimens showed an error of only about 4 to 5% in calculated modulus compared with reference values. Tests on cortical bone specimens showed modulus differences on the order of 17% compared with published values; this larger error for calculated cortical bone tissue modulus probably reflects the fact that the modulus of cortical bone tissue is in general much more variable. These tests indicated that the test apparatus was sufficiently accurate to test small, relatively compliant specimens.

Several areas of potential error in finite-element modeling were also quantified. The sensitivity of the model to changes in the position of the digitized cross sections was found to be about 5%. Changes in the positioning of the load on a given level changed the calculated results 2 to 8%, while moving the load between adjacent vertical levels resulted in changes of about 10%. Changes in specimen rotation were found to cause changes of about 5%. These sources of error were found to be generally small and represent the largest errors that might be induced in translating the specimen geometry into a finite-element model. The most significant effects were found to result from changing the representation of the epoxy meniscus. Not including the epoxy meniscus at the base of the specimen in the models, for example, resulted in changes of between 30 and 70% in predicted modulus. This indicates the importance of this feature, which models the fixation conditions, to the specimen response, and underscored the importance of creating an accurate model of the specimen and the test conditions.

III. TESTING CONSIDERATIONS

A. Specimen Geometry

One of the major difficulties in measuring the tissue modulus of individual trabeculae is dealing with the irregular shape of the available specimens. In the studies that have been performed this has been dealt with in several different ways; each method has its advantages and disadvantages. In tensile tests a uniform circular cross section was assumed for the entire specimen. While this greatly simplifies the analysis and allows a simple beam equation to be used to calculate the tissue modulus, it also introduces errors that result from the changes in the specimen cross section along its length and in the accuracy of determining an average radius. Ryan and Williams[13] and Rho et al.[14] have estimated that these effects result in errors in modulus calculations of about 10%. Irregularities in specimen geometry, particularly deviations along the axial loading direction, result in specimens that are not subjected to pure axial tension loads. In these specimens bending loads will be introduced that may also influence the specimens response.

The problems that result from irregularities of geometry can be avoided by machining specimens into a standard uniform geometry, as was done by Kuhn et al.[10] and Choi et al.[11] This is the normal practice in standard material testing procedures. The difficulty that arises from doing this with trabecular tissue is that the available material is small and inhomogeneous. As specimens are machined, voids and defects in the tissue can become more pronounced. In addition, this process can interrupt the tissue microstructure. Bone tissue is a composite material with hydroxyapatite crystals deposited on a collagen scaffolding. The tissue material properties are dependent on the properties of the hydroxyapatite and the collagen as well as the internal architecture of the scaffolding. In trabecular tissue the collagen architecture is much less aligned than in cortical bone; machining away part of a trabeculae may disrupt this internal architecture resulting in changes to the material properties of the trabecular tissue.

These problems can be circumvented by modeling the complete trabecula as was done in bending tests using the finite-element method. Finite-element modeling of the trabeculae allows the irregular shape of the specimens to be taken into account and allows specimens to be tested without disturbing their internal architecture. While finite-element modeling has the potential to represent the specimen geometry accurately, the creation of individual models for each specimen, particularly when each specimen has to be ground down in order to define its geometry, is an extremely time-consuming procedure. In addition, proper element sizes and shapes must be generated to obtain reliable results, as the accuracy of the models is highly dependent on the mesh density. Recent advances in μ-CT technology and finite-element preprocessing may make this procedure more robust and reliable by allowing models on the single trabecula scale to be scanned and a finite-element mesh generated automatically.[1-7] The speed and storage capacity of new computers and finite-element algorithms also mean that finer models can be created, eliminating problems related to poor mesh density. These advances may eventually make this procedure quick and reliable enough to allow testing of significant specimen numbers, making this method more appealing.

There is also some indication that there is a size effect in specimen testing.[11] These effects may arise due to inhomogeneties in the material properties of the tissue, increased influence of structural defects as specimen size becomes small, specimen surface-to-volume ratio, or machining effects. Choi et al.[11] have observed this size effect in cortical bone specimens, although similar results were not seen by Rho et al.[14] Nonetheless, it should be remembered that bone tissue is an inhomogeneous material and special consideration should be given to the size and shape of specimens being tested.

B. GRIPS AND EDGE EFFECTS

Another testing concern is stress concentrations due to concentrated loading and edge effects around supports and grips. These effects were probably most severe for the test geometry used by Ryan and Williams[13] where the small free length relative to the diameter of the specimen in the grip meant that edge effects could be felt over a large percentage of the specimen length. While elongation measurements in standard testing procedures are made on a subset of the specimen length away from the grips to avoid these effects, this is not a practical solution for testing small trabeculae. It should, however, be noted that stress calculations based on the applied loading probably underestimate the tissue stresses that are experienced throughout a large percentage of the specimen length.

Another problem that needs to be addressed with grips is specimen slipping. Ryan and Williams[13] noted that specimen slipping could be detected by sudden changes in the force–displacement tracings; slipping was also checked by placing a mark on the specimen where it was fixed in the grips so that any specimen movement occurring during their test could be noted after the tests. In their experience, approximately 5 to 6% of the specimens tested experienced slipping in the grips. Tests where slipping was suspected were discarded. While glue can be used to eliminate specimen slipping as done by Rho et al.,[14] the glue may be absorbed into the specimen, thus altering its mechanical properties. Rho et al.[14] used ultrasonic techniques to quantify the effect this had on specimen modulus calculations and found an approximate 4% difference between specimens before and after they were infiltrated with glue. These differences were, however, only measured on dried specimens.

In three-point bending tests, the shear contributions due to the concentrated nature of the load have been incorporated into Equation 19.2. However, Lotz et al.[16] have indicated that local plastic deformation around loading heads and supports can also have an effect on measured specimen deflection when overall displacements are small. They recommended using an experimentally determined correction factor to measure these local deformation effects. This correction factor (ϕ) is determined by testing a completely supported specimen (a specimen resting on a rigid support) in compression with a single indenter. The magnitude of local deformation can be quantified by measuring the slope of the resulting force–displacement curve (p/d):

$$\frac{1}{\phi} = \frac{p}{d} \tag{19.6}$$

This can be incorporated into the analysis by adjusting the specimen stiffness measurement (P/δ) used in Equation 19.3 according to the equation:

$$\frac{P}{\delta} = \frac{P}{\delta - (1.5)P\phi} \tag{19.7}$$

The factor of 1.5 in this equation is used for three-point bending to take into account that the two bottom supports only see half the total force of the load head so local deformation effects due to the bottom supports will be half that due to the single loading point on the top. While this effect may have an influence on three-point bending tests, it is unlikely that this effect will be as significant in cantilever beam tests. The specimen displacement relative to the applied force is much greater in cantilever bending than in three-point bending; thus, any local deformations will have a much smaller effect on measurements of the overall specimen stiffness.

Edge effects that are most significant for cantilever beam specimens are due to the meniscus that develops at the base of cantilever beam specimens when they are potted in epoxy. Although these effects can be taken into account by including the meniscus in the finite-element model, the meniscus does add to the complexity of the models and the time necessary to create and solve them. The finite-element method does take into account the stress concentrations that arise from geometric factors such as grips or material changes (provided appropriate boundary conditions are imposed), which makes it a good method for dealing with edge effects.

C. TISSUE HYDRATION

Tissue hydration has been shown to be a significant factor in tissue modulus, with dried specimens as much as 24% stiffer than wet specimens.[9] Maintaining specimen hydration is a particularly significant problem for small specimens that can dry out very quickly. Specimens should be kept frozen when in storage and every effort should be made to keep them moist throughout both preparation and testing. Kuhn et al.[10] and Choi et al.[11] kept specimens between saline-soaked filter paper to prevent dehydration. Mente and Lewis[15] kept their specimens submerged in a saline bath to keep them moist before testing. This was necessary, in part, to rehydrate specimens that dried out during preparation. Specimen drying can be a problem for testing configurations that require that the specimen be bonded to a grip or support. Specimens, for example, may need to be dried before they are glued to ensure good glue adhesion, or the specimen may dry out while the glue or epoxy sets. In these cases it is possible to rehydrate specimens by soaking them in saline, although no data exist on whether drying and rehydrating of specimens has an effect on the resulting measured tissue modulus. In general, it is prudent to avoid letting the specimens dry out if possible and to keep them moist throughout the testing procedure.

D. APPARATUS CHECKS

Because the apparatus used to test trabeculae are usually built for this single purpose, it is necessary to ensure the accuracy of the apparatus and its ability to handle the small load, and displacements that must be applied or measured, as well as the generally high compliance of the small specimens being tested. It is necessary to ensure that the compliance of the testing system is very much lower than the compliance of the specimens. Many measuring devices used to measure small loads are by nature fairly compliant and deformations in these elements may be a significant percentage of the deformation of the specimen. If there is significant compliance, or elements of the test system introduce loads to the system, these sources need to be quantified and subtracted from the specimen response. Any nonstandard test system also requires calibration and verification; this can usually be done by testing homogeneous specimens of known modulus to verify the testing procedures. The specimens chosen should be similar in size and stiffness to the trabeculae to be tested. Testing should include both the mechanical test apparatus and the equations or procedure used to analyze the results.

IV. RESULTS

Results to date (Table 19.1) indicate a modulus of trabecular bone tissue that ranges from approximately 1.0 to 8.0 GPa (for specimens tested wet). Reported values for cortical bone tissue are on the order of 20 GPa.[17] While the amount of available data is still quite small and does not provide a basis for making any statement about the modulus of trabecular bone tissue in general, these studies do suggest that trabecular bone tissue modulus is less stiff than the cortical bone tissue modulus. There are several possible explanations for the differences in these tissues. There may

TABLE 19.1
Elastic Modulus of Trabecular Bone Tissue

Source of Tissue	Condition of Test Specimen	No. Tested	Testing Method	Loading or Strain Rate	Approximate Dimensions, mm	Calculated Tissue Modulus (GPa) Mean (StD)	Ref.
Human medial tibial plateau	Dry	9	Trabecular buckling	0.1346 mm/s	$L = 1.0$–1.8 $t = 0.09$–0.14 $w = 0.25$–1.0	14.1	9
	Wet	9				11.3	
Human distal femur	Dry	4	Trabecular buckling	Unknown	$L = 2.4$–3.0 $t = 0.13$ $w = 0.8$–1.2	8.7 (3.2)	8
Human femur (dried)	Rewetted	3	Cantelever beam with FEA	Unknown	$L = 5$–10	6.2 (1.2)	15
Human tibia (fresh)		3				11.2 (10.1)	
Combined		6				8.7 (7.0)	
Human iliac crest							
63 years old	Wet	29	Three-point bending	0.81 mm/s	$L = 1.5$–2.0 $h = 0.05$–0.20 $b = 0.05$–0.20	4.2 (2.0)	10
23 years old		13				3.0 (1.6)	
Combined		42				3.8	
Bovine distal femur	Wet	38	Tension	0.01 ε/s	$L = 4.0$ $r = 0.3$	0.8 (0.4)	13
Human proximal tibia							
Vertical	Wet	13	Three-point bending	0.11 mm/s	$L = 1.5$–2.0 $h = 0.05$–0.20 $b = 0.05$–0.20	4.9 (1.8)	11
Horizontal		7				3.8 (0.5)	
Combined		20				4.6 (1.3)	
Human tibia	Dried	20	Tension	5.5 με/s	$L = 2.3$ $r = 0.09$	10.4 (3.5)	14
Human tibia	Wet	23	4-point bending	0.02 N/sec	$L = 1.5$–2.0 mm $h = 0.07$–0.140 mm $b = 0.07$–0.140 mm	5.7 (1.3)	18

be differences in the degree of mineralization of the two tissues. The microarchitecture of the tissue including the organization or orientation of the collagen fiber network and the relationship between the fiber network and the mineralization may also affect the modulus of the two tissues. Cortical bone tissue is much more organized than trabecular bone; it is built up around the osteon with concentric lamellae of mineralized collagen fibers which tend to alternate direction between the lamellae. There is no such organized structure in the trabecular tissue. Collagen orientation is more random and cement lines indicating the juncture between remodeled areas are randomly dispersed through the tissue.[18] How these architectural differences may influence the modulus is unknown, but they do suggest a structural basis for differences in tissue modulus between cortical and trabecular bone.

REFERENCES

1. Hollister, S.J., Brennan, J.M., and Kikuchi, N., A homogenization sampling procedure for calculating trabecular bone effective stiffness and tissue level stress, *J. Biomech.*, 27, 433, 1994.
2. Ladd, A.J. and Kinney, J.H., Numerical errors and uncertainties in finite-element modeling of trabecular bone, *J. Biomech.*, 31, 941, 1998.
3. Ladd, A.J., Kinney, J.H., Haupt, D.L., and Goldstein, S.A., Finite-element modeling of trabecular bone: comparison with mechanical testing and determination of tissue modulus, *J. Orthop. Res.*, 16, 622, 1998.
4. Muller, R. and Ruegsegger, P., Analysis of mechanical properties of cancellous bone under conditions of simulated bone atrophy, *J. Biomech.*, 29, 1053, 1996.
5. Muller, R. and Ruegsegger, P., Three-dimensional finite-element modeling of noninvasively assessed trabecular bone structures, *Med. Eng. Phys.*, 17, 126, 1995.
6. Ulrich, D., van Rietbergen, B., Weinans, H., and Ruegsegger, P., Finite element analysis of trabecular bone structure: a comparison of image-based meshing techniques, *J. Biomech.*, 31, 1187, 1998.
7. van Rietbergen, B., Weinans, H., Huiskes, R., and Odgaard, A., A new method to determine trabecular bone elastic properties and loading using micromechanical finite-element models, *J. Biomech.*, 28, 69, 1995.
8. Runkle, J.C. and Pugh, J., The micromechanics of cancellous bone. II. Determination of the elastic modulus of individual trabeculae by a buckling analysis, *Bull. Hosp. Joint Dis.*, 36, 2, 1975.
9. Townsend, P.R., Rose, R.M., and Radin, E.L., Buckling studies of single human trabeculae, *J. Biomech.*, 8, 199, 1975.
10. Kuhn, J.L., Goldstein, S.A., Choi, K., et al., Comparison of the trabecular and cortical tissue moduli from human iliac crests, *J. Orthop. Res.*, 7, 876, 1989.
11. Choi, K., Kuhn, J.L., Ciarelli, M.J., and Goldstein, S.A., The elastic moduli of human subchondral, trabecular, and cortical bone tissue and the size-dependency of cortical bone modulus, *J. Biomech.*, 23, 1103, 1990.
12. Timoshenko, S.P. and Goodier, J.N., *Theory of Elasticity*, 3rd ed., New York, McGraw-Hill, New York, 1970.
13. Ryan, S.D. and Williams, J.L., Tensile testing of rodlike trabeculae excised from bovine femoral bone, *J. Biomech.*, 22, 351, 1989.
14. Rho, J.Y., Ashman, R.B., and Turner, C.H., Young's modulus of trabecular and cortical bone material: ultrasonic and microtensile measurements, *J. Biomech.*, 26, 111, 1993.
15. Mente, P.L. and Lewis, J.L., Experimental method for the measurement of the elastic modulus of trabecular bone tissue, *J. Orthop. Res.*, 7, 456, 1989.
16. Lotz, J.C., Gerhart, T. N., and Hayes, W.C., Mechanical properties of metaphyseal bone in the proximal femur, *J. Biomech.*, 24, 317, 1991.
17. Cowin, S.C., The mechanical properties of cortical bone tissue, in *Bone Mechanics*, Cowin, S.C., Ed., CRC Press, Boca Raton, FL, 1989, 97.
18. Choi, K. and Goldstein, S.A., A comparison of the fatigue behavior of human trabecular and cortical bone tissue, *J. Biomech.*, 25, 1371, 1992.

20 Strain Gauge Measurements from Bone Surfaces

John A. Szivek and Vasanti M. Gharpuray

CONTENTS

I. INTRODUCTION

There are several applications for strain measurement in orthopaedic biomechanics and biomaterials research.[1] These include testing and development of prosthetic and implantable devices,[2-5] determining the mechanical properties of biological structures,[6,7] determining bone strains during physiological activities,[8-10] determining strain levels that lead to an adaptive bone remodeling response,[11-13] and validating or complementing computational simulations.[14,15] Although various strain measurement techniques such as photoelasticity, brittle coatings, holographic interferometry, and thermographic stress analysis have been established, the most common is electric resistance strain gauging.[16]

Strain gauging offers many advantages over other techniques.[17] Gauges are very sensitive and can measure strains directly. When properly protected, gauges can measure strains in a wide variety of corrosive environments and can be continuously monitored in a dynamic loading situation. The primary disadvantage of strain gauges is that they measure strain at discrete points only. One must have a good idea of the critical regions in the test specimen prior to gauge attachment and testing. In addition, strain measurement must be used in conjunction with material properties derived from separate tests to determine stresses. Thus, strain gauges are commonly used to measure strains in a few critical regions, and are used in conjunction with material properties and analytical models to draw inferences about the stress state of the bone.

The most common use for strain gauges *in vitro* has been to determine strain and stress distributions in cadaver bone under various loading conditions and with various implants in place. However, it is extremely difficult to accurately simulate muscle and joint loads in animals during physiological activities with a mechanical testing apparatus. For this reason, *in vitro* studies of animal whole bones are much less common than *in vitro* studies of human whole bones. *In vivo* strain gauging studies are more commonly used to study whole bones in animal models.

One challenge faced when performing *in vivo* strain gauging is the selection of a consistent zero strain point. Since bones are always loaded by muscles in living animals it is not possible to define a posture in which the bone strain is zero. Gauges can be used to measure strain changes relative to some established "zero" during a specific activity. In this chapter, techniques for both *in vitro* and *in vivo* strain measurement will be discussed. Additional information about errors and pitfalls that the user should be aware of and some criteria for gauge, adhesive, and protective coating selection will be provided.

II. HISTORY OF STRAIN GAUGE USE IN BIOMECHANICS

The fundamental principle underlying the electric resistance strain gauge is that when a wire is stretched, its length increases and its cross-sectional area decreases causing a change in its electrical resistance.[18] The equation relating the length change to the resistance change is

$$R = \frac{\rho L}{A} \qquad (20.1)$$

where R = resistance (ohm), ρ = a material property of the conductor called resistivity (ohm·cm), L = length of the conductor (cm), and A = cross-sectional area of the conductor (cm^2). In a properly calibrated system, one can determine the change in length of a wire by measuring its change in electrical resistance.

The first recorded use of a wire strain gauge was in 1931 when the deformation of pillars was measured by using wires stretched between them.[19] The bonded wire gauge was first used by Clark and Datwyler[20] in 1938 to measure strains during tensile impact loading and was patented by Edward Simmons in 1942.[21] Advanced fabrication techniques led to the development of foil strain gauges made of self-temperature-compensated alloys.[22] The foil is photoetched in a grid pattern onto a plastic backing which makes it easier to handle. The backing also makes attaching the foil onto the test specimen easier. The foil pattern can vary in size and shape and, if necessary, several gauges can be stacked in different orientations on top of each other to create rosettes.

Gurdjian and Lissner[23] first described the use of a strain gauge on living bone in 1944. The wire strain gauge, which was bonded with polymethylmethacrylate (PMMA) to the cranium of an anesthetized test animal, was used to collect *in vivo* bone deformation measurements. In this early study, it took 2 h for the methacrylate to cure thoroughly and the site had to be kept exposed because of the lack of waterproofing. In a review of stress analysis techniques used on bone, Evans[24] reported that he, Coolbaugh, and Lebow had strain-gauged a canine tibia and collected the first bone strains during gait.

The earliest review of gauge preparation and bonding techniques was provided by Roberts.[25] He described a number of ways to waterproof, wire, and bond strain gauges to bone in living animals. The most important suggestions from his review were that bone surfaces should be prepared by degreasing with alcohol, ether, or acetone and that a cyanoacrylate adhesive was a better choice for bonding gauges than dental cement (PMMA) or epoxy because it bonded almost instantaneously. He also recommended obtaining lead wire isolation by using wires coated with Teflon® (E.I. du Pont de Nemours and Company, Inc., Wilmington, DE) with an additional silastic layer or silastic tubing around them and using subcutaneous strain relief loops.

At about the same time, biochemical studies examining cyanoacrylates for other tissue-bonding applications showed that these adhesives are broken down quickly *in vivo*,[26] but that the butyl form lasts longer and is better tolerated than the methyl, ethyl, or propyl cyanoacrylates.[27]

Lanyon and Smith[28] were the first to publish a thorough description of gauge preparation and placement techniques as part of an *in vivo* strain gauge study. In their study, polyester-backed wire gauges were attached with isobutyl 2-cyanoacrylate to the tibiae of sheep and *in vivo* strain measurements were collected during gait. However, this study was plagued with problems caused by the electric circuitry and recording devices. An AC-based signal conditioner used in conjunction with high-resistance semiconductor gauges eliminated these problems.[29] Foil gauges were first used in 1972.[30] They were noted to be easier to place and to cause less damage to the bone and surrounding tissues.[31] Studies using foil gauges were extended to several types of animals and to humans. Gauges attached with isobutyl 2-cyanoacrylate were used to collect *in vivo* measurements from the human tibial shaft during gait.[32]

The earliest reported use of strain gauges in a human (although it was attached to a prosthesis and not directly to bone) was by Rydell in 1966.[33] In that study, strain gauges were attached to a femoral prosthesis before it was implanted. The instrumented prosthesis was used to determine the forces acting on the femoral head.

Evidence that gauges placed *in vivo* could measure physiological bone deformation was reported when strains were collected and related to simultaneous accelerometer readings[28] and bone surface electrical potential readings.[34,35] One of these studies[35] showed a linear relationship between bone surface charge and bone strain during gait. Later, optical extensometry was used during mechanical loading of freshly explanted bones from test animals which had been used for *in vivo* measurements for validation of *in vivo* strain measurement accuracy.[36] Carter et al.[37] also showed that accurate strain measurements could be collected after strain-gauged, explanted bones were soaked in saline for a week.

In vitro, strain gauges have been used for bone strain measurements since the late 1950s.[38] Lambert[39] reported that gauges could be attached directly to the surface of moist cortical bone and described methods for waterproofing the gauges and lead wires. In the Lambert study, the deformation and weight-bearing functions of the fibula and tibia were measured.

In some of these studies, bone surfaces were dried prior to bonding of gauges. In addition, procedures such as surface cleaning, scraping, degreasing, and dehydration were used prior to gauge placement. A report on gauge application to bone *in vitro* showed that techniques such as scraping and degreasing create visible surface damage to bone.[40] The authors concluded that these techniques were acceptable for *in vitro* preparations and produced good bonding. However, they are too aggressive for *in vivo* studies. The surface damage created can be expected to cause a remodeling or healing response which would alter bone properties and could recruit cells which degrade and remove the adhesive more quickly.

Around 1979, widespread interest in measurement of physiological strains and advances in strain gauge and adhesive technology led to a proliferation of bone strain measurement studies. *In vitro* procedures were used to determine the mechanical behavior of bone under various loading conditions.[41-44] They were also used to assess the effect of disease, surgical procedures, or implants on strain patterns.[3,45-47] *In vivo* strain measurements were used to compare loading pattern changes to anatomical and histological characteristics of bone,[9,12,39,48-50] to examine evolutionary aspects of bone shape,[10,49-51] and to correlate implant-induced bone shape changes with implant-induced strain changes.[52-55] Bone strains were also measured during exercise protocols in a variety of mammals and birds[56-61] and to study remodeling in microgravity environments.[62,63]

The aspect of the *in vivo* strain gauging procedure that still needs significant development is bonding. Cyanoacrylate adhesives degrade within the body's environment in as little as 2 to 3 weeks leading to measurement inaccuracies. An ongoing search for better methods of attaching strain gauges to bone *in vivo* has led to three approaches. One approach is the use of dental adhesives originally used on enamel surfaces. Page et al.[8] reported the successful use of this approach to bond gauges to femora in a dog model. The second approach which has been successfully used in animals

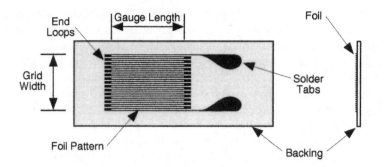

FIGURE 20.1 Schematic showing a typical strain gauge.

and humans utilizes PMMA but requires that the bone surface be abraded or drilled and roughened.[64] A more promising approach for very long-term sensor attachment is the use of calcium phosphate ceramic (CPC) particles bonded to the strain gauge sensing surface.[65-68] This approach has been successfully used to collect strain measurements after as long as 16 weeks *in vivo*.[68] In addition, recent studies[69] have shown that the bond strength of the CPC gauge interface and the bone–CPC interface remain constant for up to 9 months *in vivo*.[70]

III. COMPONENTS OF A STRAIN GAUGE MEASURING SYSTEM

Beckwith et al.[71] have outlined several factors for successful strain gauge measurement:

- Accurate operation and stability of the gauge itself;
- Selecting appropriate lead wires (and an adequate percutaneous conduit when *in vivo* monitoring is performed);
- Providing protection of the gauge from the environment;
- Utilizing a strong, stable adhesive to bond the gauge to the test specimen and a reproducible attachment technique;
- Measuring with a stable, low-noise electrical circuit to provide adequate measurement accuracy.

A good understanding of each of these factors is important, since gauge performance can be optimized for a particular environment by the correct choice of these characteristics.

IV. STRAIN GAUGE SELECTION

The first step in projects requiring strain measurement is the selection of suitable gauges. The choices to be made include (1) the foil material and resistance; (2) the backing material; and (3) the gauge length and pattern (Figure 20.1). A comprehensive examination of all gauge types available is beyond the scope of this chapter but is available in texts[72,73] and in technical literature[22,74] provided by manufacturers. However, a brief review of some criteria for appropriate gauge selection will be given.

A. FOIL GRID MATERIAL

The three most important requirements that a foil must satisfy are (1) low temperature sensitivity; (2) high strain sensitivity or gauge factor (GF); and (3) high electric resistivity.[71] Commercial gauges, which satisfy most of these requirements, are usually made of a nickel-copper alloy such as Constantan, Advance, or Monel or a nickel–chromium alloy such as Karma, Isoelastic, or Nichrome V. Table 20.1 gives the compositions and properties of some of the more commonly used alloys.

TABLE 20.1
Common Foil Grid Materials and Their Properties[22,71]

Grid Material	Composition	Gauge Factor	Resistivity ρ $\Omega.cm \times 10^{-6}$
Nichrome V	80% Nickel	2.0	108
	20% Chromium		
Constantan, Copel, Advance	45% Nickel	2.0	49
	55% Copper		
Isoelastic	55.5% Iron	3.5	112
	36% Nickel		
	8% Chromium		
	0.5% Molybdenum		
Karma	74% Nickel	2.4	130
	20% Chromium		
	3% Aluminum		
	3% Iron		
Manganin	84% Copper	0.47	48
	12% Manganese		
	4% Nickel		
Platinum-Iridium	95% Platinum	5.1	24
	5% Iridium		
Monel	67% Nickel	1.9	42
	33% Copper		

Temperature sensitivity can cause errors in strain gauge measurements because temperature fluctuations induce changes in the resistance of the gauge and GF. Thus, if the temperature of the environment changes after the gauge is installed and balanced, the indicator will register strains even in the absence of loading changes. This reading is called *thermal output* or *apparent strain*. Thermal output can be quite large when gauges are used at high temperatures but is relatively small (approximately 0.5 $\mu\varepsilon$/°F) when gauges are used between room temperature and body temperature. While this may not appear to be of concern in biomechanical testing where the temperature is held constant by body fluids, one must be aware that friction between overlying tissue and gauges can cause a localized temperature increase. To minimize thermal output, alloys are processed to reduce the temperature sensitivity of the foil material. These self-temperature-compensated (STC) gauges are available in different grades, which are based on the thermal expansion coefficient of the test material.

The sensitivity of the foil material is defined by GF, which is the ratio of the relative change in resistance to the relative change in length of the material.

$$GF = \frac{dR / R}{dL / L}$$

(20.2)

Clearly, the higher GF, the more sensitive the gauge. GF depends on the material, size and geometry of the grid, the STC number, and the temperature, and is determined experimentally for each gauge. Of the commonly available foil materials, the Isoelastic alloy usually has the highest GF (approximately 3.5), while for most other materials GF varies from 1.9 to 2.5. Unfortunately, the Isoelastic alloy is not available in STC form, and can be used only under dynamic loading conditions in which a zero reference is not required. One has to compromise between choosing the highest GF and the best STC. Constantan or Advance are good foil material choices. These materials have good thermal stability and a linear strain sensitivity over a large range of strain.[72] This makes them an ideal choice for strain measurement in biomechanics, since such gauges can be accurately calibrated over a narrow range and the calibration constant will remain the same over a much wider range.

The highest-resistance strain gauges offer the advantages of reduced heat generation within the foil and they aid in heat dissipation, provide for lead wire desensitization, and improve the signal-to-noise ratio. Since bone has poor thermal conductivity, a high-resistance gauge (i.e., 1000 or 5000 Ω) would be the best choice to minimize thermal drift. Matching of the thermal expansion coefficient of the gauge with that of the bone will also reduce errors due to thermal expansion of the gauge. Fortunately, since most testing with bone is performed with the bone and gauges immersed in body-temperature fluids (both *in vivo* and *in vitro*), thermal changes are relatively insignificant. Thus, the very high resistance gauges (i.e., greater than 1000 Ω), which are also more expensive, are not essential. Gauges are most commonly available with 120 and 350 Ω resistances. The 120-Ω gauges provide adequate measurements. In cases in which low excitation voltages and the least thermal effects are desired, higher-resistance gauges are a better choice even though gauge selection is limited and prices are higher.

B. Gauge Backing Material

The three functions of the gauge backing material are to provide ease of handling, to provide a means of attaching the foil to the test specimen, and to act as an insulator between the test material and the foil. The most common backing materials are phenolic impregnated paper, polyimide, epoxy-type plastic films, and glass fiber–reinforced epoxy-phenolic. The choice of the backing material is not completely independent of the foil and adhesive.

Most gauges are made on a polyimide backing. This is the backing material of choice for bone strain measurements because it is tough and flexible and can tolerate deformations up to 20% without experiencing any loss of integrity. Its flexibility is an asset when placing gauges on surfaces with a small radius of curvature and when collecting strains from very flexible bones.

C. Gauge Length, Width, and Pattern

Strain gauges are available with gauge lengths that range from about 0.2 to about 100 mm. When selecting a gauge length and width, it is important to remember that a gauge averages the strain it measures over its surface area. Critical regions on a test specimen may experience high strains and high strain gradients. Measurements from a strain gauge in regions with large strain gradients can be unrepresentative of the true strain (Figure 20.2). Errors in excess of 20% have been noted when relatively large gauges are placed in regions of high strain gradients.[75,76] For this reason it is critical that the narrowest grid width appropriate be selected. In addition, bone specimens often have curved surfaces, and bone properties vary as a function of position along and across the bone. Narrow gauges can help minimize measurement inaccuracies caused by these factors. When selecting small gauges, the length should also be considered carefully. Gauges less than 3 mm in length can be difficult to handle, install, and wire, and have poorer heat dissipation properties. In addition, their maximum elongation, measurement stability during static loading, and endurance during fatigue loading are poorer than those of larger gauges.[22] A compromise must often be made between a small gauge length to minimize gradient errors and a larger gauge length to minimize thermal drift errors. The same considerations should be given to gauge width selection. A smaller width should be chosen to minimize averaging errors caused by high strain gradients, while a larger width should be chosen when heat dissipation and gauge stability are considered essential.

In addition to length, width, and pattern choices, gauges are also available in single and multiple grids. Single-grid gauges (also called uniaxial gauges) are often used when the strain along one direction is of primary interest. Similarly, double-grid or biaxial gauges (i.e., gauges that have two strain sensing elements oriented perpendicular to each other) are often used when

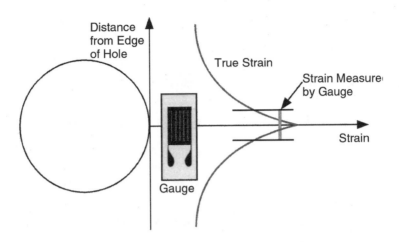

FIGURE 20.2 Schematic showing how gauge length can cause averaging errors in regions of high strain gradients. A hole in a test specimen causes a stress concentration at its edge. Since a strain gauge has a finite length, it measures an average strain over its length, and thus does not give a measure of the true strain near the hole.

the strains along two perpendicular directions are of interest. Rosette gauges, which have three or more elements, provide the most complete information about the strain state of a point on the bone. They can be used to determine strains along specific directions as well as the principal strains. Misalignment errors are less critical if rosettes are used for measuring principal strains.[76-78] However, it should be noted that accurate principal strain measurements are dependent on accurate gauge orientation measurements. As such, careful alignment of gauges should not be abandoned when rosettes are utilized. Their relative insensitivity to misalignment makes these the gauges of choice when it is difficult to align gauges accurately along specific axes or landmarks or when only peak strains are of interest. Although the alignment of the rosettes during installation is not critical, as already noted, the accurate measurement of gauge orientation is critical in order to be able to complete the strain analysis. The equations used to assess the principal strains and principal strain directions are dependent on the type of rosette utilized and can be found in many fundamental mechanics books.[72,79]

Rosettes are generally available in several different configurations (Figure 20.3) and the choice of a configuration usually depends on the proposed location of the gauge on the test specimen. Another choice that an investigator must make when using rosettes is whether to use a single-plane rosette (i.e., one in which all elements are in one plane) or a stacked rosette (i.e., one in which the elements are stacked on top of each other) (see Figure 20.3). The advantage of the single-plane rosette is that it has better heat dissipation properties and thus its measurements are more accurate when it is used on relatively flat specimens experiencing small strain gradients. Single-plane rosettes are more flexible than stacked rosettes and can be contoured to a specimen surface better. However, principal strain measurements can be extremely inaccurate when used on curved surfaces with large strain gradients because each element collects strain from a different location. The stacked rosette measures strains in different directions at a single point, and is much more suitable in areas with high strain gradients and on curved surfaces with an uneven or small radius of curvature.

D. OTHER GAUGE OPTIONS

When selecting gauges for bone strain measurements, it is valuable to select a gauge type which offers the option of large solder dots, integral strain relief tabs, and an encapsulated face. This

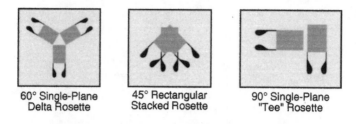

60° Single-Plane   45° Rectangular   90° Single-Plane
Delta Rosette   Stacked Rosette   "Tee" Rosette

FIGURE 20.3   Some configurations of strain gauge rosettes.

combination of options allows ease of soldering, which ultimately results in stronger, more elec-trically conductive solder joints, a sensor that is more immune to measurement errors caused by wire motion, and a more waterproof sensor wire system.

V. LEAD WIRES AND TRANSCUTANEOUS CONNECTORS

The first step in gauge preparation is wiring. This must be done on the bench top prior to gauge attachment to bone since *in situ* soldering is cumbersome for *in vitro* tests and impossible during sterile surgery. In order to minimize contamination of gauges, they should be placed on a clean glass surface. One edge of each gauge can be held in place with a tape that leaves minimal residue. An invisible Scotch® tape (3M, St. Paul, MN) can be used. The low-tack surface of a Post-it® (3M, St. Paul, MN) note leaves even less residue, although it holds the gauge less securely. If gauges without integral strain relief tabs have been purchased, it is advisable to attach strain relief tabs to the gauge (Technical Tip, TT-604, Measurements Group, Raleigh, NC) and then attach wires to the tabs. In this way any wire motion will not be transferred to the gauge.

For *in vitro* applications, any flexible, relatively low resistance wire may be used (see Section VIII). In most cases two wires are sufficient, one attached to each solder tab. Three-wire systems, which are used to provide lead wire temperature compensation, are not essential because the temperature of the testing setup is usually maintained constant. Wires used *in vivo* must satisfy some additional requirements. First, they must be very flexible so that motion of muscles does not put large stresses on the gauge–wire junction. Multiconductor cables with multistrand high-con-ductivity, low-oxygen copper wires can be obtained from Cooner Wire (Chatsworth, CA). A shielded two-conductor cable such as the NMUF 2/30-4046 SJ (Cooner Wire, Chatsworth, CA) works well for single-element gauges, or one such as NMUF 3/30-4046 SJ (Cooner Wire, Chatsworth, CA) can be used if a three-wire system is to be implemented. For small animal models the wires from this cable can be used without the shield and cable cover. The six conductor NMUF 6/30-4046 SJ (Cooner Wire, Chatsworth, CA) is a good choice for use with rosette gauges.

If wires are to be buried *in vivo* for any length of time prior to monitoring, the ends of the wires or cables can be waterproofed using the same procedure used for waterproofing gauges (discussed in Section VI). In some cases, individual wires can be led transcutaneously and left exposed for later monitoring. In rat models wires can often be left exposed in this fashion for several weeks. Connectors can then be attached at the time of monitoring and removed when monitoring is complete, leaving transcutaneous wires exposed for future monitoring sessions. If measurements are to be collected often for extended periods, transcutaneous multipin connectors may be anchored in the skin.[62] However, this requires additional surgical manipulation to place the connection system.

In cases in which a few wires will be chronically transcutaneous, it is advisable to make a small puncture through the skin with a new, fine-tipped scalpel blade. A purse string suture can be used to hold the skin closed around each wire. A drop of cyanoacrylate can be used to seal the skin–wire junction. If transcutaneous connectors are to be used, silicone flanges on the connector are valuable, allowing them to be sutured to the skin. For a connector placed in the cranium, PMMA can be used to attach it to surrounding bony tissues and the scalp can be closed around the connector. If a large number of strain gauges are to be implanted, a large number of wires must be brought out through the skin. In such cases, heat-shrinkable Teflon tubing can be used to hold all the wires together, and a percutaneous device (PMMA post with a stainless steel mesh flange) can be placed at the exit site of the wires.[80] Alternatively, an exit site for each wire has been used successfully[68] but requires that wires be kept 2 to 3 cm apart.

Connector selection is dependent on the monitoring system used to collect measurements. Widely available, inexpensive nine-pin connectors can be used to connect up to four gauges to monitoring equipment. If gauges are to be monitored using externally attached miniature radio telemetry or the connection requirements mandate the use of very small, multipin connectors, the C-46 series Konigsberg implantable seven-pin connectors (Konigsberg Instruments, Pasadena, CA) work well.

Surgical approaches will be dependent on the gauge placement site. In addition to planning the approach to reach the bone site of interest, planning to allow wire placement is essential. In small animal models, because of space constraints, it is often easier to place the wires in the positions that they will occupy at the completion of surgery before attempting to attach the gauges to bone. In all cases it will be necessary to route the wires subcutaneously to a site which the animal cannot easily reach. In most animals the best site is at the nape of the neck or the crown of the skull. With primates, additional restraints to prevent them from manually destroying wires and connectors are also needed. In these animal models an implantable telemetry system may provide the best solution. These systems are best housed in the abdominal cavity of small animals, although miniaturization has made some systems so small they can be left adjacent to the gauge site.

Another common problem is infection at transcutaneous leads. In larger animal models transcutaneous leads and transdermal connectors necessitate careful wound care to prevent infections and require protection of leads or connectors. Recent developments in implantable telemetry systems should solve these problems. However, telemetry systems are still relatively noisy compared with hard-wired measurement systems and do require the use of higher-resistance gauges to reduce bridge power requirements.

VI. PREPARATION OF GAUGES BEFORE ATTACHMENT

For the results of an *in vitro* test to be representative of the *in vivo* behavior of bone, the *in vivo* conditions must be simulated as closely as possible. Although early studies showed that there was no difference between the deformation behavior of live and dead bone,[81,82] recent studies have shown that if bone is allowed to dry, its properties change significantly.[83] For this reason, *in vitro* strain gauge measurements are generally made while the bone is kept moist or immersed in a physiological solution, and strain gauges used for *in vivo* measurements are constantly exposed to body fluids. Therefore, gauges used for both *in vitro* and *in vivo* tests must be encapsulated in a protective waterproof coating.

One of the challenges of strain measurement collection is preventing fluid infiltration into the gauge–wire junction. For short-term *in vitro* testing, this requirement can be satisfied by purchasing strain gauges with attached lead wires that are completely encapsulated. If infiltration is a problem after immersion in fluid, an additional coating of nitrile rubber may be applied. For long-term testing in saline, the gauge and gauge–wire junction should be coated with a film of Teflon. Coatings of nitrile rubber and polysulfide epoxy should be applied over the Teflon film with each coating extending beyond the previous one. It is also advisable to coat the lead wires with a thin coat of nitrile rubber. It is important to note that some of these coatings take up to 24 h to cure completely. If a gauge is installed on a bone surface prior to waterproofing, the specimen may dehydrate during the coating-curing period.

In vivo, the waterproofing technique used should not only keep wires and gauges insulated but should also produce a gauge–wire assembly that is relatively bioinert so that the tissue reaction to the waterproofed gauge is minimal. Handling of gauges during surgery also presents unique waterproofing challenges. Two drawbacks of the traditional coating materials used for waterproofing, such as epoxy and silicone, are that these materials can induce a biological response and that they create assemblies that are stiff and bulky. Loads on the gauge assemblies caused by muscles can create large interfacial shear stresses at the gauge–bone interface leading to adhesive failures. Thus, the coating must be flexible, relatively bioinert, and waterproof and must protect the gauges and wires from damage caused by handling during surgery. A multilayer coating developed by Szivek[54] has provided waterproofing for up to 16 weeks during *in vivo* strain measurement collection.[56,68] After wiring the gauge (Figure 20.4A), the first step in the coating process is to strengthen mechanically and waterproof the gauge–wire junction (Figure 20.4B) with a small bead of PMMA (Kerr Fastcure Sybron, Romulus, MI). Once the PMMA has set and dried for 4 h, the gauge–wire junction is coated with a layer of M Coat B (Measurements Group, Raleigh, NC), an air-drying nitrile rubber, and allowed to dry for an additional 24 h (Figure 20.4C). The nitrile rubber acts as a coupling agent between the next waterproofing coating and the wire insulation and manufacturer's polyimide gauge backing. A thin layer of M Coat D (Measurements Group, Raleigh, NC), an air-drying acrylic, is placed on the gauges next and allowed to dry for 24 h (Figure 20.4D). At this point an ultrafine-point permanent marker can be used to assign the gauge a number or to mark the orientation of specific elements of a rosette. The acrylic coating provides a waterproof coating on the gauge and gauge–wire junction but is brittle and easily damaged by surgical instruments. The final coating is a layer of M Coat A (Measurements Group, Raleigh, NC), an air-drying polyurethane, which is allowed to cure for 7 days (Figure 20.4E). The primary purpose of this coating is to protect the acrylic layer from surface damage.

In preparation for surgery, the wired gauges must be sterilized. Ethylene oxide sterilization assures minimum thermal damage to gauges and coatings. Sterile wired gauges should be double aerated since residual ethylene oxide trapped in the wires can leach out *in vivo* and cause tissue irritation and necrosis.

VII. ATTACHMENT OF GAUGES

A. Attachment for *In Vitro* Studies

Cyanoacrylates, such as M Bond 200 (Measurements Group, Raleigh, NC), are the most common adhesives used *in vitro*. The bone is first cleaned of all soft tissue and the periosteum is removed. Depending on the nature of the tests, specimens may be machined from the cleaned bone, or the whole bone used as is. The location on the specimen at which the gauge is to be bonded is marked and then dried thoroughly. Aggressive degreasing and scraping as suggested by Wright and Hayes[40] is not necessary for satisfactory adhesive performance. However, if the gauge is to be applied in an area containing periosteal blood vessels or in an area in which the bone is very thin, the area should be sealed and prepared for the adhesive. This is usually done by applying a thin layer of the adhesive catalyst and allowing it to dry. Then one or two drops of the adhesive are spread thinly over the bone surface and allowed to dry for about 5 min. Next the area is smoothed down with a fine grit (300 to 400) silicon-carbide paper.[43] To attach the gauge, one drop of the adhesive is placed on the prepared surface and the gauge is held against the surface for 1 min using finger pressure. This is enough to develop a strong bond, and the bone can then be returned to its saline environment. Care must be taken to align the gauge correctly during the installation. An established technique such as the one described by Wright and Hayes[40] may be used.

B. Attachment for *In Vivo* Studies

The most commonly used adhesives for *in vivo* applications are the cyanoacrylates. Isobutyl cyanoacrylate bonds quickly and, when used at relatively dry sites, may hold gauges in place for several weeks. A single-component form of this adhesive such as VetBond™ (3M Animal Care

Steps in Gauge Preparation

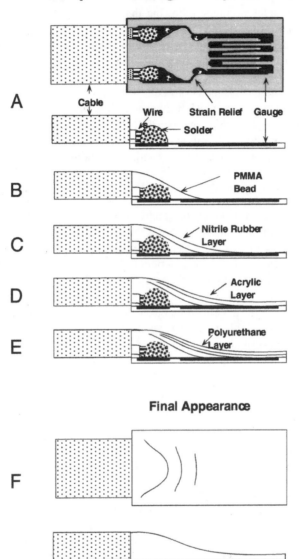

FIGURE 20.4 This series of diagrams shows the steps used to wire and waterproof a strain gauge for use *in vivo*. Note that the PMMA in B is tapered to cover the gauge–wire junction but also to maintain the flexibility of the gauge. The rubber layer should adequately cover the junction and a short region of the cable housing. The remaining two waterproofing layers should cover the junction and the entire gauge.

Products, St. Paul, MN) or an adhesive which comes with a separate accelerator such as M-Bond 200 can be used. When using the one-component system it is best to place a small amount of adhesive on the bone surface prior to gauge attachment and allow it to dry. This procedure will seal the bone surface. This region should be scraped slightly prior to gauge attachment. A drop of adhesive should then be placed on the gauge and the gauge pressed against the bone surface for 1 min. The tip of a blunt surgical instrument can be used to hold miniature gauges in place while the glue sets. Care should be taken not to let any glue get on instruments, gloves, or tissues.

One should be aware that cyanoacrylate adhesives experience biodegradation and that measurements collected from glued gauges may vary in accuracy from day to day. Adhesive degradation mandates the testing of gauge accuracy following the completion of *in vivo* measurements using some form of bench-top testing. Three approaches have been reported. The first involves loading the bones with a known load, collecting strains from the gauge which had been used for *in vivo* bone strain measurements, then replacing the gauge with a freshly glued gauge in the same location and retesting the bone.[30] The second procedure utilizes a second strain measurement technique (either optical or electronic extensometry) to collect bone strain while simultaneously collecting strain measurements from the gauge which had been used for *in vivo* bone strain measurements.[38,39] The third technique requires explanting and bench-top testing both the bone which was originally gauged and the contralateral bone.[63-68] Validity of strain comparisons to measurements from freshly attached gauges on contralateral bones, during cantilever bending, have been confirmed.[84,85]

C. PREPARATION OF CPC-COATED GAUGES FOR EXTENDED *IN VIVO* STRAIN MEASUREMENT

As noted earlier, cyanoacrylate bonding of gauges to bone *in vivo* is acceptable for short-term measurement. However, adhesive failure precludes the use of these systems for long-term measurement. CPC-coated gauges can be used instead. After wiring and waterproofing gauges using the three-stage process described earlier, gauges should be sanded with 600-grit carbide paper on their sensing surfaces. This surface is coated with a layer of 15 wt.% Udel®, a medical-grade polysulfone (Amoco, Huntington Beach, CA) dissolved in 1,1,2,2-tetrachloroethane (Eastman Kodak Company, Rochester, NY). Coated gauges must then be baked for 1 h at 90°C. This first-baked polysulfone layer is then sanded with 1200-grit carbide paper. Another coating of polysulfone is applied, followed by CPC particles sprinkled onto the moist polysulfone. A combination of an amorphous tricalcium phosphate with a particle size of 9 ± 7 mm and a microcrystalline CPC with a particle size of approximately 561 ± 85 mm (Biointerfaces, San Diego, CA) have produced an ideal combination of bone bonding and gauge–CPC bond stability *in vivo*.[42] Coated gauges will then be baked for 5 h at 90°C. Following this preparation process, gauges must be sterilized with ethylene oxide and double-aerated prior to implantation.

VIII. MEASUREMENT COLLECTION

In order to measure strains from gauges, the wire leads from the gauge must be connected to a signal conditioning and recording system. A hard-wired system can successfully be used for this purpose. However, if extensive freedom of movement is required, a radio telemetry system may be a better choice. Hard-wired systems are typically made up of a signal conditioning circuit which provides a balance capability (often in the form of a Wheatstone bridge) to offset the initial resistance of the gauge, lead wires, and connectors. They generally also contain an electronic signal calibration capability that can be used to place a known resistance into the circuit so that voltage signals from the signal conditioning circuit can be accurately converted to strains. A recording system attached to the signal conditioning circuit should be able to record the voltage changes resulting from strain changes accurately. A continuous recording device such as a multipen recorder with a broad frequency response and high slew rate can be used. Recording systems will be a function of the needs of the experiment, however. For most *in vivo* applications a recording device which can accurately monitor strain changes at sampling rates of no less than 1000 Hz should be selected. Alternatively, a digital recording system provides more data reduction and presentation flexibility.

A system that has been preconfigured such as the Measurements Group System 6000 (Measurements Group, Raleigh, NC) is a good choice if one computer is likely to be dedicated solely to strain and load measurement collection. LabView™ (Signalogic, Dallas, TX) software used in conjunction with a data acquisition board (National Instruments Corporation, Austin, TX) is a more flexible data collection system that may be a better choice if a variety of measurements from various types of test devices will be used. LabView is more difficult to configure, however, and a significant time commitment may be required to get this software configured to the specific needs of individual users. A number of other data collection systems are also available and may do an equally acceptable job. When evaluating a system for *in vivo* strain measurement collection, the sampling rate (which should not be less than 1000 Hz) and number of channels it can simultaneously accommodate are of primary consideration. Real-time strain display and the ability to monitor other equipment, such as video or electromyograms (EMGs) which could be used for limb tracking, are also valuable features to have in a hard-wired measurement system.

If the measurements to be collected require that the test animal or subject have complete freedom of movement, a radio telemetry system can provide signal conditioning and measurement transmission to a receiver and recording device. These systems are for the most part custom-made and have often been made by investigators who collect the strain measurements. Companies such as Konigsberg (Pasadena, CA), MicroStrain (Burlington, VT), and CME Telemetrix (Waterloo, Ontario, Canada) have built biomedical measurement systems in the past and have produced custom-made radio telemetry systems. The transmission signal stability and measurement reproducibility of digital radio telemetry systems are generally far superior to analog radio telemetry systems. However, currently available subminiature implantable radio transmitters suffer from slow sampling rates and remote powering challenges.

Whether the system chosen to collect measurements is a hard-wired or radio telemetry system, measurements should be checked for validity prior to measurement collection. Custom-made systems which do not have built-in signal calibration capabilities must be bench-top calibrated using an external calibration procedure. The validity of measurements made by a system can be checked by comparing strains collected from metal test specimens with well-characterized material properties against either (1) strains computed using beam theory or (2) strains measured with another device such as an extensometer.

Finally, in preparation for *in vivo* strain measurement a zero strain state must be selected. Although no concensus on an ideal point has been reached, zeroing of signals is often carried out with the test animal in a resting posture.[54] Alternatively, the zero can be selected as the strain state during swing phase[56] or when a particular parameter is at a minimum.[86] In this case the strains must be computed following measurement collection relative to the swing phase strain state.

IX. DATA ANALYSIS

Analysis of uniaxial strains in one location generally provides little information about the strain state of a bone. Multiple gauges around a bone section and along the length of a long bone offer much more information about its strain state. A linear elastic response of bone material properties in relatively uniform cross sections of long bones can be assumed at the load rates associated with gait. As such, the strain state of these bones can be interpolated from measured strains using simple beam analysis. If an implant is present, or if relatively complex regions of a bone are analyzed, finite-element analysis must be used in conjunction with strain measurements to evaluate the strain state of the bone between gauges.

Analysis of strains from rosette gauges allows evaluation of strains along each element of the gauge and also allows evaluation of maximum and minimum principal strains at the measurement location. The equations to calculate principal strains are dependent on the type of gauge used and can be found in texts that have chapters describing strain analysis.[72] Strains can also be converted into stress if an accurate value for modulus of the bone under consideration is available. One should keep in mind that bone is not isotropic and that its properties vary as a function of location. Whether single-element or rosette gauges are used for *in vivo* studies, investigators must make assumptions about the zero strain point. Careful consideration of these factors and the limitations of the *in vitro* and *in vivo* strain measurement process will provide a reasonable understanding of the deformation of bone in various situations.

REFERENCES

1. Little, E.G. and Finlay, J.B., Perspectives of strain measurement techniques, in *Strain Measurement in Biomechanics*, Miles, A.W. and Tanner, K.E., Eds., Chapman & Hall, London, 1992, 1.

2. Finlay, J.B., Bourne, R.B., Landsberg, R.P., and Andreae, P., Pelvic stresses *in vitro,* I: malsizing of endoprostheses, *J. Biomech.*, 19, 708, 1986.

3. Finlay, J.B., Bourne, R.B., Landsberg, R.P., and Andreae, P., Pelvic stresses *in vitro,* II: a study of the efficacy of metal-backed acetabular prostheses, *J. Biomech.*, 19, 715, 1986.

4. Hasenkam, J.M., Nygaard, H., Paulsen, P.K., et al., What force can the myocardium generate on a prosthetic mitral valve ring? An animal experimental study, *J. Heart Valve Dis.*, 3, 324, 1994.

5. Nagata, H., Schendel, M.J., Transfeldt, E.E., and Lewis, J.L., The effects of immobilization of long segments of the spine on the adjacent and distal facet force and lumbosacral motion, *Spine*, 18, 2471, 1993.

6. Bowman, S.M., Zeind, J., Gibson, L.J., et al., The tensile behavior of demineralized bovine cortical bone, *J. Biomech.*, 29, 1497, 1996.

7. Roth, V. and Mow, V.C., The intrinsic tensile behavior of the matrix of bovine articular cartilage and its variation with age, *J. Bone Joint Surg.*, 62, 1102, 1980.

8. Page, A.E., Jasty M., Harrigan, T. P., et al., Determination of loading parameters in the canine hip *in vivo*, *J. Biomech.*, 26, 571, 1993.

9. Hylander, W.L., Johnson K.R., and Crompton A.W., Loading patterns and jaw movements during mastication in Macaca fascicularis: a bone-strain, electromyographic, and cineradiographic analysis, *Am. J. Phys. Anthropol.*, 72, 287, 1987.

10. Swartz, M.S., Bennett, M.B., and Carrier, D.R., Wing bone stresses in free flying bats and the evolution of skeletal design for flight, *Nature*, 359, 726, 1992.

11. Lanyon, L.E. and Baggott, D.G., Mechanical function as an influence on the structure and form of bone, *J. Bone Joint Surg.*, 58, 436, 1976.

12. Goodship, A.E., Lanyon, L.E., and McFie, H., Functional adaptation of bone to increased stress: an experimental study, *J. Bone Joint Surg.*, 61A, 539, 1979.

13. Mikic, B. and Carter, D.R., Bone strain gage data and theoretical models of functional adaptation, *J. Biomech.*, 28, 465, 1995.

14. Cheal, E.J., Hayes, W.C., White, A.A., and Perren, S.M., Three-dimensional finite element analysis of a simplified compression plate fixation system, *J. Biomech. Eng.*, 106, 295, 1984.

15. Rohlmann, A., Mossner, U., Bergmann, G., and Kolbel, R., Finite element analysis and experimental investigation in a femur with hip endoprosthesis, *J. Biomech.*, 16, 727, 1983.

16. Miles, A.W. and Tanner, K.E., Eds., *Strain Measurements in Biomechanics*, Chapman & Hall, London, 1992.

17. Dabestani, M., *In vitro* strain measurement in bone, in *Strain Measurement in Biomechanics*, Miles, A.W. and Tanner, K.E. Eds., Chapman & Hall, London, 1992, 58.

18. Thompson, K., On the electro-dynamic qualities of metals, *Philos. Trans. R. Soc. London*, 146, 649, 1856.

19. Eaton, E.C., Resistance strain gauge measures stresses, *Concr. Eng. News Rec.*, 107, 615, 1931.

20. Clark, D.S. and Datwyler, G., Stress–strain relations under tension impact loading, *Proc. ASM*, 38, 98, 1938.

21. Simmons, E.E., U.S. Patent No. 2292549, 1942.

22. Measurements Group, TN-505, Technical Notes, Raleigh, NC, 1996.

23. Gurdjian, E.S. and Lissner, H.R., Mechanism of head injury as studied by the cathode ray oscilloscope: preliminary report, *J. Neurosurg.*, 1, 393, 1944.

24. Evans, F.G., Methods of studying the biomechanical significance of bone form, *Am. J. Phys. Anthropol.*, 11, 413, 1953.

25. Roberts, V.L., Strain-gauge techniques in biomechanics, *Exp. Mech.*, 19A, 1966.

26. Cameron, J.J., Boodward, S.C., Pulaski, E.J., et al., The degradation of cyanoacrylate tissue adhesives, *Surgery*, 58, 424, 1965.

27. Leonard, F., Kulkarni, R.K., Brandes, G., et al., Synthesis and degradation of poly(alkylalphacyanoacrylates), *J. Appl. Polym. Sci.*, 10, 259, 1966.

28. Lanyon, L.E. and Smith, R.N., Bone strain in the tibia during normal quadrupedal locomotion, *Acta Orthop. Scand.*, 41, 238, 1970.
29. Lanyon, L.E., Strain in sheep lumbar vertebrae recorded during life, *Acta Orthop. Scand.*, 42, 102, 1971.
30. Cochran, G.V., Implantation of strain gages on bone *in vivo*, *J. Biomech.*, 5, 119, 1972.
31. Lanyon, L.E., Analysis of surface bone strain in the calcaneus of sheep during normal locomotion, *J. Biomech.*, 6, 41, 1973.
32. Lanyon, L.E., Hampson W.G., Goodship A.E., and Shah J.S., Bone deformation recorded *in vivo* from strain gauges attached to the human tibial shaft, *Acta Orthop. Scand.*, 46, 256, 1975.
33. Rydell, N.W., Forces acting on the femoral head-prosthesis. A study of strain gauge supplied prostheses in living persons, *Acta Orthop. Scand.* 37 (Suppl. 88), 1, 1966.
34. Cochran, G.V., A method for direct recording of electromechanical data from skeletal bone in living animals. Technical notes, *J. Biomech.*, 7, 563, 1974.
35. Lanyon, L.E. and Hartman, W., Strain related electrical potentials recorded *in vitro* and *in vivo*, *Calcif. Tissue Res.*, 22, 315, 1977.
36. Baggott, D.G. and Lanyon, L.E., An independent post-mortem calibration of electrical resistance strain gauges bonded to bone surfaces *in vivo*, *J. Biomech.*, 10, 615, 1977.
37. Carter, D.R., Smith, D.J., Spengler, D.M., et al., Measurement and analysis of *in vivo* bone strains on the canine radius and ulna, *J. Biomech.*, 13, 27, 1980.
38. Hirsch, C. and Frankel, V., The reaction of the proximal end of the femur to mechanical forces, in *Biomechanical Studies of the Musculoskeletal System*, Evans, F.G., Ed., Charles C Thomas, Springfield, IL, 1961.
39. Lambert, K.L., The weight-bearing function of the fibula, *J. Bone Joint Surg.*, 53A, 507, 1971.
40. Wright, T.M. and Hayes, W.C., Strain gage application on compact bone, *J. Biomech.*, 12, 471, 1979.
41. Huiskies, R., On the modeling of long bones in structural analysis, *J. Biomech.*, 15, 65, 1982.
42. Gies, A.A. and Carter, D.R., Experimental determination of whole long bone sectional properties, *J. Biomech.*, 15, 297, 1982.
43. Finlay, J.B., Bourne, R.B., and McLean, J.A., Technique for the *in vitro* measurement of principal strains in the human tibia, *J. Biomech.*, 15, 723, 1982.
44. Kennedy, J.G., Carter, D.R., and Caler, W.E., Long bone torsion, II. A combined experimental and computational method for determining an effective shear modulus, *J. Biomech. Eng.*, 107, 189, 1985.
45. Arner, M. and Hagberg, L., Wrist flexion strength after excision of the pisiform bone, *Scand. J. Plast. Reconstr. Surg.*, 18, 241, 1984.
46. Bourne, R.B., Finlay, J.B., Papadopoulos, P., et al., *In vitro* strain distribution in the proximal tibia. Effect of varus-valgus loading in the normal and osteoarthritic knee, *Clin. Orthop.*, 188, 285, 1984.
47. Bourne, R.B., Finlay, J.B., Papadopoulos, P., and Andreae, P., The effect of medial meniscectomy on strain distribution in the proximal part of the tibia, *J. Bone Joint Surg.*, 66, 1431, 1984.
48. Lanyon, L.E. and Bourn, S., The influence of mechanical function on the development and remodeling of the tibia, *J. Bone Joint Surg.*, 61A(2), 263, 1979.
49. Rubin, C.T. and Lanyon, L.E., Limb mechanics as a function of speed and gait: a study of functional strains in the radius and tibia of horse and dog, *J. Exp. Biol.*, 101, 187, 1982.
50. Rubin, C.T. and Lanyon, L.E., Dynamic strain similarity in vertebrates; an alternative to allometric limb bone scaling, *J. Theor. Biol.*, 107, 321, 1984.
51. Hylander, W.L. and Johnson, K.R., *In vivo* bone strain patterns in the zygomatic arch of macaques and the significance of these patterns for functional interpretation of craniofacial form, *Am. J. Phys. Anthropol.*, 102, 203, 1997.
52. Carter, D.R., Vasu, R., Spengler, D.M., and Dueland, R.T., Stress fields in the unplated and plated canine femur calculated from *in vivo* strain measurements, *J. Biomech.*, 14, 63, 1981.
53. Lanyon, L.E., Paul, I.L., Rubin, C.T., et al., *In vivo* strain measurements from bone and prosthesis following total hip replacement, *J. Bone Joint Surg.*, 63A, 989, 1981.
54. Szivek, J.A., A Quantitative Study of the Effect of Strain Redistribution on Bone Remodelling, Ph.D. thesis, University of Toronto, Canada, 1984.
55. Szivek, J.A., Magee, F.P., Weng, M.S., and Johnson, E.M., Comparative *in vivo* strain measurement from a two year implanted and unimplanted canine hip, *Trans. Int. Soc. Biomater.*, Kyoto, Japan, 1988.
56. Szivek, J.A., Johnson, E.M., and Magee, F.P., *In vivo* strain analysis of the greyhound femoral diaphysis, *J. Invest. Surg.*, 5, 91, 1992.

57. Loitz, B.J. and Zernicke, R.F., Strenuous exercise-induced remodeling of mature bone: relationships between *in vivo* strains and bone mechanics, *J. Exp. Biol.*, 170, 1, 1992.

58. Biewener, A.A. and Bertram, J.E., Skeletal strain patterns in relation to exercise training during growth, *J. Exp. Biol.*, 185, 51, 1993.

59. Biewener, A.A. and Bertram, J.E., Structural response of growing bone to exercise and disuse, *J. Appl. Physiol.* 76, 946, 1994.

60. Skerry, T.M. and Lanyon, L.E., Interruption of disuse by short duration walking exercise does not prevent bone loss in sheep calcaneous, *Bone*, 16, 269, 1995.

61. Turner, C.H., Yoshikawa, T., Forwood, M.R., et al., High frequency components of bone strain in dogs measured during various activities, *J. Biomech.*, 28, 39, 1995.

62. Keller, T.S. and Spengler, D.M., *In vivo* strain gage implantation in rats, *J. Biomech.*, 15, 911, 1982.

63. Szivek, J.A., Wilson, D.L., Anderson, P.L., and DeYoung, D., Development of a model for the study of *in vivo* bone strains during normal and microgravity environments, *J. Appl. Biomater.*, 6, 203, 1995.

64. Burr, D.B., Milgrom, C., Fyhrie, D., et al., *In vivo* measurement of human tibial strains during vigorous activity, *Bone*, 18, 405, 1996.

65. Szivek, J.A., Gealer, R.G., Magee, F.P., and Emmanual, J., Preliminary development of a hydroxyapatite-backed strain gauge, *J. Appl. Biomater.*, 1, 241, 1990.

66. Maliniak, M.M., Szivek, J.A., and DeYoung, D.W., The development of hydroxyapatite coated strain gauges for long-term *in vivo* bone loading response measurements, *J. Appl. Biomater.*, 4, 143, 1993.

67. Szivek, J.A., Anderson, P.L., and DeYoung, D.W., Evaluation of factors affecting bonding rate of calcium phosphate ceramic coatings for *in vivo* strain gauge attachment, *J. Biomed. Mater. Res.*, 33, 121, 1996.

68. Szivek, J.A., Anderson, P.L., and DeYoung, D.W., *In vivo* strain measurements collected using calcium phosphate ceramic bonded strain gauges, *J. Invest. Surg.*, 10, 263, 1997.

69. Battraw, G.A., Szivek, J.A., and Anderson, P.L., Interface strength studies of calcium phosphate ceramic-coated strain gauges, *J. Biomed. Mater. Res.*, 43, 462, 1998.

70. Szivek, J.A., Battraw, G.A., and Anderson, P.L., Calcium phosphate ceramic/polysulfone/polyimide interface characteristics after 4, 6 and 9 months *in vivo*, *Trans. Surf. Biomater.*, 163, 1998.

71. Beckwith, T.G., Marangoni, R.D., and Lienhard, J.H., *Mechanical Measurements*, Addison-Wesley, New York, 1993.

72. Dalley, J.W. and Riley, W.F., *Experimental Stress Analysis*, McGraw-Hill, New York, 1991.

73. Murray, W.M. and Miller, W.R., *The Electric Resistance Strain Gauge: An Introduction*, Oxford University Press, Oxford, U.K., 1992.

74. BLH Electronics Inc., Catalogue 100-6, Canton, MA, 1998.

75. Perry, C.C., The electric resistance strain gauge revisited, *Expl. Mech.* 24, 286, 1984.

76. Pople, J., DIY strain gauge transducers, *Strain*, 16, 23, 1980.

77. Perry, C.C., Strain gauge misalignment errors, *Instrum. Control Syst.*, 42, 137, 1969.

78. Tuttle, M.E. and Brinson, H.F., Resistance foil strain gauge technology as applied to composite mechanics, *Expl. Mech.*, 24, 54, 1984.

79. Malvern, L.E., *Introduction to the Mechanics of a Continuous Medium*, Prentice-Hall, Englewood Cliffs, NJ, 1969.

80. Hiatt, M.J., *In Vivo* Strains in Bone near Transcortical Implants, Thesis, Clemson University, Clemson, SC, 1996.

81. Greenberg, S.W., Gonzalez, G., Gurdjian, E.S., and Thomas, L.M., Changes in the physical properties of bone between the *in vivo*, freshly dead and embalmed conditions, in *12th Stapp Car Crash Conference*, Society of Automotive Engineers, New York, 1968, 272.

82. Evans, F.G., *The Mechanical Properties of Bone*, Charles C Thomas, Springfield, IL, 1973.

83. Broz, J.J., Simske, S.J., Greenberg, A.R., and Luttges, M.W., Effects of rehydration state on the flexural properties of whole mouse long bones, *J. Biomech. Eng.*, 115, 447, 1993.

84. Kersey, R.C., Szivek, J.A., and Sacoman, D.M., Symmetry of biomechanical properties of canine femora, *J. Appl. Biomater.*, 5, 99, 1994.

85. Battraw, G.A., Miera, V., Anderson, P.L., and Szivek, J.A., Symmetry of biomechanical properties in rat femora, *J. Biomed. Mater. Res.*, 32, 285, 1996.

86. Bessman, E.S., Carter, D.R., McCarthy, J.C., and Harris, W.H., Accuracy enhancement of *in vivo* bone strain measurements and analysis, *J. Biomech. Eng.*, 104, 226, 1982.

21 Screw Pullout Test for Evaluating Mechanical Properties of Bone

Matthew S. Crum, Franklin A. Young, Jr., and Yuehuei H. An

CONTENTS

I. INTRODUCTION

Screw pullout testing refers to the measurement of the force required to pull out a screw inserted in a bone specimen. Analysis of the test allows determination of the optimum screw size, insertion technique, angle of penetration, and screw hole preparation method. While all of these variables play a major role in the success of the screw fixation, another parameter that must be explored is the impact of bone structure on the force required to pull the screw. This chapter primarily focuses on the effects of bone microstructure, density, and pathological conditions on the screw pullout test. The chapter introduces the methods of testing the mechanical variables of bone using "one" screw, but will not discuss the methods for testing the effects of fixation of different type screws in one "bone" (for the latter, see Chapter 36).

II. EXAMPLES

A. SCREW PULLOUT STRENGTH AND BONE STRUCTURE

The screw pullout test basically involves the insertion of screws of various sizes and at several different angles into a bone specimen. This analysis is necessary due to the heterogeneous structure of the bone. If the bone were a simple homogeneous material, the location and angle of insertion would be irrelevant. However, because bone consists of a complex column–strut arrangement of trabeculae (Figure 21.1B), the direction and location of screw penetration are vital parameters that must be considered, evaluated, and optimized.

Recently, An et al.[1,2] investigated the correlation between the angle of screw insertion and trabeculae orientation. Because more trabeculae lie in the weight-bearing, or "vertical," direction, they hypothesized that the screw would have an optimum strength at 0° to vertical (parallel to trabeculae), minimum strength at 90° (perpendicular to trabeculae), and an intermediate strength at 45° (Figure 21.1C and D). To insure that the angle of screw insertion would be the only

0-8493-0266-9/00/$0.00+$.50
© 2000 by CRC Press LLC

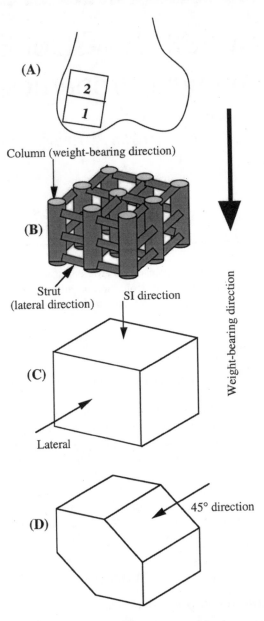

FIGURE 21.1 Illustration of a test for screw-holding powers of bovine cancellous bone from different directions. (A) The sampling site and orientation. (B) The structure of the bone block is idealized into a column-strut model. The columns indicate thicker trabeculae at the weight-bearing direction and the struts represent the trabecular connections between columns (column trabeculae). It is assumed that the columns are thicker and stronger and the struts are thinner and weaker. (C and D) The directions of screw insertion. (From An, Y.H. and Draughn, R.A., Mechanical properties and testing methods of bone, in *Animal Models in Orthopaedic Research*, An, Y.H. and Friedman, R.J., Eds., CRC Press, Boca Raton, FL, 1999. With permission.)

variable tested in the experiment, An et al. used identical screws (40 mm long × 3.5 mm thread diameter self-tapping cortical screws). The samples were small cubes (at least 2.5 × 2.5 × 4.0 cm) extracted from adult bovine femoral condyles at two different levels (Figure 21.1A). The corners of the specimens used for the 45° insertion were chamfered to ensure optimum penetration (Figure 21.1D).

Screw pullout tests were performed on the different specimens (with the screw inserted at different angles to the main trabecular direction) using a mechanical testing machine (MTS System 810, Minneapolis, MN), at a displacement rate of 1 mm/min. The load–displacement curve was obtained using a chart recorder. The slope of the linear portion of the curve (before the yield stress was achieved and permanent deformation occurred) was investigated to determine the stiffness of the bone–screw interface. From these measurements, the ultimate strength σ (MPa) was calculated using the following formula:

$$\sigma = P/\pi dh \tag{21.1}$$

where P (N) was the ultimate applied load, d (mm) was the major diameter of the screw, and h (mm) was the length of the effective threads in the screw in the cancellous bone. An ANOVA test was then used to determine the holding strengths for each of the three angles of insertion. X rays were also taken of 3-mm bone slices from the specimens for radiographic analysis. Sections 5 mm thick were then cut from the 3-mm bone slices, dehydrated, and stained for further analysis under a light microscope.

Histological analysis showed trabeculae lying in the weight-bearing direction (Figure 21.2B).[1,2] A histological image of the cross section of the specimen revealed a honeycomb-like structure, which represented the tops of the trabeculae (Figure 21.2A). The oblique orientation of trabeculae shown in Figure 21.2C represented the 45° insertion. The ANOVA clearly supported the hypothesis. The screw insertions at 0° had significantly higher strengths because they were in the weight-bearing direction (where the plates were subjected to compressive loading). Conversely, those penetrating at 90° performed the worst due to the bending moments they experienced. The 45° screws were affected by both compressive and bending loads but to a lesser extent. Hence, this orientation possessed an intermediate strength. The maximum stresses for the 0, 45, and 90° orientations were 54 ± 5.4, 43 ± 3.9, and 37 ± 5.0 MPa at applied loads of 840 ± 82, 655 ± 59, and 560 ± 76 N, respectively.

In addition, a finite-element analysis (FEA) was performed on the specimens to investigate further the bone microstructure and its impact on pullout strength.[3] A 60° section was chosen for modeling because the bone–screw samples are axisymmetric. A model consisting of 2982 elements was employed in the 0 and 90° testing. The 45° analysis involved 5964 six-noded pentahedral elements. The model was subjected to 3.6, 2.8, and 2.4 N concentrated loading at the implant surface over 39 nodes about 360°. The results clearly showed a strong correlation in strength and ultimate load between the FCA data and the measurements from the pullout test (Table 21.1). This experiment also presents a strong argument on the effects of trabeculae orientation on the ultimate pullout power of screws.

B. Effects of Vertebral Cortices and Insertion Angle on Screw Pullout Strength

A similar study was performed by Horton et al.[4] Their analysis consisted of two experiments. The first of these introduces another variable affecting the screw pullout test, unicortical vs. bicortical predrilling. Unicortical and bicortical drilling simply refer to the screw predrill depth. A 4.5-mm-diameter drill bit was used to penetrate five cadaver thoracic vertebrae to two different depths. Half of the specimens were drilled only in the first cortex (unicortical) and the other half were drilled completely through the first and second cortices (bicortical). These samples were then subjected to pullout tests. Horton et al. observed no statistical variation in screw pullout strengths between those samples subjected to bicortical rather than unicortical predrilling.

The second experiment performed by Horton et al.[4] offers more insight into the significance of screw orientation and the effects of vertebral bone structure. Using cadaver thoracic spines Horton et al. employed screw insertion at traditional midbody, superior endplate, superior oblique, and inferior oblique orientations (Figure 21.3) on 48 vertebrae. Although the 0° screw orientation

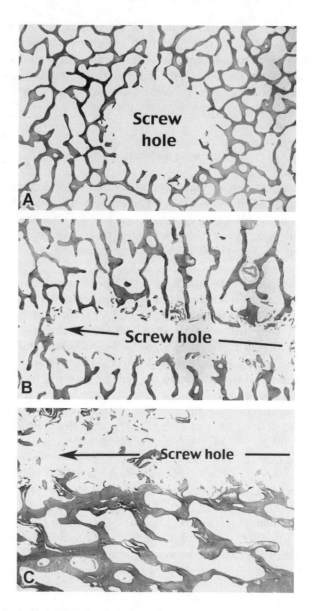

FIGURE 21.2 Histological sections showing the relations between the directions of screw insertion and trabecular orientations. (A) The axial view of 0° insertion; (B) side view of 90° insertion; and (C) side view of 45° insertion.

of An et al. (screw insertion in the weight-bearing direction) was not studied, Horton et al. did experiment with off-center drilling locations (Figure 21.3B) and insertion angles below horizontal (Figure 21.3D). Allowing all insertion techniques and preparations (with the exception of the screw angle) to remain analogous, the researchers inserted a Danek TSRH 6.5-mm-diameter vertebral screw at the various orientations until only one thread was visible between the specimen surface and screw head, indicating the same depth. The results revealed the strongest orientation to be the superior oblique and the weakest alignment to be the inferior oblique.

The poor performance of screws inserted in the traditional midbody and inferior oblique orientations can once again be attributed to the microstructure of the bone sample. By common knowledge the trabeculae are thicker and more robust at the ends of the vertebrae (Figure 21.4).

TABLE 21.1
Mechanical Parameters of the Pullout Test and FEA Results
(mean ± SEM, N = 16, ANOVA test for repeated measures)

Testing Method	Direction	Ultimate Load (N)	Stiffness (N/mm)	Strength (MPa)
Pullout test	0°	818 ± 82	2,833 ± 297	54.9 ± 5.4
	45°	649 ± 59	2,237 ± 196	42.8 ± 3.9
	90°	563 ± 76	1,955 ± 219	37.1 ± 5.0
P value		<0.0001	<0.001	<0.0001
Finite element	0°	840	18,000	53
Analysis	45°	655	16,200	43
	90°	560	14,800	37

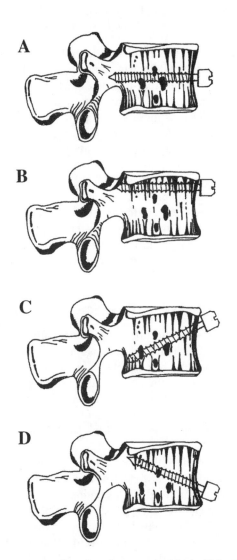

FIGURE 21.3 Different screw orientations in a vertebral body (Adapted from Horton et al.[4])

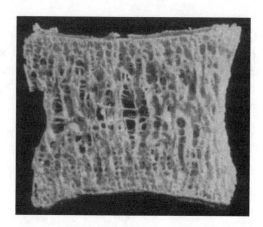

FIGURE 21.4 Macrophotograph of a vertebral section showing differences in bone density (trabeculae) between middle and end portion. (From Brien, E. and Healey, J.H., Orthopedic aspects of osteoporosis, in *Osteoporosis Diagnosis and Treatment*, Sartoris, D.J., Ed., Marcel Dekker, New York, 1996. With permission.)

The midsection of the specimen consists of looser, generally mechanically weaker trabeculae. In addition, vertebrae are thinner in the middle than at the upper and lower ends. Hence, not only are the screws being forced into less bone from a dimensional standpoint, they are also penetrating less dense bone. Therefore, the performance of screws inserted in the traditional midbody orientation will quite obviously not fare as well as those screws piercing denser and more massive portions of the vertebrae. The thicker arrangement of trabeculae at the ends of the vertebral bone would also explain why Horton et al. saw a higher pullout strength in the superior endplate orientation. Without a careful morphological evaluation of vertebral bone, however, there is no explanation for the poor performance of the inferior oblique insertion.

Clearly, based on work by Horton et al.,[4] An et al.,[1,2] and Nicholson et al.[5] at least the angle in which the screw is inserted with respect to the trabeculae orientation and the density of the bone are two determining factors on the holding power of screw fixation. However, there are additional specimen characteristics that must be taken into account. These variables include the duration and methods utilized in bone preservation as well as the overall condition, health, and age of the bone specimen.

C. EFFECTS OF PRESERVATION METHODS ON BONE SCREW PULLOUT STRENGTH

Roe et al.[6] investigated the effects of four different preservation methods on the mechanical properties of canine femoral bones. One femur of each animal was chosen as experimental and the other represented its matched control. The control specimens were cooled to 4°C and subjected to mechanical testing. The first group, aseptic collection, consisted of 15 limbs prepared for aseptic surgery with the femurs removed. The epiphyseal sections and all soft tissues were extracted and the bone was sealed in sterilized polyethylene tubing and stored at –20°C. Group 2 (ethylene oxide) was composed of 15 cleanly harvested bones dried for 18 to 24 h at room temperature, packaged in polyethylene tubing, and sterilized in 12% ethylene oxide for 2 h, aerated for 8 h, and stored at room temperature. Group 3 (chemical sterilization) contained 15 cleanly harvested femurs immersed in a methanol:chloroform solution (1 : 1) for 24 h, and moved to a filtered solution of 10 mM iodoacetic acid in 0.1 M phosphate-buffered NaCl solution for 48 h before they were finally sealed in sterilized polyethylene tubing and stored at –20°C. The fourth group (chemical sterilization and partial decalcification) consisted of 15 cleanly harvested bones immersed in a methanol:chloroform solution (1 : 1) for 4 h, then in 0.6 N hydrochloric acid solution for 24 h, and finally in filter-sterilized, 10 mM iodoacetic acid and 10 mM sodium azide in 0.1 M phosphate-buffered NaCl solution for 72 h. The bones were then stored identically to the Group 3 and 4 samples. The storage times were 1, 16, and 32 weeks for each treatment.

When subjected to compressive loading to failure the aseptically collected bones stored for 1 week were significantly stronger than the control bones. The comparison after 16 and 32 weeks was much less apparent. Similarly, there was no substantial difference in screw pullout testing for this group at 1, 16, or 32 weeks of storage. Bones sterilized in ethylene oxide withstood compressive loading slightly better than the aseptically collected specimens for 1-week-old samples, but did not fare as well after 16 and 32 weeks. Group 2 was also much weaker in the pullout test for the 32-week-old specimens. Chemically treated bones showed no variation between experimental and control lots during testing after 1 week. However, the compressive and screw pullout tests showed that the strength of the specimens decreased considerably after 16 and 32 weeks. Partially decalcified, chemically sterilized samples were considerably (48 to 82%) weaker than the control specimens for all cases.

Roe et al.[6] concluded that the mechanical properties of the bone are considerably affected by the techniques used for storage. Among the different mechanisms, the clearest is the effect of partial decalcification on the weakened mechanical properties of the bone. Other potential reasons for the changes of mechanical properties include loss of water vapor, dehydration, and enzyme activity during storage.

D. Effects of Bone Density on Screw Pullout Strength

The bones of middle-aged adults are much stronger than the soft bones of children and weak bones of the elderly. While the youthful bones will eventually grow strong, old bones are more fragile and often become susceptible to the effects of osteoporosis. Numerous studies have been performed to show the effects of osteoporosis on the strength of the bone. Osteoporosis, experienced most often by postmenopausal females, occurs when a loss of estrogen results in an imbalance between osteoblast and osteoclast production and function. The equilibrium is lost as osteoclast activity (bone resorption) overruns osteoblast production and the bone mineral density (BMD) and mechanical strength are significantly reduced.[7,8] How does one secure a screw in weak bone? The effects of osteoporotic bone on the screw pullout test are quite significant and must also be examined.

Halvorson et al.[9] studied the effects of bone mineral density and the techniques of screw insertion on the screw-holding power. Ten experimental groups were used. The first six lots were classified as untapped, 5.5 mm tap, and 6.5 mm tap for both normal and osteoporotic bone samples, respectively. The other four groups had the following characteristics: stripped and packed with bone chips (normal), osteoporotic, one screw/one hook, and one screw/two hooks.

The results of Halvorson et al.[9] clearly showed the effects of osteoporosis on bone mineral density. The average bone mineral density in normal spines (1.17 ± 0.08 g/cm^2) was significantly higher than that for the osteoporotic spines (0.08 ± 0.05 g/cm^2). The difference between healthy bone and osteoporotic bone is even more apparent in the average pullout force withstood by each specimen before fracture. The normal bones fared much better with an average pullout force of 1540 ± 361 N. The osteoporotic samples, on the other hand, withstood only 206 ± 159 N of applied force. Halvorson et al. also showed that screws inserted in 5.5 or 6.5 mm tapped holes were significantly stronger than untapped samples.

From this study the substantial impact that bone mineral density has on screw pullout strength is apparent. The bone specimens from normal spines had a pullout strength almost 7.5 times greater than the osteoporotic specimens. Because the performance of the osteoporotic samples was significantly worse than that of the normal specimens, special screws may have to be designed and employed at the bone–implant interface for victims of osteoporosis. Clinically, the bone microstructure and density of all implant recipients should therefore be inspected carefully before a screw design is chosen.

III. SUMMARY

This chapter briefly introduces several applications of testing bone mechanical strength using the screw pullout test. Other factors that influence the magnitude of the pullout force a bone specimen can experience include the application of a resin around the screw, the size of the sample and the method of fixation, as well as the dimensions of the screw (such as thread profile) and the depth of its penetration. Although these variables have significant effects on the screw pullout test, they are not directly related to the impact of the bone on the pullout test. These factors are discussed in Chapter 36 of this book.

REFERENCES

1. An, Y.H., Kang, Q., Friedman, R.J., and Young, F.A., Comparison of screw pullout strength from weight-bearing and non-weight-bearing directions in the cancellous bone of bovine tibial plateau, in *The 20th Annu. Meet. Am. Soc. Biomech.*, Atlanta, Ga, 1996, 181.
2. An, Y.H., Kang, Q., Friedman, R.J., and Young, F.A., The effect of microstructure of cancellous bone on screw pullout strength, *Trans. Soc. Biomater.*, 20, 385, 1997.
3. An, Y.H., Young, F.A., Kang, Q., and Williams, K.R., Effects of microstructure of cancellous bone on screw pullout strength, Unpublished data, 1999.
4. Horton, W.C., Blackstock, S.F., Norman, J.T., et al., Strength of fixation of anterior vertebral body screws, *Spine,* 21, 439, 1996.
5. Nicholson, P.H., Cheng, X.G., Lowet, G., et al., Structural and material mechanical properties of human vertebral cancellous bone, *Med. Eng. Phys.,* 19, 729, 1997.
6. Roe, S.C., Pijanowski, G.J., and Johnson, A.L., Biomechanical properties of canine cortical bone allografts: effects of preparation and storage, *Am. J. Vet. Res.,* 49, 873, 1988.
7. Dickenson, R.P., Hutton, W.C., and Stott, J.R., The mechanical properties of bone in osteoporosis, *J. Bone Joint Surg.,* 63B, 233, 1981.
8. Van Audekercke, R. and Van der Perre, G., The effect of osteoporosis on the mechanical properties of bone structures, *Clin. Rheumatol.,* 13 (Suppl. 1), 38, 1994.
9. Halvorson, T.L., Kelley, L.A., Thomas, K.A., et al., Effects of bone mineral density on pedicle screw fixation, *Spine,* 19, 2415, 1994.

22 Viscoelastic Properties of Bone and Testing Methods

Naoki Sasaki

CONTENTS

I. INTRODUCTION

According to Ferry, viscoelasticity of a material is defined as follows.[1] The theory of elasticity deals with mechanical properties of elastic solids, for which, in accordance with Hooke's law, stress is always directly proportional to strain in small deformations but independent of the strain rate. The theory of hydrodynamics deals with properties of viscous liquids, for which, in accordance with Newton's law, stress is always directly proportional to the strain rate but independent of the strain itself. These categories are idealizations; however, it is true that the behavior of many solids approaches Hooke's law for infinitesimal strains and the behavior of many liquids approaches Newton's law for infinitesimal rates of strain. Deviations from ideal behavior are observed under other conditions. Even if both strain and rate of strain are infinitesimal, a system may exhibit behavior that combines liquid-like and solid-like characteristics. Materials whose behavior exhibits such characteristics are called viscoelastic.

In many of the materials of interest in physics, as well as of practical importance in engineering, viscoelastic anomalies are negligible or of only minor significance. Although the foundations of phenomenological theory of linear viscoelasticity have provided valuable information about, for example, the structure of metals, the deviations from perfect elasticity here are small. In polymers, on the other hand, mechanical behavior is dominated by viscoelastic phenomena which are often truly spectacular. Each flexible threadlike polymer molecule has a number of internal degrees of freedom compared with materials containing molecules of low molecular weight and is continually changing the shape of its contour as it wriggles and writhes with its thermal energy. Rearrangements on a local scale are relatively rapid, but they are very slow on a long-range scale. Under stress, a new assortment of configurations is obtained; the response to the local aspects of the new distribution is rapid, the response to the long-range aspects is slow, and, all told, there is a very wide and continuous range of time covering the response of such a system to external stress. This distribution of response times in a system brings about the viscoelasticity of polymers.[1]

Viscoelasticity has been regarded as a characteristic feature of polymeric materials. Almost all biological materials are made of polymers. This is the reason many biological materials manifest viscoelasticity. The major constituents of bone are stiff hydroxyapatite-like mineral and pliant collagen. Because of the viscoelastic nature of collagen fibers in the bone matrix, bone itself has remarkable viscoelasticity.

However, detailed experimental works on the viscoelasticity of bone have only been carried out recently, despite the fact that it has been known for a long time that bone has viscoelasticity.[2–6] A considerable amount of work has been done on some of the mechanical properties of bone,[7] especially its strength and its modulus of elasticity. Most of the strength tests have been static, but some work has been done on the dynamic and fatigue strength of bone. Thus, at the present time, there is still little known about the viscoelastic properties of bone.

There seems to be at least three reasons viscoelastic properties of bone have not been an important subject for many investigators. The first reason is that an elastic approximation for bone had been working well for actual bone statics and a deviation of the mechanical properties of bone from elasticity was regarded as a scatter of data generally observed in biological systems. The second reason is that the biological importance of the viscoelasticity has not been recognized. It is difficult to find a situation in the lives of animals that is similar to even simple viscoelastic experiments, such as creep and stress relaxation. The third reason is the dearth of information available on how constituents of bone are mechanically combined. After knowledge about the histological structure of bone accumulated, the contribution of a collagen matrix to the mechanical properties of bone was taken into consideration. Lees[8] proposed that the mechanical properties of a collagen matrix change with mineral content. Sasaki and Yoshikawa,[6] furthermore, showed that the viscoelastic properties of bone also change as a function of mineral content.

In a viscoelastic material, some of the elastic energy generated by an external force applied to the material is dissipated as heat. All living things make use of this dissipating mechanism of energy for survival. In bone, dissipated energy may contribute to the driving force in the remodeling process of bone.[9] By elucidating the mechanism by which viscoelasticity of bone is generated, it may be possible to understand the physicochemical origin of Wolff's law.[10] In this chapter, only the viscoelastic properties of cortical bone are discussed; the mechanical properties of trabecular bone are discussed in another chapter.

II. VISCOELASTICITY AND VISCOELASTIC ANALYSIS

A. GENERAL REMARKS

Viscoelasticity as reviewed here is limited to static experiments (creep properties and stress relaxation of bone), although the dynamic mechanical properties of bone are also an important issue.

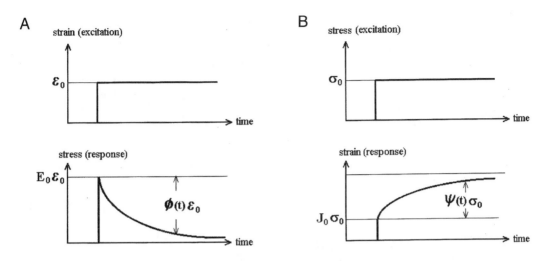

FIGURE 22.1   Stress relaxation (A) and creep measurements (B).

The ultrasonic method (a high-frequency limit of dynamic mechanical measurement) is reviewed in another chapter.

The objectives of the phenomenological viscoelasticity investigation are (1) to understand phenomenological relations between excitation and the response of the material to it in order to find a constitutive equation of the material and (2) to visualize molecular events occurring in the material during the process. For description of the constitutive equation, a relaxation function and a creep function must be determined (Figure 22.1). Both functions are defined as follows. When a step strain ε was applied to the material, the stress response $\sigma(t)$ of the material was expressed as

$$\sigma(t) = E_0[1 - \phi(t)]\varepsilon_0 = E(t)\varepsilon_0 \qquad (22.1)$$

where E_0 is the glass modulus, $\phi(t)$ is the relaxation function and $E(t)$ is the relaxation modulus. When a step stress σ_0 was applied to the material the strain response $\varepsilon(t)$ was described as

$$\varepsilon(t) = J_0[1 + \psi(t)]\sigma_0 = J(t)\sigma_0 \qquad (22.2)$$

where J_0 is the glass compliance, $\psi(t)$ is the creep function, and $J(t)$ is the creep compliance. In order to determine if these functions can be used for accurate estimation of the viscoelasticity of a material, stress relaxation and creep experiments have been performed by many investigators.

B. Viscoelastic Analysis

Analysis based on the theory of linear viscoelasticity was used to determine the relationships between material functions, $\phi(t)$, $E(t)$, $\psi(t)$, and $J(t)$, and molecular events occurring in bone from data obtained from viscoelastic experiments. The elementary process of stress relaxation is idealistically described by the so-called Maxwell element, and that of the creep process is described by the Voigt element (Figure 22.2). Debye used an exponential-type decay function to describe the time course of relaxation with a single relaxation time, as in the case of the Maxwell element. Relaxation described by an exponential decay function is called a Debye-type relaxation. Material functions for both elements are related to a single exponential type function, $e^{-t/\tau}$, where τ is a characteristic time of the process.

In the actual case of a viscoelastic material, no single element can describe the actual relaxation or creep process. Relaxation that cannot be described by a simple exponential decay is referred to

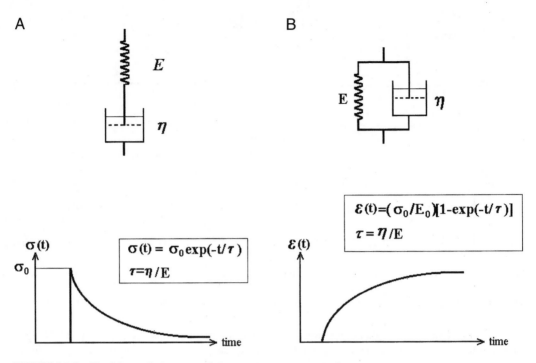

FIGURE 22.2 The Maxwell element and the elementary process of stress relaxation (A) and the Voigt element and the elementary creep process (B).

as non-Debye relaxation. There is no established method for determining the decay function for non-Debye relaxation. Combinations of Maxwell elements or Voigt elements have usually been used to describe the non-Debye-type viscoelastic properties of a material. For a more complicated case, the conventional approach to non-Debye relaxation is to consider a distribution of Debye-type relaxing elements, each with its own relaxation time.

Then the relaxation modulus $E(t)$ is expressed by the relaxation spectrum $H(\ln\tau)\,d\ln\tau$ as[1]

$$E(t) = \int_{-\infty}^{+\infty} H(\ln\tau)\exp(-t/\tau)d\ln\tau \qquad (22.3)$$

One course of mechanical analysis of a material is to obtain the relaxation spectrum from stress relaxation data.

A relaxation spectrum, however, does not contain more information than the original data, as it is simply a mathematical transform of the original, invariably non-Debye, data. It is still difficult to deduce molecular events occurring in relaxation. A number of empirical functions for non-Debye relaxation processes have been proposed and have been applied to specific samples of materials.

Recently, the universality of non-Debye-type relaxation phenomena in condensed matter has been demonstrated. This universality means that almost all of the non-Debye relaxation processes can be described by a few simple relaxation functions. Jonscher[11] and his colleagues demonstrated that relaxation of a variety of materials can be described by a combination of the power-law relation of time or frequency.[11,12] Williams and Watts[13] empirically obtained a response function which is called a stretched exponential. It was shown that this function is identical to the Kohlrausch fractional exponential function, which was first applied to estimate the stress relaxation and plastic deformation of glass fibers by Frederick Kohlrausch in 1863:[14,15]

$$E(t) \propto \exp[-(t/\tau)^{\beta}], \quad (0 < \beta \leq 1) \qquad (22.4)$$

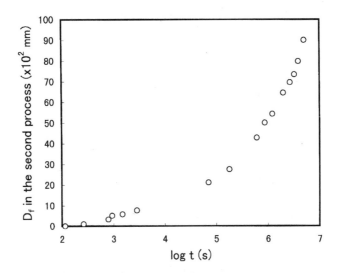

FIGURE 22.3 Creep process in bovine cortical bone. Data points were replotted from Currey.[2]

where τ is a characteristic time of the relaxation and β is a parameter describing the shape of the time dependence of the relaxation modulus. Recently, this function has been used to describe the relaxation phenomena of glass-forming amorphous polymers.[16] Several models have been proposed for explaining the relaxation phenomenon that have a relaxation function of the same type as that of Equation 22.4.[17-19]

III. VISCOELASTIC PROPERTIES OF BONE

A. CREEP PROPERTIES

In Figure 22.3, the results of creep experiments conducted by Currey[2] on cortical bone from bovine tibia and metacarpal bone have been reproduced. A cantilever bending test method was employed. According to Currey, the creep process can be divided into two subprocesses: the creep response that occurs almost immediately after stress application, and the creep response that occurs after the first process and continues for more than 10 days. The former is dominated by elastic deformation. Currey concluded that the second creep process is anelastic, not plastic. Anelasticity is a recoverable strain that appears over a certain period of time. Lakes and Saha[20] also performed creep experiments in conjunction with observations using an optical microscope. They also observed the same two creep processes. For the process that occurred after several minutes and continued for more than 10 days, they found simultaneous cement-line slippage in the micrograph. They concluded that creep that occurred over a long period of time is attributed to large-scale structural change in bone, such as cement-line slippage. A creep process that originates from a structural change in the material usually causes an unrecoverable strain. The results by Lakes and Saha contrasted with those of Currey on this point. Lakes and Saha also observed creep fracture phenomena at comparatively large stress values for the creep.[21] The difference between the results of Currey and those of Lakes and Saha may have originated from the stress values applied. A creep function was not determined in either study, but a review of their experimental data showed that creep functions in both cases could not be described by a simple exponential function. Rimnac et al.[22] empirically determined the strain rate of a steady creep process that appeared after an immediate deformation process of bovine femoral cortical bone as a function of temperature, applied stress, and the volume fraction of Haversian bone in the specimen. In a steady creep process, viscosity is dominant and the strain can be described as $\varepsilon(t) = \dot{\varepsilon}t$, where $\dot{\varepsilon}$ is a constant.

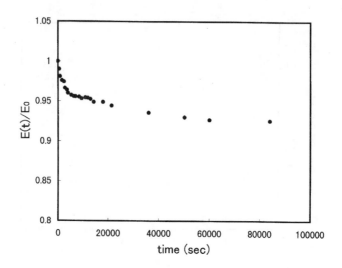

FIGURE 22.4   Stress relaxation in bovine femoral cortical bone. Data points were replotted from Lugassy and Korostoff.[23]

B. STRESS RELAXATION PROPERTIES

Figure 22.4 shows the results of stress relaxation experiments conducted by Lugassy and Korostoff[23] on bovine femoral cortical bone. With the influence of specimen orientation, the effects of loading speed and amount of deformation were examined. The general features of stress relaxation of cortical bone are rapid relaxation in the early stage of relaxation and then gradual relaxation over a long period of time. These correspond well to the characteristic feature of creep in cortical bone. In the case of relaxation over a long period of time, relaxation modulus can be described by a simple exponential decay function (Debye-type relaxation). According to Tobolsky's method,[24] which is usually applied to polymer systems, the relaxation process can be divided into two parts: an initial rapid relaxation process lasting for up to 100 min followed by a process of gradual relaxation. The relaxation time for the latter process was determined to be in the order of 10^6 s. For the former process, description of the relaxation by a simple exponential decay was found to be impossible. Instead, Lugassy and Korostoff found that the early stage of the relaxation process in bone could be described by a linear relation between the relaxation modulus $E(t)$ and the logarithm of time:

$$E(t) = a - b \log t \tag{22.5}$$

where a and b are constants that are independent of time. This equation was derived in a procedure for obtaining a relaxation time spectrum using Alfrey's approximation method. The linear relation indicates that this part of stress relaxation in bone is reminiscent of the wedge-type region of the relaxation spectrum in amorphous polymeric materials, although obtained by approximation.[25,26]

Lakes and Katz[4] presented eight decades of relaxation spectra for human tibial cortical bone and bovine femoral cortical bone from both stress relaxation and dynamic mechanical measurements. Figure 22.5 shows the relaxation spectra for human bone and bovine bone. The spectra were estimated by using Alfrey's approximation. In accordance with the results by Lugassy and Korostoff,[23] it was shown that relaxation can be described by at least two relaxation processes. For human bone, the relaxation process having a single relaxation time of about 5×10^4 sec was most remarkable, and there were several small processes on the short time-side foot of it. Lakes and Katz estimated the contribution of thermoelasticity in osteons and lamellae toward tan δ of the

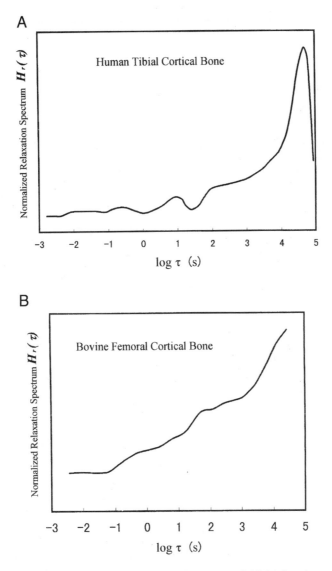

FIGURE 22.5 Normalized relaxation spectra, $H_r(t)$, with respect to initial relaxation modulus values of (A) human tibial and (B) bovine femoral cortical bone. (Adapted from Lakes and Katz.[8])

system, and they assigned the small peaks in the spectrum as contributions from the inhomogeneous structure in bone.[4] For bovine bone, there were no remarkable relaxation processes over a long duration as there are in human bone. Rather, the spectra increased monotonously with relaxation time. This difference, however, may be due to the fact that the stress relaxation measurement of bovine bone was performed only up to 5×10^4 s, and a remarkable peak may appear at a time more than 10^5 s, as was suggested by the results of Lugassy and Korostoff.[23]

As described above, the general features of stress relaxation in cortical bone are rapid, non-Debye relaxation in the early stage (process I) and gradual relaxation of the Debye type over a long period of time (process II). The total relaxation shear modulus, $G(t)$, can be described by an empirical equation such as

$$G(t)/G_0 = A_1 \, f(t/\tau_1) + A_2 \exp(-t/\tau_2) \tag{22.6}$$

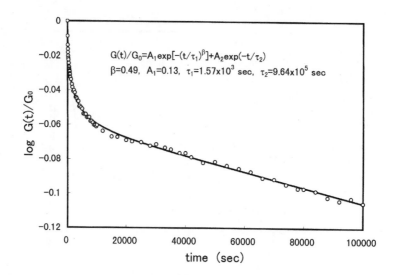

FIGURE 22.6   Stress relaxation of bovine femoral cortical bone. Data points were replotted from Sasaki et al.[27] The solid line represents values obtained from Equation 22.8.

where G_0 is the glass modulus of bone, A_1 and A_2 are the non-Debye and Debye fractions, respectively, against the relaxation as a whole, τ_2 is the relaxation time for process II, and $f(t/\tau_1)$ is the non-Debye function to be determined, where τ_1 is the relaxation time for process I. Sasaki et al.[27] proposed that process I can be described by the Kohlrausch–Williams–Watts (KWW) function:

$$f(t/\tau_1) = \exp\left[-(t/\tau_1)^\beta\right] \quad (0 < \beta \le 1). \tag{22.7}$$

Then, for all the relaxation process, the following empirical equation was presented:

$$G(t)/G_0 = A_1 \exp\left[-(t/\tau_1)^\beta\right] + A_2 \exp\left(-t/\tau_2\right) \quad (A_1 + A_2 = 1, \quad 0 < \beta \le 1). \tag{22.8}$$

Figure 22.6 shows a comparison of the experimental data points with estimated values obtained by using Equation 22.8. The results show that the equation can be used to describe accurately the relaxation process as a whole for bone.

In Figure 22.7, the relaxation curve (logarithm of averaged relaxation modulus vs. time) by Lugassy and Korostoff for bovine femur is replotted.[23,27] The data points were normalized by reference to the initial stress. In this figure, the solid curve represents values obtained from Equation 22.8 for compressive stress relaxation. The data points corresponded well to the values obtained from the equation. The parameters are listed in the figure. A combination of the KWW function and the Debye function was recently proposed to describe the relaxation phenomena in amorphous polymers.[28]

C. Determination of the Relaxation Mechanism on the Basis of the Empirical Relaxation Modulus

1. KWW-Type Relaxation

The mechanism of relaxation in bone was investigated on the basis of the empirically determined relaxation modulus. The mechanical properties of collagen fibril have been shown to be greatly affected by the water content,[29-31] ϕ (in g/g bone), while those of hydroxyapatite are thought to be unaffected. These different responses in mechanical properties to a change in water content competitively determine the mechanical properties of wet bone. Sasaki and Enyo[32] carried out torsional

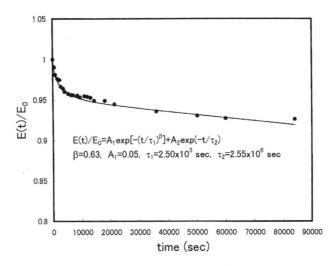

FIGURE 22.7 Fitting of values obtained from Equation 22.8 to the data obtained by Lugassy and Korostoff.[23] (Adapted from Sasaki et al.[27])

stress relaxation measurements in bone samples of various water contents. All of the obtained relaxation curves could be described by Equation 22.8. Figure 22.8 shows the water content dependence of $G(t)$ at indicated times. In the early stage, up to 10^3 s after strain application, $G(t)$ decreased with ϕ, while in the later stage, at 10^4 to approximately 10^5 s, curves of $G(t)$ – vs. ϕ almost leveled off. Thus, the collagen matrix is believed to be responsible for the relaxation of bone in the early stage. However, in the later stage $G(t)$ values are very similar, indicating that the modulus, in this stage of hydration, is not so sensitive to ϕ. This leads to a preliminary conclusion that KWW relaxation is closely related to the mechanical properties of the collagen matrix.

Figure 22.8B shows the creep process of collagen fiber in saline, as was observed by a time-resolved X-ray diffraction method where strain was determined for the Hodge–Petruska D-period.[33,34] Creeplike change in D-period strain, ε_D, corresponds well with the KWW-type stress relaxation in collagen fiber soaked in saline, as shown in Figure 22.8C.[35] The change in ε_D was found to be related to molecular rearrangement in the fiber caused by externally applied force.[36,37] Therefore, the KWW-type stress relaxation in bone is also thought to originate from a molecular rearrangement in collagen fiber in a bone matrix.

2. The Debye-Type Relaxation Process (Process II)

Because of the similarity in the time course, process II is related to the nonelastic deforming process in the creep results for bone.[20] Such a nonelastic deformation of inhomogeneous material in the solid state by an external force has been discussed generally on the basis of the concept relating to the crack nucleation and propagation. Here, process II is discussed on the basis of the microcrack nucleation concept at a stress-concentrated area, such as the tip of an osteosyte lacuna in bone. As a consequence of stress concentration around the tip of the crack, nucleation of small cracks near the tip occurs. The nucleation reduces the concentrated stress, and this can be the elementary process of stress relaxation in bone.

In general, the nucleation rate, K_n, is written as[38]

$$K_n = A \exp[-(U - \psi)/kT] \tag{22.9}$$

where A is a constant, U is the activation energy of the relaxation, ψ is the function representing the contribution of applied stress σ and then the concentrated local stress σ_L to the free energy

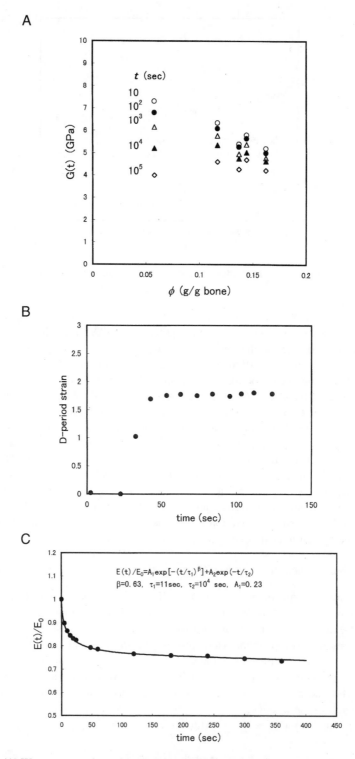

FIGURE 22.8   (A) Water content dependence of relaxation shear modulus at indicated time after the strain application. (Adapted from Sasaki and Enyo[32]) (B) Creep in the D-period of tendon collagen. Data points were replotted from Sasaki et al.[34] (C) Stress relaxation of tendon collagen. Data points were replotted from Azuma and Hasegawa.[35] The solid curve represents values obtained from Equation 22.8 fitted to the data.[34]

of the system, and k is the Boltzmann constant. On the basis of the nucleation concept, ψ is described as[39,40]

$$\psi \sim \ln \sigma_L. \tag{22.10}$$

By using this relation, the nucleation rate is rewritten as

$$K_n = A' \exp(-U/kT) \, \sigma_L^{\delta} \tag{22.11}$$

where A' and δ are constants, which are determined according to the material. As σ_L is related to the macroscopic stress σ via the stress concentration coefficient, σ_L can be estimated from the relaxation stress. When $\delta \sim 1$, the stress relaxation rate determined by the nucleation process is written as

$$K_n = - (d\sigma/dt) \propto \sigma \tag{22.12}$$

and the relaxation process then becomes the Debye type. In this case, the relaxation was confirmed empirically to be the Debye type, and δ should therefore be almost unity.

In order to establish the characterization of σ ($\propto \sigma_L$) relating to water content, the initial value of the shear modulus G_{RD}^0 ($= A_2 G_i$, G_i; initial relaxation shear modulus) for the Debye-type relaxation in bone was plotted in Figure 22.9A as a function of water content. The values have been normalized, and the modulus value for the sample with the smallest water content should therefore be unity. It is clear that G_{RD}^0 reduces monotonously and almost linearly with ϕ. The shear modulus value for collagen film has also been reported to depend almost linearly on ϕ in the range of $0.05 < \phi < 0.2$.[29] Assuming that $\sigma_L \propto G_{RD}^0(\phi) = \alpha - \gamma\phi$ (α and γ being constants that are independent of ϕ and α, $\gamma > 0$) as an empirical relation and utilizing the relation in Equation 22.11, the relaxation rate of the Debye process K_D ($\approx K_n$) can be described as

$$K_D = (a - b\phi)^{\delta} \tag{22.13}$$

where a and b are constants that are independent of ϕ. Empirically, $\delta \sim 1$, then

$$K_D \sim a - b\phi \tag{22.14}$$

This expectation can be compared with the empirical results of the authors' experiments. The relaxation time, τ_2 of the Debye process is equal to K_D^{-1}. In Figure 22.9B, the relaxation rate of the Debye relaxation, $K_D (= 1/\tau_2)$, is plotted against ϕ. K_D decreases linearly with ϕ. The results shown in this figure confirm the validity of the relation in Equation 22.14. This indicates that the effect of ϕ on τ_2 can be explained by the formulation of a crack nucleation process with the help of empirical data.

IV. METHOD OF TESTING

A. METHOD AND APPARATUS

In order to investigate the viscoelastic properties of bone, a "viscoelasticity testing machine" is not needed. For example, an Instron testing machine can be used to detect the anelasticity of bone.[23] Here, the apparatus used in past studies is described.

1. Torsion Pendulum Used by Lakes et al.[3]

Figure 22.10 shows a schematic representation of the biaxial torsion pendulum developed by Lakes et al.[3] for examining the viscoelastic nature of cortical bone. A specimen, shaped into a

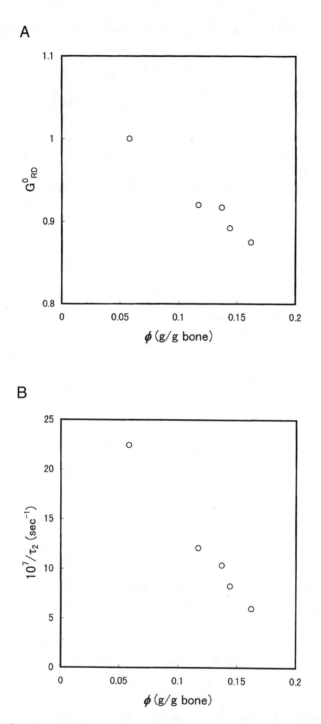

FIGURE 22.9   (A) G_{RD}^0 plotted against water content, ϕ. Data were adapted from Sasaki and Enyo.[32] (B) Relaxation rate for process II, plotted against ϕ. Data points were replotted from Sasaki and Enyo.[32]

waisted cylinder, is fixed between clamps and exposed to a slight extending force along the specimen and torsion axes. The torsional strain is generated by a torsion motor consisting of a DC magnet assembly and a driving coil rotor. One end of the rotor shaft is connected to the upper clamp, and the other end is connected to a torsional strain sensor using a linear variable

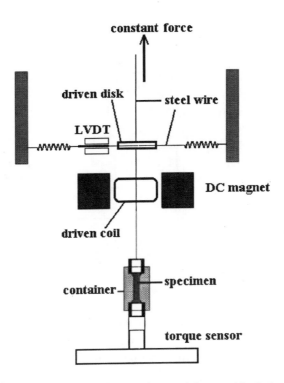

FIGURE 22.10 Schema of the torsion pendulum used by Lakes et al.[3]

differential transformer (LVDT). Torsional force is detected by a torque sensor mounted between the frame and the lower clamp of the specimen. The rise time of a step function angular displacement is electronically controlled to 60 to 100 ms for zero to final value of angle. By operating the driving coil with the output from an oscillator, dynamic mechanical measurements up to a maximum of 50 Hz are possible. Some results obtained by using this apparatus were presented in a previous section.

2. Compression Tester Used by Lugassy and Korostoff

Strain application and force detection were performed by the use of an Instron testing machine.[23] The strain value was signalized by an LVDT, which was attached to an upper ram. A specimen holder for the relaxation experiments of bone is schematically shown in Figure 22.11. A cylinder-shaped specimen was prepared for a compressive stress relaxation experiment. The specimen was placed between the upper and lower rams. The lower ram was connected to a load cell. The specimen was bathed in Ringer's solution. Some results obtained by using this apparatus were presented in a previous section.

B. SPECIMEN PREPARATION

Cortical bone specimens for viscoelastic measurements are prepared as follows. From the middi-aphysis of a long bone, rectangular plates of cortical bone are cut using a diamond saw under tap water. (The specimen must be shaped as a rectangular plate to fit the apparatus.) The plate is then shaped to a suitable size by using emery paper, and final polishing is done using apatite paste. The surface of the specimen is then observed under an optical microscope to confirm that there are no scratches. The suitable specimen size is discussed in the apparatus section. The actual size of the specimen is determined by observation using a traveling microscope.

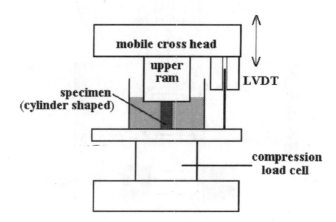

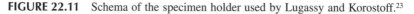

FIGURE 22.11   Schema of the specimen holder used by Lugassy and Korostoff.[23]

C. Apparatus

1. Torsion Tester

The relaxation shear modulus is usually determined by a torsion tester. Figures 22.12A and B show, respectively, a cross-sectional view and the top view of a torsion tester of the type invented by Kusano and Murakami[41] and modified for experiments on bone.[27,32] The bone specimen used in this apparatus is a plate with dimensions of $8 \times 40 \times 0.5$ mm. The torsion axis is parallel to the longer edges of the specimen plate. The suitable size of the specimen for this system is estimated according to the formula:

$$ab^3[1 - (0.63025/u)] = (3LF/G\theta), \quad u = a/b \qquad (22.15)$$

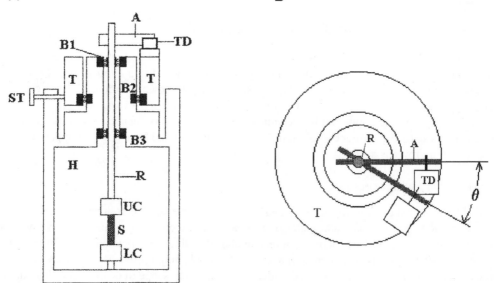

FIGURE 22.12   Schema of the torsion tester: (A) a cross-sectional view along the torsion axis and (B) a top view.

and by using the average bone modulus value G in the literature and the resolution of the sensitivity of the force sensor, where a and b are the width and thickness, respectively; and L, F, and θ are the length of the specimen, the recovering force, and torsional deformation in radians, respectively. The bone specimen, S, is set between an upper clamp, UC, and a lower clamp, LC, in a temperature- and humidity-controlled chamber, H. The temperature is controlled by an electric heater and circulation of tap water around the chamber. For the regulation of humidity, the ambient atmosphere of the specimen was exposed to saturated salt solution in the chamber. The lower clamp is fixed to the frame, and the upper clamp is connected to the force translational rod, R. A rigid arm, A, is attached to the top of the rod, and a force transducer, TD, is connected to the end of the arm. The transducer is mounted on a turntable, T. When T is rotated around the sample axis, A, R, and UC also rotate around the same axis. To achieve smooth rotation, two ball bearings (B1; NSK 6000; B2, NSK 5208) and a needle bearing (B3, 30203) are used, as shown in the figure. These bearings also enable the transducer TD to detect the recovering force generated in the bone specimen against the shearing deformation applied by the rotation of T. Torsional loading is applied within a few seconds by rotating ($\theta = 10°$ on average) the turntable, T, on which the force sensor, TD, is mounted. Shear strain is fixed by a stopper screw, ST. According to Kusano and Murakami shear-modulus values smaller than 10^{-2} GPa were obtained.[41] In the present form, shear strain is applied manually. However, by using an automatic turntable with a stepping motor, all the measurements could be automatically performed.

2. Cantilever Bending System

One of the most commonly used methods for measuring the relaxation Young's modulus of bone is cantilever bending. Figure 22.13 shows a top view of the cantilever bending system used for determining the relaxation Young's modulus function of cortical bone.[6,27] This system is also set in a temperature- and humidity-regulated chamber. The bone specimen used in this system is also a plate of similar dimensions to those of the plate used in the torsion tester. The suitable size of the specimen for this system is estimated according to the formula:

$$ab^3 = 4FL^3/Ed \qquad (22.16)$$

and by using the average bone modulus value E in the literature and the resolution of the sensitivity of the force sensor, where a and b are the width and thickness respectively, and L, F, and d are the length of the specimen, the recovering force, and the bending deformation, respectively. The sample plate, S, is fixed to one end of a clamp, C. A force transducer, TD, is mounted on the sliding table, T. Bending deformation is applied to the specimen by the probe tip of the force transducer, and the recovering force is detected while keeping the probe of the transducer perpendicular to the

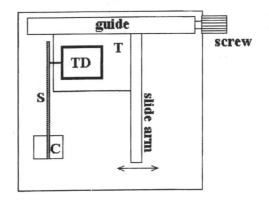

FIGURE 22.13 Schema of a cantilever bending tester.

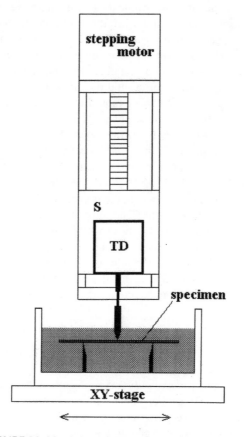

FIGURE 22.14   Schema of a three-point bending tester.

specimen plate. Deformation is applied within about 1 s. The deformation thus applied is held constant during the duration of the test. Care must be taken to ensure that the bones are not strained into the plastic deformation range. In the present form, the bending deformation is applied manually. However, by using an automatic pulse stage with a stepping motor, all measurements could be automatically performed.

3.   Three-Point Bending System

A three-point bending system is also used for determining the relaxation Young's modulus function. Figure 22.14 shows a side view of the three-point bending tester used in the author's laboratory. A force transducer, TD [LTS-1LK, Kyowa Electric Works (KEW), Japan] is mounted on a Sigma Koki (SK) auto pulse z-stage, S. The pulse stage is controlled by an SK-stage controller (Mark-12) with a terminal box (SK CSG-5151). For the force application to the specimen, the stage is lowered perpendicular to the plate surface. In order for the force to be applied just at the center of the fulcrums, the specimen holder can be moved by the XY-stage on which the holder is mounted. The suitable size of the specimen, the width and thickness, and the interfulcrum distance L of this system are estimated according to the formula:

$$ab^3 = \frac{FL^3}{4Ed} \qquad\qquad (22.17)$$

and by using the average bone modulus value E in the literature and the resolution of the sensitivity of the force sensor, where F and d are the recovering force and the bending deformation, respectively.

4. Data Acquisition

The signal from the sensor used in each apparatus is first passed to a KEW data logger UCAM 10A and then through the data logger to a personal computer. Figure 22.15 shows a block diagram of the measuring system. The data acquisition program is operated before applying the strain to the specimen and a baseline of the recovering force is detected by reading the signal value. Measurements are made at 1-s intervals for 30 min after the strain application, and then the sampling interval is increased. The measurements are performed for more than 10^5 s after strain application.

5. Fast Measurements

The three-point bending system can be used to measure the relaxation modulus in an early stage of stress relaxation in bone.[42] The results of experiments showed that there is a relaxation process in the early stage that cannot be described by the empirical relaxation modulus, Equation 22.8.

The relaxation Young's modulus was measured by three-point bending of a rectangular sample plate, as shown in Figure 22.16A. A KEW LTS-1K strain gauge transducer was used as both the deformation generator and the force sensor. The LTS-1K gauge was set on an automicrostage, which was operated by a rectangular pulse generated by a function synthesizer (Toa FS-111A) to guarantee identical deformation for a series of measurements. Bending deformation was detected by a Yokogawa Electric Works (YEW, Musashino, Japan) 3612 strain transducer with a YEW 3624-05 sensor of the noncontacting type. Over a 50-s time interval, an electric signal from the LTS-1K was passed on to a KEW DPM-613A strain amplifier, then to an Autonics S-210 autodigitizer, and finally to a personal computer using a GP-IB. The electric signal was recorded every

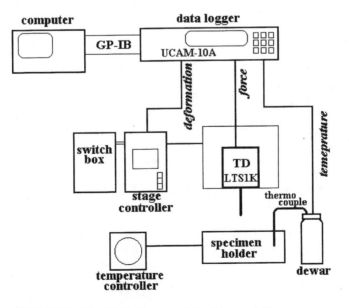

FIGURE 22.15   Block diagram of the data acquisition system.

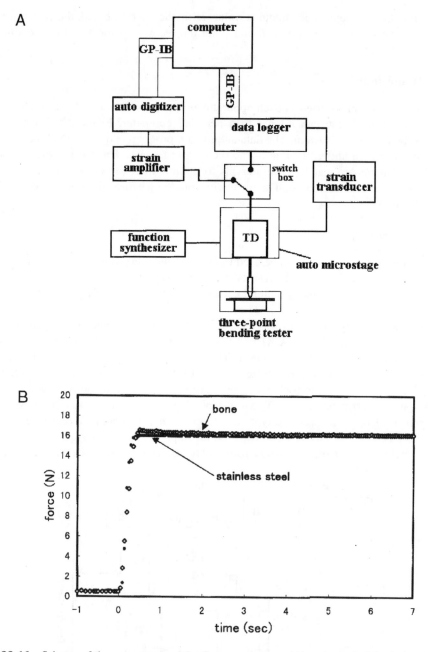

FIGURE 22.16 Schema of the apparatus used for fast measurement (A) and a typical load–time curve showing the stress response of a stainless steel plate (B).

0.05 s by the S210. From 50 s to 5×10^4 s, electric signals generated from LTS-1K were directly recorded by a KEW data logger (UCAM 10A) and finally passed on to a microcomputer. A maximum strain of less than 0.05% was applied within 0.025 s. This value is well within the frequency range examined by other authors in dynamic studies. Figure 22.16B shows the stress response from a high-carbon stainless steel plate, which can be regarded as an ideally elastic material, compared with a bone. From the stress response by the stainless steel plate, it was found that there was no overshoot in the applied strain.

V. SUMMARY AND FUTURE DIRECTIONS OF RESEARCH

Although the viscoelasticity of bone has long been regarded as a phenomenon of minor significance, the author's group found, by using a simple experimental method, that the viscoelasticity of bone is as remarkable as that of polymeric materials. However, most techniques currently used to investigate the viscoelastic properties of bone are still phenomenological ones. In order to understand molecular events occurring in the viscoelastic process, structural measurements during the process should be performed. On the other hand, mechanical measurements are methods of materials science, but bone is a living tissue. One of the biggest problems in bone mechanics is the adaptation or remodeling of bone. Recent investigations have focused on the residual stress in bone as a result of remodeling.[43] Such a residual stress, although very small compared with the forces applied to an animal in its daily life, will also be relaxed by the viscoelastic nature of bone. The longest relaxation time of bone, $\sim 10^6$ s, is roughly comparable with the remodeling cycle in bone. Further investigation of the viscoelasticity of bone may lead to an understanding of the remodeling process and mechanism of bone tissue.

REFERENCES

1. Ferry, J.D.,*Viscoelastic Properties of Polymers*, 3rd ed., Wiley & Sons, New York, 1980.
2. Currey, J.D., Anelasticity in bone and echinoderm skeletons, *J. Exp. Biol.*, 43, 279, 1965.
3. Lakes, R.S., Katz, J.L., and Sternstein, S.S., Viscoelastic properties of wet cortical bone. 1. Torsional and biaxial studies, *J. Biomech.*, 12, 657, 1979.
4. Lakes, R.S. and Katz, J.L., Viscoelastic properties of wet cortical bone. 2. Relaxation mechanisms, *J. Biomech.*, 12, 679, 1979.
5. Lakes, R.S. and Katz, J.L., Viscoelastic properties of wet cortical bone. 3. A nonlinear constitutive equation, *J. Biomech.*, 12, 689, 1979.
6. Sasaki, N. and Yoshikawa, M., Stress relaxation in native and EDTA-treated bone as a function of mineral content, *J. Biomech.*, 26, 77, 1993.
7. Currey, J.D., *The Mechanical Adaptations of Bones*, Princeton University Press, Princeton, NJ, 1984.
8. Lees, S., Sonic velocity and the ultrastructure of mineralized tissues, in *Calcified Tissue*, Hukins, D.W.L., Ed., Macmillan Press, London, 1989.
9. Levenston, M.E. and Carter, D.R., An energy dissipation-based model for damage stimulated bone adaptation, *J. Biomech.*, 31, 579, 1998.
10. Roesler, H., Some historical remarks on the theory of cancellous bone structure (Wolff's law), in *Mechanical Properties of Bone*, Cowin, S.C., Ed., American Society of Mechanical Engineers, 1981.
11. Jonscher, A.K., *Dielectric Relaxation in Solids*, Chelsea Dielectrics, London, 1983.
12. Hill, R.M. and Dissado, L.A., Relaxation in elastic and viscoelastic materials, *J. Mater. Sci.*, 19, 1576, 1983.
13. Williams, G. and Watts, D.C., Non-symmetrical dielectric relaxation behavior arising from a simple empirical decay function, *Trans. Faraday Soc.*, 66, 80, 1970.
14. Tschoegl, N.W., *The Phenomenological Theory of Linear Viscoelastic Behavior — An Introduction*, Springer-Verlag, Heidelberg, 1987.
15. Scher, H., Shlesinger, M.F., and Bendler, J.T., Time-scale invariance in transport and relaxation, *Phys. Today*, 44, 26, 1991.
16. Legrand, D.G., Olszewski, W.V., and Bendler, J.T., Anelastic response of bisphenol-A polycarbonate, *J. Polym. Sci. B Polym. Phys. Ed.*, 25, 1149, 1985.
17. Palmer, R.G., Stein, D.L., Abraham, E., and Anderson, P.W., Models of hierachically constrained dynamics for glassy relaxation, *Phys. Rev. Lett.*, 53, 958, 1984.
18. Klafter, J. and Shlesinger, M.F., On the relationship among three theories of relaxation in disordered systems, *Proc. Natl. Acad. Sci. U.S.A.*, 83, 848, 1986.
19. Ngai, K.L., Evidence for universal behavior of condensed matter at low frequencies/long times, in *Non-Debye Relaxation of Condensed Matter*, Ramakrishnan, T.V. and Lakshimi, M.R., Eds., World Science, Singapore, 1987.

20. Lakes, R. and Saha, S., Cement line motion in bone, *Science*, 204, 501, 1979.
21. Lakes, R. and Saha, S., Long-term torsional creep in compact bone, *J. Biomech. Eng.*, 102, 178, 1980.
22. Rimnac, C.M., Petko, A.A., Santner, T.J., and Wright, T.M., The effect of temperature, stress and microstructure on the creep of compact bovine bone, *J. Biomech.*, 26, 219, 1993.
23. Lugassy, A.A. and Korostoff, E., Viscoelastic behavior of bovine femoral cortical bone and sperm whale dentin, in *Research in Dental and Medical Materials*, Korostoff, E., Ed., Plenum Press, New York, 1969.
24. Tobolsky, A.V. and Murakami, K., Existence of a sharply defined maximum relaxation time for monodisperse polystyrene, *J. Polym. Sci.*, 40, 443, 1959.
25. Tobolsky, A.V., Elastoviscous properties of polysiobutylene. VI. Relation between stress relaxation modulus and dynamic modulus, *J. Am. Chem. Soc.*, 74, 3786, 1952.
26. Tobolsky, A.V., Stress relaxation studies of viscoelastic properties of polymers, *J. Appl. Phys.*, 27, 673, 1956.
27. Sasaki, N., Nakayama, Y., Yoshikawa, M., and Enyo, A., Stress relaxation function of bone and bone collagen, *J. Biomech.*, 26, 1369, 1993.
28. Wagner, H. and Richert, R., Dielectric relaxation of the electric field in poly(vinyl acetate): A time domain study in the range $10^{-3} – 10^{-6}$ s, *Polymer*, 38, 255, 1997.
29. Tanioka, A., Jojima, E., Miyasaka, K., and Ishikawa, K., Effect of water on the mechanical properties of collagen films, *Biopolymers*, 11, 1489, 1973.
30. Nomura, S., Hiltner, A., Lando, J.B., and Baer, E., Interaction of water with native collagen, *Biopolymers*, 16, 231, 1977.
31. Pineri, M.H., Escoubes, M., and Roche, G., Water-collagen interactions: calorimetric and mechanical experiments, *Biopolymers*, 17, 2799, 1979.
32. Sasaki, N. and Enyo, A., Viscoelastic properties of bone as a function of water content, *J. Biomech.*, 28, 809, 1995.
33. Hodge, J.A. and Petruska, J.A., Recent studies with the electron microscope on ordered aggregates of the tropocollagen macromolecule, in *Aspects of Protein Structure*, Ramachandran, G.N., Ed., Academic Press, New York, 1963.
34. Sasaki, N., Shukunami, N., Matsushima, N., and Izumi, Y., Time-resolved X-ray diffraction from tendon collagen during creep using synchrotron radiation, *J. Biomech.*, 32, 285, 1999.
35. Azuma, T. and Hasegawa, M., A rheological approach to the architecture of arterial walls, *Jpn. J. Physiol.*, 21, 27, 1971.
36. Sasaki, N. and Odajima, S., Elongation mechanism of collagen fibrils and force-strain relations of tendon at each level of structural hierarchy, *J. Biomech.*, 29, 1131, 1996.
37. Mosler, E., Folkhard, W., Geercken, W., et al., Stress-induced molecular rearrangement in tendon collagen, *J. Mol. Biol.*, 182, 589, 1985.
38. Yokobori, T., *An Interdisciplinary Approach to Fracture and Strength of Solids*, Wolters-Noordhoff Ltd., Groningen, the Netherlands, 1968.
39. Yokobori, T., Failure and fracture of metals as nucleation processes, *J. Phys. Soc. Jpn.*, 7, 44, 1952.
40. Yokobori, T., Creep fracture of copper as nucleation process, *J. Phys. Soc. Jpn.*, 7, 48, 1952.
41. Kusano, T. and Murakami, K., Apparatus for stress-relaxation experiments, *Bull. Res. Inst. Non-Aqueous Soln.*, 199, 1970.
42. Goto, T., Sasaki, N., and Hikichi, K., Early stage stress-relaxation in compact bone, *J. Biomech.*, 32, 93, 1999.
43. Todoh, M., Tadano, S., Shibano, M., and Ukai, T., Polychromatic X-ray measurements of anisotropic residual stress in bovine femoral bone, *Trans. Jpn. Soc. Mech. Eng. (Ser. A)*, 65, 406, 1999.

23 Observation of Material Failure Mode Using a SEM with a Built-In Mechanical Testing Device

Rong-Ming Wang and Yuehuei H. An

CONTENTS

I. INTRODUCTION

This chapter introduces a technology for potential combined testing of bone properties and observation of failure mode. There are now available low-vacuum scanning electron microscopes (LV SEM, e.g., Model: JSM-5600LV, JEOL, Tokyo, Japan) equipped with a sample loading stage and an energy dispersive X-ray spectrometer (Figure 23.1). These systems allow simultaneous observation of changes in surface morphology of a specimen under loading; fracture modes of materials under tensile, compression, and possibly bending load; measurement of mechanical parameters of the sample; and elemental analysis of chemical composition. The systems have great potential for the determination of mechanical properties and failure modes of biological materials such as bone, cartilage, or ligament. Since no data on bone, cartilage, or ligament are available from these types of instruments, the principles of the system and the potential uses are discussed using some data on inorganic materials.

A. SCANNING ELECTRON MICROSCOPY

Scanning electron microscopy (SEM) has had widespread use in biology, physics, chemistry, and materials science in recent years owing to the rapid developments in its easily operated multifunctions. With the development of computer technology, computer-controlled SEMs have been developed and applied in many fields.

In SEM, a focused electron beam is continuously scanned, in a rasterlike pattern, over the inclined surface of a specimen, causing both backscatter of some of the primary electrons, and ejection of secondary electrons. These secondary electrons are attracted to a positively charged collector, and the signal is amplified and displayed on a cathode-ray tube in which a beam spot is scanned in synchronization with the primary beam on the specimen. The magnification of the image on the screen of the cathode-ray tube can readily be controlled by varying the area of specimen

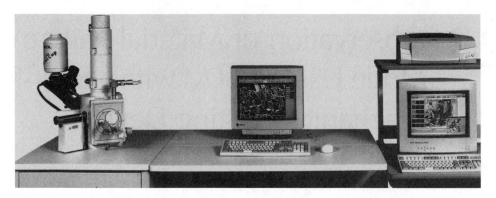

FIGURE 23.1   A JSM-5600LV and EDS combination system.

covered by the raster. The electron-optical arrangement is similar to that of the microprobe analyzer, and, for convenience in manipulating the specimen, the final (or "objective") lens must have a longer working distance, of about 20 mm. Three or more lenses are therefore commonly employed in the illuminating system.

B. LOW-VACUUM SCANNING ELECTRON MICROSCOPY

In recent years, the LV SEM has been developed, which allows specimen observation without the chemical fixation, dehydration, drying and coating needed for conventional high-vacuum SEM. The LV SEM neutralizes the charge of nonconductive specimens by utilizing ions generated by the interaction between residual gas molecules in the specimen chamber and the electrons used for observation. For this purpose, the pressure of the specimen chamber can be raised to approximately 270 Pa by using differential pumping. The use of backscattered electrons for imaging allows not only specimen surfaces but also inner structures to be observed.[1]

In the low-vacuum mode, the specimen chamber is kept in a low vacuum (high pressure) to observe a nonconductive specimen without conductive coating. Since an energy dispersive spectrometer and one channel of wavelength spectrometer can be attached to the microscope, the application of this instrument can be expanded from high-resolution morphological observation in the high-vacuum mode and nonconductive specimen observation in the low-vacuum mode for elemental analysis.

The LV SEM mode is used for observing backscattered electron images. This type of image contains both composition contrast, which shows the distribution of different substances in the specimen, and contrast caused by specimen topography. The LV SEM allows nonconductive specimens to be observed in their original state. Since there is no need to lower the accelerating voltage, the instrument allows elemental analysis with an energy dispersive X-ray spectrometer (EDS).

The LV SEM also allows the observation of specimens that contain water or are stained (biological tissues such as bone and cartilage). Even specimens that are difficult to pretreat, such as aqueous microorganisms, can be observed with an LV SEM. For this purpose, such specimens are rapidly frozen in liquid nitrogen and then freeze-dried on the standard specimen stage in the specimen chamber of an LV SEM. It is also possible to coat freeze-dried specimens for observation in the HV SEM mode, or to preserve the specimens for later observation.

C. SEM WITH AN IN-SCOPE LOADING SYSTEM

The JSM-5600LV instrument in the authors' laboratory (Beijing Institute of Aeronautical Materials) is equipped with a loading stage (or tensile stage) and an EDS (see Figure 23.1). The instrument allows observation of surface morphology with X, Y, and R (rotation) movement, and observation of

TABLE 23.1
Typical Specifications of a JEOL Tensile Stage

Specimen movement range	X = –5~+20 mm
	Y = –3~+3 mm
	T = –5°~+45°
Working distance (WD)	20 mm
Specimen size	For tension: 5(W) × 29(L) × 1(T) mm
	For compression: 5(W) × 20(L) × 1(T) mm
Tensile load	200 kg at maximum
Tensile amount	20 mm at maximum
Driving methods	Automatic or manual
Driving speed	0.05~1.0 mm/min (4-steps; 50 Hz)
	0.06~1.2 mm/min (4-steps; 60 Hz)
Alarm buzzer	Active when tension/compression range exceeded

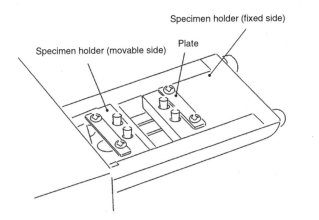

FIGURE 23.2   Diagram of the specimen holder in a JEOL tensile stage.

fracture modes of materials under tensile, compression, and possibly bending load. Most operations, such as auto-gun-alignment, autofocusing, auto-astigmatism-correction, and auto-contrast/brightness-adjustment can be controlled using a personal computer.

II. MECHANICAL LOADING WITHIN THE SEM SCOPE

The loading stage makes possible the observation of the fracture process of a material. The stage is used to observe the dynamic change in a specimen by applying tensile or compression load. The amount of load can be measured in real time with a load cell. Table 23.1 gives the typical specifications of a tensile stage.

Figure 23.2 shows a typical diagram of the specimen holder in a JEOL tensile stage, which consists of fixed and movable ends. The movable side can be controlled by a motor at a constant velocity, e.g., 0.05 mm/s, or manually controlled. The amount of load is measured in real time with a load cell. The accuracy of the cell is 1 kg.

Figure 23.3 shows a typical tensile specimen size and attachment to the stage. The width of the specimen at the center should be less than 5 mm. The size can be modified to ensure the fracture of the specimen within 200 kg load. The specimen can also be compressed in the stage. Figure 23.4 shows a typical compression specimen setup.

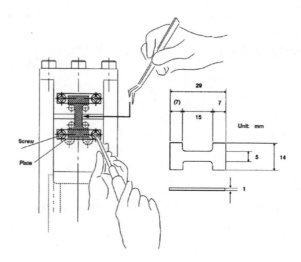

FIGURE 23.3   Schematic diagram of a tensile specimen on the loading stage.

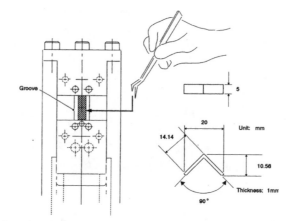

FIGURE 23.4   Schematic diagram of a compression specimen on the loading stage.

After the tension or compression specimen has been installed in the stage, the load is applied and the changes in the specimen observed. Specimen position can be changed with the stage controls if the viewing field shifts with application of load. From the observed image, the size of the area supporting the load can be calculated. Combined with the measured load, the strength and modulus values can be obtained. The fracture mode of the material can also be obtained from the observed image and EDS can be used for chemical analysis.

III. OBSERVATION OF MATERIAL FRACTURE MODE

The authors have studied the dynamic fracture of steels containing nonmetallic inclusions using the SEM-in-scope loading system. Figure 23.5 shows a typical fracture process of 38CrMoAl steel containing aluminum nitride (AlN) particles. Cracks start at sharp corners of the inclusions perpendicular to the tensile force and propagate along the interface between the inclusions and the matrix.

Xiao and Han[2] have investigated the microstructure change in a directionally solidified Ni_3Al base alloy IC6 with 0.12 wt.% Y and 0.1~0.2 wt.% Si addition. Figure 23.6 shows a typical secondary electron image of the modified alloy. A nodular precipitate with bright edge is seen in the

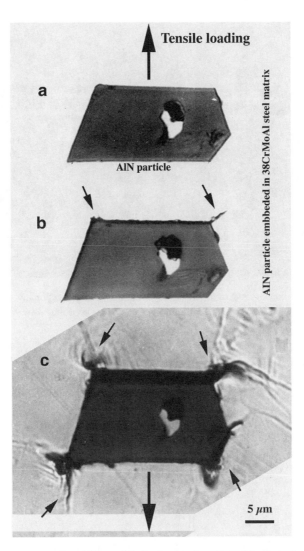

FIGURE 23.5 Fracture process of an AlN particle in the matrix of 38CrMoAl steel. (a) The morphology of AlN before tensile loading. (b) The crack initially appears at the sharp corner in AlN perpendicular to the tensile force. (c) During propagation of the crack, the interfaces between the AlN particle and the matrix separate perpendicular to the direction of the tensile load.

TABLE 23.2
Chemical Composition of the Precipitate in Figure 23.6

	Ni	Mo	Al	Si
Atom percentage (%)	40.2	47.2	2.4	10.2
Weight percentage (%)	32.6	62.5	0.9	4.0

interdendritic area. The EDS/spectrum from the nodular phase is shown in Figure 23.7. The chemical composition is summarized in Table 23.2. Combined with transmission electron microscopy (TEM) analysis, the precipitate is identified as $Mo_6(Ni_{0.75}(Si,Al)_{0.25})_7$.

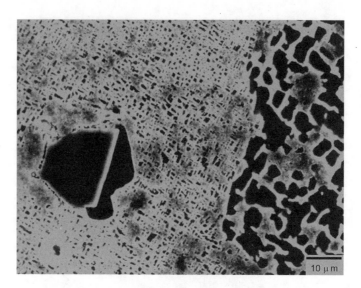

FIGURE 23.6   Typical secondary electron (backscattered) image of the directionally solidified Ni_3Al base alloy IC6 with 0.12 wt.% Y and 0.1~0.2 wt.% Si addition. (The image was contributed by Xiao, B. and Han, Y.F.)

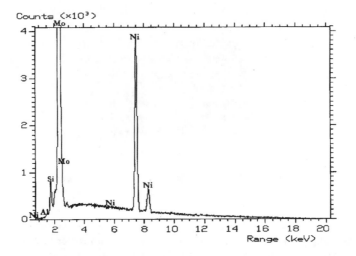

FIGURE 23.7   Energy dispersive X-ray spectrum of the nodular phase in Figure 23.6. (The graph was contributed by Xiao, B. and Han, Y.F.)

Yamashita and Kameyama[3] studied the microstructures of oil/water (O/W) emulsions using cryoscanning electron microscopy. The emulsions used in the study were oil-in-water types of surfactant-cetostearyl alcohol–water systems. A field emission SEM (FESEM) was used to investigate the microstructure of the emulsions because the procedures for specimen preparation were much simpler. A conventional method, the freeze-fracture method, was used to fracture the emulsion with a cooled knife in the sample stage of the SEM. A spherical oil droplet was revealed on the uneven fracture surface (Figure 23.8).

IV. POTENTIAL APPLICATIONS IN BONE-RELATED RESEARCH

The technology presented in this chapter has great potential for applications in bone-related research. Cortical or cancellous bone cylinders or cubes can be compressively loaded and the

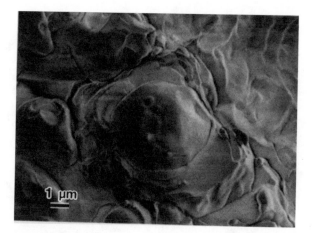

FIGURE 23.8   A cryo-SEM image of an oil/water emulsion fractured in the SEM. The partial sphere in the center is a frozen oil droplet. (From Yamashita, M. and Kameyama, K., *JEOL News,* 33E, 28, 1998. With permission.)

dynamic morphological changes during deformation and failure can be monitored. Bone can also be cut into dumbbell-shaped specimens for observation of the fracture process under tensile force. With a self-designed fixture, bending tests of bone or tensile tests of bone–implant interface specimens could also be done.

The loading stage within the scope is similar to the frame of a standard uniaxial materials testing machine. With appropriate fixtures, most tests commonly used for measuring mechanical properties of bone, tendon and ligament, skin, and fascia could be performed in the SEM. Researchers could test the mechanical properties of bone or other biological materials, observe their morphological changes under loading, and possibly collect data on chemical composition of the samples at the same time.

REFERENCES

1. Product Manual, JSM-5600LV/JSM-5600 Scanning Electron Microscopes, JEOL, Tokyo, Japan, 1998.
2. Xiao, B. and Han, Y.F., Study on precipitates due to the addition of silicon in yttrium modified Ni-Al-Mo-Cu alloy IC6, unpublished data.
3. Yamashita, M. and Kameyama, K., Cryo-scanning electron microscopy of microstructures of O/W emulsions, JEOL News, 33E, 28, 1998.

24 Ultrasonic Methods for Evaluating Mechanical Properties of Bone

Jae-Young Rho

CONTENTS

I. INTRODUCTION

Ultrasonic techniques have significant advantages over mechanical testing methods in the determination of the elastic properties of bone, in that they are able to use smaller, more simply shaped specimens.[1-6] Table 24.1 summarizes some of the differences between mechanical testing methods and the ultrasonic testing method.[6] Also, several anisotropic properties can be measured from a single specimen. Due to inhomogeneity, anisotropy, and size limitations of bone, these advantages are significant.

The elastic properties can be deduced from velocity measurements of shear and longitudinal waves propagating in particular directions in the bone specimens if the density and the elastic anisotropy of bone are specified. The relations between velocity and elastic properties follow from the theory of small-amplitude elastic wave propagation in anisotropic solids.[7,8] There are two modes of wave propagation, characterized by overall specimen geometry. The first case is referred to as bulk wave propagation, as overall specimen geometry tends to infinity. Since the cross-sectional dimension is large, the wave does not perceive the solid boundaries. The second case, where overall specimen geometry tends to 0, is called bar wave propagation.[2] In this case the entire cross section is excited by the passing wave. The bar wave velocity can be written in terms of Young's modulus directly as

$$v_{bar} = \sqrt{\frac{E}{\rho}} \ . \tag{24.1}$$

The bulk wave velocity is

$$v_{bulk} = \sqrt{\frac{k}{\rho}} \ , \tag{24.2}$$

Mechanical Testing of Bone and the Bone–Implant Interface

TABLE 24.1
Comparison between Mechanical Testing and Ultrasonic Testing Methods

	Tensile	Compressive	Bending	Ultrasonic
Specimen shape	Difficult to machine specialized shapes for mounting.	Right cylinders or cubes; parallel faces are critical.	Rectangular parallelepiped; length/cross section ratio is critical.	Cylinders or parallelepiped; parallel faces not necessarily critical; less complicated shape.
Anisotropic elastic properties	Three orthogonal specimens for three moduli; shear moduli possible if cross section is round; Poisson's ratio possible with biaxial extensometer.	Three orthogonal moduli from cube; may be possible to measure Poisson's ratio with extensometer, but as yet no reports of Poisson's ratio measured in this way.	Three orthogonal specimens for three moduli; determination of Poisson's ratio in pure bending tests; this method requires specimens with relatively large cross sections.	Three moduli, three shear moduli, six Poisson's ratios possible from a cube as small as 10 mm for cancellous bone and 5 mm for cortical bone.
Notes	If induced bending is accounted for, and if strain is measured with an extensometer, this technique can be accurate; tensile testing is most common method of measuring elasticity of engineering materials.	This technique can be accurate if faces are parallel and if strain is measured with an extensometer instead of platen motion. Compressive testing is less common for engineering materials, but ASTM standards have been written and are used for rigid plastics; the ASTM suggested specimen size is 12 × 12 × 50 mm, not cubic specimens.	For determination of elastic constants, several series of specimens with different h/l ratio are necessary. Inaccuracies occur due to specimen misalignment, friction at the load points, imprecise strain measurement, inadequate h/l ratio, and elastic-plastic deformation; the limitations imposed by theoretical considerations must be taken into account.	Actual path length is unknown unless specimen shape is simple; path length is determined by averaging the actual lengths. The velocity of propagation of an ultrasonic wave can be dependent on the frequency of oscillation. Pure longitudinal and shear waves propagate only in directions parallel to axis of material symmetry.

Source: Rho, J.Y., *Ultrasonics*, 34, 777, 1996. With permission.

where k is the bulk modulus. The bulk modulus for an isotropic material is

$$k = \frac{E}{3(1-2\nu)} \quad . \tag{24.3}$$

Here, ν is Poisson's ratio. This phenomenon refers to geometric dispersion in which the velocity of propagation depends on the external dimensions of the material in which the wave is propagated.[2,9,10] The ultrasonic technique has been used to measure both the elastic modulus of the cancellous bone structure (structural modulus) and the elastic modulus of trabecular bone material (material modulus).[11] The wavelength of the ultrasonic wave must be larger than the characteristic dimension of the material in order to measure structural modulus. Conversely, ultrasonic waves with wavelengths shorter than the characteristic dimension of the material would be less affected by the elasticity of the structure, and would propagate at velocities determined by the elasticity of trabecular material.[11]

Several investigators have assumed cortical bone specimens to be orthotropic with nine independent elastic constants.[6,12-15] Consideration must be given to the different structures of cortical and cancellous bone. Techniques for the ultrasonic velocity measurement for cortical bone have utilized frequencies between 2 and 10 MHz. These relatively high frequencies allow accurate determination of the time delay due to propagation through cortical specimens with dimensions as small as 5 mm.[2] Both cylindrical and cubic specimen shapes have been used, but cubic specimens offer the possibility of velocity measurement in several different directions. The use of ultrasound to measure the elastic properties of the porous structure of cancellous bone is a much more complex problem. Lower-frequency waves (50 to 100 kHz) of longer wavelength are necessary to determine the elastic properties of the cancellous bone structure due to its high porosity.[3,11] Porosity can be quantified by measuring the void fraction, defined as the ratio of void volume to total volume. Void fractions range from 0.5 to 0.8 for cancellous bone. A direct consequence of the large void fraction is that ultrasonic waves are much more strongly attenuated in cancellous bone than in cortical bone. In other words, the velocity of propagation of an ultrasonic wave is strongly dependent on the frequency of oscillation. The dispersive nature of cancellous bone must be analyzed carefully in order to obtain meaningful values for its elastic properties.

The shear moduli and Poisson's ratio for cancellous bone have rarely been measured using ultrasound, since bar wave propagation techniques may not be adequate to measure Poisson's ratio for the cancellous bone. Ashman et al.[2] and Rho[6] show that the bulk mode works well for the measurement of the orthotropic elastic properties of cortical bone. In the same context, bulk wave propagation in cancellous bone may provide an adequate method for measuring Poisson's ratio. Bulk wave propagation in cubic cancellous bone specimens measuring approximately 10 mm on a side may be achieved by raising the frequency of the ultrasonic waves from 50 to approximately 500 kHz. This would reduce the wavelength from approximately 40 to about 4 mm. To achieve this task, one should be careful not to increase the frequency so much as to cause continuum breakdown, where the waves begin to propagate along individual trabeculae.[16] Ultrasonic velocity measurements should be made at intermediate frequencies between 50 and 500 kHz to determine at what frequency a transition between bulk and bar waves occurs.

In a solid material, as mentioned above, ultrasonic velocity is equal to the square root of the ratio of the elastic modulus to density. Whether or not this is true in a porous material like cancellous bone is critically dependent on the wavelength of sound in relation to the bone specimen and microstructural dimensions.[11,17] Even though Ashman and Rho[11] have found good agreement between the ultrasonically determined and mechanically measured elastic modulus of cancellous bone structure, the conflicting results for high-frequency sound velocities relative to the microscopic modulus (i.e., trabecular bone material) have suggested that the theory must be modified.[17] These modifications need to deal with

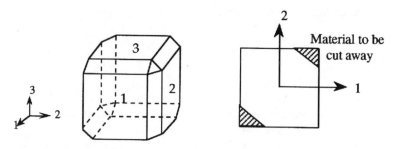

FIGURE 24.1   Cubic specimen developed by Van Buskirk et al.[14] (From Rho, J., *Ultrasonics,* 34, 777, 1996. With permission.)

cancellous bone structure and describe the relationship of high-frequency clinical measurements to bone microstructure. One reason for the conflicting results is the unknown actual path length. Ultrasonic velocity data at mixed cortical and cancellous bone sites have been reported. Langton et al.[18] suggest that the path must be linear. However, McCartney et al.[19] demonstrated a nonlinear transverse path of ultrasound in thick-walled cylinders. It is essential to know the exact path of the ultrasound beam in bone, as the determination of ultrasonic velocity is based on measuring the time of flight and the distance traveled.

II. SAMPLE PREPARATION

Cortical bone specimens are obtained from the diaphysis of long bones. Positions along the length of the bone are standardized by using external anatomical landmarks on the surface of the bone to define specimen locations. For an example, a femoral bone is placed posterior quadrant down on a flat surface. Three anatomical structures, the quadrant tubercle and the medial and lateral knee condyles, come into contact with the surface. These contact points are used to define the length of the bone. The length is then divided into any number of increments at which transverse sections are cut. The anterior, medial, posterior, and lateral quadrants are then marked on the transverse sections. Specimens can then be located with respect to these four locations on each transverse section. A three-step cutting procedure is used to fabricate cortical specimens of the desired geometry (side dimensions on the order of 5 mm). Bones are cleaned of attached muscles prior to cutting. The first step is to make rough cuts with a band saw to obtain the transverse sections along the length of the bone. Although it is easy to burn bone using a band saw, rough cutting affects an area only 1 to 2 mm into the bone from the cut.[4] In the second step, the cutting process consists of machining cubic specimens from the anterior, posterior, medial, and lateral quadrants at the several sections along the length of the bone. This is accomplished with a 1/8-in. diameter end mill while the bone is kept wet. Materials burned by the first step can be removed during this step. Since a particular geometry proposed by Van Buskirk et al.[14] is utilized to obtain all necessary velocity measurements from one specimen, the third step consists of cutting the edges of the cube off at 45° angles with a "v" using a slow-speed diamond cutter[2] (Figure 24.1). Specimens axes are aligned with the axial (x_3), the circumferential (x_2), and the radial (x_1) axes for each bone.

Cancellous bone specimens can be obtained from the ends of long bones. The inhomogeneity of cancellous bone and the fact that cancellous elastic properties are less well documented require a greater number of cancellous specimens. Location of the specimens is standardized on several 12-mm slabs using plastic templates[3] and care is taken to ensure that specimen orientation is recorded. The $10 \times 10 \times 10$ mm specimens are cut from the 12-mm sections with a slow-speed diamond wafering saw ensuring no dense epiphyseal bone is included in the $10 \times 10 \times 10$ mm cubes. Diamond wafering blades are particularly good for making smooth and parallel cuts. Specimens axes are aligned

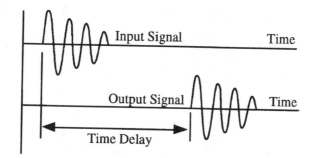

FIGURE 24.2 Graphic representation for measuring time delay with a pulse propagation method.

with the superior-inferior (x_3), medial-lateral (x_2), and anterior-posterior (x_1) axes for each bone. Bone marrow is removed from each cube with a water jet prior to analysis, and specimens are kept moist in saline at all times between testing. Individual trabeculae (0.3 mm diameter by 2 mm length) can be isolated using a stereomicroscope, scalpel, and forceps.

III. TESTING METHODS

The general method used to measure the ultrasonic wave velocities is a pulse transmission technique. The basis of this technique is the time delay of propagation between the transmitted and received ultrasonic waves. From the time delay and the thickness of the specimen, the ultrasonic velocity can be calculated. To measure ultrasonic velocities of cortical bone, a frequency of 2.25 MHz is used. To measure ultrasonic velocities of cancellous bone structure, 50 kHz is used. At 50 kHz, the wavelength of the ultrasonic wave is much longer than the characteristic dimension of the cancellous bone structure. These specific frequencies are optimized by comparing elastic properties determined ultrasonically at several frequencies for cortical or cancellous bone with those measured by mechanical testing techniques. When comparing the ultrasonically measured elastic properties with those determined mechanically, the ultrasonic strain rate is often brought up. It would appear that the strain rate is relatively high, but strain rate is change in length/original length/time. For 2.25 MHz the time is indeed short, but so is the change in length. The values of elastic properties determined ultrasonically are in fact similar to those obtained at quasi-static rates.[2,3,11]

By using a pulse generator, ultrasonic waves produced by the transducers are recorded by an oscilloscope which allows the time delay between the transmitted and received waves to be determined. The time delay for both longitudinal and shear measurements is measured from the start of the input signal to the start of the output signal. The first received point is taken to be the beginning of the output signal (Figure 24.2). Longitudinal and shear transducers of 2.25 MHz are used to measure the velocity of the cortical bone specimens and trabecular bone material (material modulus), while those of 50 kHz are used to measure the structural velocity of the cancellous bone. Coupling of the transducers to the bone is done with water for the longitudinal mode transducers and with a viscous liquid acoustic coupler for the transverse mode transducers.

The density of bone must be used in the calculation of the elastic coefficients from the wave velocities. The density range of cortical bone from 1700 to 2000 kg/m³ is determined by Archimedes' principle. The density range of the cancellous structure (often referred to as the apparent density) from 50 to 1000 kg/m³ is determined by weighing the cancellous structure after removing the bone marrow and dividing by the volume of the overall physical dimensions, including pores. The specimens are centrifuged to remove residual water from the intertrabecular spaces prior to weighing.

IV. DATA COLLECTION AND CALCULATION

Cortical bone is an inhomogeneous anisotropic, viscoelastic material. However, it is reasonable to model cortical bone as linearly elastic and anisotropic.[1,14,15,21] The constitutive equation, Hooke's law, for a linear anisotropic elastic material is

$$\sigma_i = c_{ij}\,\varepsilon_j \tag{24.4}$$

where the terms σ_i and ε_j represent components of the stress and strain tensors, respectively, and c_{ij} is the matrix of elastic coefficients. The matrix of elastic coefficients for an orthotropic material is written as follows:

$$[c_{ij}] = \begin{bmatrix} c_{11} & c_{12} & c_{13} & 0 & 0 & 0 \\ c_{12} & c_{22} & c_{23} & 0 & 0 & 0 \\ c_{13} & c_{23} & c_{33} & 0 & 0 & 0 \\ 0 & 0 & 0 & c_{44} & 0 & 0 \\ 0 & 0 & 0 & 0 & c_{55} & 0 \\ 0 & 0 & 0 & 0 & 0 & c_{66} \end{bmatrix}. \tag{24.5}$$

There are 12 nonzero components of which 9 are independent. Equation 24.4 can be rewritten in terms of the compliance matrix, s_{ij}.

$$\varepsilon_j = s_{ij}\,\sigma_i \tag{24.6}$$

The compliance matrix for an orthotropic material is expressed in terms of elastic properties such as Young's modulus, shear modulus, and Poisson's ratio and is

$$[c_{ij}]^{-1} = [s_{ij}] = \begin{bmatrix} \dfrac{1}{E_1} & -\dfrac{v_{21}}{E_2} & -\dfrac{v_{31}}{E_3} & 0 & 0 & 0 \\ -\dfrac{v_{12}}{E_1} & \dfrac{1}{E_2} & -\dfrac{v_{32}}{E_3} & 0 & 0 & 0 \\ -\dfrac{v_{13}}{E_1} & -\dfrac{v_{23}}{E_2} & \dfrac{1}{E_3} & 0 & 0 & 0 \\ 0 & 0 & 0 & \dfrac{1}{G_{23}} & 0 & 0 \\ 0 & 0 & 0 & 0 & \dfrac{1}{G_{31}} & 0 \\ 0 & 0 & 0 & 0 & 0 & \dfrac{1}{G_{12}} \end{bmatrix}. \tag{24.7}$$

where E_i is the Young's moduli in the i direction, v_{ij} is Poisson's ratio for strain in the j direction with stress applied in the i direction, and G_{ij} are the shear moduli in the i–j plane ($i, j = 1, 2,$ or 3). The matrix of elastic coefficients and the compliance matrix are symmetric; hence,

$$\frac{v_{ij}}{E_i} = \frac{v_{ji}}{E_j}. \tag{24.8}$$

TABLE 24.2
Analytical Expressions for the Inversion between the Orthotropic Matrix of Elastic Coefficients and the Orthotropic Compliance Matrix

$$c_{11} = \frac{s_{22}s_{33} - s_{23}^2}{\Delta} \qquad c_{12} = \frac{s_{13}s_{23} - s_{12}s_{33}}{\Delta} \qquad c_{44} = \frac{1}{s_{44}}$$

$$c_{22} = \frac{s_{33}s_{11} - s_{13}^2}{\Delta} \qquad c_{13} = \frac{s_{12}s_{23} - s_{13}s_{22}}{\Delta} \qquad c_{55} = \frac{1}{s_{55}}$$

$$c_{33} = \frac{s_{11}s_{22} - s_{12}^2}{\Delta} \qquad c_{23} = \frac{s_{12}s_{13} - s_{33}s_{11}}{\Delta} \qquad c_{66} = \frac{1}{s_{66}}$$

$$\Delta = s_{11}s_{22}s_{33} - s_{11}s_{23}^2 - s_{22}s_{13}^2 - s_{33}s_{12}^2 + 2s_{12}s_{23}s_{22}$$

Source: Ashman, R.B., Ph.D. dissertation, Tulane University, New Orleans, LA, 1982. With permission.

The relationship between c_{ij} and s_{ij} can be accomplished in closed form as outlined in Table 24.2. However, the matrix of elastic coefficients and the compliance matrix must be positive.[1,21] Therefore, to satisfy this requirement,

$$s_{11}, s_{22}, s_{33}, s_{44}, s_{55}, s_{66} > 0,$$

$$\begin{vmatrix} s_{11} & s_{12} \\ s_{12} & s_{22} \end{vmatrix} > 0, \quad \begin{vmatrix} s_{22} & s_{23} \\ s_{23} & s_{33} \end{vmatrix} > 0, \quad \begin{vmatrix} s_{11} & s_{13} \\ s_{13} & s_{33} \end{vmatrix} > 0, \tag{24.9}$$

and

$$\begin{vmatrix} s_{11} & s_{12} & s_{13} \\ s_{12} & s_{22} & s_{23} \\ s_{13} & s_{23} & s_{33} \end{vmatrix} > 0.$$

Similar requirements must be satisfied by the components of the matrix of elastic coefficients.

$$E_1, E_2, E_3, G_{23}, G_{31}, G_{12} > 0$$

$$(1 - \nu_{23}\nu_{32}), \quad (1 - \nu_{13}\nu_{31}), \quad (1 - \nu_{12}\nu_{21}) > 0 \tag{24.10}$$

and

$$1 - \nu_{12}\nu_{21} - \nu_{23}\nu_{32} - \nu_{31}\nu_{13} - 2\nu_{21}\nu_{32}\nu_{13} > 0.$$

These relations provide an additional check on the experimentally obtained values of the elastic coefficients. Relations between velocities and elastic coefficients for an orthotropic material are listed in Table 24.3. These relationships are the solutions of the equations of motion of elastic

TABLE 24.3
Relationships between the Measured Velocities and the Terms of the Matrix of Elastic Coefficients[2,6,14]

$$c_{11} = \rho v_1^2$$

$$c_{22} = \rho v_2^2$$

$$c_{33} = \rho v_3^2$$

$$c_{44} = \rho v_{23}^2 = \rho v_{23}^2$$

$$c_{55} = \rho v_{13}^2 = \rho v_{31}^2$$

$$c_{66} = \rho v_{12}^2 = \rho v_{12}^2$$

$$c_{12} = \sqrt{(c_{11}+c_{66}-2\rho v_{12/12}^2)+(c_{22}+c_{66}-2\rho v_{12/12}^2)} - c_{66}$$

$$c_{13} = \sqrt{(c_{11}+c_{55}-2\rho v_{13/13}^2)+(c_{33}+c_{55}-2\rho v_{13/13}^2)} - c_{55}$$

$$c_{23} = \sqrt{(c_{22}+c_{44}-2\rho v_{23/23}^2)+(c_{33}+c_{44}-2\rho v_{23/23}^2)} - c_{44}$$

Relations permitting to check the assumption of orthotropy:

$$c_{55}+c_{66} = 2\rho v_{23/1}^2$$

$$c_{44}+c_{66} = 2\rho v_{13/2}^2$$

$$c_{44}+c_{55} = 2\rho v_{12/3}^2$$

v_i: velocity of a longitudinal wave in i direction
v_{ij}: velocity of a transverse wave traveling in i direction, with particle motion in j direction
$v_{ij/k}$: velocity of a transverse wave traveling in $(i+j)/\sqrt{2}$ direction with particle motion in k direction
$v_{ij/ij}$: velocity of a transverse or longitudinal wave traveling in $(i+j)/\sqrt{2}$ direction with particle motion in the i–j plane; velocities are quasi-longitudinal or quasi-transverse

Source: Rho, J., *Ultrasonics*, 34, 777, 1996. With permission.

waves in a unbounded medium.[1,8,14] It should be noted that the velocities associated with the diagonal directions are not necessarily purely longitudinal or purely transverse.[1] The velocities measured in these directions are called quasi-longitudinal and quasi-transverse.

A total of 18 different velocities can be measured, three in each of six directions using the specimen shape developed by Van Buskirk et al.[14] shown in Figure 24.1. However, only nine velocities could be measured from tibial cortical specimens due to the thin cortex, the shape of which is shown in Figure 24.3. Two of the nine independent orthotropic elastic constants (c_{12} and c_{13}) cannot be obtained using this specimen shape, but can be obtained by relationships assuming transverse isotropy: $c_{13} = c_{23}$ and $c_{66} = \frac{1}{2}(c_{11} - c_{12})$. However, seven elastic coefficients are sufficient

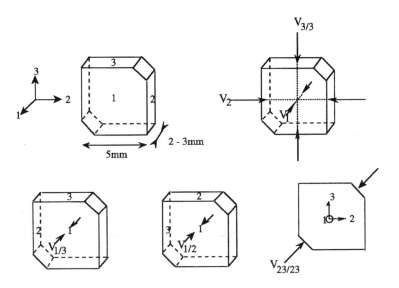

FIGURE 24.3 Specimen shapes used to obtain the necessary velocities for the calculation of the anisotropic elastic coefficients. v_i is velocity of a longitudinal wave in the i direction. v_{ij} is velocity of a transverse wave in i direction with particle motion in j direction. $v_{ij/ij}$ is velocity of a transverse or longitudinal wave in the (i + j)/$\sqrt{2}$ direction with particle motion in the i–j plane (quasi-longitudinal or quasi-transverse velocity). (From Rho, J., *Ultrasonics*, 34, 777, 1996. With permission.)

to determine whether the elastic symmetry of the material is orthotropic, transversely isotropic, or isotropic.

Cancellous bone is also considered linearly elastic and anisotropic.[22] The most straightforward relationships between velocities and elastic properties are derived for waves of long wavelength propagating in bar-shaped specimens of narrow cross section.[7] Longitudinal velocities v_i of waves propagating in the i direction and shear wave velocities v_{ij} for propagation in the i direction with particle motion in the j direction are related to Young's moduli and shear moduli by

$$E_i = \rho v_i^2 \qquad (24.11)$$

and

$$G_{ij} = \rho v_{ij}^2 = \rho v_{ji}^2 \qquad (24.12)$$

where ρ is the apparent density of the structure, E_i is the elastic modulus in the i direction, and G_{ij} is the shear modulus. Two requirements must be satisfied for correct application of Equations 24.11 and 24.12. First, the wavelength must be greater than the characteristic dimensions of the structure, if the structure is to be considered a continuum. Second, the wavelength must be larger than the cross-sectional dimensions of the specimen. Wave propagation fulfilling these requirements is often referred to as bar wave propagation. In order for an ultrasonic wave to propagate at a velocity governed by the elastic properties of the gross structure, the first requirement must be satisfied. Harrigan et al.[16] presented arguments that the 5-mm characteristic dimension is the lower limit at which cancellous bone can be considered a continuum. The 50-kHz frequency of the transmitted ultrasonic wave, with measured velocities between 1000 and 1600 m/s, predicts a wavelength (velocity/frequency) on the order of 20 mm, well above the 5-mm characteristic dimension of the cancellous structure and the 10-mm cross-sectional dimension of the specimen.

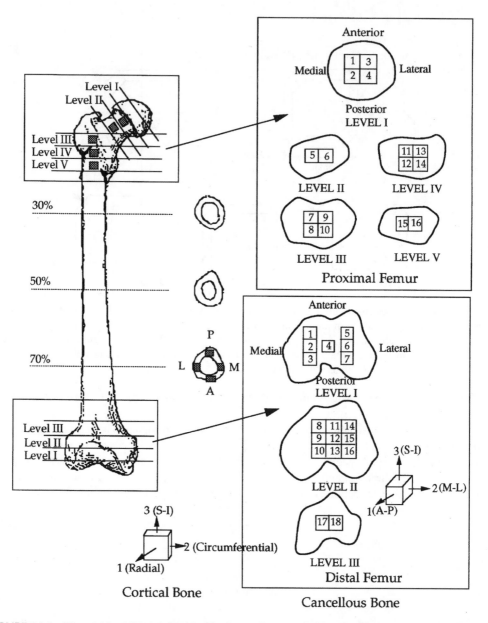

FIGURE 24.4   The position of femoral cortical and cancellous specimens. The three directions are coincident with the long axis of the bone; the one and two directions are the radial and circumferential directions for cortical bone and anterioposterial and mediolateral directions for cancellous bone, respectively.

V. RESULTS FOR MEASUREMENTS IN BONE

Eight right femorae were obtained from frozen unembalmed human cadavers. None of the individuals had a history of bone disease. Cortical bone specimens were obtained from the four specimens from each of three transverse sections at 30, 50, and 70% of total bone length (Figure 24.4). There is a greater variability along the length of a whole bone than around its circumference (the variation in the mechanical properties around the circumference being less than 10%) which could be due to a changing thickness in the longitudinal direction. The elastic moduli

TABLE 24.4
Elastic Properties (standard deviation in parentheses) of Human Femoral Cortical Bone

Elastic Properties	Minimum	Maximum	Average (SD)
E_1 (GPa)	7.4	16.2	11.6 (1.9)
E_2 (GPa)	8.1	16.4	12.2 (1.9)
E_3 (GPa)	11.4	31.9	19.9 (2.7)
G_{12} (GPa)	2.3	5.6	4.0 (0.7)
G_{13} (GPa)	3.6	6.3	5.0 (0.7)
G_{23} (GPa)	3.9	6.9	5.4 (0.7)
v_{12}	0.267	0.563	0.417 (.070)
v_{13}	0.143	0.323	0.232 (.039)
v_{21}	0.323	0.548	0.436 (.50)
v_{23}	0.147	0.302	0.225 (.032)
v_{31}	0.294	0.496	0.396 (.053)
v_{32}	0.309	0.411	0.362 (.020)
ρ (kg/m³)	1453	1996	1811 (148)

Note: The direction 3 is coincident with the long axis of the bone; the directions 1 and 2 are the radial and circumferential directions, respectively. Values of elastic properties are expressed in GPa.

TABLE 24.5
Elastic Properties (standard deviation in parentheses) of Human Proximal Femoral Cancellous Bone

Level	Position	E_1	E_2	E_3
I	1	1584 (485)	1620 (501)	2212 (663)
	2	1698 (628)	1646 (653)	2244 (760)
	3	2114 (633)	2061 (647)	2710 (745)
	4	2036 (620)	1846 (685)	2476 (760)
II	5	860 (705)	804 (706)	1453 (644)
	6	620 (326)	590 (392)	1488 (810)
III	7	299 (162)	570 (257)	902 (436)
	8	321 (357)	426 (299)	801 (297)
	9	310 (164)	482 (204)	1170 (363)
	10	261 (174)	540 (220)	753 (440)
IV	11	142 (85)	227 (193)	565 (220)
	12	175 (139)	274 (299)	622 (312)
	13	220 (144)	308 (223)	792 (453)
	14	286 (238)	366 (277)	808 (599)
V	15	257 (132)	309 (282)	764 (505)
	16	217 (196)	242 (235)	518 (282)

Note: The direction 3 is coincident with the long axis of the bone; the directions 1 and 2 are the anterioposterior and mediolateral directions, respectively. Values of elastic properties are expressed in MPa.

TABLE 24.6
**Elastic Properties (standard deviation in parentheses)
of Human Distal Femoral Cancellous Bone**

Level	Position	E_1	E_2	E_3
I	1	606 (212)	604 (267)	1627 (396)
	2	1093 (474)	1129 (526)	2328 (818)
	3	1654 (692)	1173 (485)	2676 (1037)
	4	1071 (329)	1054 (348)	1941 (511)
	5	1123 (351)	1096 (378)	2468 (911)
	6	1118 (361)	1076 (295)	2110 (517)
	7	1828 (562)	1842 (529)	3098 (1144)
II	8	420 (217)	416 (227)	1241 (338)
	9	264 (170)	280 (206)	967 (367)
	10	599 (367)	669 (392)	1516 (797)
	11	571 (435)	527 (353)	1409 (562)
	12	224 (114)	183 (122)	683 (357)
	13	312 (285)	386 (441)	810 (584)
	14	917 (460)	643 (366)	2320 (958)
	15	599 (273)	437 (269)	1487 (718)
	16	723 (535)	762 (609)	1991 (1233)
III	17	190 (161)	171 (158)	678 (454)
	18	363 (365)	285 (295)	1212 (957)

Note: The direction 3 is coincident with the long axis of the bone; the directions 1 and 2 are the anterioposterior and mediolateral directions, respectively. Values of elastic properties are expressed in MPa.

in the radial or circumferential directions correlate to the axial/longitudinal modulus, but the correlation coefficients are relatively low (0.4 and 0.2, respectively). However, all three perpendicular moduli correlated even better with the density of the material, on the order of 0.5 to 0.8. Cancellous bone specimens are obtained from both the proximal and distal femorae. Tables 24.4 through 24.6 provide the values in elastic properties of cortical and cancellous bone along the length and around the quadrant of the bone.[5] Mechanical properties vary significantly around the periphery and along the length, and there is a pronounced anisotropy of cancellous structure in the highly mechanically loaded bone. Overall, the differences between the mechanical properties in cancellous bone are much broader than those in cortical bone.

The pulse transmission ultrasonic technique has been undertaken to characterize the actual pathway and the wavelength dependence in relation to the bone specimen and microstructural dimensions.[23] From one human right tibia, 20 individual trabeculae and 20 cylindrical cancellous bone specimens are obtained. The average velocity through individual trabecular bone is 2901 ± 161 m/s (mean ± SD), while the mean velocity through cylindrical cancellous bone specimens is 2717 ± 171 m/s. Thus, the velocity through the cylindrical cancellous bone specimens is underestimated as 6.4% as much as that through individual trabeculae. As expected, the actual pathway of trabecular bone material measurement is slightly longer than the average length of the specimen. It may be postulated that ultrasonic energy has propagated along trabeculae, the shortest pathway. The wavelengths, determined from the measured velocities ranging from 2600 to 3300 m/s, are on the order of 1 mm. The 1-mm wavelength is larger than the cross-sectional dimension of the trabeculae (0.1 to 0.5 mm); hence, bar wave propagation can be applied to calculate the elastic modulus. Also, since the 1-mm wavelength is smaller than the 5-mm characteristic dimension of the structure, the wave may be considered not to be affected by the cancellous bone structure.

ACKNOWLEDGMENT

This work was supported in part by grants from the Whitaker Foundation.

REFERENCES

1. Ashman, R.B., Ultrasonic Determination of the Elastic Properties of Cortical Bone: Techniques and Limitations, Ph.D. dissertation, Tulane University, New Orleans, LA, 1982.
2. Ashman, R.B., Cowin, S.C., Van Buskirk, W.C., and Rice, J.C., A continuous wave technique for the measurement of the elastic properties of cortical bone, *J. Biomech.,* 17, 349, 1984.
3. Ashman, R.B., Rho, J.Y., and Turner, C.H., Anatomical variation of orthotropic elastic moduli of the proximal human tibia, *J. Biomech.,* 22, 895, 1989.
4. Ashman, R.B., Experimental techniques, in *Bone Mechanics,* Cowin, S.C., Ed., CRC Press, Boca Raton, FL, 1989.
5. Rho, J.Y., Mechanical Properties of Cortical and Cancellous Bone, Ph.D. dissertation, University of Texas Southwestern Medical Center, Dallas, TX, 1991.
6. Rho, J.Y., An ultrasonic method for measuring the elastic properties of human tibial cortical and cancellous bone, *Ultrasonics,* 34, 777, 1996.
7. Kolsky, H., *Stress Waves in Solids,* Dover Publications, New York, 1963.
8. Hearmon, R.F.S., *An Introduction to Applied Anisotropic Elasticity,* Oxford University Press, Oxford, U.K., 1961.
9. Nigro, N.J., Wave propagation in anisotropic bars of rectangular cross section. I. Longitudinal wave propagation. *J. Acoust. Soc. Am.,* 46, 958, 1968.
10. Thurston, R.N., Elastic waves in rods and clad rods, *J. Acoust. Soc. Am.,* 64, 1–37, 1978.
11. Ashman, R.B. and Rho, J.Y, Elastic moduli of trabecular bone material, *J. Biomech.,* 21, 177, 1988.
12. Yoon, H.S. and Katz, J.L., Ultrasonic wave propagation in human cortical bone — I. Theoretical considerations for hexagonal symmetry, *J. Biomech.,* 9, 409, 1976.
13. Yoon, H.S. and Katz, J.L., Ultrasonic wave propagation in human cortical bone — II. Measurements of elastic properties and microhardness, *J. Biomech.,* 9, 459, 1976.
14. Van Buskirk, W.C., Cowin, S.C., and Ward, R.N., Ultrasonic measurement of orthotropic elastic constants of bovine femoral bone, *J. Biomech. Eng.,* 103, 67, 1981.
15. Van Buskirk, W.C. and Ashman, R.B., The elastic moduli of bone, in *Mechanical Properties of Bone,* Cowin, S.C., Ed., AMD Vol. 45, American Society of Mechanical Engineers, New York, 1981.
16. Harrigan, T.P., Jasty, M., Mann, R.W., and Harris, W.H., Limitations of the continuum assumption in cancellous bone, *J. Biomech.,* 21, 269, 1988.
17. Martin, R.B., Determinants of the mechanical properties of bones, *J. Biomech.,* 24 (Suppl. 1), 79, 1991.
18. Langton, C.M., Ali, A.V., Riggs, C.M., et al., A contact method for the assessment of ultrasonic velocity and broadband attenuation in cortical and cancellous bone, *Clin. Phys. Physiol. Meas.,* 11, 243, 1990.
19. McCartney, R.N., Jeffcott, L.B., and McCarthy, R.N., Transverse path of ultrasound waves in thick-walled cylinders, *Med. Biol. Eng. Comput.,* 33, 551, 1995.
20. Knets, I.V., Mechanics of biological tissues: a review, *Polym. Mech.* [translation of *Mekhanika Polimerov*], 13, 434, 1978.
21. Jones, R.M., *Mechanics of Composite Materials,* McGraw-Hill, New York, 1975.
22. Carter, D.R. and Hayes, W.C., The compressive behavior of bone as a two-phase porous structure, *J. Bone Joint Surg.,* 59A, 954, 1977.
23. Rho, J.Y., Characterization of ultrasonic pathway and wavelength dependence in determining elastic properties using ultrasound method, *Med. Biol. Eng. Comp.,* 36, 57, 1998.

25 Evaluating Mechanical Properties of Bone Using Scanning Acoustic Microscopy

Charles H. Turner and J. Lawrence Katz

CONTENTS

I. INTRODUCTION

Scanning acoustic microscopy (SAM) was introduced in the early 1970s by Quate and colleagues[1] at Stanford University. Since then a number of individually constructed and commercially available reflection-mode SAMs have been developed. SAM works on the principle of having a beam of acoustic waves, generated by a piezoelectric transducer, travel through a high-quality single-crystal lens (usually sapphire) that focuses the waves onto an interface. Part of the wave is reflected back toward the source and part of the wave is transmitted across the interface (Figure 25.1). The former wave is what is analyzed to determine the mechanical properties of the reflecting surface at the interface. The fraction of the wave reflected from the interface will depend on the acoustic impedance differences of the materials comprising the interface.

Acoustic impedance, generally denoted by Z, is the product of local density (ρ) times acoustic velocity (v), i.e., $Z = \rho v$, where the units for Z are called Rayleighs, abbreviated as Rayls. Z is usually given in terms of MRayls, 1 MRayl = 10^6 kg m^{-2}s^{-1}. For optimum results a liquid medium is required to couple the acoustic lens to the material being imaged. Thus, if distilled (or deionized) water is used as the couplant fluid for studying bone, the fractional value of the reflected wave will be determined by solving the equation for the reflection coefficient r, defined as

$$r = \frac{Z_1 - Z_2}{Z_2 + Z_1} \qquad (25.1)$$

where Z_1 and Z_2 are the acoustic impedances of the water and bone, respectively. By using an average value of $Z_2 = 8$ MRayls for bone and $Z_1 = 1.5$ MRayls for water at 20°C, $r = 0.68$, or 68% of the incident sound wave will be reflected back through the same lens to the piezoelectric transducer now acting as a receiver. A graph of the reflection coefficient vs. acoustic impedance indicating the relative location of various materials is given in Figure 25.2.

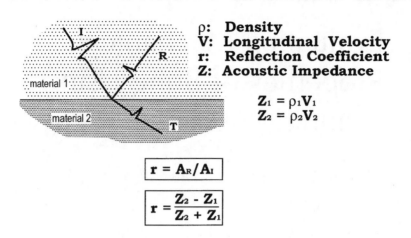

ρ: **Density**
V: **Longitudinal Velocity**
r: **Reflection Coefficient**
Z: **Acoustic Impedance**

$$Z_1 = \rho_1 V_1$$
$$Z_2 = \rho_2 V_2$$

$$r = A_R / A_I$$

$$r = \left| \frac{Z_2 - Z_1}{Z_2 + Z_1} \right|$$

FIGURE 25.1 Sketch of reflected and transmitted acoustic waves at an interface between two materials, including definition of acoustic impedance, Z, and reflection coefficient, r. A_R and A_I are the amplitudes of the reflected and incident waves, respectively.

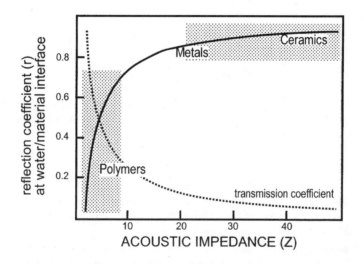

FIGURE 25.2 Plots of reflection and transmission curves for r vs. Z, indicating properties of different materials. (Adapted from Katz, J.L. and Meunier, L., *J. Biomech. Eng.*, 115, 543, 1993. With permission.)

The amplitude of the reflected wave arriving at the transducer will have been attenuated during its propagation through the water couplant; this attenuation increases with increased frequency of the acoustic wave. It is the amplitude of this attenuated wave that is stored as a voltage in the electronic system of the SAM and then displayed as a shade of gray proportional to the voltage. In the scanning mode, the lens and/or specimen raster relative to one another over a preprogrammed number of pixels resulting in an image in shades of gray (or pseudo-color) of the relative acoustic impedance properties of the material over the area being scanned.

The attenuation of the reflected beam makes it somewhat more difficult to use SAM with soft tissues whose values of Z generally are close to that of the water couplant, so that the amplitude of the signal arriving at the transducer is relatively weak, potentially limiting the ability to discriminate between aspects of the image.

Using acoustic impedance information in the SAM image to determine the mechanical properties of the material being scanned requires some intermediate steps. Generally, the mechanical properties derivable from acoustic wave propagation studies that are of interest are the technical moduli: Young's modulus, E; Bulk modulus, K; shear modulus, G; and Poisson's ratio, ν, treating the material as isotropic and homogeneous; or the elastic stiffness coefficients, C_{ij}, for an anisotropic material. In either case the constants, C, are related to density, ρ, times acoustic velocity squared, v^2, i.e., $C = \rho v^2$ as is obtained by solving the wave equation.[2] Clearly, this is closely related to the acoustic impedance $Z = \rho v$, as both depend on the density and elastic properties of the material. Thus, if one can determine the proportionality between the two it is possible to obtain the mechanical properties of the biological material from the SAM image at a much finer scale, down to micro-meters, than is possible by mechanical testing.

The spatial resolution of the lens system at high frequencies depends on the operating frequency, the coupling medium, and the quality and properties of the transducer. The equation demonstrating the relation between the spatial resolution and frequency is $v/f = \lambda$, where λ is the wavelength, f the frequency, and v the velocity of sound. The higher the frequency, the shorter the wavelength, thus the finer will be the spatial resolution. Unfortunately, the higher the frequency, the greater the attenuation of the acoustic wave into the body of the material being examined. This does limit studies of the deep interior of high-Z materials such as bone, ceramics, and metals as opposed to low-Z materials such as soft tissues and polymers. For more details on the physics of SAM see Briggs.[3]

This chapter describes several techniques for measuring the mechanical properties of bone using acoustic microscopy. The methods can be divided into low-frequency and high-frequency approaches. Low-frequency approaches use acoustic waves ranging in frequency from 30 to 100 MHz. At low frequencies, mechanical properties of bone can be measured using acoustic impedance or transmission velocity methods. The spatial resolution of these methods ranges from 30 to 100 μm. High-frequency approaches range in frequency from 100 MHz to 2 GHz. These approaches offer fine spatial resolution (as good as 0.5 μm), but at high frequencies the attenuation of the acoustic waves is very high so transmission velocity methods cannot be used. Instead, mechanical properties can be measured using acoustic impedance or x–z curves.

II. LOW-FREQUENCY STUDIES

A. ACOUSTIC IMPEDANCE METHOD

Meunier, Katz, and co-workers in Paris developed a low-frequency pulse-mode SAM for studying the mechanical properties of bone, skeletal biomaterials, and the bone–implant interface. With this instrument it was possible to obtain the amplitude of the first echo of the longitudinal sound wave reflected back into the lens from the specimen surface pixel by pixel. Using this technique Meunier et al.[4] compared their Z measurements and calculation of r with literature values of ρv for several materials. In addition, Meunier et al.[4] showed that there was excellent correlation between the SAM maps of acoustic impedance and the elastic stiffness coefficients determined using traditional bulk ultrasonic wave propagation for all four aspects (anterior, lateral, posterior, medial) of femoral cortical bone specimens from the middiaphyses from both a 25- and a 74-year-old male. The relationship between r and the elastic stiffness in gigapascals for a variety of materials, including a number of different bone specimens is shown in Figure 25.3; note that the bone data are nearly linear in the figure. Zimmerman et al.[5] studied the remodeling of femoral cortical bone around hip implants. In addition to using SAM for studying local inhomogeneities at a microstructural level, bulk ultrasonic wave propagation and histology were used to measure elastic properties and geometric characteristics, respectively.

Descriptions of additional low-frequency SAM experiments of cortical bone material properties are presented by Zimmerman et al.[6] The first describes studying the variations in SAM properties at each of the four quadrants within each cross section of femoral cortical bones at each of ten locations along the length of the bones from three elderly males and three elderly females. In

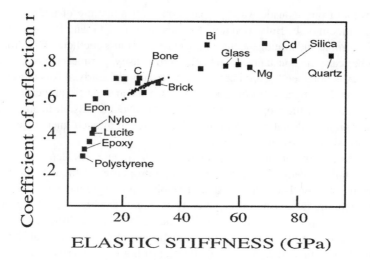

FIGURE 25.3   Reflection coefficient, r, vs. elastic stiffness for a number of materials including bone.

addition to the acoustic properties peaking at midshaft, it was found that the posterior quadrants had significantly lower acoustic impedances than the three other quadrants for the six most proximal sections. At the more distal locations the acoustic impedance values appeared to converge to one another. These findings were found to be in essential agreement with the measurements of both Ashman et al.[7] and Meunier et al.[8] of the longitudinal elastic stiffness coefficient, C_{33}, and density variations along the femur. Both the Zimmerman et al.[6] and Meunier et al.[8] studies showed that most bone sections are quite heterogeneous; i.e., even sections with very low average acoustic properties had numerous locations with high acoustic properties. Thus, the bone remodeling that may create regions of decreased elastic properties does not appear to be uniform throughout the cortical regions of bone.

Meunier et al. also performed a SAM study on human tibial cortical bone similar to their study of human femoral bone.[8] In addition to studying specimens from all four quadrants of the midshafts of 20 pairs of human femurs from both males and females of varying ages, they also studied specimens cut from six different aspects of the midshafts of tibial bones from the same cadavers from which the femoral specimens were obtained. Six aspects were used here because of the near-triangular cross section of the tibiae; this comprised one specimen from each of the three sides of the tibia and one from each corner of the triangular shape. Results similar to those cited above for the femoral specimens were observed for the tibial specimens as well.[8]

A SAM experiment studying the relationship between acoustic impedance and modulus of elasticity is described by Zimmerman et al.[6] for bovine bone. Flattened dumbbell-shaped specimens of bovine femoral bone were prepared from bone sections soaked in varying amounts of NaF. After mechanically testing each specimen to failure they were prepared for low-frequency SAM analysis. Due to the NaF treatment a wide variation of specimen densities was available, and thus it was possible to obtain a linear relationship between SAM-measured acoustic impedance and mechanical testing values of Young's moduli, with an $r^2 = 0.672$ over a range of stiffness moduli from 7.5 to 22.5 GPa. This value is lower than the $r = 0.99$ for a second-order regression between the coefficient of reflection from SAM measurements and the stiffness coefficient, along the femoral bone axis, C_{33}, from transmission measurements by Meunier et al.,[8] and the results cited above from Meunier et al.[4] However, it supports the consistency of the relationship between the acoustic impedance and mechanical properties of bone. These observations present a strong argument supporting the contention that acoustic impedance is directly related to a material property of bone. Indeed, Yoon and

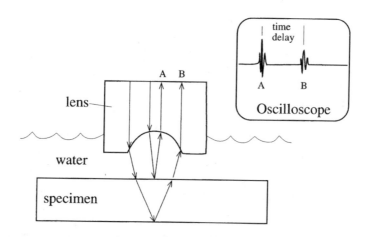

FIGURE 25.4 Acoustic velocity measurement. A specimen is cut 300 to 500 μm thick using a wire saw, submerged in distilled water, and fixed to the bottom of a chamber in a scanning acoustic microscope. A 50-MHz transducer and lens is used to generate and receive acoustic waves in pulse-echo mode. Delay time between waves reflected at the surface (A) and those reflected at the bottom of the specimen (B) are measured at five sites for each specimen. Acoustic velocity is calculated as twice the specimen thickness divided by the delay time. (From Hasegawa, K. et al., *Bone,* 16, 85, 1995. With permission.)

Katz[9] showed how the elastic stiffness coefficient, C_{ij}, for bone could be used to calculate the technical moduli, i.e., Young's, bulk, and shear moduli for Haversian bone.

For acoustic impedance measurements, specimens can be prepared either fresh or embedded, either in epoxy or polymethylmethacrylate (PMMA). Whether fresh or embedded, the specimen is cut with a diamond blade under flowing water and then polished with successively finer and finer grit, down to 0.05 μm for the high-resolution studies and of the order of 1 μm for the low-frequency studies. Ultrasonic cleaning is used to clean the surface of both bone particles and polishing debris. Specimens are kept in a fluid environment and refrigerated until being thawed slowly for the SAM studies.

B. Transmission Velocity Measurements

The preferred orientation of mineral crystals and collagen fibrils within bone give the tissue directional variation in elastic properties or anisotropy. This anisotropy can be quantified using acoustic velocity measurements. The measurement requires cross-sectional and longitudinal sections cut from a bone specimen. The thickness of these sections should be 300 to 500 μm. In previous studies[10-13] acoustic velocity was measured using a scanning acoustic microscope (UH3, Olympus, Tokyo, Japan) with a 50-MHz transducer (V-390, Panametrics, Waltham, MA). This system has a spatial resolution of about 60 μm. Velocity is measured using the pulse-echo method (Figure 25.4). As noted above, the elastic stiffness coefficient for a specimen is calculated as $C = \rho v^2$, where ρ is the density of the specimen and v is the measured acoustic velocity. The accuracy of the acoustic method was verified by measuring the elastic constants of materials with known properties (Figure 25.5). The coefficient of variation for the velocity measurement is 0.3%.[13] An anisotropy ratio (AR) can be calculated from velocities measured along the symmetry axes of the bone (e.g., longitudinal and transverse directions for a long bone).

$$AR = [V_L/V_T]^2 \tag{25.2}$$

where V_L is the longitudinal velocity and V_T is the transverse velocity.

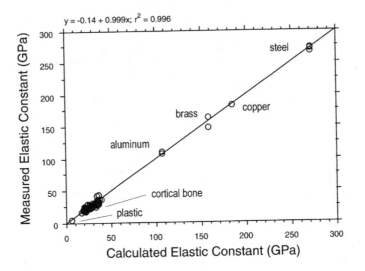

FIGURE 25.5   Verification of the acoustic method. For comparison with measured values, elastic constants of metals and plastics were calculated from mechanical properties provided by the manufacturers. The elastic constants of cortical bone (canine) were measured using a standard technique reported previously.[10] The slope of the regression line was not significantly different from one ($p > 0.8$, t-test), and the y-intercept was not significantly different from zero ($p > 0.7$, t-test). (From Turner, C.H. et al., *J. Biomech.*, 32, 437, 1999. With permission.)

The acoustic method allows anisotropy measurements of the collagen and mineral components of bone tissue. For measurement of the collagen matrix, specimens are demineralized by submerging in 10% ethylenediaminetetraacetic acid (EDTA) with 0.1 *M* Tris buffer adjusted to pH 7.4 for 72 h. This procedure removes all of the inorganic material from the bone.[13] For measurement of the bone mineral, specimens are deproteinized by submerging in 2.5% sodium hypochlorite for 72 h. This procedure removes the protein matrix from the tissue. Verification of deproteinization can be verified by subsequent demineralization, which should leave no organic residue.[13]

The fixation of bone tissue with 10% buffered formalin can affect the acoustic properties of the bone matrix. Takano et al.[12] showed that formalin fixation had no effect on the acoustically derived elastic coefficients of monkey cortical bone, either before or after deproteinization. However, formalin fixation affected the elastic coefficients of the demineralized bone. Demineralized bone was significantly stiffer in both the longitudinal and transverse directions after formalin fixation (Table 25.1). Embedding bone specimens in plastic also can affect the acoustic properties of the bone matrix. Embedding has no effects on the AR of bone but can affect the acoustic properties of demineralized bone (Table 25.2).

Initial studies of canine femoral bone[10] showed that the anisotropy of the bone matrix is considerably different from the anisotropy of the bone mineral (Figure 25.6). Similar results were observed by Takano et al.[12] for human, monkey, cow, and rat bone (Figure 25.7). In particular, the anisotropy of the collagen matrix in rat bone is nearly isotropic, AR = 1. This reflects the more random, woven nature of primary rat bone. Nevertheless, the mineral in rat bone has considerable anisotropy, indicating that mineral anisotropy and collagen anisotropy are not necessarily related.

To a great extent the anisotropy of bone tissue reflects predominant loading patterns. In a recent study, bone tissue anisotropy ratios were measured in dog radii from which the *in vivo* longitudinal strain patterns had been measured. The average AR in the posterior cortex was 1.28 ± 0.01, and the average AR in the anterior cortex was 1.43 ± 0.01 (these values are significantly different at $p < 0.0001$). Interestingly, the posterior cortex is loaded predominantly in compression and the anterior cortex is loaded in tension. Takano et al.[11] found a strong correlation between the peak *in vivo* strains and the AR (Figure 25.8).

TABLE 25.1
Effects of Formalin Fixation on Acoustic Properties of Bone before and after Demineralization or Deproteinization

	C_L (GPa)	C_T (GPa)	AR
(1) Fresh	39.21 ± 0.21	25.15 ± 0.18	1.56 ± 0.01
(2) Fixed	39.28 ± 0.34	25.32 ± 0.20	1.55 ± 0.01
(3) Fresh-demin	4.37 ± 0.02	3.70 ± 0.03	1.18 ± 0.01
(4) Fixed-demin	4.78 ± 0.05	4.01 ± 0.03	1.19 ± 0.01
(5) Fresh-deprot	23.85 ± 0.37	14.83 ± 0.34	1.62 ± 0.04
(6) Fixed-deprot	23.39 ± 0.26	14.56 ± 0.44	1.63 ± 0.04
1–2	$p = 0.96$	$p = 0.26$	$p = 0.24$
3–4 (demin)	$p < 0.001$	$p < 0.001$	$p = 0.37$
5–6 (deprot)	$p = 0.28$	$p = 0.62$	$p = 0.84$

Mean $\pm$ SEM. C_L, longitudinal elastic coefficient; C_T, transverse elastic coefficient; AR, anisotropy ratio; demin, demineralization with EDTA; deprot, deproteinization with NaOCl. p values are from paired t-tests.

TABLE 25.2
Effects of Embedding on Acoustic Properties of Rat Femoral Bone before and after Demineralization or Deproteinization

	V_L (m/s)	V_T (m/s)	AR
(1) Nonembedded	4246 ± 17	3782 ± 20	1.25 ± 0.02
(2) Embedded	4245 ± 20	3818 ± 11	1.24 ± 0.01
(3) Nonembed-demin	1752 ± 22	1718 ± 33	1.04 ± 0.04
(4) Embed-demin	1825 ± 10	1802 ± 10	1.03 ± 0.01
(5) Nonembed-deprot	3385 ± 35	2742 ± 42	1.57 ± 0.05
(6) Embed-deprot	3356 ± 24	2739 ± 21	1.51 ± 0.03
1–2	$p = 0.94$	$p = 0.12$	$p = 0.63$
3–4 (demin)	$p < 0.01$	$p < 0.05$	$p = 0.80$
5–6 (deprot)	$p = 0.50$	$p = 0.95$	$p = 0.31$

Mean $\pm$ SEM. V_L, longitudinal acoustic velocity; V_T, transverse acoustic velocity; AR, anisotropy ratio; demin, demineralization with EDTA; deprot, deproteinization with NaOCl. p values are from paired t-tests.

III. HIGH-FREQUENCY STUDIES

The initial SAM studies of the acoustic properties of osteons and osteon lamellae were reported by Katz and Meunier[15] using bovine femoral cortical bone. Specimens were prepared as described above and imaged using the burst mode at both 400 and 600 MHz in an Olympus UH3 SAM. Three important characteristic traits of osteonic bone were observed for the first time. First, adjacent

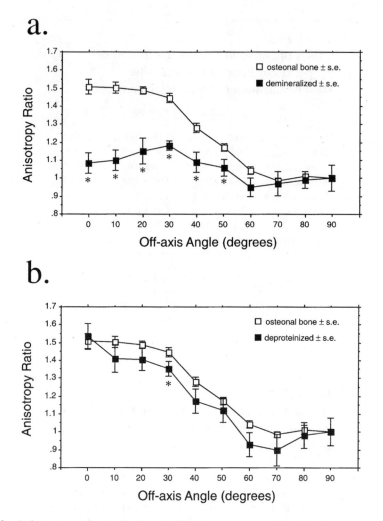

FIGURE 25.6 Anisotropy ratios (velocity divided by transverse velocity) for canine femoral bone. Demineralization (a) significantly decreased the anisotropy ratio at angles 0°, 10°, 20°, 30°, 40°, and 50°, while deproteinization (b) changed the anisotropy ratio only at 30° off-axis. Asterisks indicate significant differences ($p < 0.05$) by paired t-tests. (From Turner, C.H. et al., *Bone,* 17, 85, 1995. With permission.)

lamellae within osteons as well as in the endosteal region alternated regularly in light and dark gray levels. The gray level of a pixel is proportional to the reflection coefficient of the material at the point it is being examined; i.e., it is a measure related to the acoustic impedance of the material. The larger the reflection coefficient, the lighter the gray level; i.e., a white spot represents a larger value of Z at that pixel than does a gray spot, while a black spot would represent the lowest value of Z in the image. Such variations in gray levels on a SAM micrograph for normal bone, corresponding to variations in $Z = \rho v$, can arise due to either a change in local material density (essentially mineral content) and/or changes in elastic properties. The changes themselves can be caused by a number of factors: different orientation of apatite crystallites relative to the bone axis and/or different amount of crystallites in adjacent lamellae. Both of those factors would affect the elastic properties and thus the velocity; the latter factor only would affect the density. Therefore, a complementary technique, such as backscatter scanning electron microscopy (B-SEM) or microcomputed tomography, must be used to determine possible variations in density. This alternation in gray levels implies an alternation between relative compliancy and stiffness in adjacent lamellae. The outermost

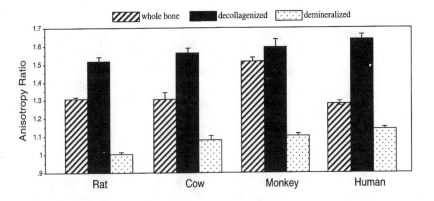

FIGURE 25.7 Anisotropy ratios (AR, means and SEM) for minerialized tissues from rat, cow, human, and monkey femora. AR is given for the mineralized tissue before and after treatment with EDTA (demineralization) and NaOCl (deproteinization). AR for mineralized tissues varied significantly among the groups ($p < 0.001$, by ANOVA). AR for demineralized tissue also varied significantly among the groups ($p < 0.001$), but AR for deproteinized tissue did not vary among the groups ($p > 0.6$). (From Takano, Y. et al., *J. Bone Miner. Res.*, 11, 1292, 1996. With permission.)

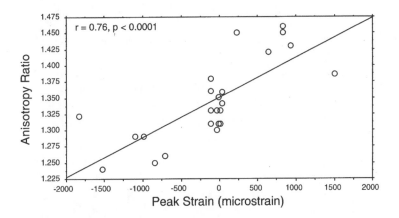

FIGURE 25.8 The anisotropy ratio of the bone tissue was strongly correlated with the measured peak longitudinal strains in the radii of dogs. Anisotropy ratio tended to be greater in regions under tensile (positive) strains and lowest in regions under compressive (negative) strains. (From Takano, Y. et al., *J. Orthop. Res.*, 17, 59, 1999. With permission.)

lamella of each osteon in an image always had a dark gray level, indicating that it was a more compliant lamella. Also, the outermost lamella of adjacent abutting osteons always exhibited essentially the same dark gray level to the degree that the osteons appeared to interdigitate (blend) at their borders. The B-SEM micrographs showed that the osteons are structurally distinct even though they overlap in acoustic impedance (and thus essentially in elastic properties). This will be illustrated in the following discussion of similar SAM observations made with human femoral cortical bone specimens prepared in the same manner described above.

Figure 25.9A is a SAM micrograph of the same specimen of human femoral cortical bone, cut transversely to the bone axis, described in previous studies by Katz and Meuiner,[15,16] using a 600 MHz burst-mode lens (120° aperture angle). Clearly, the same three observations made with the canine femoral cortical bone are made here, i.e., alternating gray levels, outermost lamellae dark,

A

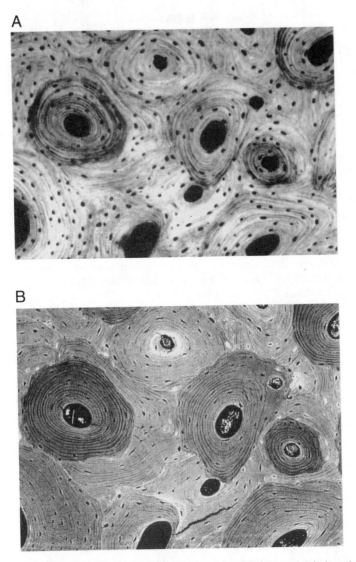

B

FIGURE 25.9   (A) 600 MHz burst-mode (aperture angle 120°, full scale *x* dimension is 1 mm) SAM micrograph of a portion of human femoral cortical bone cut transverse to the bone axis. (B) B-SEM micrograph of the same region shown in Figure 25.4a. The clear delineation of individual Haversian structures is observed here.

and interdigitation of the gray levels of the outermost lamellae of adjacent abutting osteons. Figure 25.9B is a backscatter SEM of the same area shown in Figure 25.9A. It is clear here as well that the adjacent abutting osteons are separated as opposed to the interdigitation (overlap or blending) of gray levels seen on Figure 25.9A. The interpretation of the gray levels in the B-SEM is as follows: the lighter the pixel, the higher the relative density; the darker the pixel, the lower the relative density. This apparent "blending" of the acoustic (and therefore elastic) properties of the outermost lamellae of adjacent abutting osteons may also impact on the modeling of bone as a hierarchical structure–materials composite.[17] Instead of requiring a compliant interface (matrix) between stiff hollow fibers (osteons) in the model, it may be that each osteon provides its own compliant "matrix" via the outermost lamellae, which thus provides the net effect of osteons (stiff solid hollow cylinders) interfacing with one another through the interdigitating compliant properties of the adjacent abutting outermost lamellae.

A

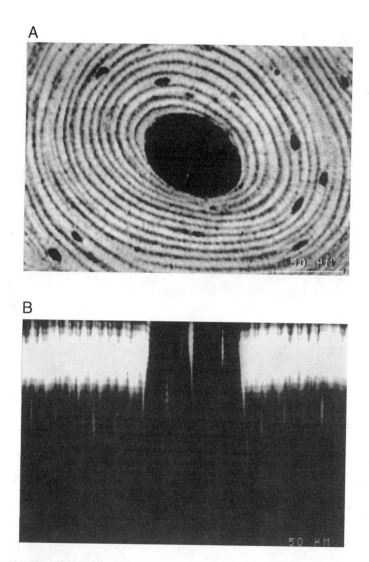

B

FIGURE 25.10 (A) 600-MHz burst-mode (aperture angle 120°, full scale x dimension is 250 μm) SAM micrograph of the dark Haversian system seen in the upper left-hand guadrant of Figure 25.9A clearly showing the variations in gray levels of alternate lamellae. (B) x–z SAM image along the line through the midpoint on Figure 25.10A (full scale x is 250 μm; full scale z is 50 μm). The level white band shows the sample was flat and well aligned perpendicular to the lens. Slight incursions in the flat surface reflect, in part, polishing artifacts and changes in material properties.

Figure 25.10A is a 600-MHz burst-mode (120° aperture; full-scale x dimension 250 μm) of the dark osteon seen in the upper left-hand region of Figure 25.9A; the alternation of gray levels in adjacent lamellae is clearly delineated. Figure 25.10B is the x–z SAM image along a line through the midpoint of Figure 25.10A (full-scale x dimension is 250 μm; full-scale z is 50 μm). x–z images are obtained as follows: the lens is vibrated along the x direction (left to right) while the stage is held stationary at a location along the y direction (front to back). The lens is lowered (defocused) to a specific depth below the surface (the z direction) and then scans upward in z while the lens vibrates in x. The resulting image is an acoustic interference profile in the x–z plane providing additional information about the acoustic properties of the material at each pixel along the x line. The level nature of the top of the broad band shows that the specimen surface is perpendicular to

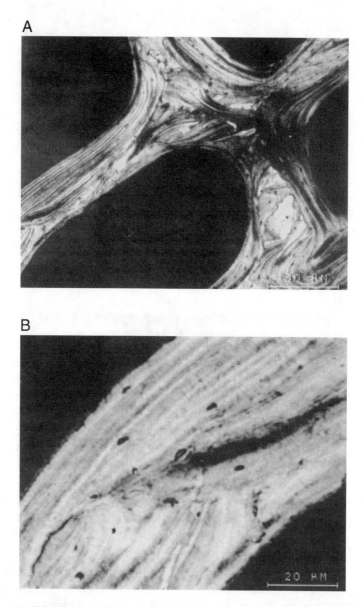

FIGURE 25.11 (A) 600-MHz burst-mode (aperture 120°, full scale x dimension is 250 μm) SAM micrograph of a trabecular portion of a specimen of sheep femoral condyle showing clearly the same alternations in gray levels in the lamellar structure as observed in the osteonic lamellae of Figure 25.10A. (B) 600-MHz burst-mode (aperture angle 120°, full scale x dimension 100 μm) SAM of the lower left-hand quadrant of Figure 25.11A. The disruption of the lamellar structure and properties at the tip of the lunate-shaped defect is observed.

the lens, a necessary condition to ensure that experimental artifacts are minimized. The slight incursions in the broad band reflect a combination of property differences and possible polishing artifacts. The separation between the solid broad white band and the scattered narrower white lines below is related to the average subsurface longitudinal acoustic velocity.

The x–z image is a generalized example of a form of interference pattern between longitudinal and surface waves generated when a lens whose aperture angle is greater than a critical angle is defocused and raised while the specimen is motionless. The signal that is produced as the lens is raised is known as a $V(z)$ curve. Spectral analysis (Fourier transform) of this $V(z)$ curve will provide the Rayleigh wave velocity for high-Z materials such as ceramics and metals. However, for bone because of the high attenuation due to porosity, and "because the low Rayleigh velocity puts the Rayleigh angle outside the useful aperture angle of a water-coupled lens,"[3] it has not proved possible to obtain a Rayleigh wave velocity. However, Briggs also points out that "with care, at higher resolution in reflection, lateral longitudinal waves can be made to perform a role very similar to that of the Rayleigh waves in stiffer materials."[3] This last condition is made use of in analyzing the x–z curves.

The same alternations in lamellae gray levels in cortical Haversian bone is observed in trabecular bone. Figure 25.11A is a 600-MHz burst-mode (120° aperture; full scale x dimension 250 μm) of cancellous bone from a sheep femoral condyle. Figure 25.11B is a SAM micrograph taken with the same lens, over a scan range of 100 μm in the x dimension, of the region surrounding the lunate-shaped defect seen in the lower left-hand corner of Figure 25.11A. In addition to the same gray level alternations in adjacent lamellae, the effect of the defect on the structural organization and properties is also clearly delineated. Similar observations of the alternation in lamella gray levels have recently been made in trabecular bone from a human femoral condyle.[18]

REFERENCES

1. Lemons, R.A. and Quate, C.F., Acoustic microscope-scanning version, *Appl. Phys. Lett.*, 24, 163, 1974.
2. Beyer, R. and Lechter, S., *Physical Ultrasonics*, Academic Press, New York, 1969.
3. Briggs, G.A.D., *Acoustic Microscopy*, Clarendon Press, Oxford, 1992.
4. Meunier, A., Katz, J.L., Christel, P., and Sedel, K., A reflection scanning acoustic microscope for bone and bone-biomaterials interface studies, *J. Orthop. Res.*, 6, 770, 1988.
5. Zimmerman, M.C., Meunier, A., Katz, J.L., and Christel P., The evaluation of cortical bone remodeling with a new ultrasonic technique, *IEEE Trans. Biomed. Eng.*, 37, 433, 1990.
6. Zimmerman, M.C., Harten, R.D., Shieh, S.J., et al., Techniques and applications of scanning acoustic microscopy in bone remodeling studies, in *Oxford Textbook of Orthopaedic Trauma*, J.A. Buckwalter et al., Eds., Oxford University Press, in press.
7. Ashman, R.B., Cowin, S.C., van Buskirk, W.C., and Rice, J.C., A continous wave technique for the measurement of the elastic properties of cortical bone, *J. Biomech.*, 17, 349, 1984.
8. Meunier, A., Riot, O., Katz, J.L., et al., Inhomogeneities in anisotropic elastic constrants of cortical bone," *IEEE 1989 Ultrasonic Symposium*, IEEE, New York, 1015, 1989.
9. Yoon, H.S. and Katz, J.L., Ultrasonic wave propagation in human cortical bone. II. Measurement of elastic properties and microhardness, *J. Biomech.*, 9, 459, 1976.
10. Turner, C.H., Chandran, A., and Pidaparti, R.M., The anisotropy of osteonal bone and its ultrastructural implications, *Bone*, 17, 85, 1995.
11. Takano, Y., Turner, C.H., Forwood, M.R., et al., Elastic anisotropy and collagen orientation of osteonal bone are dependent on the mechanical strain distribution, *J. Orthop. Res.*, 17, 59, 1999.
12. Takano, Y., Turner, C.H., and Burr, D.B., Mineral anisotropy in mineralized tissues is similar among species and mineral growth occurs independently of collagen orientation in rats: results from acoustic velocity measurements, *J. Bone Miner. Res.*, 11, 1292, 1996.
13. Hasegawa, K., Turner, C.H., Recker, R.R., et al., Elastic properties of osteoporotic bone measured by scanning acoustic microscopy, *Bone*, 16, 85, 1995.
14. Turner, C.H., Rho, J., Takano, Y., et al., The elastic properties of trabecular and cortical bone tissues are similar: results from two microscopic measurement techniques, *J. Biomech.*, 32, 437, 1999.
15. Katz, J.L. and Meunier, A., Scanning acoustic microscope studies of the elastic properties of osteons and osteon lamellae, *J. Biomech. Eng.*, 115, 543, 1993.
16. Katz, J.L. and Meunier, A., Material properties of single osteons and osteonic lamellae using high frequency scanning acoustic microscopy, in *Bone Structure and Remodeling*, Odgaard, A. and Weinans, H., Eds., World Scientific Publishing, Singapore, 1995, 157.
17. Katz, J.L., On the anisotropy of Young's modulus of bone, *Nature*, 283, 105, 1980.
18. Bumrerraj, S., M.S. project, Department of Biomedical Engineering, Case Western Reserve University, Cleveland, OH, May, 1999.

26 Peripheral Quantitative Computed Tomography for Evaluating Structural and Mechanical Properties of Small Bone

José Luis Ferretti

CONTENTS

I. INTRODUCTION

Quantitative computed tomography (QCT) technology offers many opportunities for the investigation of bone biomechanics because it determines some indicators of bone properties that are

TABLE 26.1
Major pQCTs on the Market

Machine and Characteristics	Sample Diameter, mm	Voxel Max Size, μm	Max SV Path, mm	Min Slice Thickness
XCT 960, research option, good for large bones	88	90–690	120	2.50 mm
XCT Research SA, formerly 960 A, wide size–thickness range, variable slice capacity, avoids repositioning	90	90–500	180	0.75 mm
XCT Research M, narrower, softer X-ray beam, higher and controlled resolution	50	70–500	180	0.55 mm
XCT Microscope, higher mechanical precision, smaller source–center distance, special for thin cortical shells, quasi-histomorphometric scan, three-dimensional network reconstruction	50	30–300	180	0.13–0.50 mm
Scanco μ-CT 20, ultrahigh definition, static histomorphometry allowed, three-dimensional network reconstruction, no bone densitometry allowed	17	8–14	50	30 μm

relevant to bone strength, namely, the mass, the mechanical quality, and the spatial distribution of bone material.[1-11]

Peripheral QCT was developed as a small-field, high-resolution extension of the existing QCT systems,[12-15] to measure the peripheral skeleton with a substantial improvement of the image definition. Currently available pQCT machines perform transverse scans of a wide size range of regions of interest, from large body segments such as the whole human head, neck, or thigh, to tiny excised bones such as mouse femurs or vertebrae. The gantry size of the machines limits the size of the specimen or body segment to be studied.

Stratec/Norland (Pforzheim, Germany) produces the widest range of pQCT machines in the market. These were developed from the original, XCT-960 model (the only pQCT device with FDA approval by 1993[15,16]), which allowed a "research option" for studying relatively small bones. Some of these models are especially adapted for that purpose. The XCT Research SA (SA refers to small animals) is designed to study bones of animals ranging in size from sheep or primates to rats *in vivo* or *in vitro*, and the high-resolution XCT Research M (M refers to mouse) is used to study specimens ranging from mice to ferrets, even *in vivo*. A special achievement, the XCT Microscope, was also developed for quasi-histomorphometric analysis of small excised bones at a very high resolution, up to allowing the measurement of individual trabeculae. Scanco Medical AG (Bassersdorf, Switzerland) produces ultrahigh-resolution (microtomographic) machines[17,18] as the μ-CT-20, which is able to analyze two- and three-dimensional histomorphometrical images of trabecular bone specimens but cannot determine bone density values. Some disadvantages of the high-resolution equipment are the high cost and the long determination time. Table 26.1 shows some distinctive characteristics of the equipment described.

II. WHAT IS A pQCT MACHINE?

A basic pQCT machine consists of two major components: a scanner unit and a control/analysis computer system. The scanner unit contains (1) a source that emits a very narrow X-ray beam; (2) a detector of the emitted radiation fixed at a short distance from the source, which can measure the intensity of the radiation and the attenuation produced by the tissues studied; and (3) a mechanical system allowing radial, transverse, and axial displacements of the source–detector couple in order to achieve different scanning positions of the bone (Figure 26.1A). The bone sample

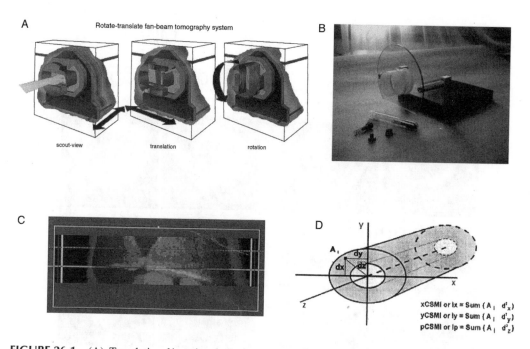

FIGURE 26.1 (A) Translational/rotational displacements of a pQCT machine (XCT-960). (Courtesy of Stratec Medizintechnik GmbH, Germany.) (B) Standard support and tube provided for positioning rodent limbs and excised long bones for a pQCT measurement in the XCT-960 A. (C) Example of a pQCT scout-view (human radius). (Courtesy of Stratec Medizintechnik GmbH, Germany.) (D) Didactical representation of the meaning and calculation of the rectangular (related to x and y axes, relevant to bending analyses) and polar versions (related to z axis, relevant to torsional analyses) of the cross-sectional moments of inertia of a bone diaphysis (see Equation 26.2).

is centrally located between the source and the detector with the aid of special supports adapted to *in vivo* or *in vitro* conditions (Figure 26.1B). As a first step, when the measurement is started, successive transverse displacements of the source–detector couple, repeated after small axial displacements, produce a computed radiograph or scout-view of the bone piece along its longitudinal axis, resembling a standard densitometric (DEXA) picture (Figure 26.1C). Reference points on the screen allow selection of any convenient position along the bone axis. At that point, a series of transverse measurements are then performed after successive, partial rotation displacements of the couple until completion of a 180° excursion (translate/rotate mechanism).

The computer system controls the complete scanning procedure and integrates the information obtained into a composed image of the bone "slice," the tomographic scan that is shown on the screen (Figure 26.2), and analyzes that scan as described below. The scan is integrated by the computer system through a complex procedure known as "backprojection with filtration." The complete field scanned is divided into a number of tiny square areal units (pixels). As the tomographic bone slice has a predetermined, constant thickness, the pixels actually represent the bases of volume units which are more properly referred to as "voxels." The number of voxels per field is a fixed characteristic of each type of machine. The operator can change the size of the field, but not the number of voxels in the field. Therefore, the smaller the field selected, the smaller the voxels and the greater the information contained per unit of field area (i.e., the resolution of the machine), and vice versa. For the earlier Stratec machines the voxel resolution was $1/128$ of the variable scanning diameter.[15] The new machines provide 1024×1024 voxels. Some improvements such as automatic contextual segmentation algorithms to identify bone compartments[19] or post-processing of the images in a separate workstation with a region grow and skeletonization step[20] may approach some histomorphometric assessments of bone structure.

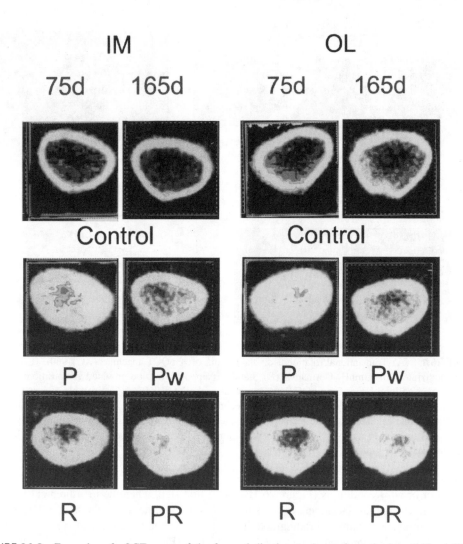

FIGURE 26.2 Examples of pQCT scans of the femoral distal metaphyses from the immobilized (IM) or overloaded legs (OL) of rats otherwise untreated or given anabolic doses of hPTH(1-38) for 75 days (P), withdrawn with no other treatment (Pw), or sequenced by risedronate (PR,R) during further 90 days[30,31,40] obtained with an adapted XCT-960 machine.

III. WHAT DOES pQCT MEASURE?

As an essentially absorptiometric technique, the pQCT measures only the attenuation of the radiation passing through the whole tomographic slice. This is the information from which the scan is performed. The magnitude of the attenuation depends on both the mass and the number of electrons in the atoms of the elements present in the tomographic slice, so that bone minerals are most relevant for such measurement. The attenuation is expressed in cm^{-1} units as the linear attenuation coefficient (μ, a variable depending on the absorbing material) of the relationship between the intensities (I_o, I) of the emitted radiation before and after absorption, according to the equation

$$I = I_o \cdot D^{-\mu d} \tag{26.1}$$

where D is the density of the absorber in g/cm^3, and d is its layer thickness in cm.

The integration algorithm calculates the attenuation coefficient value corresponding to every particular voxel. This is a correlate of the amount (content) of absorbing matter in the voxel. However, the machine is unable to assess the absolute "mineral density" value of each voxel as a direct measurement. A special hydroxyapatite phantom is provided for this purpose and provides a particularly stable reference that does not require calibration too frequently.[21] The phantom allows the machine to transform the attenuation coefficients of every voxel into the "volumetric mineral content" (vBMC) and "volumetric mineral density" (vBMD = vBMC/voxel volume) data that are provided as the outcome. The machine is also able to assign different, default (rainbow scheme) or customizable voxel colors to successive ranges of attenuation/density values. Thus, the integrated image of the bone slice can be given a "semiquantitative" densitometric aspect (see Figure 26.2).

The machines are arranged for assigning automatically a zero attenuation/density value to every voxel in the image corresponding to a measurement of pure fat.[22] Therefore, any above-zero attenuation measured for a given voxel should represent a certain content of matter denser than the fat it contains. Regardless of whether that corresponds to a soft or a hard (mineral-containing) tissue, or a mixture of both, the automatic reference to the phantom scale forces the machine to take and express that value as a "mineral content." The energy of the radiation used is specifically selected in order to minimize the error involved in such estimations of "mineral," as well as to optimize the "separation" of bone from soft tissues. On summing up the individual values assigned to each voxel, the machine can determine the mineral mass or vBMC and the vBMD of the whole-bone slice or of a selected region of it. The vBMD represents the vBMC/bone volume relationship of the region and is usually expressed in mg/cm^3.

It is critical to interpret correctly what kind of "bone density" the machine assesses. No available absorptiometric device can measure the "true" density of an ideal piece of pure "solid," absolutely pore-free bone substance (a hardly available specimen, if ever!). The established value of about 1.9 g of matter/cm^3 of solid tissue volume for such a material could only be estimated by calculation from what is known about its fractional composition. Practically, assuming it to be 58% matrix + 42% mineral, the following approximate estimation can be derived.

$$\text{Matrix density} = 1.0 \text{ g/cm}^3 \times 0.58 \qquad = 0.58 \text{ g/cm}^3$$

$$\text{Mineral density} = 3.2 \text{ g/cm}^3 \times 0.42 \qquad = 1.34 \text{ g/cm}^3$$

$$\text{Specific density of the solid bone matter} = 1.92 \text{ g/cm}^3$$

(matrix + mineral composite)

What is actually measurable in practice is the density of the whole bone including all hard substance, cells, vessels, marrow, etc. This is known as the "apparent" or Archimedean bone density. This concept is valid for the full range of bone porosity of either woven or lamellar, cortical or trabecular bone tissue, and also applies to bones as organs or to whole skeletons. The pQCT machines assess only this aspect of bone density in the bone slice. Moreover, they merely compare the absorptiometric data to a phantom scale of volumetric mineral densities. For that reason their outcome (vBMD) is expressed as a mineral mass per volume unit of whole-bone tissue.

Despite that limitation, the vBMD value could be regarded as a noninvasive indicator of the mechanical quality (specific stiffness, or elastic modulus) of the "solid" bone tissue. In fact, it represents at least one (the mineral amount per unit volume) of the most relevant determinants of that property. In support of that assumption, a close correlation between the chemically assessed "vBMD" (ash content per unit of bone volume) and the mechanically determined elastic modulus of the "solid" (cortical) bone tissue has been verified repeatedly.[23-25]

It has also been demonstrated that the pQCT-assessed vBMD is more representative of the actual bone material quality than the "areal" bone mineral density (BMD) expressed as a mass of mineral per (square) unit of projected bone area provided by DEXA.[1-9,26,27] A further advantage of the pQCT-assessed vBMD values is that they are independent of the rotation of the bone slice during the measurement, as well as (to some extent) of the bone size or shape. In addition, the information provided by the pQCT determinations can be processed by the machine in order to (1) distinguish between trabecular and cortical bone in many instances,[3,22,28,29] and (2) calculate a number of variables which describe many aspects of bone architecture,[4-11,22,29-40] as commented below.

The machine is "blind" concerning the type of tissue under measurement in each voxel because the vBMD is calculated from the attenuation coefficient value of the whole voxel, which reflects its bulk mineral mass content. In other words, voxels with trabecular bone of relatively low porosity and high "true" mineral density could not be distinguished from those containing cortical bone with relatively high microporosity if both of them show a similar attenuation coefficient. This pitfall gives rise to the so-called partial volume effect which is discussed below.

However, both the distinction between bone- and no-bone-containing voxels and the histological limitation between trabecular and cortical tissue are usually clear enough in practice to overcome the above inconveniences. The menu of operator-defined modes provided by the "Special Analysis Software" in the Norland/Stratec machines deals generally quite well with that purpose, as described below.

IV. HOW DOES A pQCT MACHINE OPERATE?

Before starting the measurement, the operator must check the apparatus through the quality assurance steps, and then adjust the measurement parameters such as bone length, voxel size, number of steps in the scout-view scan, position of the reference line, number of sites to measure, and their distances to the reference line. These procedures vary for the different machines.

Some recommendations have to be followed concerning the management of the samples. As attenuation values for air are lower than for fat, it is convenient to avoid any interference from the air that may surround or be inside the bone sample, which would produce "negative density" values. Although this may not be relevant for in vivo or whole-limb studies, it is recommended that operators (1) avoid measuring dried bones containing some air within the pores, as well as (2) immerse the fresh bones into water in tubes (see Figure 26.1B) during any in vitro determination. Freezing the samples should not interfere the absorptiometric determinations, provided that air was not allowed to go into the bone cavity. However, it is not advisable to freeze the bones for long periods of time (say, more than 1 month) if investigators also aim to perform mechanical testing on the same samples.

Positioning the sample is critical for the measurement. Some special devices as limb clamps for in vivo studies (see Figure 26.1B) can be provided on request, but special supports or cradles usually would have to be prepared by each laboratory according to the particular aim of the study. The software helps to improve the reproducibility by detecting the same region of interest from one measurement to the next by testing the number of voxels.[15,16] The reproducibility of the determinations concerning repositioning should be assessed by calculating the corresponding coefficients of variation, for which quite low values have been reported.[26,27,41,42]

Different field/voxel sizes can be conveniently selected according to the bone studied in order to optimize the resolution of the measurement. Ideally, the bone slice should fit within the scanned field allowing just a minimal margin all around. Care should be taken to prevent the bone image from reaching the margins of the field; otherwise important sources of errors in the measurement could be introduced.

The first step of the determination is to obtain the scout-view, which is automatically made by the machine, and to define the scan sites on the screen. This can be arranged either symmetrically or asymmetrically concerning the starting reference line. However, there is a length limitation for the scout analysis (see Table 26.1) that restricts the performance of multiple slices in a single measurement. Following the scout-view, a single command initiates the whole CT measurement automatically under screen control to detect the misplacement of the sample within the field. The image obtained is then displayed, ready for analysis (see Figure 26.2). Special tools ("Loop" functions) help when performing the standardized or customized analysis of the images. The most critical requisite for performing a good analysis (and hence that most subjected to discussion and further elaboration in the future) is the image definition concerning both the boundary between the bone section and the surrounding tissues and the one between the cortical and trabecular bone regions.

The Special Analysis Software in the Norland/Stratec machines (reference is made here to the newest available versions, 5.20 for XCT 960 A and 5.40 for XCT SA) allows customizing the methods (Modes) for separating (1) the soft tissue from the outer edge of the bone (ContMode); (2) the trabecular region from the cortical shell within the ContMode-defined bone to obtain a trabecular and a "cortical-subcortical" value (PeelMode); and (3) the cortical bone from the trabecular bone to obtain a cortical bone value (CortMode), as follows.

A. CONTMODE

A preselected or user-defined attenuation threshold (the THBD threshold) causes the machine to eliminate automatically any voxel with an attenuation value below that level. A 0.5 cm^{-1} THBD value is recommended for that purpose (at this point it is possible to set the attenuation thresholds directly in milligrams per cubic centimeter as a resource to standardize the procedure for the different machines). As the machine automatically works centripetally in this mode until a complete bone perimeter is defined from the outside, every soft tissue surrounding the bone is removed that way (ContMode 1). For relatively large, regularly shaped bones, a couple of iterative contour-detection procedures can also test the neighboring voxels with respect to either default or user-defined thresholds. This algorithm can be additionally activated in order to optimize the selection of a particular voxel as a boundary one (ContModes 2 and 3).

B. PEELMODE

Working now from the outside bone edge in, this algorithm concentrically peels away an operator-defined percent of the outside area of the bone (usually 55% for the human radius; different values should be tried for animal bones). This default procedure (PeelMode 1) peels away (1) the outside cortical shell; (2) an inner area that is part cortical and part trabecular; and (3) a small portion of the inner area that is purely trabecular. It works well when the trabecular region is regularly shaped and hence the remaining, inner region can be considered to be purely trabecular.

PeelMode 1 may be unsatisfactory otherwise, including when the trabecular bone area must be analyzed as completely as possible. In these cases an operator-defined, inner attenuation threshold (the THBD2 threshold) should be selected (proposedly, 0.63 cm^{-1} for rat bones) to separate a "trabecular" (attenuation values lower than threshold) and a "cortical-subcortical" region (values higher than threshold). A filtering process is used to ignore any high-attenuation voxel isolated within the trabecular area as well as in areas that are not continuous (PeelMode 2). If the operator wants also to eliminate the "subcortical" region as completely as possible, an additional peeling of the remaining area down to an indicated percentage can be ordered (PeelMode 3). An additional percentage of peeling can also be performed as an attempt to eliminate completely any high-density voxel inside the trabecular area which could influence the trabecular density (PeelMode 4).

When the cortical shell is well defined in the scan, the cortical/trabecular boundary can also be iteratively defined by testing the maximal attenuation gradient between the successive voxels working from the outside in, perpendicularly to the tangents to every voxel on the outer bone edge. This way the trabecular/cortical boundary is defined as a continuous chain of selected, high-slope voxels around a complete circle (PeelMode 5). This procedure works well for *in vivo* rat studies. Additional peeling as in PeelModes 3 and 4 can also be commanded (PeelModes 6 and 7). These modes may be useful when PeelMode 5 worked well for performing serial studies or if a low resolution had to be employed, respectively.

Abnormalities such as a coupling of a high attenuation value and a low trabecular density, or a high-density pocket within a low-trabecular-density region, can be identified by displaying the highest attenuation coefficient in trabecular bone, which allows one to see the density shifts (PeelMode 20).

C. CortMode

The cortical shell can be separated by selecting an adequate threshold (the THCRT2 threshold; a 0.93 cm^{-1} value is recommended for rat bones, but in skeletally immature animals — younger than 9 months — it should be lowered to around 0.76 cm^{-1}). The machine will automatically peel away every voxel showing an attenuation value below the selected one, i.e., the "trabecular" bone region (CortMode 1). When working at low resolutions, the remaining voxels showing a comparatively low attenuation with respect to their neighbors can also be additionally peeled away in order to ignore any low-density point within the cortical area (CortMode 2). An iterative contour detection algorithm, analogous to that employed in PeelMode 5 for the trabecular region, can also be employed to define the cortical shell from both the outer and inner sides (CortMode 3). This procedure may work well for lower resolutions such as those employed in *in vivo* studies. The cortical region can also be defined after setting the outside bone edge by CortMode 1, working in, selecting a maximal attenuation for the inner threshold first and then lowering it until the whole cortex is displayed (CortMode 4). In many instances, the selected modes succeed in defining the trabecular and cortical regions of interest (ROIs), which are shown on the screen. Then, special functions as CalcBD and CortBD yield the results of total, trabecular, cortical-subcortical, and cortical vBMD (in mg/cm^3) and the cross-sectional areas of the corresponding bone portions (in mm^2) as determined.

A two-color histogram represents the proportional distribution for total and trabecular voxels (the latter are characterized as those featuring within the trabecular region defined by the PeelMode) according to their attenuation values. The greater the accumulation of trabecular voxels in the "low-attenuation" region of the histogram, the better the boundary definition achieved between the trabecular and cortical ROIs. By modifying the selected thresholds the operator can improve that definition up to a certain limit. Bone images could, hence, be classified as apparently "well" or "poorly" defined concerning the sharpness (or the reliability) of the trabecular/cortical boundary. The standard analyses of cortical and trabecular bone provided by the machines obviously refer to the first case.

Nevertheless, whatever the method employed for defining the cortical and trabecular regions, the outcome will always be affected by the partial volume effect (PVE).[22,43] The PVE is a source of error in the determination of the bone areas derived from the unavoidable inclusion of voxels that are not filled with mineralized tissue. It derives from the "blindness" of the machine as commented above and may lead to underestimation of the regional vBMD measurements that may exceed 15%. By optimizing the above modes, as well as by selecting the smallest voxel sizes available, the PVE can be minimized, although it raises a severe limitation for the analyses of relatively thin cortical shells unless the definition achieved was actually very high.

The only way to test the PVE interference in the interpretation of the pQCT data is by measuring bones of the same kind but of different size and cortical thickness. On plotting the assessed cortical vBMD data (y) against the cortical thickness (x), a constant (horizontal) relationship for the greater values of the latter will be observed; however, toward the lowest end of the range the points should tend to shift to the lower-left region of the graph. This would point out the existence of the PVE and allow measurement of its relative significance.

V. WHAT KIND OF VARIABLES AND BONE PROPERTIES ARE MEASURED BY pQCT?

Many bone variables can be measured by pQCT in different long bones from small animals, principally in the midshafts (in order to correlate the data with those of bending tests[37]) in the metaphyseal regions (where trabecular bone and remodeling are present in most species[44]), in femoral necks, and, tentatively, in vertebral bodies and hemimandibles, too. The available data can be classified as follows according to their relevance as indicators of the different aspects of bone mechanical quality, namely, "mass," "apparent density," architectural design, and structural stiffness and strength.

A. INDICATORS OF BONE "MASS"

The vBMC of the trabecular, cortical, and total bone regions (0.6 to 1.9% *in vitro* and *in vivo* precision, 1.7 to 3.2% with repositioning with the XCT 960 A), as well as the cortical bone area (1.3 to 2.4%, and average 3.8%, respectively), reflect the amount of mineralized tissue in the corresponding parts of the bone section.[17,45] Close correlations have been found between the pQCT and histomorphometrically assessed values of cortical area and other variables in rat tibiae and femorae.[40,42] These indicators, especially those for cortical bone, should be regarded as relevant to bone strain and structural stiffness and strength in longitudinal compression.[46-52] The trabecular bone area (as arbitrarily defined by the above modes) is not directly suitable for a proper biomechanical estimation of bone quality. The total bone area (calculated as the whole "solid" section area within the outer edge of the bone, regardless of the inner tissue structure) should only provide information on bone size.

B. INDICATORS OF BONE "APPARENT DENSITY"

The vBMD of the trabecular region can be measured very precisely (0.4 to 0.6% in rats *in vitro* and *in vivo*, 2.9% with repositioning[8]) and with a high statistical power, especially at the distal-femoral and proximal-tibial metaphyses. Changes can be detected within a few weeks after gonadectomy or treatment with raloxifene or PTH in small groups of rodents, much sooner than when employing DEXA.[8,9,27,28,41,53-55] Rather than to represent a true "material property," the trabecular vBMD should be regarded as a correlate of the structural stiffness and strength of the trabecular network, i.e., a mechanical quality indicator expressed at the tissue level of complexity.[56,57]

The vBMD of the cortical region (0.6 to 1.9% precision *in vitro* and *in vivo*, 3.3% with repositioning[8,10,53]), represents the "true" vBMD of the solid bone substance. Therefore, it may be regarded as indicative of one of the chief determinants of the intrinsic stiffness (elastic modulus) of the "solid" bone tissue.[7,23-25] Moreover, it has been shown to correlate well with the bone-breaking force in femoral diaphyses and necks of rats and mice and in the human radius.[11,29,51] However, especially when measuring thin cortices at low resolutions, PVE-derived errors in the cortical area measurements (not in the vBMC determination) may lead to underestimation of the vBMD.[22,41,51,58] High-resolution techniques should overcome this problem.[17] Changes in the cortical vBMD are much slower than those in the trabecular density.[8]

No directionality could be ascribed to these "qualitative" indicators because bone material or structural anisotropy is disregarded by the absorptiometric determinations. The total vBMD of the slice (a combination of the trabecular and cortical vBMDs) should not be an indicator of any particular bone mechanical property, analogously to the areal BMD provided by DEXA.[20]

C. INDICATORS OF BONE ARCHITECTURAL QUALITY

The equatorial and polar second moments of inertia of the cross-sectional bone area (xCSMI, pCSMI; CV = 6.4% with the XCT-960 A in mice) are relevant to long-bone stiffness and strength in bending and torsion, respectively.[1-7,29-37,39,47,52,59,60] The Norland/Stratec machines calculate the CSMIs of the total or cortical bone areas as

$$\text{CSMI} = \Sigma \ (A_i \cdot d_i^2) \tag{26.2}$$

where A_i is the area of an individual voxel within the bone section and d_i is the distance from the center of that area to the reference, bending (x, y) or torsion (z) axis (see Figure 26.1D). As seen from the formula, the CSMI values (given in mm^4) increase linearly with bone mass (A), but are also exponentially proportional to the distance (d^2) of the bone material from the reference axis. Therefore, the equatorial and polar CSMIs are true indicators of the bending or torsional stiffness/strength of the assayed long bone, respectively, regardless of the bone material quality.[7,10,11]

The machines can also measure the cross-sectional diameters, endosteal and periosteal perimeters, and average cortical thickness. These variables may help to evaluate the modeling-derived changes provoked by growth or by anabolic or anticatabolic treatments.[8] However, they do not affect the quality of the architectural design or the mechanical competence of long bones as much as do the CSMIs.[1-3,7]

D. INDICATORS OF WHOLE-BONE QUALITY

The mechanical properties of the whole bones as measured by pQCT exceed the possibilities of standard densitometry.[5-8,48] The structural stiffness and strength of long hollow tubular structures are generally proportional to the product CSMI $\times E$ (E being the elastic modulus of the material of which the structure is made[61]). The elastic modulus can only be assessed mechanically, but it could be reasonably estimated by the apparent mineral density of the "solid" bone.[23-25] Hence, on replacing E by the pQCT-assessed vBMD of the cortical bone in Equation 26.2, the authors' group developed the so-called bone strength index (BSI) as the product

$$\text{BSI} = \text{xCSMI} \cdot \text{cortical vBMD} \tag{26.3}$$

The author's group has shown that this BSI correlates strongly with the actual three-point bending strength (breaking force) in a large sample of rat femur shafts, regardless of bone size and experimental conditions (Figure 26.3).[5] Conversely, weak correlations were observed between the breaking force and the DEXA-assessed, areal BMD of the central diaphyseal region of the same bones. This is evidence of the greater ability of the tomographic BSI to describe the bone strength in the assayed conditions. Besides this BSI (xBSI), the pQCT machines also calculate its bending "y" and "torsion" versions (yBSI, pBSI, for which a mechanical validation is still needed), by using the yCSMI or the pCSMI (see Figure 26.1D) instead of the xCSMI in Equation 26.3, respectively.

The BSI concept should not be freely generalized to the analysis of any bone region or method of deformation. Specially adapted formulae should be derived in order to achieve further, suitable BSIs for every method of bone deformation applied to every skeletal region of interest.[5,11] The Norland/Stratec machines provide also another kind of BSI for long bones, the stress/strain index (SSI),[62,63] calculated as

$$\text{SSI} = \frac{\text{pCSMI} \cdot \text{cortical vBMD}_i}{d_{\text{Mx}} \cdot \text{vBMD}_{\text{Mx}}} \tag{26.4}$$

where d_{Mx} is the maximal distance from a voxel to the polar (z) axis in the image, and vBMD$_{\text{Mx}}$ is the maximal value the cortical vBMD could theoretically assume (i.e., 1200 mg/cm^3). This SSI was proposed to reflect the long-bone strength more generally than the above BSIs and as such it should be validated in future investigations. These BSIs or SSIs do not take into account any other

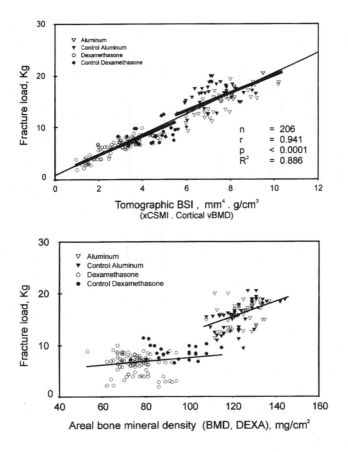

FIGURE 26.3 Upper: Close, linear correlation between a BSI (x) assessed from pQCT scans of the midshafts and the actual fracture load in bending (y) of 206 femurs from rats of different ages and sizes,[5] treated with dexamethasone[8,36] or aluminum hydroxide,[65] or studied as controls. Lower: Lack of correlation of the DEXA-assessed BMD of the central diaphyses with the same indicator of bone strength of the same bones. (From Feretti et al., *Bone*, 18, 2, 97, 1996. Reproduced by permission of Elsevier Science.)

relevant factors to bone material quality. They ignore the many microstructural determinants, including fatigue damage, that may also affect the mechanical ability of the bone tissue. Those indexes may be useful, however, provided that these factors can be assumed to remain unaffected by the assayed treatments.

VI. HOW CAN THE RAW INFORMATION PROVIDED BY pQCT BE APPLIED?

The standard information provided by pQCT studies in animals may be used for descriptive purposes.[64] However, it can also be used for other purposes,[4,6,7,45,60] as the following examples suggest.

A. Analysis of the Pathogenesis of Some Experimental Effects on Bone Biomechanics

Data from separate pQCT evaluations of trabecular and cortical bone and the material and architectural properties of bones can be correlated with those from biomechanical studies in order to investigate the pathogenesis of any change in the whole-bone quality. Figure 26.4, upper, shows the ovariectomy (OX)-induced impairment and the alendronate-induced protection of the bending strength in rat

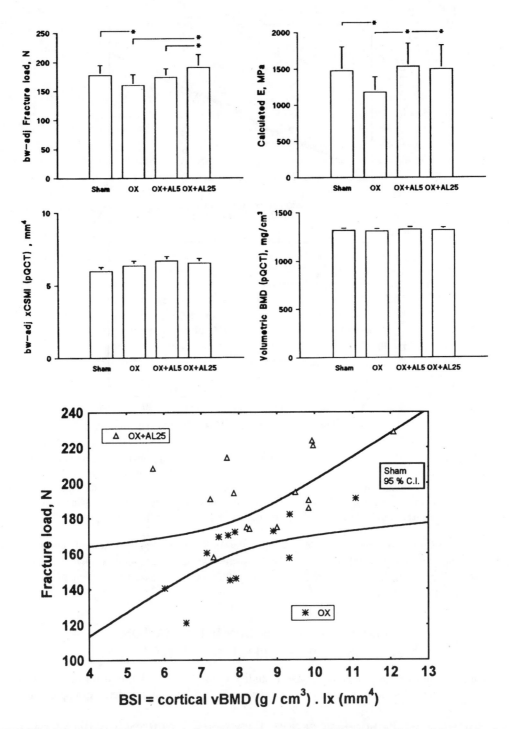

FIGURE 26.4 Upper: Effects of peripubertal ovariectomy alone (OX) or immediately followed by 5 or 25 μg/kg sc 2/week of alendronate for 6 months on the diaphyseal strength (fracture load) and architecture (body-weight adjusted CSMI, Ix) and the material quality (calculated elastic modulus, E) and vBMD of cortical bone of rat femurs.[65,66] Asterisks express the statistical significance of the intergroup differences. Lower: Correlation between the breaking force and the pQCT-assessed BSI of the bones from the OX- and 25-μg-alendronate-treated animals of the same experiment. Values for sham controls are represented by their 95% C.I.

femurs.[65,66] This effect must have resulted from changes in cortical material quality or in the diaphyseal architecture, or both. The lack of changes in the pQCT-assessed diaphyseal CSMIs in any group ruled out bone architecture as a source of such an effect. Parallel changes in the elastic modulus of the cortical tissue pointed to bone material quality as the cause of the observed variation in the whole-bone quality. However, the cortical vBMD did not vary between groups. Therefore, the changes in bone material quality must be ascribed to effects on some of the mineralization-unrelated, microstructural components of bone tissue that are known to affect bone material quality.

In support of that conclusion, the correlation between the measured breaking force and the calculated BSI of the same bones showed that bones from both the OX and risedronate-protected rats varied in opposite directions from the natural association between these variables (Figure 26.4, lower). The reason for that behavior should be a change in some factor(s) relevant to bone material quality that the BSI calculation disregarded (i.e., unrelated to bone mineralization). Findings like this may help to explain some differences between drug effects on fracture incidence and on the DEXA-assessed areal BMD in human studies.

B. ANALYSIS OF THE MECHANOSTAT STATUS BY MEANS OF "DISTRIBUTION/QUALITY" CURVES

An opposite behavior of parameters of material quality (E) and architectural cross-sectional design (CSMIs) of femur shafts from growing rats of two different lines have been described.[1,3] This reflected a normalization of the bone strength to the body weight of the animals, due to a feedback regulation of diaphyseal modeling by a function of the bone strain history (Frost's "mechanostat" theory).[7,45,67-73] The negative hyperbolic functions describing that relationship were called "distribution/quality" curves.[4,6,7] It was also found that the same interrelationships could be shown by plotting the CSMIs vs. the vBMD of the cortical bone as a correlate of the mechanical indicator, E, in many instances.[1-3,29-36,65,66,74,75]

The effects of some treatments on the control of bone quality by the mechanostat can be described by such graphs in a useful way. On the one hand, displacements of the points along the curve showing no departure from the normal relationship would reflect an indemnity of the mechanostatic control. On the other, any shift of the data to the upper-right or to the lower-left of the graph should indicate an anabolic (or anticatabolic) or a catabolic (or antianabolic) shift of the mechanostat set point,[4,6,7] respectively. In this way the effects of many treatments on rat bones have been described.[29-36,39,65,66,74,75] As examples, a negative interaction of dexamethasone and a positive influence of anabolic PTH alone or combined with risedronate on bone mechanostat are summarized.

Dexamethasone administration to growing rats reduced all material (vCtBMD), architectural (CSMIs), and mechanical properties (breaking force) of femur shafts in a dose-dependent fashion.[36,39] Figure 26.5a shows the antianabolic shift induced to the bone mechanostat set point. A three-dimensional representation (Figure 26.5b) shows the combined, dose-dependent, negative influence of changes in both vCtBMD and CSMI on bone strength.

Low, intermittent doses of hPTH(1-38) given for 75 days to rats with a right hind limb immobilization and a mechanical overloading of the other leg enhanced all femur CSMI, vCtBMD, and bending breaking strength.[30,31,40] The distribution/quality curves (Figure 26.5c) showed that these effects (1) reflected an anabolic interaction with the mechanostat set point; (2) were of a transient nature; (3) were maintained by a sequential administration of a remodeling inhibitor, the bisphosphonate olpadronate (an anti-catabolic interaction); and (4) were potentiated by the mechanical overload.

C. ANALYSIS OF THE ARCHITECTURAL EFFICIENCY OF BONE MATERIAL DISTRIBUTION WITHIN BONE DIAPHYSES

This interesting feature of bone modeling can be assessed by plotting any of the CSMIs (y) vs. the cortical area of the same scan (x; Figure 26.6a). The higher the slope of the correlation, the better

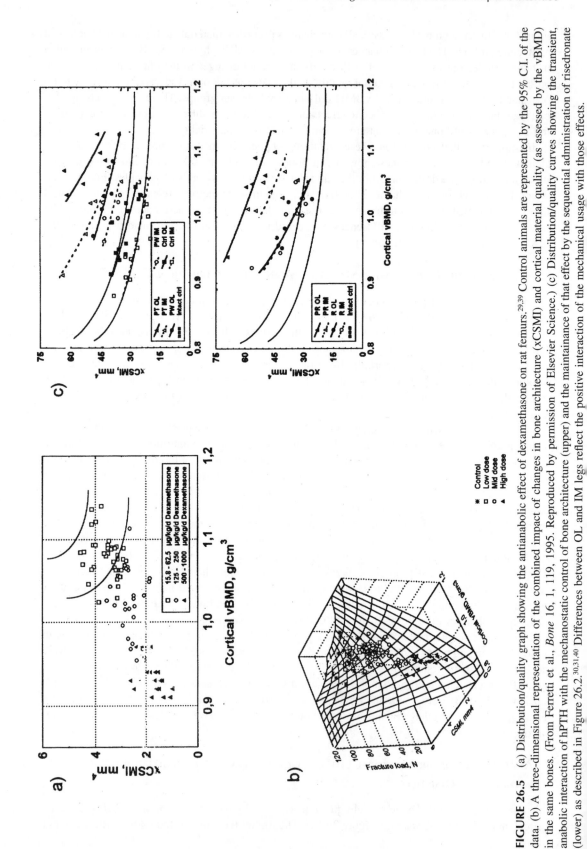

FIGURE 26.5 (a) Distribution/quality graph showing the antianabolic effect of dexamethasone on rat femurs.[29,39] Control animals are represented by the 95% C.I. of the data. (b) A three-dimensional representation of the combined impact of changes in bone architecture (xCSMI) and cortical material quality (as assessed by the vBMD) in the same bones. (From Ferretti et al., *Bone* 16, 1, 119, 1995. Reproduced by permission of Elsevier Science.) (c) Distribution/quality curves showing the transient, anabolic interaction of hPTH with the mechanostatic control of bone architecture (upper) and the maintainance of that effect by the sequential administration of risedronate (lower) as described in Figure 26.2.[30,31,40] Differences between OL and IM legs reflect the positive interaction of the mechanical usage with those effects.

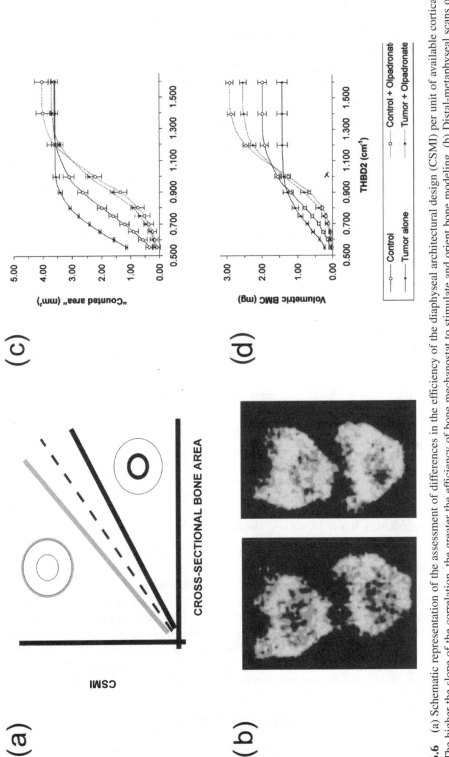

FIGURE 26.6 (a) Schematic representation of the assessment of differences in the efficiency of the diaphyseal architectural design (CSMI) per unit of available cortical material.[38] The higher the slope of the correlation, the greater the efficiency of bone mechanostat to stimulate and orient bone modeling. (b) Distal-metaphyseal scans of the femurs from hypercalcemic, tumor-transplanted mice untreated (left) or treated with olpadronate (right) obtained with an XCT-960 A showing the impossible distinction between "trabecular" and "cortical" bone.[76] (c) Distribution curves of the counted voxels of cross-sectional area (CSA). (d) the vBMC of the animals from the same study, throughout the available range of THBD2 thresholds.

the architectural design that the same bone mass achieved. This method allowed a description of gender-related differences in the design of human bones[38] and is most suitable for analyzing the interactions of the mechanical usage of the limb with the effects of treatments on bone architecture and strength in animal models.

D. ANALYSIS OF THRESHOLD-DEFINED ROI's WHEN CORTICAL AND TRABECULAR BONE ARE INDISTINGUISHABLE

When the distinction between cortical and trabecular bone is difficult but still possible, one should use the function Loop, working first at a fixed THBD, ContMode and CortMode and varying the THBD2 to measure the "trabecular" bone. A second Loop should then be made at a fixed THBD, ContMode, THBD2, and Cortmode and varying the THCRT2 to measure the "cortical" bone. The software allows changing the ROI and the methods of analysis of the images as desired while working with a given image. However, the parameters selected to perform the image itself cannot be changed *a posteriori*, so one has to be careful when setting the conditions at which the image is made. On following the above procedure, when a treatment blunts any distinction between cortical and trabecular bone, its effects can be properly analyzed by displaying the changes in the bone variables (y) along the whole range of attenuation thresholds (x) at which the machine is able to work, so the effects are described as differences between the distribution curves of the assessed variables in the "threshold-defined" ROI's. The resulting "type of bone" is thus defined by the vBMD of the corresponding ROI, and the effects can be described according to the THBD2 threshold range at which they were most evident in each group.

As an example, the author's group failed to define the olpadronate-induced protection of metaphyseal bone of tumor-implanted, hypercalcemic mice as related to pQCT-assessed changes in trabecular tissue by performing the traditional pQCT measurements in PeelMode 1 (Figure 26.6b). However, on varying the THBD2 threshold (PeelMode 2; Figure 26.6c) it was possible to show that the differences between the tumor- and olpadronate-induced effects varied widely,[76] so one could conclude that (a) the tumor reduced the bone mass and made the "cortical bone" undetectable, and (b) olpadronate increased bone mass above normal values by protecting that "trabecular bone" from remodeling. Those conclusions could not have been derived from standard pQCT determinations at a fixed THBD2 threshold. This novel pQCT application is proposed as a useful tool in skeletal research, avoiding many false negative results.

E. ANALYSIS OF MUSCLE/BONE INTERRELATIONSHIPS

The ability of pQCT machines to measure also the cross-sectional muscle areas allows evaluation of some muscle/bone interrelationships that are essential for assessing the state of bone mechanostat in different experimental conditions. In human studies, a close, linear relationship has been shown between bone CSMIs or BSIs (y) and the force or the pQCT-assessed, cross-sectional area of the regional muscles (x) in normal men and women. The slope of that relationship changed significantly after menopause (Figure 26.7, top).[45,60,62,63,77] This offers the basis for distinguishing between disuse osteopenias (in which the mechanostat is still working properly) and true osteoporosis (in which the mechanostat set point is offset, most commonly because of an endocrine disorder; Figure 26.7, bottom).[60,67,68] The field is open for a wide variety of animal studies concerning this attractive proposal.

VII. CONCLUDING REMARKS

Many new opportunities are open to future research that uses pQCT in animal models. pQCT can provide exclusive information concerning many biomechanical aspects of bone that are highly specific to the skeletal region studied. For that reason, special recommendations should be followed in future studies. They should avoid the understandable temptation to (1) extrapolate the pQCT

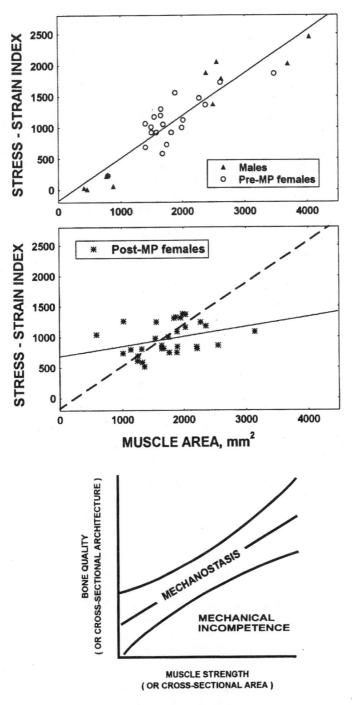

FIGURE 26.7   Top: Muscle/bone interrelationships as described in humans by the correlation between the tibial SSI and the cross-sectional muscle area of the calf of normal males and premenopausal females.[77] Center: The same data from postmenopausal females depart significantly from the above correlation. Bottom: Schematic representation of zones of normal "mechanostasis" (i.e., muscle/bone interrelationships under normal control by bone mechanostat) and "biomechanical incompetence" (because of a shift in the bone mechanostat set point), as derived from the evidence shown in the analogous graphs at the left. According to Frost's principles,[78] this proposal (which can be tested employing animal models) should help to achieve a tomographic differentiation between osteopenias and osteoporoses.

data of a given skeletal region to a different site and (2) compare the pQCT performance with those of other techniques that measure different aspects of bone mass — as the standard densitometry does — especially if these are inadequately taken as "gold standards."

REFERENCES

1. Ferretti, J.L., Spiaggi, E., Capozza, R., et al., Interrelationships between geometric and mechanical properties of long bones from three rodent species with very different biomass. Phylogenetic implications, *J. Bone Miner. Res.*, 7(S2), S423, 1992.
2. Ferretti, J.L., Capozza, R., Mondelo, N., and Zanchetta, J., Interretionships between densitometrical, geometric and mechanical properties of rat femurs. Inferences concerning mechanical regulation of bone modeling, *J. Bone Miner. Res.*, 8, 1389, 1993.
3. Ferretti, J.L., Capozza, R., Mondelo, N., et al., Determination of femur structural properties by geometric and material properties as a function of body weight in rats. Evidence of a sexual dimorphism, *Bone*, 14, 265, 1993.
4. Ferretti, J.L., Perspectives of pQCT technology associated to biomechanical studies in skeletal research employing rat models. *Bone*, 17(4S), 353S, 1995.
5. Ferretti, J.L., Capozza, R., and Zanchetta, J., Mechanical validation of a tomographic (pQCT) index for the noninvasive assessment of rat femur bending strength, *Bone*, 18, 97, 1996.
6. Ferretti, J.L., Noninvasive assessment of bone architecture and biomechanical properties in animals and humans employing pQCT technology, *J. Jpn. Soc. Bone Morphom.*, 7, 115, 1997.
7. Ferretti, J.L., Biomechanical properties of bone, in *Bone Densitometry and Osteoporosis*, Genant, H.K., Guglielmi, G., and Jergas, M., Eds., Springer, Berlin, 1998, 143.
8. Gasser, J.A., Assessing bone quantity by pQCT, *Bone*, 17, 145S, 1996.
9. Gasser, J.A., Quantitative assessment of bone mass and geometry by pQCT in rats *in vivo* and site specificity of changes at different skeletal sites, *J. Jpn. Soc. Bone Morphom.*, 7, 107, 1997.
10. Jämsä, T., Jalovaara, P., Peng, Z., et al., Comparison of three-point bending test and peripheral quantitative computed tomography analysis in the evaluation of the strength of mouse femur and tibia, *Bone*, 23, 155, 1998.
11. Jämsä, T., Tuukkanen, J., and Jalovaara, P., Femoral neck strength of mouse in two loading configurations: method evaluation and fracture characteristics, *J. Biomech.*, 31, 723, 1998.
12. Börner, W., Grehn, S., and Moll, E., Messung der Absorption des Fingerknochens mit einem I^{125}-Profiscanner. Quantitative Methode zur Erkennung der Osteoporose, *Fortschr. Röntgenstr.*, 110, 378, 1969.
13. Rüegsegger, P., Elsasser, U., Anliker, M., et al., Quantification of bone mineralization using computed tomography, *Radiology*, 121, 93, 1976.
14. Schneider, P. and Berger, P., Bone density determination using quantitative computed tomography and a special purpose scanner, *Nuklearmediziner*, 2, 145, 1988.
15. Schneider, P. and Reiners, C., Peripheral quantitative computed tomography, in *Bone Densitometry and Osteoporosis*, Genant, H.K., Guglielmi, G., and Jergas, M., Eds., Springer, Berlin, 1998, 349.
16. Guglielmi, G., Schneider, P., Lang, T., et al., Quantitative computed tomography at the axial and peripheral skeleton, *Eur. Radiol.*, 7(S2), S332, 1997.
17. Kinney, J.H., Lane, N., and Haupt, D., in *vivo* three-dimensional microscopy of trabecular bone, *J. Bone Miner. Res.*, 10, 264, 1995.
18. Müller, R., Hildebrand, T., and Rüegsegger, P., Non-invasive bone biopsy: a new method to analyse and display the three-dimensional structure of trabecular bone, *Phys. Med. Biol.*, 39, 145, 1994.
19. Helterbrand, J.D., Higgs, R., Iversen, P., et al., Application of automatic image segmentation to tibiae and vertebrae from ovariectomized rats, *Bone*, 21, 401, 1997.
20. Gordon, C.L., Webber, C., Adachi, J., and Christoforou, N., in *vivo* assessment of trabecular bone structure at the distal radius from high-resolution computed tomography images, *Phys. Med. Biol.*, 41, 495, 1996.
21. Rüegsegger, P. and Kalender, W., A phantom for standardization and quality control in peripheral bone measurements by pQCT and DEXA, *Phys. Med. Biol.*, 38, 1963, 1993.

22. Augat, P., Gordon, C.L., Lang, T., et al., Accuracy of cortical and trabecular bone measurements with peripheral quantitative computed tomography (pQCT), *Phys. Med. Biol.*, 43, 2873, 1998.

23. Burstein A. H., Zika, J., Heiple, K., and Klein, L., Contribution of collagen and mineral to the elastic-plastic properties of bone, *J. Bone Joint Surg.*, 57A, 956, 1975.

24. Currey, J.D., The mechanical consequences of variation in the mineral contents of bone, *J. Biomech.*, 2, 1, 1969.

25. Currey, J.D., The effect of porosity and mineral content on the Young's modulus of elasticity of compact bone, *J. Biomech.*, 21, 131, 1988.

26. Sato, M., Comparative X-ray densitometry of bones from ovariectomized rats, *Bone*, 17(4S), 157S, 1995.

27. Sato, M., Kim, J., Short, L., et al., Longitudinal and cross-sectional analyses of raloxifene effects on tibiae from ovariectomized aged rats, *J. Pharmacol. Exp. Ther.*, 272, 1252, 1995.

28. Breen, S.A., Millest, A., Loveday, B., et al., Regional analysis of bone mineral density in the distal femur and proximal tibia using peripheral quantitative computed tomography in the rat *in vivo*, *Calcif. Tissue Int.*, 58, 449, 1996.

29. Ferretti, J.L, Gaffuri, O., Capozza, R., et al., Dexamethasone effects on structural, geometric and material properties of rat femur diaphyses as described by peripheral quantitative computerized tomography (pQCT) and bending tests, *Bone*, 16, 119, 1995.

30. Capozza, R.F., Ferretti, J.L., Ma, Y.F., et al., Tomographic (pQCT) and biomechanical effects of hPTH(1-38) on chronically immobilized or overloaded rat femurs, *Bone*, 17(4S), S233, 1995.

31. Capozza, R.F., Aplicación de Recursos Originales Biomecánicos, Radio-densitométricos e Histomor-fométricos a la Evaluación de los Efectos Óseos de la Parathormona, Ph.D. thesis, University of Buenos Aires, Buenos Aires, 1998.

32. Cointry, G.R., Mondelo, N., Zanchetta, J., et al., Intravenous olpadronate restores ovariectomy-affected bone strength. A mechanical, densitometric and tomographic (pQCT) study, *Bone*, 17(4S), S373, 1995.

33. Cointry, G.R., Estudio de la Curva Completa de Efectos de Bisfosfonatos de Tercera Generación sobre la Biomecánica, Densitometría e Histomorfometría en Huesos de Rata, Ph.D. thesis, University of Buenos Aires, Buenos Aires, 1997.

34. Ferretti, J.L., Lin, B., Ke, H., et al., Geometric, material, structural and histomorphometric properties of femurs and tibiae of ovariectomized rats as affected by leg immobilization or overloading, *Calcif. Tissue Int.*, 54, 349, 1994.

35. Ferretti, J.L., Mondelo, N., Peluffo, V., et al., Sub-chronic effects of high doses of mildronate on femur densitometric (DEXA), tomographic (pQCT) and mechanical properties in young rats, *Bone Miner.*, 25(S2), S12, 1994.

36. Ferretti, J.L., Mondelo, N., Capozza, R., et al., Effects of large doses of olpadronate (dimethyl-pamidronate) on mineral density, cross-sectional architecture, and mechanical properties of rat femurs, *Bone*, 16(4S), 285S, 1995.

37. Ferretti, J.L., Frost, H. M., Gasser, J., et al., Perspectives in osteoporosis research: its focus and some insights from a new paradigm, *Calcif. Tissue Int.*, 57, 399, 1995.

38. Ferretti, J.L., Zanchetta, J., Capozza, R., et al., The premenopausal accumulation of bone material per unit muscle mass in women would be of little mechanical relevance, *Osteoporosis Int.*, 8(S3), 37, 1998.

39. Gaffuri, O.H., Desarrollo y Aplicación de Recursos Biomecánicos, Densitométricos e Histomorfo-métricos a la Evaluación Farmacológica del Efecto de los Glucocorticoides de Uso Clínico Corriente, Ph. D. thesis, University of Buenos Aires, Buenos Aires, 1994.

40. Ma, Y.F., Ferretti, J.L., Capozza, R., et al., Effects of on/off anabolic hPTH and remodeling inhibitors on metaphyseal bone of immobilized rat femurs. Tomographical (pQCT) description and correlation with histomorphometric changes in tibial cancellous bone, *Bone*, 17(4S), S321, 1995.

41. Breen, S.A., Loveday, B., Millest, A., and Waterton, J., Stimulation and inhibition of bone formation: use of peripheral quantitative computed tomography in the mouse *in vivo*, *Lab. Anim.*, 32, 467, 1998.

42. Mühlbauer, R.C., Schenk, R., Chen, D., et al., Morphometric analysis of gastrectomy-evoked osteopenia, *Calcif. Tissue Int.*, 62, 323, 1998.

43. Links, J.M., Beach, L., Subramaniam, B., et al., Edge complexity and partial volume effects, *J. Comput. Assist. Tomogr.*, 22, 450, 1998.

44. Frost, H.M. and Jee, W.S.S., On the rat model of human osteopenias and osteoporoses, *Bone Miner.*, 18, 227, 1992.

45. Frost, H.M., Ferretti, J.L., and Jee, W.S., Some roles of mechanical usage, muscle strength, and the mechanostat in skeletal physiology, disease, and research, *Calcif. Tissue Int.*, 62, 1, 1998.

46. Brinckmann, P., Biggemann, M. and Hilweg, D., Prediction of the compressive strength of human lumbar vertebrae, *Clin. Biomech.*, 4(S2), S1, 1989.

47. Crenshaw, T.D., Peo, E., Lewis, A., and Moser, B., Bone strength as a trait for assessing mineralization in swine. A critical review of techniques involved, *J. Anim. Sci.*, 53, 827, 1981.

48. Faulkner, K.G., Gluer, C., Majumdar, S., et al., Noninvasive measurements of bone mass, structure, and strength. Current methods and experimental techniques, *Am. J. Roentgenol.*, 157, 1229, 1991.

49. Hansson, T., Roos, B., and Nachemson, A., The bone mineral content and ultimate compressive strength of lumbar vertebrae, *Spine*, 5, 46, 1980.

50. Hayes, W.C., Piazza, S., and Zysset, P., Biomechanics of fracture risk prediction of the hip and spine by quantitative computed tomography, *Radiol. Clin. North Am.*, 29, 1, 1991.

51. Louis, O., Boulpaep, F., Willnecker, J., et al., Cortical mineral content of the radius assessed by peripheral pQCT predicts compressive strength on biomechanical testing, *Bone*, 16, 375, 1995.

52. Turner, C.H. and Burr, D.B., Basic biomechanical measurements of bone. A tutorial, *Bone*, 14, 595, 1993.

53. Jerome, C.P., Johnson, C., and Lees, C., Effect of treatment for 6 months with human parathyroid hormone 1-34 peptide in ovariectomized cynomolgus monkey (*Macaca fascicularis*), *Bone*, 17(4S), 415S, 1995.

54. Rosen, H.N., Tollin, S., and Balena, R., Differentiating between orchidectomized rats and controls using measurements of trabecular bone density: a comparison among DXA, histomorphometry, and peripheral quantitative computerized tomography, *Calcif. Tissue Int.*, 57, 35, 1995.

55. Takada, M., Engelke, K., Hagiwara, S., et al., Accuracy and precision study *in vitro* for peripheral quantitative computed tomography, *Osteoporosis Int.*, 6, 207, 1996.

56. Mosekilde, Li., Mosekilde, Le., and Danielsen, C., Biomechanical competence of vertebral trabecular bone in relation to ash density and age in normal individuals, *Bone*, 8, 79, 1987.

57. Mosekilde, Li., Danielsen, C., and Gasser, J., The effect on vertebral bone mass and strength of long term treatment with antiresorptive agents (estrogen and calcitonin), human parathyroid hormone (1-38), and combination therapy, assessed in aged ovariectomized rats, *Endocrinology*, 134, 2126, 1994.

58. Fujii, Y., Miyauchi, A., Takagi, Y., et al., Fixed ratio between radial cortical volume and density measured by peripheral quantitative computed tomography (pQCT) regardless of age and sex, *Calcif. Tissue Int.*, 56, 586, 1995.

59. Burr, D.B. and Martin, R.B., The effects of composition, structure and age on the torsional properties of the human radius, *J. Biomech.*, 16, 603, 1983.

60. Ferretti, J.L., Schiessl, H., and Frost, H. M., On new opportunities for absorptiometry, *J. Clin. Densitom.*, 1, 41, 1998.

61. Baker, J. L. and Haugh, C., Mechanical properties of bone: a review, *Trans. Am. Soc. Agric. Eng.*, 22, 678, 1979.

62. Schiessl, H., Ferretti, J.L., Tysarczyk-Niemeyer, G., and Willnecker, J., Noninvasive bone strength index as analyzed by peripheral quantitative computed tomography (pQCT), in *Paediatric Osteology. New Developments in Diagnostics and Therapy*, Schönau, E., Ed., Elsevier, Amsterdam, 1996, 141.

63. Schiessl, H., Ferretti, J.L., Tysarczyk-Niemeyer, G., et al., The role of the muscles to the mechanical adaptation of bone, in *Advances in Osteoporosis*, Vol. 1, Lyritis, G.P., Ed., Hylonome, Athens, 1998, 53.

64. Beamer, W.G., Donahue, L., Rosen, C., and Baylink, D.J., Genetic variability in adult bone density among inbred strains of mice, *Bone*, 18, 397, 1996.

65. Chiappe, A., Iorio, B., Alvarez, E., et al., Alendronate protects rat femur against the negative impact of ovariectomy. A densitometric (DXA), tomographic (pQCT) and biomechanical study, *Bone*, 17, 601, 1995.

66. Chiappe, A., Efectos del Alendronato sobre la Estructura y la Biomecánica Ósea, Ph.D. thesis, University of Buenos Aires, Buenos Aires, 1998.

67. Burr, D.B. and Martin, R.B., Mechanisms of bone adaptation to the mechanical environment, *Triangle (Sandoz)*, 31, 59, 1992.

68. Carter, D.R., Mechanical loading history and skeletal biology, *J. Biomech.*, 20, 1095, 1987.

69. Frost, H.M., Ed., *The Intermediary Organization of the Skeleton,* Vols. I and II, CRC Press, Boca Raton, FL, 1986.

70. Frost, H.M., The mechanostat: a proposed pathogenetic mechanism of osteoporoses and the bone mass effects of mechanical and nonmechanical agents, *Bone Miner.*, 2, 73, 1987.
71. Frost, H.M., Structural adaptations to mechanical usage (SATMU): 2. Redefining Wolff's law: the bone modeling problem, *Anat. Rec.*, 226, 403, 1990.
72. Lanyon, L.E., Functional strain in bone tissue as an objective, and controlling stimulus for adaptive bone remodelling, *J. Biomech.*, 20, 1083, 1987.
73. Rubin, C.T., McLeod, K., and Bain, S., Functional strains and cortical bone adaptation. Epigenetic assurance of skeletal integrity, *J. Biomech.*, 23, 43, 1990.
74. Cointry, G.R., Negri, A., Vázquez, S., et al., Densitometric, tomographic (pQCT), histomorphometric and biomechanical changes produced by chronic aluminum intoxication in rat femurs and tibiae, *Bone Miner.*, 25(S2), S13, 1994.
75. Ferretti, J.L., Effects of bisphosphonates on bone biomechanics, in *Bisphosphonate on Bones*, Bijvoet, O.L., Canfield, R., Fleisch, H., and Russel, R., Eds., Elsevier, Amsterdam, 1995, 211.
76. Parma, M., Schneider, P., Piccinni, E., et al., Threshold-defined ROI analysis of bisphosphonate effects on bone structure in tumor-implanted mice employing pQCT, *Bone*, 23(5S), S479, 1998.
77. Roldán, E.J., Pérez Lloret, A., and Ferretti, J.L., Olpadronate: a new amino-bisphosphonate for the treatment of medical osteopathies, *Expert Opinion Invest. Drugs*, 7, 1521, 1998.
78. Frost, H.M., Defining osteopenias and osteoporoses. Another view (with insights from a new paradigm), *Bone*, 20, 385, 1997.

27 Computer Modeling for Evaluating Trabecular Bone Mechanics

Rakesh Saxena and Tony S. Keller

CONTENTS

0-8493-0266-9/00/$0.00+$.50
© 2000 by CRC Press LLC

I. INTRODUCTION

A knowledge of mechanical properties of trabecular bone is essential in understanding problems of age-related bone fracture, prosthesis loosening, and bone remodeling. Over the years, researchers have attempted, both experimentally and theoretically, to relate bone mechanical properties (stiffness, strength) to bone physical properties (bone density, bone volume, bone architecture, etc.). Numerous experimental studies have shown that both apparent modulus and strength have a power-law relationship with apparent density, and that the elastic mechanical properties of bone improve as the apparent density increases.[1-5] The elastic properties of bone are also dependent upon a number of the factors including anatomical site, tissue heterogeneity, architecture, loading direction, and age. Other bone material properties, tissue modulus and Poisson's ratio, also have a direct impact on the apparent modulus and strength. In the past, research in this field has utilized *in vivo*, *in vitro*, and simple mathematical modeling techniques.

More recently, powerful computers with large memory, speed, and multiple processors combined with efficient imaging schemes have made it possible to perform large-scale, anatomically precise three-dimensional (3D) numerical modeling of trabecular bone. Such 3D models of trabecular bone are usually analyzed by finite-element (FE) stress analysis. The advantages of computer modeling of trabecular bone are as follows:

1. Physical properties can be related to mechanical properties noninvasively.
2. Parametric studies can be performed very easily (for example, variations of Poisson's ratio value on apparent modulus).
3. Precise 3D modeling can be used to quantify bone architecture.
4. Heterogeneity and anisotropy can be addressed by analyzing 3D models from different anatomical sites and by varying the loading direction, respectively.
5. Tissue modulus can be predicted.

Computer modeling of trabecular bone not only provides an alternative method to obtain correlations between bone physical properties and mechanical properties, but also allows one to study experimental artifacts such as bone–platen friction and local damage and increased compliance associated with cut surfaces of bone. Such artifacts can be problematic in mechanical tests, since they are well-known sources of measurement error.

A schematic illustration of the key steps involved in computer modeling of trabecular bone is shown in Figure 27.1. These are image array acquisition, image processing, volume of interest (VOI) selection, surface mesh generation, FE volume mesh generation, FE analysis, and morphological analysis. Each of these processes is summarized in the following sections. Various stages of the modeling and analysis process will be illustrated with a simple unit cell model of trabecular bone. Special sections identified as "Plates" are used to highlight modeling and analysis processes applied to the trabecular bone unit cell model.

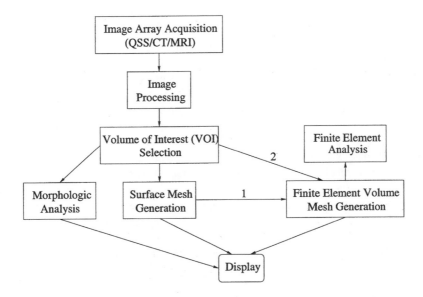

FIGURE 27.1 Schematic illustration of the steps used to generate and analyze a three dimensional model of trabecular bone (1 = > smooth surface tetrahedral mesh and 2 = > voxel based brick/tetrahedral mesh).

II. IMAGE ARRAY ACQUISITION

Image rendering is basically data visualization, and requires two-dimensional (2D) data sets which are transformed into a set of graphic primitives. Biological data are generally acquired using medical imaging hardware or histological techniques. Image data obtained using medical imaging hardware is in the form of planar or 2D slices of the patients' anatomy. There are several noninvasive medical imaging techniques which can be used to gather 3D data, including for example, X-ray, tomography, radionuclide imaging, ultrasound, and magnetic resonance imaging. Most of these noninvasive imaging methods are based on the principles of probing fundamental properties of matter through mechanical or electromagnetic waves.

Information obtained from quantification of these properties is utilized in reconstructing a 2D image, which allows one to visualize various tissues in the body in some manner. For example, an attenuation in X-ray intensity proportional to the tissue density leads to different gray levels of the image on photographic film. On the other hand, water content variations inherent in different biological tissues result in different resonant peaks in magnetic resonance imaging.

In this chapter the most common histological and noninvasive techniques for acquisition of bone image data, i.e., quantitative serial sectioning and serial grinding (QSSG), computed tomography imaging (CT and μ-CT), and magnetic resonance imaging (MRI), will be discussed in more detail.

A. QUANTITATIVE SERIAL SECTIONING AND SERIAL GRINDING (QSSG)

Quantitative serial sectioning and serial grinding are histological techniques and therefore require removal of a specimen of bone tissue from the body. One of the essential elements of images derived from QSSG and other imaging techniques is adequate contrast between the tissue of interest (e.g., bone) and surrounding tissues (e.g., marrow, ligaments, muscle, etc.). Good contrast or physical dissimilarity between bone and the surrounding tissues is important so that the feature of interest (i.e., bone) can be extracted from the image background. Noisy or otherwise poorly contrasted images make feature extraction (contouring in 2D, surface rendering in 3D) extremely difficult and may lead to an inaccurate description of the anatomy.

To enhance contrast and facilitate feature extraction in trabecular bone one needs to replace the bone marrow with some medium which is dissimilar in color value from bone. For this purpose, the marrow is removed from the bone using a high-pressure water jet, defatted in acetone (24 h), bleached in dilute ammonia solution (24 h), and dried (100°C for 1 h). This produces a trabecular bone specimen which is chalk-white in appearance (Figure 27.2A). The cleaned and dried specimen is then embedded in black-pigmented epoxy resin. A low-speed centrifuge can be used to facilitate infiltration of the resin throughout the porous network of trabeculae. This results in a histological preparation which has excellent contrast between bone and marrow spaces (Figure 27.2B), and from which the bone features can be accurately extracted using a process called thresholding (Figure 27.2C).

In order to capture the bulk architecture of the bone, the specimen is serially sectioned using a microtome (Figure 27.2D) or serially ground using a Computer Numerically Controlled (CNC) milling machine.

The surface of each slice is then recorded using a frame capture camera connected to a computer frame grabber, with care taken to ensure that each slice is spatially registered in an identical manner so that image distortion between adjacent slices is minimized. This is readily accomplished by fixing the recording device (charged-coupled device or CCD camera) over the specimen.

Plate 27.1 — QSSG APPLIED

A specimen of human (60-year-old male) L4 vertebral trabecular bone (9 × 9 × 9 mm) was removed from the vertebral centrum using an Isomet™ low-speed diamond saw (Buehler, Lake Bluff, IL). The specimen had an apparent density of 0.3 g/cm³ (ρ_a = bone mass/bulk volume) and bone volume fraction (V_f = bone volume/bulk volume) of 11%. The specimen was embedded in a black polyester resin and was serially sliced along the superior-inferior axis at 20-μm intervals using a Reichert-Jung® polycut E microtome (Leica Microsystems, Inc., Deerfield, IL). Then, 16-bit color video images of each sectioned surface were recorded at an image resolution of 20 mm/pixel, using a CCD camera and a PC image capture card (TARGA™ 16 graphic board, Truevision, Inc., Indianapolis, IN). MIPS (Map and Image Processing Software) program (MicroImages, Inc., Lincoln, NE) was used to create a 3D binary image array comprising of 201 serial (20 × 20 μm) resolution slices.[6] This process is summarized in Figure 27.2.

B. COMPUTED TOMOGRAPHY (CT)

In conventional radiography, X rays diverging from a source pass through the body projecting an image of the skeleton, organs, air spaces, and any existing tumors onto a sheet of film. However, this technique has certain limitations, namely, a 3D object is projected onto a 2D plane. Thus, many planes are superimposed onto one, and the depth information is lost. Also, conventional X rays cannot differentiate between soft tissues. The tomography (the Greek word *tomo* means a cut section) technique overcomes the limitation of depth loss by taking an X-ray projection of a single plane. This is done by simultaneously moving the X-ray source in one direction and photographic film in the opposite direction. Thus, if the patient's body can be regarded as a series of planes parallel to the film, there is only one plane that remains stationary with respect to the film as the film moves; hence, only this plane remains sharply focused and the other planes are blurred.

In 1917, Radon[7] proved that a 2D or 3D object can be reconstructed uniquely from the infinite set of all its projections. Based on this principle, techniques have been developed to reconstruct images from projections. In CT a 2D image is reconstructed by multiple projections of a single plane. CT offers much greater sensitivity and so enables soft tissue to be differentiated from hard tissue. In conventional quantitative CT (QCT), the images have an out-of-plane resolution of 1000 to 2000 μm and an in-plane resolution of approximately 500 μm. Such image resolutions are incapable of resolving trabecular bone structures, which can be 150 μm in diameter and smaller.

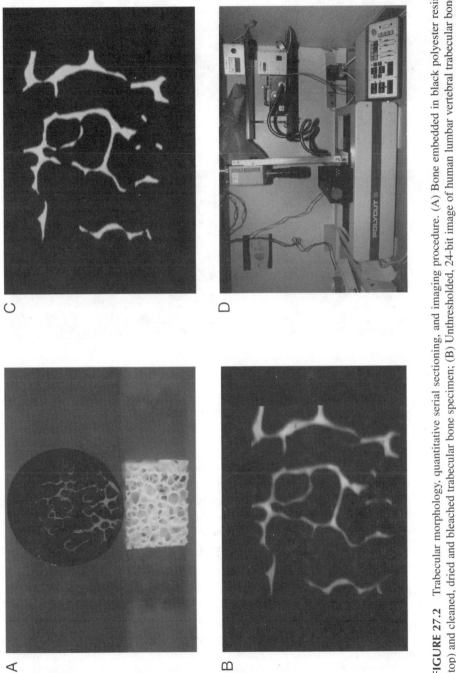

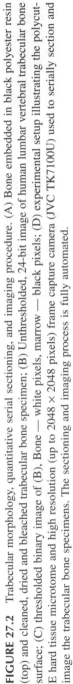

FIGURE 27.2 Trabecular morphology, quantitative serial sectioning, and imaging procedure. (A) Bone embedded in black polyester resin (top) and cleaned, dried and bleached trabecular bone specimen; (B) Unthresholded, 24-bit image of human lumbar vertebral trabecular bone surface; (C) thresholded binary image of (B), Bone — white pixels, marrow — black pixels; (D) experimental setup illustrating the polycut-E hard tissue microtome and high resolution (up to 2048 × 2048 pixels) frame capture camera (JVC TK7100U) used to serially section and image the trabecular bone specimens. The sectioning and imaging process is fully automated.

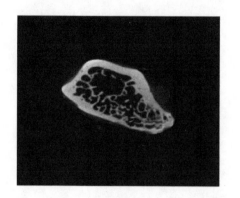
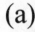

(a)

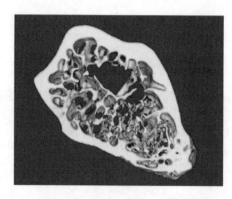
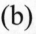

(b)

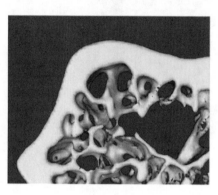

(c)

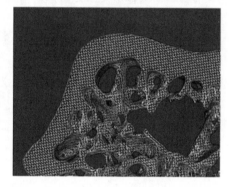

(d)

FIGURE 27.3 XCT images (256 × 256 pixels, 22 × 22 μm resolution) and FE mesh of mouse femur: (a) slice 160 from a set of 234 slices at 20 μm increments; (b) TBMAS volumetric rendering; and (c) detail; (d) the FE mesh.

Indeed, a study investigating the morphology of the lumbar vertebral centrum indicated that the optimal image resolution for human trabecular bone was 25 μm or better.[8] More recently, peripheral QCT (pQCT) and micro-CT (μ-CT) imaging techniques have been developed which can provide high-resolution images of small specimens of trabecular bone. In μ-CT, resolutions of 20 μm are possible (Figure 27.3). The advantages of μ-CT are it is nondestructive, less time-consuming than QSS, and has better resolution. By using μ-CT techniques it is also possible to obtain *in vivo* images of rodent skeletal tissues.

C. MAGNETIC RESONANCE IMAGING (MRI)

This technique is based on the principle of nuclear magnetic resonance (NMR). According to this principle, resonant peaks are obtained from a material placed in an electromagnetic field as energy is absorbed by spin flips of protons. These resonant peaks provide a unique energy signature of a particular substance. When the human body is subjected to a strong magnetic field, the NMR signal is due predominantly to water protons. Hence, water content differences in various tissues can be detected by flips of protons present in the fluid-containing tissues. The energy signature can be processed into an X-ray-like image. MRI has the advantage of being able to penetrate bony and air-filled structures with negligible attenuation and with minimal artifacts. Also, unlike conventional X-ray and computed tomography, MRI uses nonionizing radiation and is minimally invasive. Formerly, MRI was used mainly for imaging the brain and the spinal cord. However, with the advent of faster computers and imaging techniques, MRI has been extended to the chest and abdomen where thorax and blood vessel motion artifacts had previously limited the application of this technique.

III. IMAGE PROCESSING

Historically, pictures, images, maps, and charts have been made of paper and ink or film. Prior to the computer revolution, scientists used stereology tools (which have been around since the early 1950s and 1960s) to analyze 2D data sets obtained photographically from scanning electron microscopes and other available histological tools. In the case of X-ray films, CT scans, and MRI scans, microcomputers have turned paper and film into 2D and 3D image processing and graphical information systems. A desktop computer can manipulate 2D and 3D images to make their storage, retrieval, and interpretation easier and more accurate for researchers and technicians alike.

Today sophisticated image processing techniques (many of which were originally developed for military applications) greatly simplify the task of displaying, converting, and interpreting complex trabecular bone data sets derived from QSSG, CT, and MRI techniques.

A. DATA TYPES

Three-dimensional image data of an object obtained using QSSG/QCT/MRI techniques generally comprise a series of planar or 2D arrays of a single data type. A single, related, 2D grouped set of numbers of a single data type is defined as a raster or raster object. Each number represents the value of some parameter (color, attenuation coefficient, etc.), and its position in the group represents its relative position to the other values. A raster format, therefore, breaks an image into a grid of equally spaced pieces called pixels and records color information for each pixel. Most image processing software packages can display images from raster objects of any data type (1 to 64 bit integers or floating point numbers, typically 8, 16, or 24 bit). For example, if every pixel is 12 bits, then the color value will be an integer number between 0 and 4095 ($2^{12} - 1$). If every pixel is 1 bit, then the image is binary (0 or 1) or black and white.

One of the main problems with image files is the variety of standard and proprietary file formats in use. The format of a file is very important because it allows interchange of files between people and programs. Image files normally contain a header which includes the file format version, a description of data (bits per pixel, spatial dimensions) and the structure of the data (compressed or not), followed by the data section. The simplest file format for storage of image data is a simple integer array which, as the name implies, simply contains a bitmap or row × column array of digital encoded information and no header. Other standard bitmap file formats which contain header information include TARGA (.TGA, Truevision Inc., Indianapolis, IN) and TIFF (.TIF, tag image file format, Adobe Developer Association, Mountain View, CA). File size is also an important consideration when working with images. Assuming, for example, a raster object comprising a 512 × 512 pixel array where every pixel is encoded with 12 bits, then the size of a simple integer array file will be 524,288 bytes (512 kilobytes) since each pixel must be saved in 2-byte words; 8-bit pixel data can be stored as 1-byte words, which reduces the bitmap file size to 262,144 bytes (256 kilobytes). Simple array, TARGA, and TIFF files, can be compressed to reduce file size, and recent developments in data compression have enabled bitmap file sizes to be drastically reduced, often as much as 90%.

B. DISPLAYING RASTERS

The ability to display meaningfully or numerically represent a raster object of a given data type is one of the most important elements of image processing. Indeed, if one wishes to extract quantitative information accurately from a raster object (trabecular bone features, for example), then good contrast or dissimilarity between elements in the raster is an essential and prerequisite requirement for the object. As described in Section II.A of this chapter, the first step in acquiring a raster object representation of a histological sample of bone is to ensure that there is good contrast between the bone and background (marrow spaces) prior to capturing the image. One can also "tune" signals associated with CT and MRI systems in order to obtain higher-contrast raster objects. Moreover, it is possible to numerically alter the contrast of the raster object after the image has been captured. Many software packages (TBMAS, Musculoskeletal Research Laboratory, Burlington, VT; NIH Image, Scion Corporation, Frederick, MD; MIPS, MicroImages, Inc., Lincoln, NE; and others) enable the user to modify a raster object digitally using standard contrast methods such as linear, normalized, equalized, or logarithmic contrast enhancement. Such digital processes can improve the contrast of the raster object,[9] but it is always a good idea to start with the best possible contrast image.

C. DATA CONVERSION AND FEATURE EXTRACTION

Before one can perform morphological and/or FE analyses of trabecular bone, planar (2D) or multiplanar (3D) raster objects must be converted into binary or vector representations. Thus, some method to separate the object(s) of interest is required. This process is called feature extraction and involves isolating areas in raster images into surface features based on similarities and differences associated with the raster data values. In the case of trabecular bone, extraction of the trabecular bone features from the surrounding marrow spaces is of principal interest. Feature extraction is generally a semiautomated process which involves thresholding or setting a data conversion separation limit such that any value above the designated limit or threshold is assigned a 1 value (in binary thresholding, a "1") and any incoming value below or equal to the limit is assigned another value (in binary thresholding, a "0") (Plate 27.2). Thus, thresholding of 2 or higher-bit raster images generates a binary raster. Binary rasters are particularly useful for identifying features such as edges, which is an important step in raster-to-vector conversion. Binary rasters are also a standard input file format for stereologic analysis which is used to quantify bone morphology. Raster-to-vector conversion (creation of surface and volumetric meshes) and quantification of bone morphology (structural properties) are described later in this chapter.

Plate 27.2 — IMAGE PROCESSING APPLIED: THRESHOLDING

A typical unthresholded section of a small region of trabecular bone is shown in Figure 27.4a. A binary representation of the trabecular bone was produced using an iterative thresholding algorithm that determined the optimal color level separating the bone and marrow. The threshold optimization procedure consisted of computing a color histogram of the captured image (Figure 27.4c) and applying an iterative scheme (Figure 27.4d) that provided increasingly cleaner extractions of the bone. A convenient threshold to start the algorithm could be $T_o = (P_B + P_M)/2$, where P_B and P_M correspond to the peaks of bone and marrow, respectively. The iterative scheme converged to an optimal color threshold level ($P_{opt} = 76$) after four iterations. By using the optimal color threshold value, each pixel in the original, unthresholded image was assigned to a black (0, marrow) or white (1, bone) color value based upon whether its value was less than or greater than P_{opt}, respectively. The resulting thresholded image is shown in Figure 27.4b.

D. VOLUME OF INTEREST SELECTION

A smaller volume of interest (VOI) within a larger volume is often desired and can be selected by specifying its size and location within the raster array. Reasons for selecting a smaller volume are as follows:

1. Regions near the edges are usually not defined clearly.
2. The maximum size of the VOI is limited by computing resources available.

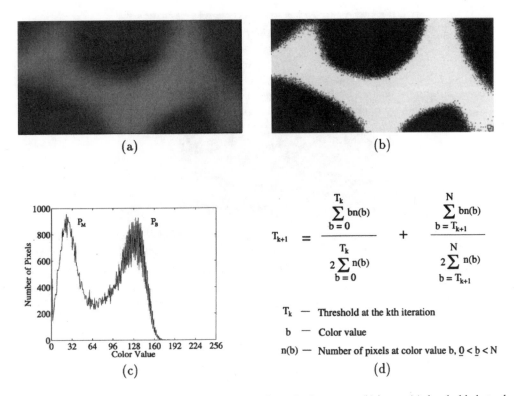

$$T_{k+1} = \frac{\sum\limits_{b=0}^{T_k} bn(b)}{2\sum\limits_{b=0}^{T_k} n(b)} + \frac{\sum\limits_{b=T_{k+1}}^{N} bn(b)}{2\sum\limits_{b=T_{k+1}}^{N} n(b)}$$

T_k — Threshold at the kth iteration

b — Color value

$n(b)$ — Number of pixels at color value b, $\underline{0} < \underline{b} < N$

FIGURE 27.4 (a) Unthresholded image of a section of vertebral centrum; (b) image (a) thresholded at color value = 76; (c) the color histogram; (d) the iterative thresholding algorithm.[10]

Plate 27.3 — IMAGE PROCESSING APPLIED: VOI SELECTION

A small $1.5 \times 1.5 \times 2.0$ mm subvolume or "unit cell" of trabecular bone is used to illustrate basic image rendering, FE mesh generation, FE stress analysis, and morphological analyses applied to trabecular bone (detailed in the following sections of this chapter). Note, however, that a larger VOI should be used in order to satisfy continuum requirements.[11] A general rule of thumb is to select a volume comprising five intertrabecular distances. A custom program, *Trabecular Bone Morphology and Analysis System* (TBMAS),[12] was used to select the VOI (Figure 27.5).

E. RASTER-TO-VECTOR CONVERSION AND IMAGE RENDERING

Raster data is a useful format for displaying planar or 2D data, but is less useful for visualization of multiplanar or 3D data arrays. Moreover, computer-aided design (CAD) and FE mesh generation packages rely on a vector description of an object. Thus, it is desirable to convert raster data into vector data. Raster-to-vector conversion is relatively straightforward in 2D, but is much more complicated for 2D structures, particularly nonhomogeneous, porous, open-cell lattice structures such as trabecular bone.

Raster-to-vector conversion or image rendering involves converting the raster object (pixels) into an object comprising nodes, lines, and polygons (vector). One of the simplest vector file formats consists of a list of nodes followed by a list of elements (connectivity). For example, a simple $1 \times 1 \times 1$ unit cube is represented in vector format as follows:

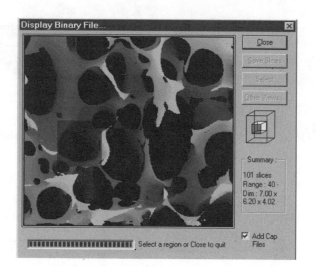

FIGURE 27.5 Volume selector tool used to select a volume of interest (1.5 mm × 1.5 mm × 2.0 mm shaded region) from the 20 μm voxel resolution dataset (7.00 mm × 6.20 mm × 4.02 mm volume). (From Saxena, R. et al., *Comput. Methods Biomech. Biomed. Eng.*, 2, 287, 1999. With permission.)

```
/* x, y, and z coordinates of 8 vertices */
0 0 0
1 0 0
1 1 0
0 1 0
0 0 1
1 0 1
1 1 1
0 1 1
/* Connectivity information of 12 triangles that comprise the cube surface */
1 2 5
6 5 2
2 3 6
7 6 3
3 4 8
8 7 3
5 4 1
4 5 8
4 2 1
4 3 2
5 6 8
6 7 8
```

In the unit cube example, the numeric values of the vertices and elements are space-delimited integer values. Comma- and tab-delimited integers and real numbers can also be used. Standard vector formats include stereo lithography (STL), initial graphics exchange specification (IGES), drawing exchange format (DXF), and many others.

There are two main types of image rendering — *surface rendering* and *volume rendering*. Surface rendering, as the name suggests, describes only the surface of an object and not the interior. However, if one is interested in looking inside an object, for example at various tissues inside a skull, this is done by volume rendering.

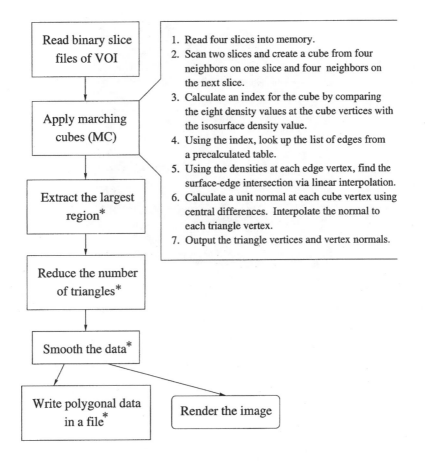

FIGURE 27.6 Surface mesh generation on VTK (* indicates optional steps).

Lorensen and Cline[13] proposed a surface rendering technique to create an isosurface from a discrete 3D raster data set called *marching cubes* (MC). The MC algorithm involved spanning the 3D raster data set by a 3D volume consisting of eight-node voxels (volume cells) and then determining how the isosurface (3D contour of constant scalar value) data intersect the 12 edges of each cube by checking the value at each of the eight cube vertices. An intersection between the isosurface and the edge is implied only if the isosurface values lies between the two vertex values of any edge. Figure 27.6 shows the main steps in an MC-based surface mesh generation scheme.

The Visualization ToolKit (VTK)[14] is a powerful graphic package that utilizes the MC algorithm to generate a triangular surface mesh separating regions of different isodensities (surfaces of constant density values). The code can written in either C, C++, or Tcl.

Plate 27.4 — IMAGE PROCESSING APPLIED: IMAGE RENDERING (Figure 27.7)

Tcl Code
 # Get the interactor ui
source vtkInt.tcl;
source colors.tcl;
 # Create the render master
vtkRenderMaster rm;
set renWin [rm MakeRenderWindow];
set ren1 [$renWin MakeRenderer];
set iren [$renWin MakeRenderWindowInteractor];

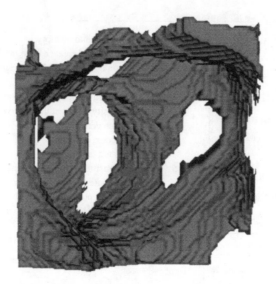

FIGURE 27.7   The surface mesh model of the unit cell ($1.5 \times 1.5 \times 2.0$ mm^3) of trabecular bone (20,545 nodes and 41,544 triangles). (From Saxena, R. et al., *Comput. Methods Biomech. Biomed. Eng.*, 1999. With permission.)

```
# A virtual light for 3D rendering
vtkLight lgt;
# Read the binary slice data
vtkVolume16Reader v16;
v16 SetDataDimensions 77 77;
[v16 GetOutput] SetOrigin 0.0 0.0 0.0;
v16 SwapBytesOn;
v16 SetFilePrefix "data/trab/z60im";
v16 SetImageRange 0 101;
v16 SetDataAspectRatio .02 .02 .02;
# Apply marching cubes (MC) algorithm
vtkMarchingCubes iso;
iso SetInput [v16 GetOutput];
# Specify the isosurface value for tissue
iso SetValue 0 1;
# Merge duplicate points and remove
# degenerate primitives
vtkCleanPolyData clean;
clean SetInput [iso GetOutput];
# Apply connectivity to extract largest
# region
vtkPolyConnectivityFilter connect;
connect SetInput [clean GetOutput];
connect ExtractLargestRegion;
# Reduce the number of triangles in a mesh
vtkDecimate deci;
deci SetInput [clean GetOutput];
# Adjust point positions using Laplacian
# smoothing
vtkSmoothPolyFilter smooth;
smooth SetInput [deci GetOutput];
# Map vtkPolyData to graphics primitives
vtkPolyMapper isoMapper;
```

```
isoMapper SetInput [connect GetOutput];
isoMapper ScalarsVisibleOff;
# Represent an object in a rendered scene
vtkActor isoActor;
isoActor SetMapper isoMapper;
set isoProp [isoActor GetProperty];
eval $isoProp SetColor 0.286 0.843 1.;
# Write vtk polygonal data
vtkPolyWriter writer;
writer SetInput [connect GetOutput];
writer SetFilename trab_z60im_out;
writer Write;
# Add the actors to the renderer,
# set the background and size
$ren1 AddActors isoActor;
$ren1 AddActors textActor;
$ren1 SetBackground 0 0 0;
$ren1 AddLights lgt;
$renWin SetSize 600 600;
$ren1 SetBackground 1 1 1;
$renWin DoubleBufferOff;
set cam1 [$ren1 GetActiveCamera];
$cam1 Elevation 0;
$cam1 SetViewUp 0 1 0;
$cam1 Zoom 1.0;
$cam1 Azimuth 0;
eval lgt SetPosition [$cam1 GetPosition];
eval lgt SetFocalPoint [$cam1 GetFocalPoint];
# Render the image
$iren SetUserMethod {wm deiconify .vtkInteract};
$renWin Render;
puts "Done";
```

IV. FINITE ELEMENT VOLUME MESHING

The FE method is a convenient numerical technique to analyze a complex structure of trabecular bone for which a closed-form solution using analytical methods is impossible. In recent years, detailed 3D FE models of trabecular bone have been investigated.[15-17] In these FE models (usually constructed from CT raster arrays), trabecular bone is represented by a 3D array of identical eight-node brick elements also called voxels. The main advantages of voxel-based FE models are (1) voxel models can be generated extremely fast, and (2) very efficient stress analysis schemes can be implemented using voxel elements. However, voxel elements lead to jagged edges due to protruding vertices of the cubes at the surface, which results in errors in the computation of local stresses and strains.

More recently, volumetric modeling of trabecular bone has been accomplished using four-node tetrahedral elements.[18,19] Using the marching cubes principle, Müller and Rüegsegger[18] developed a volumetric marching cubes (VOMAC) algorithm. When applied to a 3D discrete data set VOMAC generates tetrahedrons, in contrast to the MC approach which generates surface triangles. Thus, instead of defining a triangle surface configuration for every voxel, a tetrahedron subvolume is assembled inside the enclosed volume by the VOMAC algorithm. By using this technique the bone surface can be represented more accurately; however, the mesh generation time required is much longer.

Differences in apparent moduli derived from the two approaches have been shown to range from 2 to 27.5% for a simplified 2D model of a plate with a centered hole.[20] In general, however, the apparent mechanical behavior of trabecular bone can be predicted reasonably well by large-scale, voxel-based FE (LS-FE) schemes.[21,22]

The trabecular bone unit cell will be modeled and analyzed using both voxel and surface meshing schemes.

A. SMOOTH SURFACE TETRAHEDRAL FE MESH MODELING

For the unit cell trabecular bone example, the surface mesh was created using a custom FE mesh generator 3dMesh.[23] 3dMesh generates four-node tetrahedral elements from a surface mesh input file. 3dMesh is a grid-based system that deploys a uniform volume mesh spanning the domain (Figure 27.8a). The domain node material classification is determined using a boundary-line crossing routine.[24] Each domain node, D, is the local origin of the vector, $\mathbf{E}$. This $\mathbf{E}$ vector is oriented in the positive x-direction with a magnitude equal to the length of the body diagonal of the model. This length ensures that the end point of $\mathbf{E}$ lies outside the domain. Every time $\mathbf{E}$ intersects a boundary element, the counters of the two materials associated with that boundary element are incremented. After all the boundary elements are checked for intersection with $\mathbf{E}$, the material counter showing an odd number of crossings dictates the material zone of node D. If all the counters are even, then the node is external to the domain and it is classified with a 0 (Figure 27.8b). The external material boundary counter, material 0, is not included in the analysis. Areas of special interest (bone surfaces in this example) are specified for mesh refinement. The important features of 3dMesh are as follows:

1. *Gauge Size*: The default mesh gauge size is a user specified parameter which corresponds to an edge length of a tetrahedron.
2. *Refinement*: Refinement about the bone surfaces is performed by creating a bounding rectangular parallelepiped about each surface platelet or triangle. A refinement length parameter is specified by the user. Each bounding parallelepiped is enlarged in all directions by this refinement length. All existing volume tetrahedrons whose centroid lies within any expanded parallelepiped get tagged for refinement. Each tagged tetrahedron is subdivided into eight smaller tetrahedrons. These refined elements get knitted into the parent mesh such that the mesh remains consistent and contiguous (Figure 27.8c).
3. *Multiple Materials*: The algorithm can handle multiple material regions including, for example, bone marrow elements.
4. *FE Surface Mesh*: The FE surface mesh can also be generated for comparison to the input surface (VTK mesh). Several noncommercial (CUBIT, QMG, GENIE++) and commercial (ALGOR, ANSYS, MARC) mesh generators are currently available. A list describing and comparing various mesh generators is located at: <http://www.andrew.cmu.edu/user/sowen/softsurv.html>.

B. VOXEL-BASED FE MESH MODELING

Brick FE meshes, in which the elements are eight-node cubes, can be generated directly from a 3D voxel data set (Figure 27.9). The first step is to assign the voxel dimensions. For example, a $100 \times 100 \times 100$ mm voxel will have 5^3 or 125 pixels if the data set has a resolution of 20 mm in all three directions. Next, the data set is divided into a 3D cubic grid consisting of voxels of identical shapes and sizes. Each voxel in the data set is then checked to determine if it is "bone" or "not bone" (i.e., marrow). A common criterion is that if more than half of the volume (i.e., more than 50% of the pixels in the voxel) are bone pixels, then the voxel is considered to be "bone"; otherwise, the voxel is assigned to marrow. This is a straightforward method and a brick mesh can be generated extremely fast — a few seconds compared with a few hours for a smooth surface FE mesh of similar size and resolution. Note that a tetrahedral mesh can be generated directly from the brick mesh by creating five tetrahedra from each brick element.

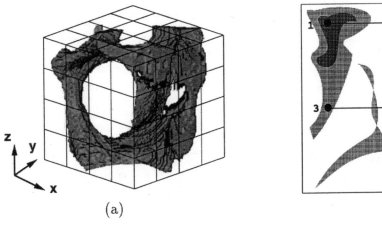

(a)

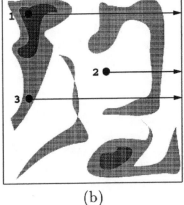

(b)

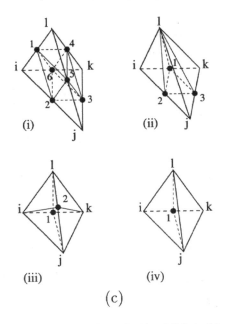

(c)

FIGURE 27.8   Generation of smooth tetrahedral FE mesh using 3dMesh: (a) a node grid bounds the surface mesh of the unit cell; (b) node classification scheme; and (c) mesh refinement. (i) Each tetrahedron has six midside nodes added and is refined into eight elements; breakdown pattern for tetrahedron containing (ii) three; (iii) two; and (iv) one midside node.

An important step after (or during, depending upon the algorithm) the FE meshing procedure is to extract the largest region. This step ensures that small regions not connected to the largest region are removed. Unconnected regions would produce singularities during FE analysis. A good check for the validity and quality of surface generation and FE mesh generation schemes is to compute the bone volume fraction (V_f or BVF) and surface area (A_s) at each step and compare it with the original value. Also, the aspect ratio (the ratio between the longest to shortest dimensions of the element) of elements in FE mesh should not be too high. The optimum aspect ratio at any location within the grid depends largely upon the difference in rate of change of displacements in different directions. If displacements vary at about the same rate in each direction, the closer the

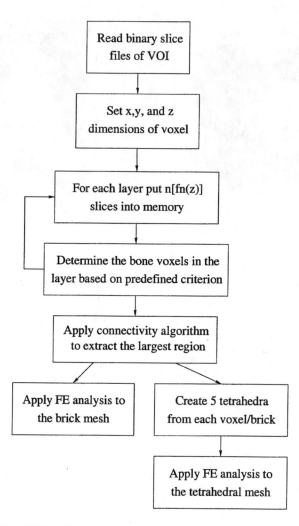

FIGURE 27.9   Voxel-based FE mesh generation.

aspect ratio to unity, the better the quality of the solution.[25] As a general rule, the aspect ratio should be kept below 10 for deformation analysis and below 3 for stress analysis.[26]

Plate 27.5 — FE MESH GENERATION APPLIED: TETRAHEDRAL AND VOXEL ELEMENTS

Figure 27.10a shows a $1.5 \times 1.5 \times 2.0$ mm 3dMesh tetrahedral FE model generated from the trabecular bone subvolume created by the VOI routine. Initially, the mesh is created by dividing the bone volume into equal-size hexahedrons (eight-node cubes). Each cube is then broken down into five tetrahedra. As the meshing algorithm progresses, however, the size of the tetrahedra may vary. The size of tetrahedral elements can also be varied by specifying alternate mesh density in a local region. The maximum number of elements that can be generated by 3dMesh is limited only by machine memory. The four-node tetrahedral meshes were generated by 3dMesh on a 200-MHz Silicon Graphics Challenger system with 256 MB memory. An eight-node brick element FE mesh was generated directly from the binary image files selected using the VOI routine. The FE mesh consisted of 52,293 nodes and 37,126 brick elements (Figure 27.10b). The mesh had a resolution of 20 μm, and the model had a $V_f = 7.05\%$.

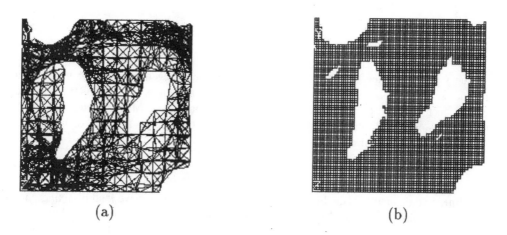

(a)

FIGURE 27.10 FE models of unit cell of trabecular bone: (a) a coarse tetrahedral model (810 nodes, 1710 tetrahedrons); (b) the voxel-based brick model (52,293 nodes, 37,126 bricks).

V. FE STRESS ANALYSIS

A. ANALYSIS ASSUMPTIONS

The most common FE analysis is linear static. A linear static analysis involves computation of stresses, displacements, and strains due to static loads. The term *static* implies that the loads do not change with time. This means that the effects of inertia and damping forces are considered insignificant. The term *linear* refers to the case when nonlinearities due to plasticity, large deflection, large strain, in-plane effects, contact surfaces, creep and relaxation effects can be either linearized or ignored. Often, the material is assumed to be isotropic (no directional dependence) and homogeneous (properties do not vary spatially within the structure). An isotropic material has only two independent constants appearing in the constitutive stress–strain relations. These two constants are Young's modulus (E) and Poisson's ratio (ν). For the case of a uniaxial compression test, these two constants appear as follows:

$$\varepsilon_{xx} = \frac{1}{E} \sigma_{xx} \tag{27.1}$$

$$\varepsilon_{yy} = \varepsilon_{zz} = \frac{1}{E} \left(-\nu \sigma_{xx} \right) \tag{27.2}$$

where ε and σ are the strain and stress, respectively.

Young's modulus gives a measure of the stiffness of the material. For trabecular bone the tissue modulus (E_t) has been reported to vary from 1 to 20 GPa.[27] For comparison, E varies between 197 GPa and 207 GPa for steel and steel alloys and is about 70 GPa for aluminum. A tensile load on the specimen causes a lateral contraction, whereas a compressive load causes a lateral extension — this is called the *Poisson effect*. Poisson's ratio relates the lateral or transverse deformations (ε_{yy}, ε_{zz}) to axial or longitudinal deformations (ε_{xx}) in a uniaxial test as follows:

$$\varepsilon_{yy} = -\nu \varepsilon_{xx} \tag{27.3}$$

The positive definiteness of strain energy puts a limit on these two constants:

$$E > 0 \tag{27.4a}$$

and

$$-1 < \nu < 1/2 \qquad\qquad (27.4b)$$

The value $\nu = 1/2$ implies elastic incompressibility, whereas negative values of ν are virtually unknown, except for special cellular solids such as reentrant foams.[28] Values of ν for trabecular bone have been reported to range from zero to just less than one.[29] Most structural FE analyses assume a Poisson's ratio value of 0.3. Poisson's ratio for steels varies between 0.265 and 0.305, and cork has a Poisson's ratio close to zero.

B. THE UNIAXIAL COMPRESSIVE TEST

Using a linear, static analysis, the FE model is subjected to a compressive load by fixing one face and applying displacement boundary condition to the opposite face. The trabecular bone tissue is generally assumed to have a uniform tissue modulus of $E_t = 5$ to 10 GPa. The choice of the tissue modulus E_t (10 GPa) is arbitrary since the actual tissue modulus can be estimated by simply scaling the apparent modulus (E_a) obtained from FE analysis to the E_a obtained experimentally. This will be covered in a later section.

Whereas the tissue modulus is a material property, the apparent modulus is defined as

$$E_a = \frac{\Sigma RF}{A_f \varepsilon} \qquad\qquad (27.5)$$

where E_a is the apparent modulus, ΣRF is the total reaction force, A_f is the area of the face of the unit cell upon which the displacement boundary conditions are applied, and ε is the applied strain (typically 1%). To calculate the apparent modulus, only the reaction force on the bone is generally considered. This is a reasonable assumption since the trabecular bone tissue is much stiffer than other constituents present (e.g., marrow).

C. BOUNDARY CONDITIONS

To compare the results of FE analysis to results obtained experimentally, it is important to ensure that the boundary conditions (BCs) used for the FE model accurately represent the experimental test setup. For example, to simulate a 1% strain compression test with zero friction between the test platens and the bone, the nodes on one face of the FE model should be prescribed using a displacement corresponding to 1% strain ($\varepsilon = 0.01$), while the displacements of the nodes on opposite face should be constrained *only* in the loading direction. The remaining model nodes should be unconstrained.

D. FE ALGORITHM

The main computation in a linear displacement-based FE analysis is to solve the following set of linear simultaneous equations:

$$[K]\{U\}=\{R\} \qquad\qquad (27.6)$$

where $[K]$ is the global stiffness matrix, $\{U\}$ is the unknown displacement vector, and $\{R\}$ is the applied load vector. A nonstationary iterative scheme such as preconditioned conjugate gradient (PCG) method can be efficiently implemented to solve Equation 27.6. The advantage of this method is that it converges to the solution very fast. A preconditioner such as the diagonal preconditioner (main diagonal of $[K]$) accelerates the solution convergence. However, if the main diagonal of $[K]$ does not have much variability as when all the voxels are of identical shape and size, another preconditioner known as incomplete Cholesky (IC) factorization should be used. The number of computations per iteration are greater for IC factorization, but this extra work is more than repaid by a reduction in the iteration count.[30]

Many commercial FE packages are readily available. Cosmos/M (Structural Research and Analysis Corp., V.2.0, Los Angeles, CA) can analyze models with up to 256,000 nodes/elements, and requires a minimum of 128 Megabytes of RAM (random access memory). For smaller models (up to 64,000 node/elements) the memory required is 32 Megabytes. Other commercial packages include ADINA, ANSYS, PATRAN, NASTRAN, and MARC. A World Wide Web address that lists a number of popular packages is <http://skyscraper.fortunecity.com/copland/949/fem-info/femsivu1.htm>.

E. VALIDATION OF FE MODEL: CONVERGENCE

A continuous structure has infinite degrees of freedom. On the other hand, an FE model of the same structure will have *finite* degrees of freedom; hence, an FE model will be stiffer than the original structure. As the number of elements in the FE model is increased, it becomes less stiff and closer to the original structure. However, increasing the number of elements also increases the computational cost. Hence, the minimum number of elements should be determined for a *desired* accuracy. One criterion for determining the minimum number of elements (or FE model resolution) is the convergence of apparent modulus. Another important numeric quantity is von Mises stress, which gives a measure of deformation energy in a structure as follows:

$$\sigma_{VM} = \frac{1}{3}\sqrt{\left(\sigma_1 - \sigma_2\right)^2 + \left(\sigma_2 - \sigma_3\right)^2 + \left(\sigma_3 - \sigma_1\right)^2} \tag{27.7}$$

$$U_{def} = \frac{3}{2} - \frac{1+v}{E}\sqrt{\left(\sigma_{VM}\right)^2} \tag{27.8}$$

where σ_{VM} is the von Mises stress (Equation 27.7), U_{def} is the deformation energy, and σ_i, $i = 1,2,3$, are the principal normal stresses. The von Mises stress can also be used to determine the validity and convergence of the FE model, and is often used as a yield failure criterion. Another common failure criterion is called the Tresca criterion.

F. VALIDATION OF FE MODEL: FE ANALYSIS

The validity of the FE analysis scheme can be checked using the following equation.[17]

$$\frac{\bar{\sigma}_t}{\sigma_a} = \frac{1}{V_f} \tag{27.9}$$

where $\bar{\sigma}_t$ is the average tissue stress, σ_a is the apparent stress ($\sigma_a = \Sigma RF/A_f$), and V_f is the bone volume fraction (BVF).

Plate 27.6 — FE STRESS ANALYSIS APPLIED: TETRAHEDRAL MODEL CONVERGENCE

Figures 27.11a and b and show the tetrahedral FE model of the unit cell and the deformed structure, respectively. An FE model should be able to capture the anatomical details of the original specimen and should also satisfy some convergence criterion. In order to determine the appropriate mesh resolution required, nine FE models with increasing mesh resolutions were generated from the *same* MC triangular

TABLE 27.1
Details of Nine FE Models

Label	No. of Nodes	No. of Tetrahedrons	Mesh Density (No. of Tetrahedrons per mm³ of Bone Volume)
A-1	810	1,700	3,911
A-2	1,891	4,456	10,251
A-3	2,522	6,208	14,281
A-4	3,839	10,208	23,483
A-5	5,402	15,056	34,635
A-6[a]	7,642	22,450	51,645
A-7	9,820	30,346	69,809
A-8	13,040	41,337	95,093
A-9	15,641	50,897	117,085

[a] The convergent model chosen for detailed analysis.

Source: Saxena, R. et al., *Comput. Methods Biomech. Biomed. Eng.,* 2, 287, 1999. With permission.

surface mesh model (Table 27.1 and Figure 27.11). Figure 27.12a shows how the resolution improves as the number of elements in the FE mesh is increased. Since the mesh resolution is proportional to the cube root of the number of elements, the rate of improvement decreases with an increase in the number of elements. The constant of proportionality between mesh resolution and number of elements will depend upon the bone volume fraction. As the mesh resolution of the FE models was varied from 32 to 107 μm, the discrepancy in the BVF was found to be about 2%. In this example the tetrahedral mesh generation time increases *linearly* as the number of tetrahedral elements are increased.

By using COSMOS/M linear static analysis, each FE unit cell model was subjected to a compressive load by fixing one face and applying a 1% strain $\varepsilon = 0.01$) to the opposite face. The trabecular bone was assumed to have a constant tissue modulus of 10 GPa. The computational time for the linear static analysis exhibited a bimodal solution time with respect to the number of elements. The computational time increased significantly for models with more than 25,000 elements.

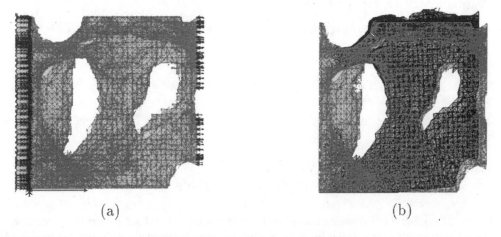

(a)   (b)

FIGURE 27.11   (a) Undeformed FE 4-node, tetrahedral mesh of unit cell shown with constrained (left) and displaced nodes (model A-6) and (b) deformed FE mesh (displacement magnification 5×). (From Saxena, R. et al., *Comput. Methods Biomech. Biomed. Eng.,* 2, 287, 1999. With permission.)

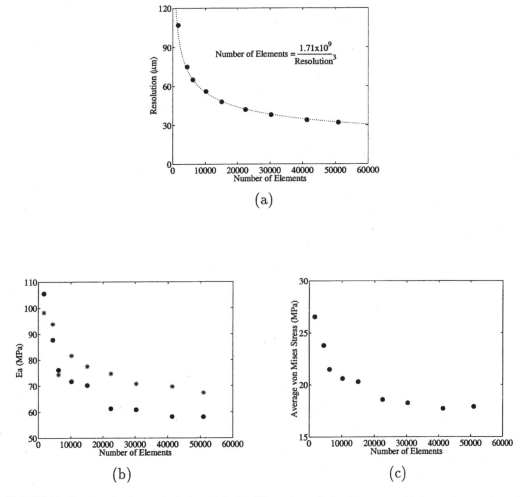

FIGURE 27.12 Results for tetrahedral models: (a) FE mesh resolution improves with increasing number of tetrahedrons. (b) Convergence plot and directional dependence of apparent modulus. Approximately 22,000 elements produced a converged result. This corresponds to a mesh density of about 50,000, four-node tetrahedral elements for the $1.5 \times 1.5 \times 2.0$ mm³ (9.66% bone volume fraction) model examined. (c) The average (over all the tetrahedra) von Mises stress showed similar convergence characteristics as the apparent modulus. (a and c, from Saxena, R. et al., *Comput. Methods Biomech. Biomed. Eng.*, 2, 287, 1999. With permission.)

Figures 27.12b and c show the dependence of apparent modulus and average von Mises stress on the number of tetrahedral elements. Both plots converge for a model with about 22,000 elements. For the converged model (A-6), an apparent modulus value of 61 MPa is obtained, which corresponds to a mesh resolution of 42 μm or a mesh density of approximately 50,000 elements/mm³ of bone tissue volume. Figure 27.12b shows apparent modulus plots obtained for compressive strains applied in two perpendicular directions denoted by (*) and (o). Note that the moduli values in the two directions are different, and indicate that the unit cell has different stiffnesses in the two directions. The convergence trend, however, is similar in the two cases.

For the convergent FE model (A-6), the ratio $\bar{\sigma}_t/\sigma_a$ is 12.427 and $1/V_f$ is 12.421 which provides additional validation for the FE model and the computational scheme.

The actual experimental apparent modulus value of the original specimen ($11 \times 11 \times 11$ mm) was 173 MPa.[31] In this case, the discrepancy between the experimental and numerical results is likely due to a number of factors, most notably the assumption of a 10-GPa constant isotropic tissue modulus and specimen size. As mentioned earlier, the tissue modulus of trabecular bone has been reported to vary from 1 to 20 GPa. Therefore, the apparent modulus for a linear analysis will lie in the range of 6 to 120 MPa. Furthermore, only a small subvolume ($1.5 \times 1.5 \times 2.0$ mm^2) of the original one cubic centimeter ($10 \times 10 \times 10$ mm^3) mechanical test specimen was analyzed. Moreover, this subvolume had a bone volume fraction of 9.66% compared with 11% in the original experimental test specimen, and would therefore be expected to yield a lower apparent stiffness. Assuming a cubic relationship between E and density, one can compute a density adjusted E value for the numerically analyzed subvolume. In this case, the adjusted value is 90 MPa, which is closer to the experimental value (173 MPa).

G. COMPUTATION OF STRESSES AND STRAINS

Besides computing the apparent modulus, another important objective of FE analysis is to determine the local stresses and strains. Noteworthy in this regard is the fact that a very small apparent strain may cause large local stresses and strains. Such stress and strain concentrations are hypothesized to result in local failure of the trabecular bone lattice.[17-19] In addition, these local stresses and strains are very important parameters from the point of view of bone remodeling. Normalized local stress or stress intensity is given by

$$\sigma_{int} = \frac{\sigma_{xx}}{\sigma_a} \tag{27.10}$$

Similarly, normalized local strain or strain intensity is given by

$$\varepsilon_{int} = \frac{\varepsilon_{xx}}{\varepsilon_{applied}} \tag{27.11}$$

Strain shapes can also be calculated using Lode's parameter (LP):[32]

$$LP = \frac{2\varepsilon_2 - \varepsilon_1 - \varepsilon_3}{\varepsilon_1 - \varepsilon_3} \tag{27.12}$$

where $\varepsilon_i = \ln(1 + e_i)$, $i = 1, 2, 3$, are principal logarithmic strains and e_i, $i = 1, 2, 3$, are the principal strains. Negative values of LP represent local constriction and positive values represent local flattening.

Plate 27.7 — FE STRESS ANALYSIS APPLIED:
STRESS–STRAIN INTENSITY AND POISSON'S RATIO

For the model with a mesh density of 50,000 elements/mm^3 (FE model A-6), the normal stress varied from –400 MPa (extreme compressive value) to 100 MPa (extreme tensile value). Compared with the computed compressive apparent stress value (0.6 MPa), these stress values indicate that while the apparent stress is quite low, the local tissue stresses are very high — almost 200 times in tension and 600 times in compression (Figure 27.13a). A similar finding was evident in the strain plot where local strains were seen to vary from 0.5% (extreme tension) to nearly –4.0% (extreme compression) and indicates that the local compressive strains are four times the applied strain (Figure 27.13b). These findings agree with previous studies.[17]

There was less than a 5% variation in the apparent modulus when Poisson's ratio values were varied between 0.1 and 0.4 (Figure 27.13c). Poisson's ratio values greater than 0.4, however, had a much more marked effect on the apparent modulus for which there was a roughly 25% increase for a corresponding increase in Poisson's ratio. This analysis (linear static, axial compression) indicates that the structural

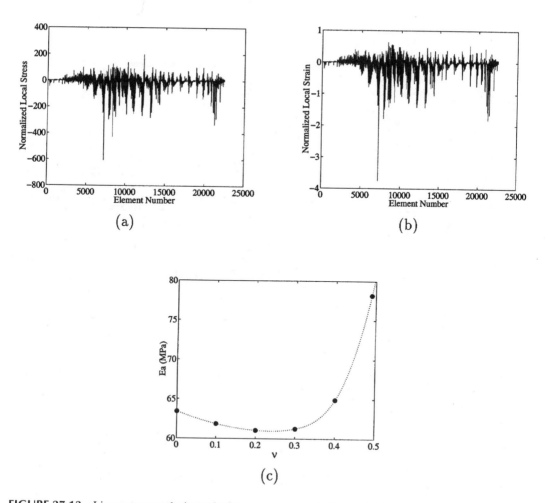

FIGURE 27.13   Linear stress analysis results for convergent tetrahedral model (A-6): (a) local stress intensity; (b) local strain intensity; (c) dependence of apparent modulus on Poisson's ratio. (From Saxena, R. et al., *Comput. Methods Biomech. Biomed. Eng.*, 2, 287, 1999. With permission.)

stiffness of trabecular bone is relatively insensitive to Poisson's ratio values less than or equal to 0.4. However, the choice of Poisson's ratio for values greater than 0.4 appears to be much more critical from the standpoint of model predictions. The result of FE analyses are dependent upon other factors, including the choice of boundary conditions and element type.

Plate 27.8 — FE STRESS ANALYSIS APPLIED: TETRAHEDRAL vs. BRICK MODEL

The stress intensity and strain intensity values were significantly higher for tetrahedral elements than for brick elements. Figure 27.14a shows the variation in Lode's parameter (LP) values obtained for the tetrahedral and brick element meshes. Both models show a similar LP trend, and the majority of elements were associated with positive LP values. Positive LP values indicate that the 1% applied compressive strain resulted in more flattening than constriction of the elements.

A frequency histogram of the local stress values in the load direction is shown in Figure 27.14b. A symmetric peak at zero stress value indicates the presence of both tensile and compressive stresses in response to bending of the trabecular struts. The smaller peak in the negative stress region corresponds to elements that are mainly axially compressed in the load direction. Note that there were a significantly lower number of brick elements that experienced compressive stresses.

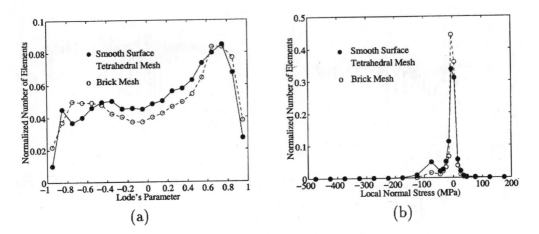

FIGURE 27.14 Comparison of tetrahedral and brick models: (a) variation of LP values for the two mesh models; (b) frequency plot of local normal stress. Normalized Number of Elements = Number of Elements/ Total Number of Elements.

H. DETERMINATION OF TISSUE MODULUS

The experimental tissue modulus of trabecular bone (E_t^{exp}) can be estimated by scaling the FE determined value (E_a^{FE}) to the apparent modulus obtained experimentally (E_a^{exp}). Assuming similar specimen geometry and similar boundary conditions, the tissue modulus is obtained as follows:

$$E_t^{exp} = \frac{E_a^{exp}}{E_a^{FE}} E_t^{FE} \qquad (27.13)$$

VI. MORPHOLOGIC ANALYSIS

The term *morphology* refers to the study of form and structure of an organism. It was mentioned earlier that the mechanical properties (apparent modulus and strength) of trabecular bone are strongly related to the apparent density. Typically, the mechanical properties are related to density using a power function ($y = ax^b$).[2-6,27] However, the value of the exponent (b) may vary significantly and power functions relating modulus and strength to apparent density generally only explain 60 to 80% of the variance in the data.[5] The unexplained variance has been hypothesized to be due to variations in the architecture of the trabecular bone lattice. Therefore, a central objective of morphological analysis is to obtain additional structural indexes which can be used to improve predictions of bone mechanical properties. In the following sections, several standard methods to quantify the architecture of a trabecular bone are presented.[33-38]

A. THE MEAN INTERCEPT LENGTH (MIL) METHOD

In the MIL method, the number of intersections between a linear grid and bone–marrow interface are counted as a function of the orientation of the grid (Figure 27.15a). The MIL function is given by

$$MIL(\omega) = \frac{L}{I(\omega)} \qquad (27.14)$$

where L is the total line length, I is the number of intersections, and ω is the orientation of the grid. Whitehouse[35] showed that the MIL plotted as a radius at the angle of measurement fit the

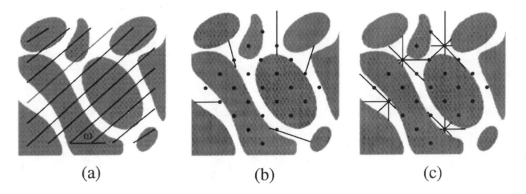

(a)   (b)   (c)

FIGURE 27.15 Principles for determining architectural anisotropy: (a) MIL measurement; (b) VO measurement; and (c) SVD and SLD measurement.

equation of an ellipse very closely. Harrigan and Mann[36] generalized this result in 3D to an ellipsoid and defined a material anisotropy tensor (M) given by

$$1/L^2 = n \cdot M \cdot n \tag{27.15}$$

where n is the unit vector, in the direction in which the measurement was made.

Cowin[39] defined a fabric tensor (H) which is related to M by

$$H = M^{-1/2} \tag{27.16}$$

Along any particular direction H will increase with an increase in modulus value in that direction. Thus, the extreme maximum and extreme minimum values of H correspond to the extreme maximum and extreme minimum values of modulus.

Plate 27.9 — MORPHOLOGICAL ANALYSIS APPLIED: MIL METHOD

The MIL method was applied to compute the morphological parameters of the trabecular bone unit cell model. By using a 3D version of the directed secant method, the binary image of the unit cell was scanned by a 3D test grid at randomly determined orientations (θ and ϕ — rotations about x-axis and z-axis, respectively) using analysis specifications given in Table 27.2. The intersections were recorded when the binary value of the current voxel differed from that of the previous voxel. Morphological and anisotropy parameters were then computed from intersection data using on the parallel plate model (see Table 27.2). The locus of the end points of the MIL vectors issuing from a common center was plotted and fitted to an ellipsoid of general formula:

$$An_1^2 + Bn_2^2 + Cn_3^2 + Dn_1n_2 + En_1n_3 + Fn_2n_3 = 1/L^2 \tag{27.17}$$

where $A \ldots F$ are the ellipsoid coefficients and n_i are the direction cosines of the MIL vector L. Equation 27.17 is identical to Equation 27.15. The material anisotropy tensor $[M]$ is given by

$$[M] = \begin{bmatrix} A & D & E \\ D & B & F \\ E & F & C \end{bmatrix} \tag{27.18}$$

TABLE 27.2
MIL Results for Unit Cell Model of Trabecular Bone[12]

Analysis Specifications

Total grid size	$77 \times 77 \times 98$
Sphere centered at	(38, 38, 49)
Sphere radius	37
Number of MIL rotations	144
Pixel size (mm^3/voxel)	$0.02 \times 0.02 \times 0.02$

Volume

Bone volume (BV) (mm^3)	0.16
Total volume (TV) (mm^3)	1.70
BV/TV (BVF)	0.0939

Intersections

Test line spacing (mm)	0.020
Number of test lines	4281
Average test line length (mm)	28.17
Total number of intersections	798109
Number of intersections per test line length (mm^{-1})	1.5477

Morphology Parameters

Bone surface/bone volume (BS/BV) (mm^{-1})	32.9464
Trabecular thickness (mm)	0.0607
Trabecular number (mm^{-1})	1.5477
Trabecular spacing (mm)	0.5854

Anisotropy Parameters — Experimental

Principal MILs (mm)	0.2411, 0.1994, 0.1063
Mean MIL (mm)	0.1268
SD of MIL (mm)	0.0305
Kurtosis	0.8397
Skew of MILs	0.9703
Orientation 1, (°)	(11.38, 55.59)
Orientation 2, (°)	(154.69, 151.05)
Orientation 3, (°)	(61.91, 123.43)
Degree of anisotropy MIL 1	0.3230
Degree of anisotropy MIL 2	0.0940
Degree of anisotropy MIL 3	–0.4169

A multivariate linear least-square fitting technique was used to fit the data by solving the linear system

$$[N]\{X\} = \{R\} \tag{27.19}$$

where N contains the projection data constituting of n_i, X is the column vector of the ellipsoid coefficients, and R is a column vector of $1/L^2$. The solution is formulated as

$$\{X\} = \frac{[N]^T\{R\}}{[N]^T[N]} \tag{27.20}$$

The resulting 3D ellipsoid is obtained by fitting Equation 27.17 to the locus of experimental MIL vectors, and is illustrated in Figure 27.16.

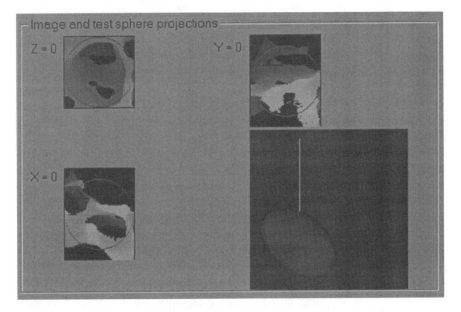

FIGURE 27.16 MIL data fitted to an ellipsoid.

B. THE VOLUME ORIENTATION (VO) METHOD

In the VO method, a local volume orientation is defined at a point. The local VO can be described as the orientation of the longest intercept length through the point as shown in Figure 27.15b. A statistic of a sample of local volume orientations is given by an orientation matrix called the VO fabric tensor (V).

C. THE STAR VOLUME DISTRIBUTION (SVD) METHOD

This method is related to both the VO method and the star volume method (Figure 27.15c). The star volume is defined as the average unobscured volume at any point, and is given mathematically as

$$\overline{v_V} = \frac{1}{3}\pi L^3 \tag{27.21}$$

A star volume component is defined as the volume at a particular orientation ω at a point given by

$$\overline{v_V}(\omega) = \frac{1}{3}\pi L^3(\omega) \tag{27.22}$$

An SVD fabric tensor (S) is described based on the variation of the star volume component with orientation.

D. THE STAR LENGTH DISTRIBUTION (SLD) METHOD

Instead of computing the volume as in the SVD method, the length is computed in the SLD method. The star length component (s) is given by

$$s(\omega) = \frac{1}{n}\sum_{i=1}^{n} L_i(\omega) \tag{27.23}$$

where the SLD fabric tensor is denoted by L.

TABLE 27.3
Correlations between Compliance Components
Obtained from the FE Analyses and Those
Predicted from MIL, VO, SVC, and SLD

	MIL	VO	SVD	SLD
$\dfrac{1}{E_1}$	0.968	0.973	0.974	0.980
$-\dfrac{v_{ij}}{E_i}$	0.924	0.959	0.958	0.957
$\dfrac{1}{G_{ij}}$	0.967	0.981	0.982	0.982

Source: van Rietbergen, B. et al., *J. Orthop. Res.*, 16, 23, 1998.

van Rietbergen et al.[40] performed a 3D FE analysis of trabecular bone specimens obtained from the single vertebral body of a whale, and computed the corresponding fabric tensors using the above four methods. Compliance matrices (inverse of stiffness) were computed from the fabric tensors. These were compared with the compliance constants determined from the FE analysis and excellent correlations were found (Table 27.3). Correlations for volume-based fabric measures were found to be slightly better than for MIL-based measures of fabric.

VII. SUMMARY

Recent advances in imaging techniques, 3D visualization software, and efficient FE analysis algorithms have made it possible to perform large-scale investigations of the apparent mechanical behavior of trabecular bone. FE analysis results indicate that small values of apparent strains can lead to very large values of local stresses and strains in the trabecular bone lattice. Such stress and strain concentrations are hypothesized to produce local failures. The effects of architecture on the apparent mechanical properties of trabecular bone can be studied utilizing 2D and 3D morphologic analysis techniques on the 3D models of the trabecular bone. By utilizing both experimental and numeric approaches, the tissue modulus value can be estimated. In the future, higher-resolution CT images and efficient FE mesh generation schemes will make anatomically precise numerical analysis a routine and powerful tool to study the mechanical behavior of complex lattice structures such as trabecular bone.

REFERENCES

1. McElhaney, J.H., Fogle, J.L., Melvin, J.W., et al., Mechanical properties of cranial bone, *J. Biomech.*, 3, 495, 1970.
2. Carter, D.R. and Hayes,W.C., The compressive behavior of bone as a two-phase porous structure, *J. Bone Joint Surg.*, 59-A, 954, 1977.
3. Gibson, L.J., The mechanical behavior of cancellous bone, *J. Biomech.*, 18, 317, 1985.
4. Rice, J.C., Cowin, S.C., and Bowman, J.A., On the dependence of the elasticity and strength of cancellous bone on apparent density, *J. Biomech.*, 21, 155, 1988.
5. Keller, T.S., Predicting the compressive mechanical behavior of bone, *J. Biomech.*, 27, 1159, 1994.
6. Zhu, M., Keller, T.S., Moeljanto, E., and Spengler, D.M., Multiplanar variations in the structural characteristics of cancellous bone, *Bone*, 15, 251, 1994.

7. Radon, J., On the determination of functions from their integrals along certain manifolds, *Ber. Verh. Saechs. Akad. Wiss. Leipzig, Math. Phys. Kl.*, 69, 262, 1917.
8. Keller, T.S., Moeljanto, E., Main, J.A., and Spengler, D.M., Distribution and orientation of bone in the human lumbar vertebral centrum, *J. Spinal Dis.*, 5, 60, 1992.
9. Hall, E.L., *Computer Image Processing and Recognition*, Academic Press, New York, 1979.
10. Trussell, H.J., Comments on "Picture thresholding using an iterative selection method," *IEEE Trans. Syst. Man Cybern.*, 9, 311, 1979.
11. Harrigan, T.P., Jasty, M., Mann, R.W., and Harris, W.H., Limitations of the continuum assumption in cancellous bone, *J. Biomech.*, 21, 269, 1988.
12. Keller, T.S., *Trabecular Bone Morphology and Analysis System* (*TBMAS*), Department of Mechanical Engineering, the University of Vermont, Burlington, 1998.
13. Lorensen, W.E. and Cline, H.E., Marching cubes: a high resolution 3D surface construction algorithm, *Comput. Graphics*, 21, 163, 1987.
14. Schroeder, W., Martin, K., and Lorensen, B., *The Visualization Toolkit — An Object-Oriented Approach to 3D Graphics*, Prentice-Hall, Upper Saddle River, NJ, 1997.
15. Fyhrie, D.P., Hamid, M.S., Kuo, R.F., and Lang, S.M., Direct three-dimensional finite element analysis of human vertebral cancellous bone, *Trans. Orthrop. Res. Soc.*, 17, 551, 1992.
16. Hollister, S.J., Brennan, J.M., and Kikuchi, N., A homogenization sampling procedure for calculating trabecular bone effective stiffness and tissue level stress, *J. Biomech.*, 27, 433, 1994.
17. van Rietbergen, B., Weinans, H., Huiskes, R., and Odgaard, A., A new method to determine trabecular bone elastic properties and loading using micromechanical finite-element models, *J. Biomech.*, 28, 69, 1995.
18. Müller, R. and Rüegsegger, P., Three-dimensional finite-element modelling of noninvasively assessed trabecular bone structures, *Med. Eng. Phys.*, 17, 126, 1995.
19. Saxena, R., Keller, T.S., and Sullivan, J.M., A three-dimensional finite element scheme to investigate the apparent mechanical properties of trabecular bone, *Comput. Methods Biomech. Biomed. Eng.*, 2, 287, 1999.
20. Guldberg, R.E. and Hollister, S.J., Finite element solution errors associated with digital image-based mesh generation, *ASME Bioeng. Conf.*, 28, 147, 1994.
21. Jacobs, C.R., Davis, B.R., Rieger, C.J., et al., Accurate quantification of cancellous bone tissue modulus can be made using experimentally measured apparent stiffness and large-scale finite-element modeling, *Trans. ORS*, 23, 111, 1998.
22. van Rietbergen, B., Ulrich, D., Pistoia, W., et al., Prediction of trabecular bone failure parameters using a tissue failure criterion, *Trans. ORS*, 23, 550, 1998.
23. Sullivan, J.M., Jr., Charron, G., and Paulsen, K.D., A three-dimensional mesh generator for arbitrary multiple material domains, *Finite Elem. Anal. Des.*, 25, 219, 1997.
24. Lo, S.H., A new mesh generation scheme for arbitrary planar domains, *Int. J. Num. Meth. Eng.*, 21, 1403, 1985.
25. Desai, C.S. and Abel, J.F., *Introduction to the Finite Element Method*, Van Nostrand Reinhold, New York, 1972.
26. Spyrakos, C.C., *Finite Element Modeling in Engineering Practice*, West Virginia University Press, Morgantown, 1994.
27. Rho, J.Y., Ashman, R.B., and Turner, C.H., Young's modulus of trabecular and cortical bone material: ultrasonic and microtensile measurements, *J. Biomech.*, 26, 111, 1993.
28. Lakes, R., Foam structures with a negative Poisson's ratio, *Science*, 235, 1038, 1987.
29. Keaveny, T.M., Borchers, R.E., Gibson, L.J., and Hayes, W.C., Theoretical analysis of the experimental artifact in trabecular bone compressive modulus, *J. Biomech.*, 26, 599, 1993.
30. Golub, G.H. and Ortega, J.M., *Scientific Computing and Differential Equations: An Introduction to Numerical Methods*, Academic Press, San Diego, CA, 1992.
31. Zhu, M., Keller, T.S., and Spengler, D.M., Effects of specimen load-bearing and free surface layers on the compressive mechanical properties of cellular materials, *J. Biomech.*, 27, 57, 1994.
32. Lode, W., Versuche über den Einfluss der mittleren Hauptspannung auf das Fliessen des Metalle Eisen, Kaupfer, and Nickel, *Z. Phys.*, 36, 913, 1926.
33. Weibel, E.R. and Elias, H.E., *Quantitative Methods in Morphology*, Springer, Berlin, 1967.
34. Underwood, E.E., *Quantitative Stereology*, Addison-Wesley, Reading, MA, 1970.

35. Whitehouse, W.J., The quantitative morphology of anisotropic trabecular bone, *J. Microsc.*, 101, 153, 1974.

36. Harrigan, T.P. and Mann, R.W., Characterization of microstructural anisotropy in orthotropic materials using a second rank tensor, *J. Mater. Sci.*, 19, 761, 1984.

37. Kuo, A.D. and Carter, D.R., Computational methods for analyzing the structure of cancellous bone in planar sections, *J. Orthop. Res.*, 9, 918, 1991.

38. Odgaard, A., Three-dimensional methods for quantification of cancellous bone architecture, *Bone*, 20, 315, 1997.

39. Cowin, S.C., *Bone Mechanics*, CRC Press, Boca Raton, FL, 1989.

40. van Rietbergen, B., Odgaard, A., Kabel, J., and Huiskes, R., Relationships between bone morphology and bone elastic properties can be accurately quantified using high-resolution computer reconstructions, *J. Orthop. Res.*, 16, 23, 1998.

Section III

Methods of Mechanical Testing of the Bone–Implant Interface

28 Factors Affecting the Strength of the Bone-Implant Interface

Brodie E. McKoy, Yuehuei H. An, and Richard J. Friedman

CONTENTS

I. INTRODUCTION

The modern era of total joint arthroplasty began in the 1960s with Sir John Charnley's development of total hip replacement consisting of a stainless steel femoral head articulating with a polyethylene acetabular implant, both secured to supporting bone by polymethylmethacrylate (PMMA) cement.

Now, 40 years later, 15- to 20-year success rates close to 90% are being reported for total hip and total knee arthroplasty. The high success rate of this early technique of fixation makes it the gold standard to which all subsequent methods should be compared. Infection and material failure presented early problems; however, these complications have been greatly reduced, and the surgeries have gained widespread popularity with consistently reliable results.

Despite great strides in the development of better component designs, biomaterials, and surgical techniques, the life span of cemented total joint-arthroplasty is limited, among other things, by the long-term mechanical properties of PMMA and polyethylene debris. The clinically significant loosening rates of cemented implants, especially in younger, active persons, have led many investigators to pursue methods of cementless fixation. New biomaterials and innovative designs are two promising approaches which will improve this type of fixation.

As research and development of cementless fixation continues, a great deal of attention is being focused on the bone–implant interface and the factors affecting its strength. Several methods of achieving implant fixation with long-term stability have been introduced, including biological fixation, achieved with ingrowth into a porous coating; press-fit fixation, in which a nonporous-coated implant is surrounded by fibrous tissue; and chemical fixation, where a bioactive ceramic chemically bonds to surrounding bone. All of these approaches have merit and each approach has its proponents and detractors.[1] Early results with each method have been promising, but only time will reveal long-term complications and rates of success.

Not only do the implant and local conditions affect the bone–implant interface, but numerous other factors exist which may have an impact on long-term fixation in either a positive or negative way. Modalities such as radiation, hormones, and various medications have the potential to interfere with implant fixation. Numerous growth factors have been studied and used in tumor and spinal surgery to promote bone ingrowth. Some of these growth factors used locally may enhance bonding between the prosthesis and bone. Surgical technique as well as various patient factors including age and lifestyle also affect the all-important bone–implant interface.

II. IMPLANT AND LOCAL FACTORS

A. IMPLANT SURFACE CONFIGURATIONS

The primary function of the bone–implant interface is to provide a safe and effective load transfer from the prosthesis to the bone. Cementless implants may be fixed to bone by both osseointegration and bone ingrowth. Branemark[2,3] originally coined the term *osseointegration* in the dental literature to refer to the intimate contact of bone tissue with the surface of a titanium implant.[2] The term bone ingrowth refers to the actual bone formation within the porous structure of the implant.[4,5] The surface configurations of the implant play a role in initial stability and type of fixation achieved.[6]

Porous-coated surfaces are used to obtain biological fixation in cementless surgery. In recent years, these have become increasingly popular in young, active patients.[7,8] Several different porous surfaces have been developed with slight differences in the strength of fixation to bone. Friedman et al.[9] compared the histological and mechanical characteristics of arc-deposited titanium implants in rabbits to one layer cobalt–chromium beads, three layers of cobalt–chromium beads, plasma-sprayed cobalt–chromium, and uncoated titanium alloy (Figure 28.1). The physiological response to a porous-coated implant is similar to the healing cascade of cancellous bone defects, with newly formed tissue filling in the void spaces of the porous material.[10,11] The initial stability of the prosthesis determines the clinical success by allowing bony ingrowth instead of fibrous tissue. This bony ingrowth gives significant strength to the bone–implant interface. The shear strength at the bone–implant interface after ingrowth equals or exceeds trabecular bone.[12-15] Galante found bone ingrowth at 6 weeks in wire mesh surfaces to be as stable as a bone cement interface.[13]

Too much relative motion between the implant and host bone and the quality of the initial press-fit in an uncemented arthroplasty are important factors leading to ingrowth of fibrous connective tissue

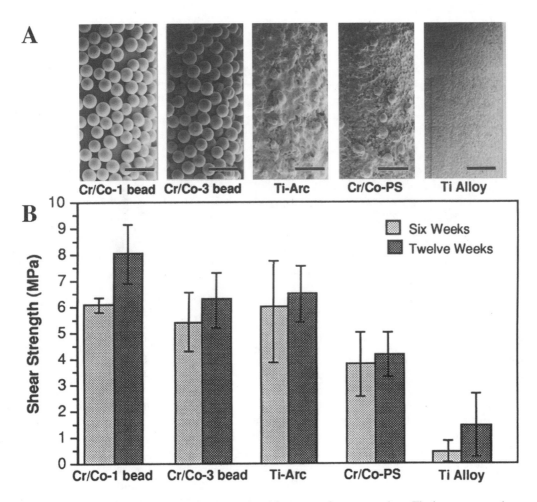

FIGURE 28.1 (A) Scanning electron micrographs of five types of porous coatings. The bar represents 1 mm. Cr/Co-1 = one layer of cobalt–chromium beads, Cr/Co-3 = three layers of cobalt–chromium beads, Ti-Arc = arc-deposited titanium, Cr/Co-PS = plasma-sprayed cobalt chromium, and Ti alloy = grit-blasted titanium alloy. (B) Shear strengths of the same implants at 6 and 12 weeks. Bar denotes SD of mean. (From Friedman R.J., et al. *J. Orthop. Res.*, 14, 456, 1996. With permission.)

rather than bone into porous surfaces.[16,17] The ingrowth of bone is necessary for initial stability and subsequent long-term fixation.[18,19] Micromotion of as little as 100 to 500 μm between bone and implant is sufficient to inhibit bone ingrowth and result in a fibrous membrane forming between the two, resulting in a mechanically unstable implant.[20]

Porous coatings used to promote bone ingrowth include both ceramics and metals. Currently, the majority of implants use porous metal surfaces, created either by sintering cobalt–chrome powder or beads or by diffusion bonding of titanium wire mesh.[21,22] In addition, plasma spraying material onto metal surfaces is another method used to produce a porous-like surface. The surface of implants manufactured in this manner is highly textured, but the actual porosity is limited.[23,24]

Pore sizes have been extensively studied and found to affect the strength of fixation. Several investigators have studied pore sizes of less than 100 μm and found that increasing pore size correlated with increasing strength of fixation.[25,26] One study showed no relationship between pore sizes in the range of 150 to 400 μm and interface shear strength.[27,28] From these and other studies, it can be concluded that the optimal range for pore size to obtain maximal strength at the bone–implant interface is from 100 to 400 μm.

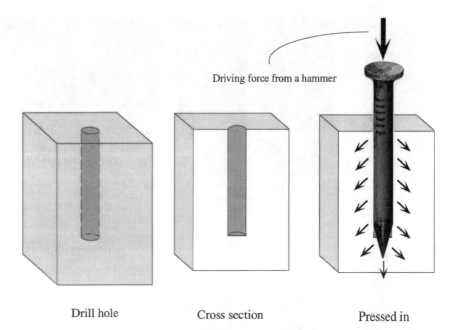

Driving force from a hammer

Drill hole   Cross section   Pressed in

FIGURE 28.2 A nail driven into a block of wood with a predrilled hole is an example of "press-fit." Carpenters predrill holes to prevent the wood from splitting when nailed. (Adapted from Blaha, J. D., Press-fit femoral components, in *The Adult Hip*, Callaghan, J. J., et al., Eds., Lippincott-Raven, Philadelphia, 1998.)

Biegler et al.[29] studied the effects of porous coating and loading conditions on femoral stem stability. This group examined the bone prosthesis–interface behavior under different load types using finite-element analysis. Torsional loads such as stair climbing were found to contribute to a greater degree of implant micromotion than stance loading. It was concluded that contact at the bone–implant interface was more dependent on load type than either surface coating or implant geometry.

Smooth surface implants have been used in cemented arthroplasties. Some investigators have used the term *press-fit* to describe the fixation of a smooth prosthesis without porous ingrowth or cement. However, press-fit is an engineering term which denotes a mechanical joining of two parts based on contact pressure. As Figure 28.2 illustrates, a nail driven into a block of wood is an example of press-fit.[30] Thus, either a smooth or porous structure can be "press-fit" by the true meaning. A fibrous tissue may form around smooth implants in cementless surgery largely as a result of low initial stability.[31] It is this intervening tissue that may weaken the bone–implant interface. Lee et al.[6] compared initial stability of uncemented porous-coated and smooth implants in synthetic femurs. This group found that porous-coated implants had greater initial stability with less axial micromotion compared with smooth implants. These findings suggest that surface configuration plays a major role in initial stability and thus strength of the bone–implant interface.

Impaction bone-grafting has been studied by several investigators in different models with varying results. Segawa et al.[32] found tibial components placed with impaction grafting to have greater micromotion and less initial stability. Meding et al.[33] found worrisome results in femoral stems fixed with cement and impaction grafting. However, several groups have shown increased initial stability and strength of the bone–implant interface.[34-36] Longer-term *in vivo* studies should be undertaken to evaluate the compaction technique and results.

Grooves and other surface modifications have been studied in cementless press-fit techniques as well as cemented techniques.[37,38] These prostheses rely on a macrointerlock with bone or cement. Wang et al.[39] found that as surface roughness increased there was a corresponding increase in interfacial shear strength. This group also showed surface finish to be more important in stem–cement interface shear strength than cement interface porosity.[40] Many investigators feel these

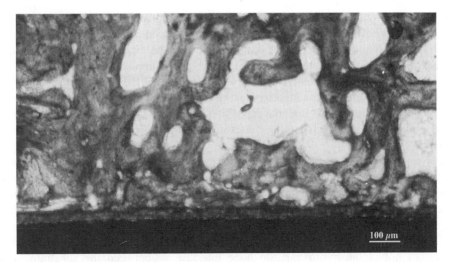

FIGURE 28.3 Photomicrograph of an implant coated with hydroxyapatite. Note the intimate union of trabecular bone and the prosthesis with the 50-μm hydroxyapatite layer.[48]

types of surface configurations may be superior to porous coating for two reasons: (1) some retrieval data show that less than 30 to 60% of porous coated specimens are occupied by bone and (2) these configurations do not lessen the fatigue strength as porous coatings might. The initial strength of the bone–implant interface appears to be good with these surface modifications. However, there is considerable debate concerning the lasting implant stability.

B. IMPLANT SURFACE COATINGS

Various surface coatings have been extensively studied and can markedly affect the strength of the bone–implant interface. Chemical fixation is a technique where bioactive ceramics chemically bond to surrounding bone.[41] Ceramics are a group of materials made from fine powder. In the biomaterials literature, ceramics comprise all nonmetallic and inorganic materials. Oxide ceramics and calcium phosphate ceramics are the two materials most often used in joint arthroplasty.

Oxide ceramics have found a use in joint surgery as femoral head components which articulate with a polyethylene acetabular component and acetabular liners. In contrast, calcium phosphate ceramics have been used as bone substitution material and coatings for joint prostheses.[42] Tricalcium phosphate and hydroxyapatite are the two most common calcium phosphate ceramics used.

Hydroxyapatite has been studied for over 20 years and is referred to as a bioactive ceramic because of the biological response it generates after implantation.[43] The biocompatibility of this substance has been documented in many *in vivo* and *in vitro* studies.[44,45] Originally studied for dental and oral surgery applications, hydroxyapatite has been used to coat metal prostheses to provide a chemical bond between the implant and bone.[46,47] This coating allows an intimate union between the bone and prosthesis as seen in Figure 28.3.[48]

Many methods have been developed to apply hydroxyapatite powder to a metal surface. The technique of plasma spraying has been used most extensively.[49] This is done by introducing the hydroxyapatite powder into a flame that directs the particles for deposit on the metal surface. Ion sputtering, dip-coating-sintering, and hot isostatic pressing are other coating methods being investigated.

Any coating applied to a metal may affect the fatigue strength of that metal. Thin coatings, between 30 and 90 μm, are recommended, because they do not affect the mechanical properties of the substrate metal.[50] Mechanical testing of the coating applied to metal has demonstrated that the mechanical properties of the coating are greatly improved in shear and tension, with shear increased three to four times.[51] The hydroxyapatite may form a chemical bond with the titanium or chromium-cobalt alloy to which it is applied.[50]

The mechanical advantages of hydroxyapatite-coated implants have been studied in various animal models.[52] When hydroxyapatite-coated implants are compared with noncoated devices of the same design, the maximum fixation strength is shown to be increased and the time required to achieve adequate fixation strength is shortened.[53,54] Thus, the implant forms a faster and stronger bond to surrounding bone. Histological studies have confirmed these findings. Sections through the bone–implant interface of a hydroxyapatite-coated implant show increased amounts of bone–implant contact through preferential deposition of new bone both on the surface of the implant as well as on the host bed.[55] This interface does not contain a fibrous tissue membrane as seen in some smooth implants.

Numerous other studies have documented that hydroxyapatite coatings increase the amount of bone ingrowth and osseointegration.[56,57] The maximal interface strength with these coatings is achieved at 6 weeks, compared with 12 to 16 weeks for porous ingrowth. The strength of the interface itself has been shown to increase more than threefold with hydroxyapatite coating.

The strength of the bone–implant interface with hydroxyapatite coating has been investigated by several groups. Mechanical testing to failure in shear has demonstrated that failure occurs in the bone, but not at the hydroxyapatite–bone interface or between the substrate metal and hydroxyapatite.[58] The strong bond made to bone and the increase in ultimate strength are secondary to the fact that hydroxyapatite is osteophilic and provides a scaffolding on which bone can proliferate and bond.[59] Small gaps between the implant and coating or defects in the coating did not alter these findings.[60]

Hydroxyapatite coating can also alter the strength of the bone-implant interface by its ability to fill defects. This bioactive coating has been shown to fill in defects up to 2 mm in size with bony ingrowth.[61,62] Thus, hydroxyapatite increases the contact between the prosthesis and bone, leading to a greater interface stability. In contrast, a fibrous membrane will form in porous material if the gap is greater than 300 mm, leading to a much weaker interface.[63]

Numerous investigations have been carried out to test the strength of hydroxyapatite prostheses in the canine model.[64,65] These implants withstood higher compression, shear, and tensile forces than did noncoated controls. In addition, the bonding occurred in a shorter time. Bone scans performed at 6 months showed an equilibrium between implant integration and bone metabolism. Histological examination also showed superior results, with no intervening fibrous tissue between the bone and hydroxyapatite coating. Again, close apposition between the bone and implant were not required to obtain a stable interface.

Another type of coating applied in arthroplastic surgery using cement is a precoating of the implant with PMMA. Mounting evidence points to the cement mantle as being the reason for failures in these types of fixations. Debonding at this interface appears to be a key problem.[66] To circumvent this, many groups have begun precoating stems with cement which allows a chemical bond to the cement mantle. This technique markedly improves the strength of the interface.

Bone marrow cells seeded in a bone filler have been shown to have osteoconductive properties *in vivo*.[67] This bone tissue engineering is in the early stages of development. In the future, this may prove useful in reconstruction surgery to treat large bone defects or to coat prostheses to promote increased bone ingrowth into porous surfaces.

C. IMPLANT GEOMETRY

Implant geometry varies between different manufacturers. The effect of different geometric patterns on implant stability and strength of the bone–implant interface has been evaluated.[68,69] For cemented prostheses, sharp edges should be avoided as these produce stress risers that may initiate a fracture of the cement mantle. Noncircular shapes, such as rounded rectangles and ellipses, help improve rotational stability of the implant with the cement mantle. The implant should fill at least 80% of the cross section of the medullary canal with an optimal cement mantle of 4 mm proximally and 2 mm distally.[70] Implants that allow these dimensions of cement in neutral placement lessen the chance of localized weakness and fracture of the cement mantle. For cementless fixation, geometry is important as well. The size and shape of femoral components should be optimal to provide both axial and rotational stability.

Schneider et al.[71] evaluated the degree of micromotion with different geometric-shaped femoral components. Three straight and one curved prostheses were submitted to *in vitro* tests in autopsy specimens. Dynamic axial and torsional loads were applied. They found micromotion at the bone–implant interface was smallest for the curved and highest for the straight femoral components. Initial stability allows less micromotion and increases the bond between the prostheses and the host bone. Prosthesis stability was found by Kelysey and Goodman[72] to be more important to surgeons than ease of implantation and removal or cost.

The geometry of acetabular cups influences stability. Ries et al.[73] studied the effect of cementless cup geometry on strain distribution and press-fit stability. This group found a nonhemispheric cup to provide greater stability. The gradual transition from a hemisphere at the dome to a larger peripheral dimension maximized peripheral strains. The geometry of all implanted components on both sides of the joint is important in stability of the prosthesis.

D. Material Properties of Implant

The material properties of the implant play a critical role in the life and strength of the bone–implant interface. The properties of the material strongly influence the design choices as well as the eventual device performance. These properties are specific to each material used in joint surgery.

Corrosion, the electrochemical dissolution of a metal, is one such property. Particles can be generated by corrosion.[74] A second property, fretting, refers to small cyclic motions, usually less than 100 µm, of one surface relative to another. These two processes may be synergistic. Fretting can disrupt the oxide films which protect cobalt–chrome and titanium-based alloys from corrosion. This disruption may dramatically accelerate the corrosion rate.

Modular implants demonstrate fretting corrosion.[75] Modular implants often have different metals in contact with each other. Levine and Staehle[75] reported that corrosion rates were increased when Co–Cr–Mo was coupled with Ti–Al–V vs. when it was coupled to itself. Another study reported less corrosion of Ti–Al–V when coupled with Co–Cr–Mo than with itself.[76] The amount of corrosion a metal undergoes is specific to the metal itself. Fretting corrosion leads to the generation of particles which may cause aseptic loosening and weakening of the bone–implant interface.

Another property of the implant which affects interface strength is the strength of the implant. Implant fractures can cause motion and failure leading to decreased stability.[77,78] In comparing different materials, the fatigue life is important. This is defined as the number of cycles needed to cause failure at a fixed cyclic stress. Sandborn et al.[79] evaluated a unicompartmental knee implant retrieved after 11 years *in situ*. The specimen was a cast stainless steel femoral component which had a fracture 1 cm from the anterior tip. Microscopic analysis showed a high inclusion content and inhomogeneous grain size which likely contributed to the fracture.

E. Quality of Cement and Cementing Procedures

Since the early days of Sir John Charnley, the cemented prosthesis still remains the gold standard of fixation techniques. The cement used in arthroplasty is PMMA. This acrylic cement as well as the methods used to prepare it have undergone extensive research in recent years. Both the quality of cement as well as the cementing procedure affect the strength of the bone–implant interface.

A great deal of information has accumulated regarding the factors that either adversely affect or enhance the use of PMMA. The cementing techniques have gone through several generations of improvement. The most current techniques are referred to as third generation and include (1) canal plugging; (2) reduced cement porosity; (3) canal preparation; and (4) cement column pressurization.[80]

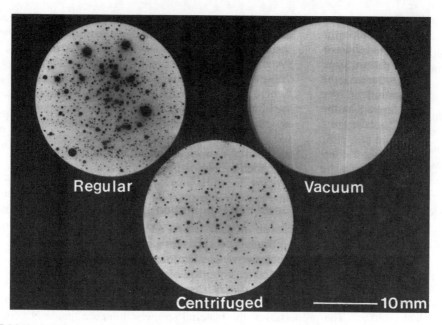

FIGURE 28.4   Polished stained cement specimens hand-mixed, centrifuged, and vaccum-mixed demonstrating amount of porosity present. (From Wixson, R.L., *J. Arthroplasty*, 2, 144, 1987. With permission.)

The presence of porosity in cement has been shown by many investigators to cause a decrease in strength.[81-83] Porosity reduction has been shown to improve the fatigue life of PMMA. Cement porosity can be decreased to less than 1% by mixing in a vacuum of approximately 500 mmHg. Centrifugation also decreases the porosity considerably (Figure 28.4).[84] Both of these techniques require additional equipment but they are easily performed and provide an increase of 10 to 20% in strength. Cement column pressurization also has been shown to increase strength by up to 20% by reducing porosity.

The quality of the cement is another important factor in strength. Any impurities will affect the fatigue strength of the compound. However, PMMA in general has not improved significantly when compared with the original cement used by Charnley. Much of the quality problems arise with cement preparation and insertion of the mixture. Canal lavage helps to clear the area of unwanted debris. Inclusion of blood or tissue can cause up to a 77% loss of strength in the cement.[85] All of these methods improve the cement and help to strengthen the interface in cemented prosthesis.

The analysis of the interfaces in cement prosthesis is complex. No true prosthesis-to-bone interface exists because of the intervening PMMA. Instead, two interfaces are present, one between the prosthesis and the cement and the other between the cement and the bone. This added variable makes individual interface analysis difficult. Because of this, the strength of the cement is studied most exhaustively and is considered by some to be an expanded interface.

F. PARTICULATE DEBRIS

Osteolysis, or periprosthetic bone loss, is a significant cause of decreased strength of the bone–implant interface. This condition is usually recognized roentgenographically either as diffuse cortical thinning or as focal cystic lesions (Figure 28.5). The pathogenesis of focal osteolysis has not been fully elucidated. In 1977, Wilbert and Semlitsch[86] were among the first to suggest that a macrophage response to particulate debris was an important factor leading to aseptic loosening. The nature of the interface between the host and the implant was described by Goldring et al.[87] They described a synovial-like membrane at the bone–cement interface in patients with a loose

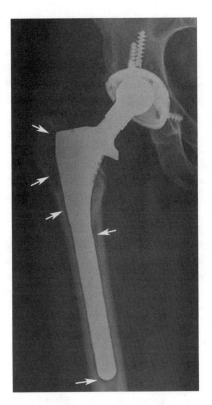

FIGURE 28.5 AP radiograph of the right hip of a patient with a total joint arthroplasty demonstrating radiotranslucent periprosthetic osteolysis around the femoral component (see arrows).

total hip prosthesis. Large amounts of prostaglandin E2 (PGE2) and collagenase were found in this membrane which was believed to produce bone resorption. Many investigators have since studied these intercellular mediators and their relationship to aseptic loosening.[88-90]

The generation of particulate debris and its migration into the synovial cavity and periprosthetic space stimulates macrophage recruitment and proliferation. This is followed by phagocytosis and secretion of various cytokines and intercellular mediators like interleukin-1 (IL-1) and prostaglandin E2 (PGE2). These substances, in turn, stimulate osteoclastic bone resorption.

The particles may originate from various sites. In acetabular components, particles may come from the articular surface of ultrahigh molecular weight polyethylene (UHMWPE), the nonarticular side of UHMWPE, at the metal shell or at the fixation screws. In the femoral component, the stem, porous coating, articular surface, and modular connection may all be the culprit. In addition, surgical tools, bone, remnants from the surface processing of the prosthetic device, and the catalyst used in the processing of UHMWPE can all be sources of particulate debris. The predominant particle appears to be UHMWPE, mostly from the articular surface.

The plethora of literature on particulate debris and its relationship to periprosthetic loosening illustrates its importance. Osteolysis around the implant significantly weakens the bone–implant interface. As research continues in this area, understanding of the interaction of this debris and its relationship to the bone–implant interface will continue to increase.

G. IMPLANT DESIGN AND STRESS SHIELDING

An engineering-related problem of design in arthroplasty is stress shielding which might eventually undermine the mechanical stability of the prosthesis. Implants are made from metallic materials which are usually an order of magnitude, or more, stiffer than the bone which they contact. This leads to a large percentage of the load normally transmitted by the bone being borne by the prosthesis instead. This shielding can lead to bone disuse atrophy.[91,92] Bone remodeling is very sensitive to stress.

In designing implants, the modulus of elasticity is a key component. A decrease in the modulus leads to a decrease in stress in the stem and an increase in stress transmitted by the bone. In addition, increasing the length and cross-sectional diameter of the stem increase the stress in the stem and result in an increase in stress shielding. The bending stiffness of a stem is proportional to the fourth power of the diameter, so a small increase in diameter leads to a large increase in rigidity.

Several investigators have identified the proximal medial cortex as the area most affected by stress shielding in both cemented and cementless implants.[93,94] Because of this finding, some cemented femoral components have been designed with a collar to load this medial area axially.[95] However, the role of a collar in preventing loosening has not been clearly established. In cementless components, a collar is more controversial because it may prevent complete seating of the implant.

In the acetabulum, ultrahigh-weight polyethylene causes peak stress to develop in the pelvic bone. However, a metal-backed design with a polyethylene liner reduces the areas of high stress and causes a more uniform distribution. The preservation of subchondral bone and thick-walled cups leads to decreased peak stress levels and may cause stress shielding in this area. The implant designs mentioned above play a crucial role in stress shielding and bone remodeling which determine the strength of the bone–implant interface.

III. MEDICATIONS AND OTHER LOCAL FACTORS

A. SYSTEMIC HORMONES

Systemic hormone deficiencies may significantly alter the strength of the bone–implant interface. The hormone studied most extensively has been estrogen.[96] Total joint arthroplasties are often performed in postmenopausal women so this issue is of extreme importance.

Martin et al.[96] studied the effects of estrogen deficiency in the growth of tissue into porous titanium implants. In this study five dogs were ovariectomized and five dogs received a sham operation. Later, 4 months after the operation, titanium implants were placed in the humerus of each dog; 2 months later the implants were harvested and pushout tests and histological studies were performed. The pushout strength of the implants from the ovariectomized dogs was 31% less than the controls. The estrogen-deficient dogs had increased fibrous tissue on histological exam.

Increased fibrous tissue at the bone–implant interface in estrogen deficiency is a key determinant to the decreased strength. Numerous investigators have implicated fibrous tissue in the failure of implants.[97,98] Not only are implants which rely on bone ingrowth affected by estrogen deficiencies, but cemented and press-fit implants are as well. The latter two of these implants rely on healthy, dense bone to form a strong fixation. Deficiencies in estrogen cause an osteoporotic bone which may not be suitable for fixation. The effects of estrogen and other systemic hormones at this level are tremendous. Clearly, more work needs to be done to define better the exact effects of hormones on the bone–implant interface.

B. NONSTEROIDAL ANTI-INFLAMMATORY DRUGS

Porous-coated implants rely on bone ingrowth to achieve implant stabilization. There is a concern that the use of certain medications, including nonsteroidal anti-inflammatory drugs (NSAIDS), may adversely affect bone ingrowth.[99] Indomethacin, a commonly prescribed NSAID, is a potent inhibitor of fracture healing and bone remodeling in therapeutic doses.[100–102] On a histological basis, the process of bone ingrowth is similar to fracture healing and factors that inhibit one may inhibit the other. NSAIDS are used clinically to inhibit heterotopic ossification. In addition, they are often administered for postoperative pain control, inflammatory arthritis, gout, and osteoarthritis.

Keller et al., using a rabbit model with quantitative histomorphometry, showed that indomethacin, compared to a placebo, caused a significant decrease in the amount of ingrowth into a porous titanium cylinder at 8 weeks, independent of pore size.[103] Follow-up studies with porous-coated chromium–cobalt cylinders in the same animal model showed that therapeutic dosages of indomethacin, aspirin, and ibuprofen all cause a statistically significant decrease in bone ingrowth, as compared with a control group.[104] A dose–response effect was found for the first two NSAIDS, with a greater inhibitory effect resulting from high doses. Longo et al.[105] found the same results with Naproxen.

Cook et al.[106] also studied the effects of indomethacin on fixation and found the adverse effects in interface shear strengths only at early periods. This group evaluated the specimens at longer postoperative intervals and determined the effects to be transient and minimal. Based on their findings, this group felt the possible benefits of postoperative use of NSAIDS, such as indomethacin, outweigh the minimal risk of transient decrease in attachment strength.

Until the mechanism of inhibition of bone ingrowth by NSAIDS is better defined and understood, caution should be exercised when using these medications immediately after surgery in patients with a porous-coated implant. If bone is inhibited from filling the pores, then fibrous tissue will develop and fill this area instead. Once this has occurred, it is unlikely that bone will be able to replace the fibrous tissue when the inhibitory medicines are withdrawn. As previously stated, fibrous tissue weakens the interface between the implant and bone and can lead to early failure.[108]

C. IRRADIATION

Not only is indomethacin used to prevent heterotopic bone formation in patients undergoing an uncemented hip replacement, but irradiation is an alternative method. Of patients undergoing these surgeries, 10 to 15% may develop heterotopic bone which can be prevented with 1000 rads of cobalt irradiation.[109] Although this treatment has been shown to be effective, recent studies suggest that it may weaken the interface of a porous-coated implant.

Wise et al.[110] implanted porous titanium fiber metal plugs in dogs which were subsequently radiated with 10 Gy given in four daily fractions of 2.5 Gy. Pullout strength tests of the irradiated implants were performed at 6 weeks survival. A 19% reduction was found in irradiated implants compared with controls. Metabolic activity monitored with bone scans was also significantly reduced in the irradiated extremity compared with the nonirradiated side. No histological evaluations of the bone–implant interface were performed.

Similar results have been produced by other investigators.[111-112] By using similar implants in dogs, dosages of 1000 rads were found to decrease the fixation strength early on by inhibiting bone ingrowth. Histological and mechanical tests documented these findings. A dose-dependent effect on ingrowth was found. The strength of the interface at 2 and 4 weeks was unchanged when the treatment consisted of only 500 rads; however, the amount of bone formation was slightly decreased.

While studies are being performed to look at the effects of lower single doses, the long-term effects of irradiation on the bone–implant interface are not known. Recommendations for patients who are felt to require postoperative irradiation are for cemented arthroplasty or shielding of porous-coated implants to minimize effects to the interface. Further studies are needed to help clarify the long-term effects of irradiation on the strength of the bone–implant interface.

D. ELECTROMAGNETIC OR ELECTRICAL STIMULATION

In both experimental and clinical settings, electrical osteogenesis has been reported to be effective on bone healing of nonunion or ununited fractures.[113-115] Several investigators have looked at the effect of electromagnetic stimulation on bone ingrowth into porous implants.[116] By using canine models, an acceleration of bone ingrowth by electrical stimulation has been demonstrated.[117-119]

This increase in bony ingrowth undoubtedly leads to greater stability and strength at the bone–implant interface.

Shinizu et al.[120] evaluated the effect of pulsing electromagnetic fields on bone ingrowth into porous hydroxyapatite and porous tricalcium phosphate implants in rabbit tibiae. They quantitated the biological response using a scanning electron microscope. The morphometrical findings in the hydroxyapatite pores showed a much greater amount of bone ingrowth in the pulsing electromagnetic field group compared with the controls at 3 to 4 weeks postimplantation. However, no significant difference was found in the tricalcium phosphate pores.[120] Histological findings supported the morphometric data. The differences in the two materials tested were felt to be secondary to the differences in pore sizes of the two ceramics.

Several investigators have studied electrical fields to stimulate bone ingrowth.[121] In a double blind study, Schutzer et al.[122] evaluated the effects of capacitively coupled electrical fields on bone ingrowth into porous-surfaced prosthesis in dogs. The electrical field was induced by an external source delivering voltage through skin electrodes. No significant growth into bone was seen at the end of 6 weeks.

Electromagnetic stimulation appears to have a positive effect on the bone–implant interface. The increased bone ingrowth caused by these forces is most striking at 3 to 4 weeks after surgery. Capacitively coupled electrical fields have not been shown to improve ingrowth. Additional studies are required to delineate the biochemical mechanisms by which increased osteogenesis may be promoted by electromagnetic stimulation.

E. LOCAL USE OF GROWTH FACTORS OR HORMONES

Growth factors, such as platelet-derived growth factor (PDGF), fibroblast growth factor (FGF), epidermal growth factor (EGF), and transforming growth factor β (TGF-β), are found in all tissues and regulate cell-to-cell metabolism. These naturally occurring proteins are mitogenic and chemotactic for the mesenchymal cells which contribute to new bone formation. These factors may accelerate and/or enhance bone ingrowth into porous implants leading to increased strength at the bone–implant interface.[123] Preliminary studies in a dog model have demonstrated that the percentage of bone ingrowth into a porous titanium implant coated with equal amounts of PDGF, EGF, and TGF-β is almost doubled.

Friedman et al.[124] have shown TGF-β, PDGF, and EGF in combination increase the rate of fracture healing in rats. Increased bone, cartilage, fibrous tissue, and callous area were seen at 1 week postoperative in rats receiving growth factor compared with controls. This indicates an accelerated rate of fracture repair. Because the process of fracture healing and bone ingrowth are similar, these growth-promoting factors may play a role in the long-term fixation of porous coated implants.

Lynch et al.[125] demonstrated an increased bone ingrowth to dental implants stimulated with PDGF and IGF-1 (insulin growth factor 1) in dogs. These implants were press-fit into the root canal. Recently, three separate groups have shown TFG-β adsorbed to ceramic-coated implants inserted into trabecular bone of dogs can stimulate anchorage, bone ingrowth, and gap healing of implants.[126-128] However, mechanical pushout tests showed no difference in fixation strength. Wang et al.[129] found basic FGF (bFGF) to promote ingrowth into porous structures coated with hydroxyapatite.

Several recent studies have evaluated the effects of growth hormone on bone ingrowth, but with conflicting results. Guicheux et al.[130] found that human growth hormone increased bone ingrowth. However, Blom et al.[131] found that human growth hormone inhibited bone formation in grooves coated with calcium phosphate. Morberg et al.[132] felt negative results reported may have been secondary to antibody formation against the growth hormone injected. This group used transgenic mice overexpressing bovine growth hormone and found increased bone-to-metal contact. From these findings, it was felt that systemic administration of growth hormone in humans may improve implant integration into bone.

More research needs to be done in this area. Only growth factors from the TGF-β superfamily (TGF-βs and bone morphogenetic proteins) and bFGF have been demonstrated to possess substantial *in vivo* bone stimulatory capacity. A major challenge for the clinical use of these growth factors is an appropriate delivery system which lasts long enough (2 weeks) and has no side effects on bone formation. However, these proteins will undoubtedly play a large role in cementless fixation in the future because of their positive effect at the bone–implant interface.

F. Other Factors

Mechanical vibration, ultrasound, and biphosphonates are several other modalities that may affect bone ingrowth but have not been extensively studied. Usui et al.[133] studied the effects of mechanical vibration on bone ingrowth into porous hydroxyapatite implant and fracture healing in a rabbit model. The effects of 20 and 60 min vibration per day was evaluated. They found that the mechanical vibration used in the study had a beneficial effect on callous volume, but did not appear to promote bone ingrowth into the porous implant.

Low-intensity ultrasound has been shown to be an effective means of accelerating fracture healing.[134,135] Tanzer et al.[136] used a canine model to determine if noninvasive ultrasound could influence the rate or extent of growth into a porous-coated implant. Porous-coated transcortical implants were inserted bilaterally into the femur of dogs. One femur served as a control and the contralateral side received daily ultrasound for 2, 3, or 4 weeks. The ultrasound-stimulated implants showed an 18% increase in bone ingrowth compared with the control side in the first 2 to 3 weeks. Further animal and clinical study is needed to assess the clinical application for noncement porous implants.

Biphosphonates have been demonstrated to block the action of osteoclasts and inhibit wear debris-mediated bone resorption in a canine model. Recently, Shanbhag et al.[137] have shown that biphosphonates can enhance the net bone formation in canine total hip components. This finding coupled with the ability of biphosphonates to inhibit osteolysis may prove to be invaluable in the long-term stability of total joints. Each of the modalities mentioned needs additional animal and clinical testing to determine its efficacy.

IV. *IN VITRO* FACTORS

A. Storage before Testing

In mechanical testing of bones, specimens often have to be frozen and thawed. Several investigators have found no significant effects on the mechanical properties of bones frozen at –20°C for less than 9 months and then thawed to 22°C (room temperature).[138,139] In fact it has been shown that multiple freezing–thawing cycles do not significantly affect the properties of bone.[140,141] Kang et al.[142] studied the effects of multiple freezing–thawing cycles on bovine tibial cancellous bone. They found these cycles did not affect the ultimate indentation load or stiffness of the bone. However, they suggest that bone specimens should be frozen and thawed in saline.

Thus far, no published data could be found on the effects of freezing on the mechanical properties of the bone–implant interface. Some may infer from previous work cited that storage will have little affect on the bone–implant interface, but this needs to be documented in animal models.

B. Specimen Preparation

In order to study properly the mechanical properties of the bone–implant interface, specimen preparation must be precise and adequate. The results obtained are only as good as the method used to obtain them. Implants are inserted into bone at various angles and orientations although they were aimed at certain directions. When harvesting the implant to test on a mechanical testing system, such as pushout test or pullout test, it is important that the removal cuts be made perpendicular to the implant and followed by precise fine cuts and grinding. If this is not done properly, it will not be possible to align the implant in the loading direction. Loading forces must be applied parallel to the implant to get a true biomechanical measure of the strength of the bone–implant interface. If the force applied to the implant is oblique, then erroneous data will be obtained.

Hartman et al.[143] evaluated the effects of pretreatment sterilization and cleaning methods on material properties and osseoinductivity. The implants were analyzed with electron spectroscopy. Argon radiofrequency glow discharge and ultraviolet chamber–treated implants were associated with rapid bone ingrowth and maturation of new bone. Conventional steam sterilization was associated with less new bone ingrowth. These different methods of implant sterilization affect bone ingrowth into porous substances and thus the strength of the bone–implant interface.

V. SURGICAL AND HOSPITAL FACTORS

A. SURGICAL SKILL

The fixation strength of an implant either cemented or uncemented is highly dependent upon the technical skill of the operating surgeons. Better long-term results are found in major medical centers where more surgeries are performed each year. Total joint arthroplasties are technical surgeries with much room for operator error. The constant evolution of information and skills required demands that the practicing orthopaedic surgeon stay up-to-date.

A thorough preoperative evaluation and radiographs are essential for a successful outcome. A skillful surgeon begins with both. Careful patient evaluation prevents catastrophic or even fatal complications. Radiographs enable the surgeon to determine the correct size prosthesis for the best fit. Poorly fitting prosthesis leads to motion which will weaken the bone–implant interface.

Many surgical approaches and techniques are used in arthroplasty. Surgeons should individualize the operation according to their clinical and educational experiences. Specific techniques for implantation vary according to the type of skeletal fixation, shape of femoral component, length of stem, and assembly of any modular components. The surgeon should be thoroughly familiar with all instrumentation prior to the procedure.

Numerous aspects of total joint arthroplasty require exacting skill. For example, while reaming the medullary canal for a cementless implant, care must be taken not to penetrate the femoral cortex. Skill is also required in positioning the acetabular cup.[144] Malposition of the cup may cause the neck of the femoral component to impinge on the margin of the socket and transfer excess stress to the cup which may lead to loosening. In cemented surgeries, surgical skill is necessary in the preparation and insertion of cement. Improperly prepared cement can lead to increased porosity and weakness at the bone–cement–implant interfaces. Also, skill is needed in centering the prosthesis to obtain a uniform cement mantle. Cracks may develop if the mantle is not uniform. These are only a few of the many aspects of joint arthroplasty which require surgical skill to ensure a strong bone–implant interface.

B. COMPLICATIONS

Infections and dislocations are two complications which may affect the long-term stability of the prosthesis. Postoperative infections can be catastrophic. Bacteria may grow in the biofilm on biomaterials making eradication difficult. Approximately 1% of all total hip arthroplasties become infected within 1 year.[145] Both acute and chronic infections often present a treatment dilemma. Component loosening can sometimes be seen on X-ray examination in chronic infections. This loosening weakens the bone–implant interface.

Dislocations are another complication seen after total hip arthroplasty. The incidence is close to 3%.[146,147] Several risk factors have been documented, including (1) history of previous surgery;

(2) posterior approach; (3) faulty positioning of components; (4) inadequate soft tissue tension; and (5) noncompliance. Dislocations may initially cause pain and swelling. If found quickly, the bone–implant interface will not be affected. However, the joint mechanics may be altered if the joint remains dislocated for extended periods of time, thus affecting the strength of the bone–implant interface.

C. POSTOPERATIVE CARE

Many different rehabilitation programs are accepted for postoperative care. Regaining motion and function and returning to independent living are vital elements. Postoperatively in hip arthroplasty, the hip is placed in approximately 15° of abduction with a pillow, and the leg is stabilized so rotation does not occur.[148] Most patients can begin limited mobilization on the first postoperative day. On the second day after the operation, patients are allowed to sit on the side of the bed and begin gait training.

Time to weight-bearing differs depending on the type of fixation used. With cementless, porous ingrowth implants, many recommend limited weight-bearing for 6 to 8 weeks.[149] If implants were cemented, weight-bearing as tolerated is permitted. Failure to follow these recommendations may weaken the bone–implant interface and affect the stability of the implant.

Sun[150] studied the effects of load bearing on bone ingrowth into porous-coated implants in rabbits. Sun found stimulation of load bearing benefited bone ingrowth and no weight-bearing resulted in fibrous tissue forming in pores after 12 weeks. These results point to the importance of some bearing in porous-coated implants. However, full weight-bearing may be detrimental, causing a failure of fixation.

Patients are often discharged when they are able to get up and out of bed on their own. This may be as early as postoperative day 3 to 6. Patients should receive printed instructions to take home. Any positions of instability noted in the operating room should be supplied to the patient. All of these specifics are aimed at ensuring stability at the bone–implant interface in order to have a successful outcome.

VI. PATIENT FACTORS

A. AGE

Age is a primary determinant of whether a surgeon will use a cemented or cementless fixation. The effect of age on cementless fixation is of paramount importance. Bone and mineral metabolism are known to change with age.[151] Most studies of biological fixation are carried out in young animals, or animals of unknown age, to show osseointegration of an implant. Very few studies have evaluated how these implants are fixed in the elderly and the consequences of aging on the bone–implant stability. Since most orthopaedic implants are placed in aged skeletons, this is a matter of utmost importance.

Magee et al.[152] evaluated bone ingrowth into transcortical porous-coated plugs in old (6.6 years) and young (2.3 years) greyhounds. Gender and ovarian status were not considered. Regardless, this group reported low interface shear stress in older animals. In another study, Nakajima et al.[153] studied implant fixation in young and old mongrel dogs. Age was defined based on teeth wear and again gender and ovarian status were not considered. This group found a significantly inferior callus quality in old dogs in the early postoperative period (3 to 6 weeks).

In contrast, Eckhoff et al.[154] evaluated bone ingrowth in hydroxyapatite-coated and uncoated implants in young and old sheep. These animals were of known age and reproductive status. Surprisingly, they found comparable fixation of implants in the young and old sheep. This group felt age was not a dominant factor in the development or failure of implant osseointegration. A case report supporting this study was presented by Soballe et al.[155] The case is a retrieval of a hydroxyapatite-coated femoral prosthesis from a 98-year-old osteoporotic female 12 weeks after implantation. Histological analysis of the specimen showed a large amount of bone in direct contact with the prosthesis despite age, gender, and presence of osteoporosis in the patient.

Due to the conflicting reports of the effects of age on bone–implant strength, further study is needed in this area. All of the previous studies have involved animals of different breeds with numerous variables. It is hoped, in the near future, that studies may document findings in humans.

B. Lifestyle

Lifestyle of the patient is a consideration when deciding on the type of implant to use in joint arthroplasty. Most surgeons will choose a biologically fixed implant in more active individuals. One reason for this is that if revision surgery must be done, uncemented prostheses are much easier to work with. Patients who are not active tend to be elderly and a cemented prosthesis is a better choice. The activity of the patient will determine the amount of stress put on the bone–implant interface. Large amounts of stress may lead to failure. However, some stress is needed for bone to remain healthy and not atrophy. Thus, the lifestyle of the patient is not only important in choosing the type of fixation but also in ultimate strength of the bone–implant interface.

C. Inflammation (Rheumatoid and Other Inflammatory Conditions)

Few studies have been carried out to study the effects of inflammation on bone ingrowth. An et al.[48] evaluated the interface between implanted cylinders with three different surface textures in the distal femur of rabbits following the induction of inflammatory arthritis. Inflammatory arthritis was induced with injections of carrageenan to the knee joint. The contralateral knee joint was used as a control. This group found the thickness and number of trabeculae less on the arthritic side of all three texture types compared with controls. Mechanical testing also showed the shear strength of the interface was weaker on the inflammatory side. From these findings, they concluded that inflammatory arthritis may influence the quality of local bone and thus compromise the bone apposition and mechanical stability of the interface between implant and bone. Branemark and Thomsen[156] found similar trends in rabbit models.

Inflammation from many different clinical conditions affects the longevity of implanted prosthesis. Dorr et al.[157] reported a higher failure rate for implants in patients with inflammatory conditions of the hip. Numerous problems such as infection are commonly seen in chronic inflammatory diseases. This may be due to the disease itself or partly because of the medications many of these patients take. Steroids are commonly prescribed for many patients with these disorders.

Rheumatoid arthritis is a common disease in orthopaedic patients. Poss et al.[158] reported an increased risk of complications in patients with this condition. In their study, 96% of patients with rheumatoid arthritis clinically improved after total hip replacement. However, 40% of patients had subsidence of the femoral component and 78% increased radiolucency of the acetabular component at 6 to 10 years after surgery. Infection rate was also doubled in the rheumatoid group vs. the osteoarthitic controls.

Rheumatoid arthritis patients often have an activity-limiting disease. This limitation of stress at the bone–implant interface may in fact lead to a longer implant survivorship compared with other conditions such as osteoarthritis. Sochart and Porter[159] reviewed 226 Charnley low-friction arthroplasties in 161 patients with congenital dislocation of the hip, osteoarthritis, and rheumatoid arthritis. They found rheumatoid arthritis patients had the lowest prevalence of loosening and revision of the acetabular component.

Systemic lupus erythematosis (SLE) is another chronic, multisystemic inflammatory disorder usually affecting women in their second or third decade. Hanssen et al.[160] evaluated hip arthroplasty in patients with SLE and found an increased rate of wound complications and deep infections. In another study, Huo et al.[161] found loosening of femoral and acetabular components to be a problem. Based on these and other studies, reamed uncemented or hybrid total hip arthroplasties are recommended for this patient population.

These clinical studies show the numerous problems in patients with inflammatory conditions who have arthroplasty. The increased rate of infection and associated problems in these patients undoubtedly affect the bone–implant interface. Further research is needed in this area to define better the mechanisms and its significance.

D. OSTEOPENIA 45 OR OSTEOPOROSIS

Osteopenia and osteoporosis afflict many patients, particularly the elderly. Since total joint arthroplasty is often performed in this age group, the effects of these conditions on implant stability is significant. These conditions may ultimately affect the bone–implant interface and success of the implant. Several investigators have evaluated osteoporosis and its effects on osseointegration.[162,163] Fujimoto et al.[164] evaluated the effects of osteoporosis on osseointegration of titanium implants in rabbits. Osteoporosis was created in these animals by administering steroids. Bone density was used to evaluate osteoporosis in these models. These investigators found a significantly lower removal torque in the osteoporotic group than in controls.

In another study, Mori et al.[165] studied the reaction of bone–implant interface in osteoporotic animal models. The experimental model consisted of a rabbit which was ovariectomized and fed a low-calcium diet. Dual energy X-ray absorptiometry was used to document the bone mineral density.[166] In this study, new bone formation was delayed in the osteoporotic animals but did occur after 12 weeks. From this they concluded that osseointegration occurs in osteoporotic bone but the healing period is extended. Thus, conditions affecting the density and quantity of bone are important factors in the bone–implant interface strength.

VII. SUMMARY

As the number and sophistication of orthopaedic implants is growing, a great deal of research is focusing on the bone–implant interface. The factors affecting the strength of this interface are important not only to surgeons implanting the prosthesis but also to researchers studying the biomechanical properties of various artificial components. As discussed, numerous factors have proved to have a significant impact either positive or negative on the strength of the interface.

Various implant surface configurations, coatings, geometric designs, and implantation techniques affect the final stability of the prosthesis. Medications commonly used by surgeons, such as NSAIDs or hormones, may decrease the bony ingrowth into porous implants. Patient factors including age, lifestyle, and osteoporosis also can dramatically affect the strength of the bone–implant interface. In addition, appropriate storage and specimen preparation can influence the data obtained in mechanical testing of this area.

It is the responsibility of the surgeon and the scientist to be cognizant of the numerous factors affecting the strength of the bone–implant interface. Continued research, especially mechanical testing, needs to be done to clarify further as well as discover new factors that play a role in the strength of the bone–implant interface.

REFERENCES

1. Park, J.B., Orthopaedic prosthesis fixation, *Ann. Biomed. Eng.*, 20, 583, 1992.
2. Branemark, P.I., Osseointegration and its experimental background, *J. Prosthet. Dent.*, 50, 399, 1983.
3. Branemark, P.I., Zarb, G.A., and Albektsson, T., *Tissue Integrated Prostheses: Osseointegration in Clinical Dentistry*, Quintessence, Chicago, 1985.

4. Sumner, D.R. and Galante, J.O., Bone ingrowth, in *Surgery of the Musculoskeletal System*, Evarts, C.M., Ed., Churchill Livingstone, New York, 1990, 151.

5. Sumner, D.R., Klenapfel, H., and Galante, J.O., Metallic implants, in *Bone Grafts: From Basic Science to Clinical Application*, Habal, M.B. and Reddi, A.H., Eds., W.B. Saunders, Philadelphia, 1993, 619.

6. Lee, T.Q., Danto, M.I., and Kim, W.C., Initial stability comparisons of modular hip implants in synthetic femurs, *Orthopedics*, 21, 885, 1998.

7. Jarcho, M., Calcium phosphate ceramics as hard tissue prosthetics, *Clin. Orthop.*, 157, 259, 1981.

8. Jarcho, M., Kay, J.F., Gumaer, K.L., et al., Tissue, cellular and subcellular events at a bone–ceramic hydroxyapatite interface, *J. Bioeng.*, 1, 79, 1992.

9 Friedman, R.J., An, Y.H., Ming, J., et al., Influence of biomaterial surface texture on bone ingrowth in the rabbit femur, *J. Orthop. Res.*, 14, 455, 1996.

10. Bobyn, J.D., Pilliar, R.M., Cameron, H.U., and Weatherly, G.C., The optimum pore size for the fixation of porous-surfaced metal implants by the ingrowth of one, *Clin. Orthop.*, 150, 263, 1980.

11. Young, F.A., Spector, M., and Kresch, C.H., Porous titanium endosseous dental implants in Rhesus monkeys: microradiography and histological evaluation, *J. Biomed. Mater. Res.*, 13, 843, 1979.

12. Galante, J. and Rostoker, W., Fiber metal composites in the fixation of skeletal prostheses, *J. Biomed. Mater. Res. Symp.*, 4, 43, 1973.

13. Galante, J., Rostoker, W., Lueck, R., and Ray, R.D., Sintered fiber metal composites as a basis for attachment of implants to bone, *J. Bone Joint Surg.*, 53A, 101, 1971.

14. Heck, D.A., Nakajima, I., Kelly, P.J., and Chao, E.Y., The effect of load alteration on the biological and biomechanical performance of a titanium fiber-metal segmental prosthesis, *J. Bone Joint Surg.*, 68A, 118, 1986.

15. Galante, J., Laing, P.G., and Lautenschlager, E., Biomaterials, *AAOS Instr. Course Lect.*, 24, 1, 1975.

16. Aspenberg, P., Goodman, S., Toksvig-Larsen, S., et al., Intermittent micromotion inhibits bone ingrowth. Titanium implants in rabbits, *Acta Orthop. Scand.*, 63, 141, 1992.

17. Friedman, R.J., Advances in biomaterials and factors affecting implant fixation, *AAOS Instr. Course Lect.*, 41, 127, 1992.

18. Branson, P.J., Steege, J.W., Wixson, R.L., et al., Rigidity of internal fixation with uncemented tibial knee implants, *J. Arthroplasty*, 4, 21, 1989.

19. Soballe, K., Hansen, E., Rasmussen, H., et al., Hydroxyapatite coating enhances fixation of porous coated implants, *Acta Orthop. Scand.*, 61, 299, 1990.

20. Soballe, K., Hansen, E.S., Rasmussen, H., et al., Tissue ingrowth into titanium and hydroxyapatite-coated implants during stable and unstable mechanical conditions, *J. Orthop. Res.*, 10, 285, 1992.

21. Kohn, D.H. and Ducheyne, P., A parametric study of the factors affecting the strength of porous coated Ti-6Al-4V implant alloy, *J. Biomed. Mater. Res.*, 24, 1483, 1990.

22. Takeuchi, M.J., Kelman, D.C., and Smith, T.S., The effects of sintering heat treatments on the fatigue strength of Ti-6Al-7NB, *Trans. Soc. Biomater.*, 14, 291, 1991.

23. Kelman, D.C., Takeuchi, M.J., and Smith, T.S., Effect of metallic plasma sprayed coatings on high cycle fatigue, *Trans. Soc. Biomater.*, 14, 290, 1991.

24. Kummer, F.J., Ricci, J.L., and Blumenthal, N.C., RF plasma treatment on metallic implant surfaces, *J. Appl. Biomater.*, 3, 39, 1992.

25. Robertson, D.M., Pierre, L., and Chehal, F., Preliminary observations of bone ingrowth into porous material, *J. Biomed. Mater. Res.*, 10, 335, 1976.

26. Weish, R.P., Pilliar, R.M., and Macnab, I., Surgical implants. The role of surface porosity in fixation to bone and acrylic, *J. Bone Joint Surg.*, 53A, 963, 1971.

27. Bobyn, J.D, Pilliar, R.M., Cameron, H.U., and Weatherly, G.C., The optimum pore size for the fixation of porous-surfaced metal implants by the ingrowth of bone, *Clin. Orthop.*, 150, 263, 1980.

28. Cook, S.D., Walsh, K.A., and Haddad, R.J., Jr., Interface mechanics and bone growth into porous Co-Cr-Mo alloy implants, *Clin. Orthop.*, 193, 163, 1985.

29. Biegler, F.B., Reuben, J.D., Harrigan, T.P., et al., Effect of porous coating and loading conditions on total hip femoral stem stability, *J. Arthroplasty*, 10, 839, 1995.

30. Shigley, J.E., *Mechanical Engineering Design*, 3rd ed., McGraw-Hill, New York, 1977.

31. Vernon-Roberts, B. and Freman, M.A.R., The tissue response to total joint replacement prostheses, in *The Scientific Basis of Total Joint Replacement*, Swanson, S.A.V. and Freeman, M.A.R., Eds., John Wiley, New York, 1977, 86.

32. Segawa, H., Lew, W.D., Bourgeault, C., et al., Micromotion study of the preparation method of the proximal tibia for primary tibial components, *Trans. Orthop. Res. Soc.*, 24, 866, 1999.

33. Meding, J.B., Ritter, M.A., Keating, E.M., and Faris, P.M., Impaction bone-grafting before insertion of a femoral stem with cement in revision total hip arthroplasty. A minimum two-year follow-up study, *J. Bone Joint Surg.*, 79A, 1834, 1997.

34. Green, J.R., Nemzek, J.A., Arnoczky, S.P., et al., The effect of bone compaction on early fixation of porous-coated implants, *J. Arthroplasty*, 14, 91, 1999.

35. Yu, L., Clark, J.G., Dai, Q.G., et al., Improving initial mechanical fixation of porous coated femoral stem by a cancellous bone compaction method, *Trans. Orthop. Res. Soc.*, 24, 863, 1999.

36. Chareancholvanich, K., Bechtold, J.E., Soballe, K., et al., Compaction of existing cancellous bone in the primary setting enhances interfacial shear strength *in vivo*, *Trans. Orthop. Res. Soc.*, 24, 865, 1999.

37. Feighan, J.E., Goldberg, V.M., Dawy, D., et al., The influence of surface-blasting on the incorporation of titanium-alloy implants in a rabbit intramedullary model, *J. Bone Joint Surg.*, 77A, 1380, 1995.

38. Goldberg, V.M., Stevenson, S., Feighan, J., and Davy, D., Biology of grit-blasted titanium alloy implants, *Clin. Orthop.*, 319, 122, 1995.

39. Wang, J.S., Taylor, M., Flivik, G., and Lindgren, L., Influence of stem roughness on the static shear strength of the stem-cement interface, *Trans. Orthop. Res. Soc.*, 24, 872, 1999.

40. Wang, J.S., Flivik, G., Taylor, M., and Lindgren, L., Stem-cement interface shear strength is influenced by stem surface finish but not cement interface porosity, *Trans. Orthop. Res. Soc.*, 24, 871, 1999.

41. Nakamura, T., Yamamuro, T., Higashi, S., et al., A new glass ceramic for bone replacement: evaluation of its bonding ability to bone tissue, *J. Biomed. Mater. Res.*, 19, 685, 1985.

42. Uamamuro, T., Hench, L., and Wilson, J., Eds., *CRC Handbook of Bioactive Ceramics*, Vols. 1 and 2, CRC Press, Boca Raton, FL, 1990.

43. Pazzaglia, U.E., Brossa, F., Zatti, G., et al., The relevance of hydroxyapatite and spongious titanium coatings in fixation of cementless stems. An experimental comparative study in rat femur employing histological and microangiographic techniques, *Arch Orthop. Trauma Surg.*, 117, 279, 1998.

44. Lemons, J.E., Hydroxyapatite coatings, *Clin. Orthop.*, 235, 220, 1988.

45. Lemons, J.E., Bioceramics: is there a difference? *Clin. Orthop.*, 261, 153, 1991.

46. Davies, J.E., Ed., *The Bone–Biomaterial Interface*, University of Toronto Press, Toronto, 1991.

47. Hench, L.L. and Paschal, H.A., Direct chemical bond of bioactive glass ceramics to bone and tissue, *J. Biomed. Mater. Res.*, 4, 25, 1973.

48. An, Y.H., Friedman, R.J., Jiang, M., et al., Bone ingrowth to implant surfaces in an inflammatory arthritis model, *J. Orthop. Res.*, 16, 576, 1998.

49. de Groot, K., Geesink, R.G., Klein, C.P., et al., Plasma sprayed coatings of hydroxylapatite, *J. Biomed. Mater. Res.*, 21, 1275, 1987.

50. Geesink, R.G., de Groot, K., and Klein, C.P., Chemical implant fixation using hydroxylapatite coatings, *Clin. Orthop.*, 25, 147, 1987.

51. Cook, S.D., Thomas, K.A., Kay, J.F., et al., Hydroxyapatite–coated titanium for orthopaedic implant applications, *Clin. Orthop.*, 232, 225, 1988.

52. Soballe, K., Hansen, E.S., Helle, B.R., et al., Tissue ingrowth into titanium and hydroxyapatite-coated implants during stable and unstable mechanical conditions, *J. Orthop. Res.*, 10, 285, 1992.

53. Thomas, K.A, Kay, J.F., Cook, S.D., et al., The effect of surface macrotexture and hydroxylapatite coating on the mechanical strengths and histologic profiles of titanium implant materials, *J. Biomed. Mater. Res.*, 21, 1395, 1987.

54. Thomas, K.A., Cook, S.D., Kay, J.F., et al., Attachment strength and histology of hydroxylapatite coated implants, *Biomater. Med. Devices Artif. Organs*, 14, 73, 1986.

55. Cook, S.D., Thomas, K.A., Kay, J.F., et al., Hydroxyapatite-coated porous titanium for use as an orthopaedic biologic attachment system, *Clin. Orthop.*, 230, 303, 1988.

56. Richardson, D.C., The response of cancellous and cortical canine bone to hydroxylapatite coated titanium rods, *Trans. Soc. Biomater.*, 12, 176, 1989.

57. Magee, F.P., Kay, J.F., and Hedley, A.K., Interface strength and histology of hydroxylapatite coated and surface textured titanium, *Trans. Soc. Biomater.*, 12, 173, 1989.

58. Manley, M.T., Kay, J.F., Uratsuji, M., et al., Hydroxylapatite coatings applied to implants subjected to functional loads, *Trans. Soc. Biomater.*, 10, 210, 1987.

59. Lemons, J.E., Hydroxyapatite coatings, *Clin. Orthop.*, 235, 202, 1988.

60. Cook, S.D. and Thomas, K.A., Coating defects in hydroxylapatite coated implants, *Trans. Soc. Biomater.*, 12, 172, 1989.

61. Noble, P.C., Alexander, J.W., Lindahl L.J., et al., The anatomic basis of femoral component design, *Clin. Orthop.*, 235, 148, 1988.

62. Soballe, K., Hansen, E.S., Rasmussen, H.B., et al., Enhancement of osteopenic and normal bone ingrowth into porous coated implants by hydroxyapatite coating, *Trans. Orthop. Res. Soc.*, 14, 554, 1989.

63. Harris, W.H., White, R.E., McCarthy, J.C., et al., Bony ingrowth fixation of the acetabular component in canine total hip arthroplasty, *Clin. Orthop.*, 176, 7, 1983.

64. Thomas, K.A., Cook, S.D, Haddad, R.J., et al., Biologic response to hydroxylapatite– coated titanium hips, *J. Arthroplasty*, 4, 43, 1989.

65. Mahomed, N., Maistrelli, G., and Fornasier, V., Interfacial shear strength of hydroxyapatite coated hip implants, *Orthop. Trans.*, 14, 710, 1990.

66. Schmalzried, T.P., Kwong, L.M., Jasty, M., et al., The mechanism of loosening of cemented acetabular components in total hip arthroplasty, analysis of specimens retrieved at autopsy, *Clin. Orthop.*, 274, 60, 1992.

67. de Bruijn, J.D., van den Brink, I., Mendes, S., et al., Bone induction by implants coated with cultured osteogenic bone marrow cells and *in vitro* formed bone matrix, *Trans. Orthop. Res. Soc.*, 24, 888, 1999.

68. Jarvis, W.C., Biomechanical advantages of wide-diameter implants, *Compend. Contin. Educ. Dent.*, 18, 687, 1997.

69. Alfaro-Adrian, J., Gill, H.S., and Murray, D.W., The influence of prosthetic design on migration. A study of Charnley and Exeter THR with RSA, *Trans. Orthop. Res. Soc.*, 24, 919, 1999.

70. Canale, S.T., Ed., *Campbell's Operative Orthopaedics*, Mosby, St. Louis, MO, 1998, 308.

71. Schneider, E., Christian, K., Eulenberger, J., et al., Comparative study of initial stability of cementless hip prostheses, *Clin. Orthop.*, 248, 200, 1989.

72. Kelsey, D. and Goodman, S.B., Design of the femoral component for cementless hip replacement: the surgeon's perspective, *Am. J. Orthop.*, 26, 407, 1997.

73. Ries, M.D., Harbaugh, M., Shea, J., and Lambert, R., Effect of cementless acetabular cup geometry on strain distribution and press-fit stability, *J. Arthroplasty*, 12, 207, 1997.

74. Jacobs, J.J., Gilber, J.l., and Urban, R.M., Corrosion of metal implants, in *Advances in Operative Orthopaedics*, Vol. 2, Staufer, R.N., Ed., Mosby, St. Louis, MO, 279, 1994.

75. Levine, D.L. and Staehle, R.W., Crevice corrosion in orthopaedic implant metals, *J. Biomed. Mater. Res.*, 11, 553, 1977.

76. Budinski, G.K., Tibological properties of titanium alloys, *Wear*, 151, 203, 1991.

77. Woolson, S.T., Milbauer, J.P., Bobyn, J.D., et al., Fatigue fracture of a forged cobalt–chromium–molybdenum femoral component inserted with cement. A report of ten cases, *J. Bone Joint Surg.*, 79A, 1842, 1997.

78. Trousdale, R.T., Berry, D.J., Jacob, J., and Gilbert, J.L., Fracture of an acetabulum component inserted without cement, *J. Bone Joint Surg.*, 79A, 901, 1997.

79. Sandborn, P.M., Cook, S.D., Kester, M.A., and Haddad, R.J., Jr., Fatigue failure of the femoral component of a unicompartmental knee, *Clin. Orthop.*, 222, 249, 1987.

80. Miller, J.J., *Review of Orthopaedics*, 2nd ed., W.B. Saunders, Philadelphia, 1996.

81. Bayne, S.C., Lautenschlager, E.P., Greener, E.H., and Myer, P.R., Jr., Degree of polymerization of acrylic bone cement, *J. Biomed. Mater. Res.*, 9, 27, 1975.

82. Cameron, U.H., Mills, R.H., Jackson, R.W., and Macnab, I., The structure of polymethylmethacrylate cement, *Clin. Orthop.*, 100, 287, 1974.

83. Haas, S.S., Brauer, G.M., and Dickson, G., A characterization of polymethylmethacrylate bone cement, *J. Bone Joint Surg.*, 57A, 380, 1975.

84. Wixson, R.L., Lautenschlager, E.P., and Novak, M.A., Vacuum mixing of acrylic bone cement, *J. Arthroplasty*, 2, 144, 1987.

85. Gruen, T.A., Markolf, K.L., and Amstutz, H.C., Effects of laminations and blood entrapment on the strength of acrylic bone cement, *Clin. Orthop.*, 119, 250, 1976.

86. Willert, H.G. and Semlitsch, M., Reactions of the articular capsule to wear products of artificial joint prostheses, *J. Biomed. Mater. Res.*, 11, 157, 1977.

87. Goldring, S.R., Schiller, A.L., Roelke, M., et al., The synovial-like membrane at the bone–cement interface in loose total hip replacements and its proposed role in bone lysis, *J. Bone Joint Surg.*, 65A, 575, 1983.

88. Goodman, S.B., Chin, R.C., Chiou, S.S., et al., A clinical pathologic biochemical study of the membrane surrounding loosened and non–loosened total hip arthroplasties, *Clin. Orthop.*, 244, 182, 1989.

89. Apple, A.M., Sowder, W.G., Hop, C.N., and Herman, J.H., Production of mediators of bone resorption by prosthesis associated pseudomembranes, *Trans. Orthop. Res. Soc.*, 13, 362, 1988.

90. Mather, S.E., Emmanuel, J., Magee, F.P., et al., Interleukin and prostaglandin E2 in failed total hip arthroplasty, *Trans. Orthop. Res. Soc.*, 14, 489, 1989.

91. Chrisman, O.D. and Snook, G.A., The problem of refracture of the tibia, *Clin. Orthop.*, 60, 217, 1968.

92. Dencker, H., Refracture of the shaft of the femur, *Acta Orthop. Scand.*, 35, 16, 1964.

93. Engh, C.A., Hip arthroplasty with a Moore prosthesis with porous coating — a five year study, *Clin. Orthop.*, 176, 52, 1983.

94. Engh, C.A., Bobyn, J.D., and Glassman, A.H., Porous coated hip replacement. A study of factors governing bone ingrowth, stress shielding, and clinical results, *J. Bone Joint Surg.*, 69A, 45, 1987.

95. Manley, P.A., Vanderby, R., Jr., Kohles, S., et al., Alterations in femoral strain, micromotion, cortical geometry, cortical porosity, and bony ingrowth in uncemented collared and collarless prostheses in the dog, *J. Arthroplasty*, 10, 63, 1995.

96. Martin, R.B., Paul, H.A., Bargar, W.L., et al., Effects of estrogen deficiency on growth of tissue into porous titanium implants, *J. Bone Joint Surg.*, 70A, 4, 1988.

97. Paul, H.A. and Bargar, W.L., Histologic changes in the dog femur following total hip replacement with current cementing techniques, *J. Arthroplasty*, 1, 5, 1986.

98. Rose, R.M., Martin, R.B., Orr, R.B., and Radin, E.C., Architectural changes in the proximal femur following prosthetic insertion: preliminary observations of an animal model, *J. Biomech.*, 17, 241, 1984.

99. Newman, N.M. and Ling, R.S., Acetabular bone destruction related to non–steroidal anti–inflammatory drug, *Lancet*, 2, 11, 1985.

100. Keller, J., Bayer-Kristensen, I., Bak, B., et al., Indomethacin and bone remodeling. Effect on cortical bone after osteotomy in rabbits, *Acta Orthop. Scand.*, 60, 119, 1989.

101. Ro, J., Sudmann, E., and Martin, P.F., Effect of indomethacin on fracture healing in rats, *Acta Orthop. Scand.*, 47, 588, 1976.

102. Longo, J.A., Hedley, A.K., Weinstein, A.M., et al., Comparative effects of EHDP, radiation therapy and indomethacin on bone ingrowth in rabbits, *Trans. Soc. Biomater.*, 8, 161, 1985.

103. Keller, J.C., Trancik, T.M., Young, F.A., et al., Effects of indomethacin on bone ingrowth, *J. Orthop. Res.*, 7, 28, 1989.

104. Trancik, T., Mills, W., and Vinson, N., The effect of indomethacin, aspirin, and ibuprofen on bone ingrowth into a porous–coated implant, *Clin. Orthop.*, 249, 113,.1989.

105. Longo, J.A., Magee, F.P., Van De Wyngaerde, D.P., et al., Naproxen and skeletal implant interfaces, in *Interfaces in Medicine and Mechanisms*, William, K.R., Toni, A., Middleton, J., and Pallotti, G., Eds., Elsevier, New York, 1991.

106. Cook, S., Barrack, R., Dalton, J.E., et al., Effects of indomethacin on biological fixation of porous coated titanium implants, *J. Arthroplasty*, 10, 3, 1995.

107. Engh, C.A., Glassman, A.H., and Suthers, K.E., The case for porous coated implants, the femoral side, *Clin. Orthop.*, 261, 63, 1990.

108. Skriptz, R. and Aspenberg, P., Tensile bond between bone and titanium: a reapproval of osseointegration, *Acta Orthop. Scand.*, 69, 315, 1998.

109. Ayers, D.C., Pellegrini, V.D., and Evarts, C.M., Prevention of heterotopic ossification in high–risk patients by radiation therapy, *Clin. Orthop.*, 263, 87, 1991.

110. Wise, M.W., Robertson, I.D., Lachiewicz, P.F., et al., The effects of radiation therapy on the fixation strength of an experimental porous–coated implant in dogs, *Clin. Orthop.*, 261, 276, 1990.

111. Sumner, D.R., Turner, T.M., Pierson, R.H., et al., Effects of radiation on fixation of non-cemented porous-coated implants in a canine model, *J. Bone Joint Surg.*, 72A, 1527, 1990.

112. Chin, H.C., Frassica, F.J., Markel, M.D., et al., The effects of therapeutic doses of irradiation on experimental bone graft incorporation over a porous-coated segmental defect endoprosthesis, *Clin. Orthop.*, 289, 254, 1993.

113. Basset, C.A.L., Pilla, A.A., and Pawluk, R.J., A nonoperative salvage of surgically resistant pseudar-throses and non-unions by pulsing electromagnetic fields, *Clin. Orthop.*, 124, 128, 1977.

114. Basset, C.A.L., Caulo, N., and Kort, J., Congenital "pseudarthroses" of the tibia. Treatment with pulsing electromagnetic fields, *Clin. Orthop.*, 154, 136, 1981.

115. Basset, C.A.L., Mitchell, S.N., and Gaston, S.R., Treatment of ununited tibial diaphyseal fractures with pulsing electromagnetic fields, *J. Bone Joint Surg.*, 63A, 511, 1981.

116. Ijiri, K., Matsunaga, S., Fukuyama, K., et al., The effect of pulsing electromagnetic field on bone ingrowth into a porous coated implant, *Anticancer Res.*, 16, 2853, 1996.

117. Park, J.B. and Kenner, G.H., Effect of electrical stimulation on the tensile strength of the porous implant and bone interface, *Biomater. Med. Devices Artif. Organs*, 3, 233, 1975.

118. Park, J.B. and Kenner, G.H., Effect of electrical stimulation on the interfacial tensile strength and amount of bone formation, *Biomater. Med. Devices Artif. Organs*, 4, 225, 1976.

119. Weinstein, A.M., Klawitter, J.J., Cleveland, T.W., and Amoss, D.C., Electrical stimulation of bone growth into porous Al_2O_3, *J. Biomed. Mater. Res.*, 10, 231, 1976.

120. Shinizu, T., Zerwekh, J.E., Videman, T., et al., Bone ingrowth into porous calcium phosphate ceramics: influence of pulsing electromagnetic field, *J. Orthop. Res.*, 6, 248, 1988.

121. Ducheyne, P., Ellis, L.Y., Pollack, S.R., et al., Field distributions in the rat tibia with and without a porous implant during electrical stimulation: a parametric modeling, *IEEE Trans. Biomed. Eng.*, 39, 1168, 1992.

122. Schutzer, S.F., Jasty, M., Bragdon, C.R., et al., A double-blind study on the effects of a capacitively coupled electrical field on bone ingrowth into porous-surfaced canine total hip prostheses, *Clin. Orthop.*, 260, 297, 1990.

123. Canalis, E., Effects of growth factors on bone cell replication and differentiation, *Clin. Orthop.*, 193, 246, 1985.

124. Friedman, R.J., Acurio, M.T., Davis, R., et al., Effects of growth factors and indomethacin of fracture healing, *Trans. Orthop. Res. Soc.*, 17, 421, 1992; *Orthop. Trans.*, 16, 514, 1992.

125. Lynch, S.E., Buser, D., Hernandez, R.A., et al., Effects of platelet derived growth factor/insulin like growth factor 1 combination on bone around titanium dental implants: results of a pilot study in beagle dogs, *J. Periodontol.*, 62, 710, 1991.

126. Lind, M., Overgaurd, S., Soballe, K., et al., Transforming growth factor beta enhances fixation of ceramic coated implants, *Trans. Orthop. Res. Soc.*, 192, 1995.

127. Sumner, D.R., Turner, T.M., Durchio, A.F., et al., Enhancement of bone ingrowth by transforming growth factor beta, *J. Bone Joint Surg.*, 77A, 1135, 1995.

128. Martin, L., Soren O., Boonsri, O., et al., Transforming growth factor beta stimulates bone ongrowth to weight loaded tricalcium phosphate coated implants, *J. Bone Joint Surg.*, 78B, 3, 1996.

129. Wang, J.S. and Aspenberg, P., Basic fibroblast growth factor promotes bone ingrowth in porous hydroxyapatite, *Clin. Orthop.*, 333, 252, 1996.

130. Guicheux, J., Gauthier, O., Aguado, E., et al., Growth hormone-loaded macroporous calcium phosphate ceramic: *in vitro* biopharmaceutical characterization and preliminary *in vivo* study, *J. Biomed. Mater. Res.*, 40, 560, 1998.

131. Blom, E.J., Verheij, J.G., de Blieck-Hogervorst, J.M., et al., Cortical bone ingrowth in growth hormone-loaded grooved implants with calcium phosphate coatings in goat femurs, *Biomaterials*, 19, 263, 1998.

132. Morberg, P.H., Isaksson, O.G., Johansson, C.B., et al., Improved long-term bone–implant integration. Experiments in transgenic mice overexpressing bovine growth hormone, *Acta Orthop. Scand.*, 68, 344, 1997.

133. Usui, Y., Zerwekh, J.E., Vanharanta, H., et al., Different effects of mechanical vibration on bone ingrowth into porous hydroxyapatite and fracture healing in a rabbit model, *J. Orthop. Res.*, 7, 559, 1989.

134. Kristiansen, T.K., Ryaby, J.P., McCabe, J., et al., Accelerated healing of distal radius fractures with the use of specific, low intensity ultrasound, *J. Bone Joint Surg.*, 79A, 961, 1997.

135. Heckman, J.D., Ryaby, J.P., McCabe, J., et al., Acceleration of tibial fracture-healing by noninvasive, low-intensity pulsed ultrasound, *J. Bone Joint Surg.*, 76A, 26, 1994.

136. Tanzer, M., Harvey, E., Kay, A., et al., Effect of noninvasive low intensity ultrasound on bone growth into porous-coated implants, *J. Orthop. Res.*, 14, 901, 1996.

137. Shanbhag, A.S., May, D., Kovach, C., et al., Enhancing net bone formation in canine total hip components with biphosphonates, *Trans. Orthop. Res. Soc.*, 24, 255, 1999.

138. Panjabi, M.M., Krag, M., Summers, D., et al., Biomechanical time-tolerance of fresh cadaveric human spine specimens, *J. Orthop. Res.*, 3, 292, 1985.

139. Roe, S.C., Pijanowski, G.J., and Johnson, A.L., Biochemical properties of canine cortical bone allografts: effects of preparation and storage, *Am. J. Vet. Res.*, 49, 873, 1988.

140. Linde, F. and Sorensen, H.C., The effect of different storage methods on the mechanical properties of trabecular bone, *J. Biomech.*, 26, 1249, 1993.

141. Sedlin, E.D. and Hirsch, C., Factors affecting the determination of the physical properties of femoral cortical bone, *Acta Orthop. Scand.*, 37, 29, 1966.

142. Kang, W., An, Y.H., and Friedman, R.J., Effects of multiple freezing–thawing cycles on ultimate indentation load and stiffness of bovine cancellous bone, *Am. J. Vet. Res.*, 58, 1171, 1997.

143. Hartman, L.C., Meenaghan, M.A., Schaaf, N.G., and Hawker, P.B., Effects of pretreatment sterilization and cleaning methods on materials properties and osseoinductivity of a threaded implant, *Int. J. Oral Maxillofac. Implants*, 4, 11, 1989.

144. Adler, E., Stuchin, S.A., and Kummer, F.J., Stability of press-fit acetabular cups, *J. Arthroplasty*, 7, 295, 1992.

145. Fitzgerald, R.H., Total hip arthroplasty sepsis, prevention and diagnosis, *Orthop. Clin. North Am.*, 23, 259, 1992.

146. Khan, M.A., Brakenbury, P.H., and Reynolds, I.S., Dislocations following total hip arthroplasty, *J. Bone Joint Surg.*, 63B, 214, 1981.

147. Kristiansen, B., Jorgensen, L., and Holmich, P., Dislocations following total hip replacement, *Arch. Orthop. Trauma Surg.*, 103, 375, 1985.

148. Canale, S.T., Ed., *Campbell's Operative Orthopaedics*, Mosby, Philadelphia, 1998, 296.

149. Nercessian, O.A. and Joshi, P.R., General principles of surgical technique, in *The Adult Hip*, Callaghan, J.J., Rosenberg, A.G., and Rubash, H.E., Eds., Lippincott-Raven, Philadelphia, 1998, 951.

150. Sun, Y., [The effects of early stage load-bearing on bone ingrowth of porous coated implant in rabbits], Chung Hua I Hsueh Tsa Chih (Taipei), 72, 265, 1992.

151. Syftestad, G.T. and Urist, M.R., Bone aging, *Clin. Orthop.*, 16, 288, 1982.

152. Magee, F.P., Long, J.A., and Hedley, A.K., The effect of age on the interface between porous coated implants and bone, *Orthop. Trans.*, 13, 455, 1989.

153. Nakajima, I., Dai, K.R., Kelly, P.J., and Chao, E.Y., The effect of age on bone ingrowth into titanium fiber-metal segmental prosthesis: an experimental study in a canine model, *Orthop. Trans.*, 6, 296, 1985.

154. Eckhoff, D.G., Turner, A.S., and Aberman, H.M., Effect of age on bone formation around orthopaedic implants, *Clin. Orthop.*, 312, 253, 1995.

155. Soballe, K., Gotfredsen, K., Brockstedt-Rasmussen, H., et al., Histologic analysis of a retrieved hydroxyapatite-coated femoral prosthesis, *Clin. Orthop.*, 272, 255, 1991.

156. Branemark, R. and Thomsen, P., Biomechanical and morphological studies on osseointegration in immunological arthritis in rabbits, *Scand. J. Plast. Reconstr. Hand Surg.*, 31, 185, 1997.

157. Dorr, L.D., Takei, G.K., and Conaty, J.P., Total hip arthroplasties in patients less than 45 years old, *J. Bone Joint Surg.*, 65A, 474, 1983.

158. Poss, R., Maloney, J.P., Ewald, F.C., et al., Six- to eleven-year results of total hip arthroplasty in rheumatoid arthritis, *Clin. Orthop.*, 182, 109, 1984.

159. Sochart, D.H. and Porter, M.L., The long-term results of Charnley low-friction arthroplasty in young patients who have congenital dislocation, degenerative osteoarthritis, or rheumatoid arthritis, *J. Bone Joint Surg.*, 79A, 1599, 1997.

160. Hanssen, A.D., Cabanela, M.E., and Michet, C.J., Jr., Hip arthroplasty in patients with systemic lupus erythematosis, *J. Bone Joint Surg.*, 69A, 807, 1987.

161. Huo, M.H., Salvati, E.A., Brone, M.G., et al., Primary total hip arthroplasty in systemic lupus erythematosis, *J. Arthroplasty*, 7, 51, 1992.

162. Dorr, L.D., Arnala, I., Faugere, M.C., and Malluche, H.H., Five-year post-operative results of cemented femoral arthroplasty in patients with systemic bone disease, *Clin. Orthop.*, 259, 114, 1990.

163. Hayashi, K., Uenoyama, K., Mashima, T., and Sugioka, Y., Remodelling of bone around hydroxyapatite and titanium in experimental osteoporosis, *Biomaterials*, 15, 11, 1994.

164. Fugimoto, T., Niimi, A., and Ueda, M., Effects of steroid-induced osteoporosis on osseointegration of titanium implants, *Int. J. Oral Maxillofac. Implants*, 13, 183, 1998.
165. Mori, H., Manabe, M., Kurachi, Y., and Nagumo, M., Osseointegration of dental implants in rabbit bone with low mineral density, *J. Oral Maxillofac. Surg.*, 55, 351, 1997.

29 Implant Pushout and Pullout Tests

Aivars Berzins and Dale R. Sumner

CONTENTS

I. INTRODUCTION

Pushout and pullout tests are commonly used to test the *ex vivo* mechanical competence of biological fixation of orthopaedic and dental implants via evaluation of the shear strength of the bone–implant interface. One of the reasons these tests are widely used is the relative simplicity of the test protocol, which usually requires a uniaxial materials testing machine to be operated under displacement control using a simple support jig for the pushout test or a hookup system for the pullout test.

The most common applications for these tests include testing for the effects of implant material, surface texture, cross-sectional geometry, porosity, and surface composition in the context of cementless fixation by bone ingrowth or bone apposition to the implant. Other studies have investigated the effects of the presence of a bone graft, bone graft substitutes, or anabolic growth factors on or in the space around the implant. Several studies have utilized pushout or pullout tests to address the effects of anti-inflammatory and anticoagulant medication, irradiation, bisphospho-nates, and local electrical stimulation on the strength of the bone–implant interface. There are a number of studies where pullout tests have been used to test fixation strength of orthopaedic devices, including screws used for adjuvant fixation of artificial joints or spinal hardware and intramedullary rods for fracture fixation. A few studies have used pushout tests to test either the cement–bone or cement–metal interfaces in cemented joint replacement.

The purpose of this chapter is to provide a practical guide to conducting these tests. The list of citations is extensive, but not exhaustive. In addition to the specific papers cited herein, there are a number of reviews covering topics beyond the scope of this chapter, including animal models,[1] factors known to augment or inhibit cementless fixation,[2,3] and certain aspects of implant design.[4] This review has limited its citations to peer-reviewed journal articles. Several groups have multiple publications using the same technique. For these groups, representative papers have been cited.

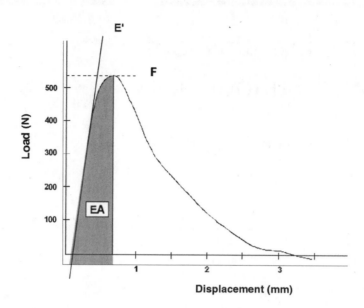

FIGURE 29.1   A typical load–displacement curve from a pushout or pullout test. F = the maximum force applied to the implant during the test; E′ = apparent shear stiffness (the slope of the load–displacement curve in its linear region); EA = energy absorption to failure. (Modified from Søballe, K. et al., *J. Arthroplasty,* 6, 307, 1991. With permission.)

II. FEATURES SHARED BY PUSHOUT AND PULLOUT TESTS

Both types of tests are usually used on cylindrical implants that had been implanted *in vivo* and left *in situ* for various lengths of time. In general, the retrieved specimens are tested either in the fresh condition or after having been frozen because histological processing methods (e.g., fixation in formalin) alter the mechanical properties of bone and soft tissue. Whether tested fresh or frozen, the specimens should not be allowed to dry out during the test.

With both pushout and pullout tests, a load is applied to the implant via a device connected to the crosshead of the materials testing machine and a force–displacement curve is recorded (Figure 29.1). This curve typically shows the force along the vertical axis and the position of the crosshead along the horizontal axis. The test is run until the bone–implant interface fails, easily recognized as a sudden displacement of the implant within the host bone. The most commonly calculated end point of these tests is the ultimate shear strength of the interface (σ_u). Its value is calculated by dividing the maximum pushout or pullout force (F_{max}) by the nominal interface area (A):

$$\sigma_u = F_{max}/A \tag{29.1}$$

For a cylindrical implant,

$$A = \pi DL \tag{29.2}$$

where D is the outer diameter of the cylindrical implant and L is the length of the implant in contact with bone. For transcortical implants, the value of L is measured on the specimen, usually at multiple points. For implants cut into slab sections, the value of L is simply the thickness of the slab. For pullout specimens L is usually the length of the implant (or in the case of porous-coated implants, the length of the porous-coating region). Thus, the results are usually reported in terms of force per unit area (i.e., the maximum shear stress). As a simplified measure for relative comparisons of two implants with the same test conditions, geometry, and nominal bone contact area, one can simply use F_{max}. Certain authors also report the results in terms of the yield strength, i.e., the force at which the load–deformation curve becomes nonlinear.

In addition to the ultimate shear strength of the interface, quantities called the "apparent shear stiffness," the "apparent elastic modulus," or the "interface stiffness" have been calculated as either

$$\Delta F/d \tag{29.3}$$

or as

$$(\Delta F/A)/d \tag{29.4}$$

where d is the displacement. These calculations are based on the assumption that the interface is infinitely thin. However, shear depends upon an angular deformation and the interface must therefore have a finite thickness.[5,6] The definition of this thickness is somewhat arbitrary, but in reality is represented by the difference in the diameter of the implant and, for pushout tests, the diameter of the hole in the support jig (i.e., the clearance listed in Table 29.1, see below). An exact formula for calculating the interface shear modulus in pullout tests has recently been derived and validated,[5] and would work equally well for pushout tests:

$$G = F((\ln R_2 - \ln R_1)/2\pi dL) \tag{29.5}$$

where G is the interface shear modulus, F is the applied force, R_1 is the radius of the implant, R_2 is the radius of the support hole, and d and L are as defined above (see also Reference 6). Energy absorption at the interface to failure can be measured as the area under the force–displacement curve.

It must be understood that the introduction of the displacement measure, as recorded from the crosshead of the materials testing machine, leads to the potential for a systematic error related to the compliance of the testing setup. Thus, the compliance of the setup should be tested first in order to adjust the displacement readings. This is probably more critical for pullout tests than for pushout tests because the test setup tends to be less rigid with pullout tests (see below). An alternative method to using the displacement at the crosshead is to take measurements from a transducer in close proximity to the interface.[5]

In addition, the rate of displacement could affect the results because bone is a viscoelastic material. On the one hand, Shirazi-Adl et al.[7] found that the pullout force of screws from polyurethane models was not dependent on the displacement rate, which was varied from 0.6 to 600 mm/min in their study. On the other hand, Raab et al.[8] showed a clear strain rate dependence in their system for testing the implant–bone–cement interface. Specifically, there was minimal effect for strain rates varying from 10^{-3}/s to 10^{-1}/s (roughly, a displacement rate of 1 to 100 mm/min for the implants tested), but an increasingly significant effect at faster strain rates.

III. FACTORS SPECIFIC TO PUSHOUT TESTS

Typical anatomical locations for pushout specimens are the cortex of femur, tibia, or mandible. In the long bones, this implant placement is often referred to as "transcortical." Occasionally, specimens placed in a trabecular bone bed are tested with this method. After retrieval the specimen is prepared for analysis. For the transcortical implants, this involves trimming or machining of bone so that the specimen can be properly placed in the testing jig (Figure 29.2). For the implants placed in trabecular bone, a slab section is usually prepared. With both types of implants, the specimen is placed on a support jig with clearance for the implant.

TABLE 29.1
Summary of Test Conditions for Pushout Tests

Ref.	Year	Related Refs.	Implant Size (mm)ᵃ	Support Clearance (mm)	Displacement Rate (mm/mm)	Outputs
28	1971	29	3.2 × 12.7	NA	0.5	Shear strength
30	1972		6.35 × 6.35	0.127	0.127	Shear strength at yield, max. shear strength
31	1973		4.5–6.4 × 4.8–6.4	NA	1.27	Shear strength
32	1976		4.8 × 10	NA	5	Shear strength
33	1976		9 × 20	Minimal	1.27	Shear strength
34	1978		~5 × 2	NA	NA	Shear strength
35	1980		4.5 × 9	0.25	0.5	Shear strength
36	1980		6.5 × 8	1.9	1.27 or 0.5	Shear strength
37	1981		10 × 4	NA	1.27	Shear strength, interface stiffness
38	1981		6.4 × 6.45	NA	0.0498	Shear strength, apparent elastic modulus
8	1981	39	6.4 × 12.8	0 ?	1ᵇ	Critical value of the strain energy release rate
40	1982		10.5–12.5 × 20	NA	25.4	Shear strength
19	1984		6 × ~8	NA	1.2	Shear strength, interface stiffness (repetitive loading/load control)
41	1985		4.75 or 5 × 10	NA	0.5	Shear strength
42	1985		6 × ~9	NA	12.7	Shear strength, interface stiffness (repetitive loading/load control)
43	1985	44,45	6 × ~9	0.4	1.27	Shear strength, shear stiffness
9	1985		6 × ~8	0.15	0.127	Shear strength, shear stiffness (repetitive loading/load control)
46	1986		8–12.7 × 6.35	NA	127	Shear strength, interface stiffness, energy to failure
47	1989		5 × 10	NA	0.1	Shear strength
48	1990	26,49–53	6 × 4	0.5	5	Shear strength, apparent shear stiffness, energy absorption

54	1992	27	5.95 × 9	0.15	1.27	Shear strength
55	1992		6.3 × ~6.5	NA	25.4	Shear strength
11	1993		6 × 13	1	0.5	Shear strength
56	1993		4.76 × 12	NA	0.2	Shear strength
57	1993		2.5 × 20	NA	1	Shear strength, energy absorption
58	1995		5.5 × 8	1.025	1	Shear strength
59	1995		6.8 × 10 or 15	NA	0.5	Shear strength
60	1995		4 × 15	NA	1	Shear strength
61	1995		5.95 × 22	0.15	1.3	Shear strength
62	1995		6 × 13	0.5	0.5	Shear strength
63	1995	64	2.8 × 6	NA	1	Shear strength
10	1995		2–3 × 5 conical shape	~1.5	0.5	Shear strength
65	1995		6.5 or 6.6 × 24c	NA	0.05	Shear strength
66	1996		7–15 × 10	NA	0.25	Maximum force
67	1996		10 × 6	0.15	1.27	Shear strength
68	1997		5.3 × 5.35	NA	1	Holding strength, holding stress
69	1997		6.4 × 5	NA	0.5	Shear strength
70	1997		6 × 20	~1.0	0.5	Shear strength
71	1998		8 × 10 × 4	0.5	0.5	Shear strength
72	1998	73	4 × 9 or 10	NA	2	Pushout force

NA = information was not available from the publication.

a Some implants were sectioned before testing; therefore, only the tested size is listed (outside diameter × length).

b Calculated from a reported strain rate of 1.3×10^{-3}/s, assuming the original length was 12.8 mm.

c Estimated from a radiograph in the manuscript (exact value not specified).

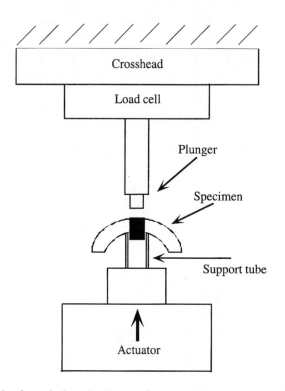

FIGURE 29.2   Schematic of a typical mechanical test fixture used in pushout tests. The support tube has an inner diameter greater than the diameter of the implant, creating a clearance. (Modified from Cook, S.D. et al., *J. Arthroplasty,* 10, 351, 1995. With permission.)

Accurate alignment among the plunger, the specimen, and the support jig is crucial to prevent the implant from jamming within its track of exit. Thus, additional features of the support fixture can be incorporated to allow for self-alignment of the longitudinal axis of the specimen with the longitudinal axis of the plunger. In cases where a slab section containing part of the original implant is tested, it is important to have accurate cutting jigs so that the slab section can be cut perpendicular to the long axis of the implant. Another important test condition is perfect seating of the specimen on the support fixture. Machining the base of the specimen to assure ideal fit and alignment with the support jig has been used in several studies.[9-11] In addition, the specimen can be affixed to the support jig by cementing.[11]

As noted, the strength of fixation is calculated as the ultimate shear stress of the interface. This simplified stress calculation assumes a uniform stress distribution at the interface. In reality, however, the stress distribution along the interface is not uniform. Thus, it becomes crucial to avoid comparisons between two implants with dissimilar interface stress distributions, i.e., implants with different geometries or testing conditions that could affect the distribution of the interface stresses.

In order to establish grounds for standardization of these tests, two theoretical studies have addressed the influence of pushout test conditions using the finite-element method. Harrigan et al.[12] investigated the effect of irregular stress distribution due to stress concentration in the region between the base of the specimen and the support fixture. They concluded that pushout test results depend heavily on uniform support of the specimen (i.e., close apposition of two flat surfaces).

Dhert et al.[13] addressed a number of pushout test variables, including clearance of the implant within the hole in the support jig, the elastic modulus of the implant, cortical thickness (length of the implant), and diameter of the implant. By analyzing stress distributions at the interface, they found that the clearance of the hole is the most critical parameter, followed by the elastic modulus of the implant. Based on this finite-element study, these authors recommended a clearance of at least 0.7 mm to minimize nonuniform stress distribution and to compare only those implants which are made from materials with similar elastic moduli. According to this finite-element study, variations in the length and diameter of the implants did not significantly affect the interface stress distribution and, thus, could be neglected. However, it should be noted that implants with a larger length-to-diameter ratio would tend to be less stable during the test and more prone to develop misalignment with the axis of the applied pushout force.

A wide range of implant sizes and testing conditions have been used in pushout tests (see Table 29.1). Many of these appear to have been conducted in contrast to the recommendations from the theoretical studies. Thus, caution is needed when comparing results among investigators or when exact values are needed for modeling interface conditions, as might be done in a finite-element analysis of a hip or knee replacement. Comparisons within a study are probably valid.

IV. FACTORS SPECIFIC TO PULLOUT TESTS

Typical implants used with pullout tests are cylindrical; however, there have been reports about implants with elliptical[14] or trapezoid[15] shapes and combined conical–cylindrical shapes.[16] Unlike the implants for the pushout test protocol, the pullout implants are usually placed in anatomical locations allowing for significant contact with cancellous bone by being aligned with the long axis of the bone in the proximal or distal femur, proximal tibia, or proximal humerus. The greatest advantage of the pullout test setup is that the presence of either a flexible linkage[17] or an X–Y slide table[16,18] allows the specimen to self-align during the test, thus eliminating concerns about potential misalignment between the axes of the implant and the pullout force. In a typical pullout test, the bone part of the specimen is potted in a self-hardening polymer cement and attached to the materials testing machine (Figure 29.3). A pulling rod is then attached to the implant, usually via a threaded piece on the implant, and the implant is pulled out, typically under displacement control of the material testing machine.

Similar to the reports on pushout tests, there are a wide variety of test conditions for pullout test protocols with a potential to bias the test results (Table 29.2). After testing a number of pullout conditions using polyurethane foam and cadaver bones, Shirazi-Adl et al.[7] found that material arrangements and boundary conditions can substantially alter the pullout force. Thus, comparisons of results of pullout tests with different design arrangements should be approached with caution. Berzins et al.[5] used polyurethane foam to test for the effects of implant geometry using combinations of three diameters (5 to 9.7 mm) and three lengths (15 to 48 mm) for a total of nine implant sizes. It was found that the interface shear modulus was significantly affected by the length of the implants, but the ultimate fixation strength was unaffected by implant diameter and length in the range studied.

V. DEVELOPMENT OF NONDESTRUCTIVE AND OTHER TEST MODES

Because the standard pushout and pullout tests are destructive, the ability to examine the intact interface after the test is lost. In the presence of accurate direct displacement monitoring at the interface, it is possible to develop a nondestructive pushout or pullout protocol to measure the interface shear modulus.[5,19] To date, the accuracy of measuring the shear modulus nondestructively has now been validated using a model system (polyurethane foam),[5] supporting the concept of using a nondestructive test to characterize the mechanical and morphological properties of the intact interface in the same specimen.[19] In addition, the shear modulus of the interface may prove to be more reflective of the type of tissue at the interface than the ultimate shear strength.

Torque tests have been reported by several groups (Table 29.3). These tests have the theoretical advantage of a uniform stress field at the interface, but the experimental setup is more elaborate than that required for a pushout or pullout test. The recent paper by Brånemark et al.[6] provides a

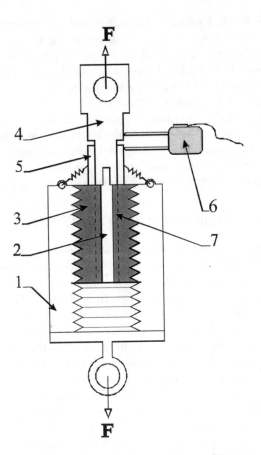

FIGURE 29.3 Schematic of a mechanical test fixture used in a pullout test in which the investigators calculated the interface shear modulus (longitudinal cross section). *Note:* 1 = aluminum mold, 2 = cylindrical implant, 3 = foam model (bone, in a biological sample), 4 = extended yoke, 5 = sliding sleeve held against the foam (bone) surface by springs, 6 = extensometer, 7 = foam (bone) layer in which the interface shear modulus is measured, F = tensile force applied to the setup (Modified from Berzins, A. et al., *J. Biomed. Mater. Res.*, 34, 337, 1997. With permission.)

useful description of how interfacial shear strength and the torsional shear modulus can be calculated. Another test method has been to test the tensile bonding strength of cortical bone to a transcortical implant.[20]

Finally, a method for testing the fatigue properties of the interface between an implant and bone cement was described nearly 20 years ago[8] and a method for testing the fatigue properties of porous surfaces was described nearly 15 years ago,[21] but to the authors' knowledge the fatigue properties of the cementless bone–implant interface have received little attention.[7,22] With the growing interest in the role of fatigue on bone remodeling in general[23,24] and the probable importance of the fatigue properties of the bone supporting an implant for the long-term maintenance of a biological interface,[25] one can only presume that more effort along these lines will be made in the future.

ACKNOWLEDGMENTS

Research was supported by NIH Grants AR16485 and AR42862.

TABLE 29.2
Summary of Test Conditions for Pullout Tests

Ref.	Year	Related Refs.	Implant Size (mm)^c	Displacement Rate (mm/mm)	Outputs
17	1971		9.52 × 12.7	12.7	Shear strength
74	1972		9 × 50	125	Shear strength
75	1973		22.225 staples	1.27	Maximum force
76	1977		8.5 or 9 × 85	2,700	Shear strength
77	1980		Plate pulloff test (exact dimensions not given)	0.5	Fixation (tensile) strength
78	1984		~4.7 × 19	50	Maximum force
79	1985		5 × 10	60	Shear strength
80	1986		3.2 × ~40	12.7	Shear strength
81	1987	82,83	10 × 50	0.25	Shear strength
84	1990		10 × 5 × 5 (rectangular)	NA	Shear strength
85	1990		10 × 17	90.6 kgf/s (load control)	Maximum force
86	1992		7 × 30	0.25	Shear strength
87	1992		2.65 × NA	1.52	Maximum force
14	1993		~4 × NA (cylindrical or elliptical)	2	Shear strength
88	1994		5 × 25	2	Shear strength
7	1994		5.75 to 8.75 ≤ 40	9.6	Pullout force
18	1995		5 × 10	2	Shear strength
16	1995		NA	3	Shear strength
15	1995		7 × 10 × 5 (trapezoid)	2	Shear load, duration of peak
89	1995	90	Pedicle screws and hooks	0.5	Maximum force
91	1995		6.5 × 55	10	Maximum force
92	1996		6.25–7 × 30–40	60	Pullout force
93	1997		3.25–5 × 12	2	Pullout force, shear strength
5	1997		5–9.7 × 15–48	0.25	Shear strength, shear modulus
6	1997	94	2 × NA	0.5	Pullout load
95	1998		~3.1 × 6	0.5	Pullout load
96	1998		5 × 25	2	Shear strength

NA = information was not available from the publication.

[a] Some implants were sectioned before testing; therefore, only the tested size is listed (outside diameter × length).

TABLE 29.3
Summary of Test Conditions for Torque Tests

Ref.	Year	Related Refs.	Size of Tested Implant,^{a} mm	Displacement Rate	Outputs
30	1972		6.35 × 9.525	NA	Maximum torque
97	1988	98,99	16 × ~30	15°/min	Torsional stiffness, maximum torque, energy absorption
100	1992	14	4 × 10	57°/min	Torsional shear strength, energy absorption
101	1995		3.5 × 10	NA	Removal torque
6	1997	94	2 × NA	2°/min	Break point torque, maximum torque
102	1997		3.75 × 10	na	Failure torque
95	1998		~3.1 × 6	2°/min	Yield torque, maximum torque, rotation at yield, rotation at maximum

NA = information was not available from the publication.

[a] Some implants were sectioned before testing; therefore, only the tested size is listed (outside diameter × length).

REFERENCES

1. Sumner, D.R., Turner, T.M., and Urban, R.M., Animal models of bone ingrowth and joint replacement, in *Animals Models in Orthopedic Research,* An, Y.H. and Friedman, R.J., Eds., CRC Press, Boca Raton, FL, 1999, 407.

2. Kienapfel, H. and Griss, P., Fixation by ingrowth, in *The Adult Hip,* Callaghan, J.J., Rosenberg, A.G., and Rubash, H., Eds., Lippincott-Raven, Philadelphia, 1998, 201.

3. Sumner, D.R., Bone ingrowth: implications for establishment and maintenance of cementless porous-coated interfaces, in *Orthopaedic Knowledge Update: Hip and Knee Reconstruction,* Callaghan, J.J., Dennis, D.A., Paprosky, W.G., and Rosenberg, A.G., Eds., American Academy of Orthopaedic Surgeons, Rosemont, IL, 1995, 57.

4. Pilliar, R.M., Porous-surfaced metallic implants for orthopedic applications, *J. Biomed. Mater. Res.,* 21(A1), 1, 1987.

5. Berzins, A., Shah, B., Weinans, H., and Sumner, D.R., Nondestructive measurements of implant–bone interface shear modulus and effects of implant geometry in pullout tests, *J. Biomed. Mater. Res.,* 34, 337, 1997.

6. Brånemark, R., Ohrnell, L.O., Nilsson, P., and Thomsen, P., Biomechanical characterization of osseointegration during healing: an experimental *in vivo* study in the rat, *Biomaterials,* 18, 969, 1997.

7. Shirazi-Adl, A., Dammak, M., and Zukor, D.J., Fixation pullout response measurement of bone screws and porous-surfaced posts, *J. Biomech.,* 27, 1249, 1994.

8. Raab, S., Ahmed, A.M., and Provan, J.W., The quasistatic and fatigue performance of the implant/bone–cement interface, *J. Biomed. Mater. Res.,* 15, 159, 1981.

9. Thomas, K. A. and Cook, S. D., An evaluation of variables influencing implant fixation by direct bone apposition, *J. Biomed. Mater. Res.,* 19, 875, 1985.

10. Wie, H., Hero, H., Solheim, T., et al., Bonding capacity in bone of HIP-processed HA-coated titanium: mechanical and histological investigations, *J. Biomed. Mater. Res.,* 29, 1443, 1995.

11. Hayashi, K., Inadome, T., Mashima, T., and Sugioka, Y., Comparison of bone–implant interface shear strength of solid hydroxyapatite and hydroxyapatite-coated titanium implants, *J. Biomed. Mater. Res.,* 27, 557, 1993.

12. Harrigan, T.P., Kareh, J., and Harris, W.H., The influence of support conditions in the loading fixture on failure mechanisms in the pushout test: a finite element study, *J. Orthop. Res.,* 8, 678, 1990.

13. Dhert, W.J., Verheyen, C.C., Braak, L.H., et al., A finite element analysis of the pushout test: influence of test conditions, *J. Biomed. Mater. Res.,* 26, 119, 1992.

14. Cook, S.D., Salkeld, S.L., Gaisser, D.M., and Wagner, W.R., An *in vivo* analysis of an elliptical dental implant design, *J. Oral Implantol.,* 19, 307, 1993.

15. Li, Z., Kitsugi, T., Yamamuro, T., et al., Bone-bonding behavior under load-bearing conditions of an alumina ceramic implant incorporating beads coated with glass-ceramic containing apatite and wollastonite, *J. Biomed. Mater. Res.,* 29, 1081, 1995.

16. Maruyama, M., Hydroxyapatite clay used to fill the gap between implant and bone, *J. Bone Joint Surg.,* 77B, 213, 1995.

17. Galante, J., Rostoker, W., Lueck, R., and Ray, R.D., Sintered fiber metal composites as a basis for attachment of implants to bone, *J. Bone Joint Surg.,* 53A, 101, 1971.

18. Dean, J.C., Tisdel, C.L., Goldberg, V.M., et al., Effects of hydroxyapatite tricalcium phosphate coating and intracancellous placement on bone ingrowth in titanium fibermetal implants, *J. Arthroplasty,* 10, 830, 1995.

19. Anderson, R.C., Cook, S.D., Weinstein, A.M., and Haddad, R.J., An evaluation of skeletal attachment to LTI pyrolytic carbon, porous titanium, and carbon-coated porous titanium implants, *Clin. Orthop.,* 182, 242, 1984.

20. Park, J.B., Salman, N.N., Kenner, G.H., and Von Recum, A.F., Preliminary studies on the effects of direct current on the bone/porous implant interfaces, *Ann. Biomed. Eng.,* 8, 93, 1980.

21. Manley, M.T., Kotzar, G., Stern, L.S., and Wilde, A., Effects of repetitive loadings on the integrity of porous coatings, *Clin. Orthop.,* 217, 293, 1987.

22. Lim, T.-H., An, H.S., Hasegawa, T., et al., Prediction of fatigue screw loosening in anterior screw fixation using dual energy X-ray absorptiometry, *Spine,* 20, 2565, 1995.

23. Burr, D.B., Martin, R.B., Schaffler, M.B., and Radin, E.L., Bone remodeling in response to *in vivo* fatigue microdamage, *J. Biomech.*, 18, 189, 1985.

24. Martin, B., Mathematical model for repair of fatigue damage and stress fracture in osteonal bone, *J. Orthop. Res.*, 13, 309, 1995.

25. Sumner, D.R., Bone remodeling of the proximal femur, in *The Adult Hip,* Callaghan, J.J., Rosenberg, A.G., and Rubash, H., Eds., Lippincott-Raven, New York, 1998, 211.

26. Søballe, K., Hansen, E.S., Brockstedt-Rasmussen, H., et al., Fixation of titanium and hydroxyapatite-coated implants in arthritic osteopenic bone, *J. Arthroplasty*, 6, 307, 1991.

27. Cook, S.D., Barrack, R.L., Dalton, J.E., et al., Effects of indomethacin on biologic fixation of porous-coated titanium implants, *J. Arthroplasty*, 10, 351, 1995.

28. Welsh, R.P., Pilliar, R.M., and MacNab, I., Surgical implants: the role of surface porosity in fixation to bone and acrylic, *J. Bone Joint Surg.*, 53A, 963, 1971.

29. Cameron, H.U., Pilliar, R.M., and MacNab, I., The rate of bone ingrowth in porous metal, *J. Biomed. Mater. Res.*, 10, 295, 1976.

30. Predecki, P., Auslaender, B.A., Stephan, J.E., et al., Attachment of bone to threaded implants by ingrowth and mechanical interlocking, *J. Biomed. Mater. Res.*, 6, 401, 1972.

31. Nilles, J.L., Coletti, J.M., and Wilson, C., Biomechanical evaluation of bone-porous material interfaces, *J. Biomed. Mater. Res.*, 7, 231, 1973.

32. Robertson, D.M., St. Pierre, L., and Chahal, R., Preliminary observations of bone ingrowth into porous materials, *J. Biomed. Mater. Res.*, 10, 335, 1976.

33. Weinstein, A.M., Klawitter, J.J., Cleveland, T.W., and Amoss, D.C., Electrical stimulation of bone growth into porous Al_2O_3, *J. Biomed. Mater. Res. Symp.*, 10, 231, 1976.

34. Young, S.O., Park, J.B., Kenner, G.H., et al., Dental implant fixation by electrically mediated process. I. Interfacial strength, *Biomater. Med. Dev. Artif. Organs,* 6, 111, 1978.

35. Bobyn, J.D., Cameron, H.U., Pilliar, R.M., and Weatherly, G.C., The optimum pore size for the fixation of porous-surfaced metal implants by the ingrowth of bone, *Clin. Orthop.*, 150, 263, 1980.

36. Ducheyne, P., Hench, L.L., Kagan, II, A., et al., Effect of hydroxyapatite impregnation on skeletal bonding of porous coated implants, *J. Biomed. Mater. Res.*, 14, 225, 1980.

37. Clemov, A.J., Weinstein, A.M., Klawitter, J.J., et al., Interface mechanics of porous titanium implants, *J. Biomed. Mater. Res.*, 15, 73, 1981.

38. Colella, S.M., Miller, A.G., Stang, R.G., et al., Fixation of porous titanium implants in cortical bone enhanced by electrical stimulation, *J. Biomed. Mater. Res.*, 15, 37, 1981.

39. Ahmed, A., Raab, S. and Miller, J.E., Metal/cement interface strength in cemented stem fixation, *J. Orthop. Res.*, 2, 105, 1984.

40. Rhinelander, F.W., Stewart, C.L., Wilson, J.W., et al., Growth of tissue into a porous, low modulus coating on intramedullary nails: an experimental study, *Clin. Orthop.*, 164, 293, 1982.

41. Brooker, A.F. and Constable, D., Bone ingrowth into titanium grooves: a comparison of surfaces for biologic fixation, *Adv. Orthop. Surg.*, 125, 1985.

42. Cook, S.D., Walsh, K.A., and Haddad, R.J., Interface mechanics and bone growth into porous Co-Cr-Mo alloy implants, *Clin. Orthop.*, 193, 271, 1985.

43. Thomas, K.A., Cook, S.D., Renz, E.A., et al., The effect of surface treatments on the interface mechanics of LTI pyrolytic carbon implants, *J. Biomed. Mater. Res.*, 19, 145, 1985.

44. Thomas, K.A., Kay, J.F., Cook, S.D., and Jarcho, M., The effect of surface macrotexture and hydroxylapatite coating on the mechanical strengths and histologic profiles of titanium implant materials, *J. Biomed. Mater. Res.*, 21, 1395, 1987.

45. Cook, S.D., Thomas, K.A., Kay, J.F., and Jarcho, M., Hydroxyapatite-coated porous titanium for use as an orthopedic biologic attachment system, *Clin. Orthop.*, 230, 303, 1988.

46. Heck, D.A., Nakajima, I., Kelly, P.J., and Chao, E.Y., The effect of load alteration on the biological and biomechanical performance of a titanium fiber-metal segmental prosthesis, *J. Bone Joint Surg.*, 68A, 118, 1986.

47. Oonishi, H., Yamamoto, M., Ishimaru, H., et al., The effect of hydroxyapatite coating on bone growth into porous titanium alloy implants, *J. Bone Joint Surg.*, 71B, 213, 1989.

48. Søballe, K., Hansen, E.S., Brockstedt-Rasmussen, H., et al., Hydroxyapatite coating enhances fixation of porous coated implants: a comparison in dogs between press fit and noninterference fit, *Acta Orthop. Scand.*, 61, 299, 1990.

49. Søballe, K., Hansen, E.S., Brockstedt-Rasmussen, H., et al., Bone graft incorporation around titanium-alloy and hydroxyapatite-coated implants in dogs, *Clin. Orthop.*, 274, 282, 1992.

50. Søballe, K., Hansen, E.S., Brockstedt-Rasmussen, H., et al., Gap healing enhanced by hydroxyapatite coating in dogs, *Clin. Orthop.*, 272, 300, 1991.

51. Lind, M., Overgaard, S., Ongpipattanakul, B., et al., Transforming growth factor-β stimulates bone ongrowth to weight-loaded tricalcium phosphate coated implants, *J. Bone Joint Surg.*, 78B, 377, 1996.

52. Lind, M., Overgaard, S., Nguyen, T., et al., Transforming growth factor-β stimulates bone ongrowth: hydroxyapatite-coated implants studied in dogs, *Acta Orthop. Scand.*, 67, 611, 1996.

53. Overgaard, S., Lind, M., Glerup, H., et al., Porous-coated vs. grit-blasted surface texture of hydroxyapatite-coated implants during controlled micromotion, *J. Arthroplasty*, 13, 449, 1998.

54. Cook, S.D., Thomas, K.A., Dalton, J E., et al., Hydroxylapatite coating of porous implants improves bone ingrowth and interface attachment strength, *J. Biomed. Mater. Res.*, 26, 989, 1992.

55. Luckey, H.A., Lamprecht, E.G., and Walt, M.J., Bone apposition to plasma-sprayed cobalt-chromium alloy, *J. Biomed. Mater. Res.*, 26, 557, 1992.

56. Wang, B.C., Lee, T.M., Chang, E., and Yang, C.Y., The shear strength and the failure mode of plasma-sprayed hydroxyapatite coating to bone: the effect of coating thickness, *J. Biomed. Mater. Res.*, 27, 1315, 1993.

57. Shen, W.J., Chung, K.C., Wang, G.J., et al., Demineralized bone matrix in the stabilization of porous-coated implants in bone defects in rabbits, *Clin. Orthop.*, 293, 346, 1993.

58. Friedman, R.J., Bauer, T.W., Garg, K., et al., Histological and mechanical comparison of hydroxya-patie-coated cobalt-chrome and titanium implants in the rabbit femur, *J. Appl. Biomater.*, 6, 231, 1995.

59. Rashmir-Raven, A.M., Richardson, D.C., Aberman, H.M., and DeYoung, D.J., The response of cancellous and cortical canine bone to hydroxylapatite-coated and uncoated titanium rods, *J. Appl. Biomater.*, 6, 237, 1995.

60. Hetherington, V.J., Lord, C.E., and Brown, S.A., Mechanical and histological fixation of hydroxyla-patite-coated pyrolytic carbon and titanium alloy implants: a report of short-term results, *J. Appl. Biomater.*, 6, 243, 1995.

61. Callahan, B.C., Lisecki, E.J., Banks, R.E., et al., The effect of warfarin on the attachment of bone to hydroxyapatite-coated and uncoated porous implants, *J. Bone Joint Surg.*, 77A, 225, 1995.

62. Inadome, T., Hayashi, K., Nakashima, Y., et al., Comparison of bone–implant interface shear strength of hydroxyapatite-coated and alumina-coated metal implants, *J. Biomed. Mater. Res.*, 29, 19, 1995.

63. Li, J., Fartash, B., and Hermansson, L., Hydroxyapatite-alumina composites and bone-bonding, *Biomaterials*, 16, 417, 1995.

64. Li, J., Liao, H., Fartash, B., et al., Surface-dimpled commercially pure titanium implant and bone ingrowth, *Biomaterials*, 18, 691, 1997.

65. Eckhoff, D.G., Turner, A.S., and Aberman, H.M., Effect of age on bone formation around orthopaedic implants, *Clin. Orthop.*, 312, 253, 1995.

66. Berzins, A., Sumner, D.R., Wasielewski, R.C., and Galante, J.O., Impacted particulate allograft for femoral revision total hip arthroplasty: *in vitro* mechanical stability and effects of cement pressuriza-tion, *J. Arthroplasty*, 11, 500, 1996.

67. Walenciak, M.T., Zimmerman, M.C., Harten, R.D., et al., Biomechanical and histological analysis of an HA coated, arc deposited CPTi canine hip prosthesis, *J. Biomed. Mater. Res.*, 31, 465, 1996.

68. Vemuganti, A., Siegler, S., Abusafieh, A., and Kalidindi, S., Development of self-anchoring bone implants. II. Bone–implant interface characteristics *in vitro*, *J. Biomed. Mater. Res.*, 38, 328, 1997.

69. Lewis, C.G., Jones, C.L., and Hungerford, D.S., Effects of grafting on porous metal ingrowth, *J. Arthroplasty*, 12, 451, 1997.

70. Nakashima, Y., Hayashi, K., Inadome, T., et al., Hydroxyapatite-coating on titanium arc sprayed titanium implants, *J. Biomed. Mater. Res.*, 35, 287, 1997.

71. Vercaigne, S., Wolke, J.G., Naert, I., and Jansen, J.A., Histomorphometrical and mechanical evaluation of titanium plasma-spray-coated implants placed in the cortical bone of goats, *J. Biomed. Mater. Res.*, 41, 41, 1998.

72. Ogiso, M., Yamamura, M., Kuo, P.T., et al., Comparative pushout test of dense HA implants and HA-coated implants: findings in a canine study, *J. Biomed. Mater. Res.*, 39, 364, 1998.

73. Ogiso, M., Yamashita, Y., and Matsumoto, T., Microstructural changes in bone of HA-coated implants, *J. Biomed. Mater. Res.*, 39, 23, 1998.

74. Lembert, E., Galante, J., and Rostoker, W., Fixation of skeletal replacement by fiber metal composites, *Clin. Orthop.*, 87, 303, 1972.

75. Cameron, H.U., Pilliar, R.M., and MacNab, I., The effect of movement on the bonding of porous metal to bone, *J. Biomed. Mater. Res.*, 7, 301, 1973.

76. Ducheyne, P., DeMester, P., and Aernoudt, D., Influence of a functional dynamic loading on bone ingrowth into surface pores of orthopedic implants, *J. Biomed. Mater. Res.*, 11, 811, 1977.

77. Bobyn, J.D., Pilliar, R.M., Cameron, H.U., et al., The effect of porous surface configuration on the tensile strength of fixation of implants by bone ingrowth, *Clin. Orthop.*, 149, 291, 1980.

78. McLaughlin, R.E., Reger, S.I., Bolander, M., and Eschenroeder, H.C., Enhancement of bone ingrowth by the use of bone matrix as a biologic cement, *Clin. Orthop.*, 183, 255, 1984.

79. Barth, E., Ronningen, H., and Solheim, L.F., Comparison of ceramic and titanium implants in cats, *Acta Orthop. Scand.*, 56, 491, 1985.

80. Berry, J.L., Geiger, J.M., Moran, J.M., et al., Use of tricalcium phosphate or electrical stimulation to enhance the bone–porous implant interface, *J. Biomed. Mater. Res.*, 20, 65, 1986.

81. Rivero, D.P., Skipor, A.K., Singh, M., et al., Effect of disodium etidronate (EHDP) on bone ingrowth in a porous material, *Clin. Orthop.*, 215, 279, 1987.

82. Rivero, D.P., Fox, J., Skipor, A.K., et al., Calcium phosphate-coated porous titanium implants for enhanced skeletal fixation, *J. Biomed. Mater. Res.*, 22, 191, 1988.

83. Sumner, D.R., Turner, T.M., Pierson, R.H., et al., Effects of radiation on fixation of non-cemented porous-coated implants in a canine model, *J. Bone Joint Surg.*, 72A, 1527, 1990.

84. Ducheyne, P., Beight, J., Cuckler, J., et al., Effect of calcium phosphate coating characteristics on early post-operative bone tissue ingrowth, *Biomaterials*, 11, 531, 1990.

85. Wise, M.W., III, Robertson, I.D., Lachiewicz, P.F., et al., The effect of radiation therapy on the fixation strength of an experimental porous-coated implant in dogs, *Clin. Orthop.*, 261, 276, 1990.

86. Kienapfel, H., Sumner, D.R., Turner, T.M., et al., Efficacy of autograft and freeze-dried allograft to enhance fixation of porous coated implants in the presence of interface gaps, *J. Orthop. Res.*, 10, 423, 1992.

87. Chae, J.C., Collier, J.P., Mayor, M.B., et al., Enhanced ingrowth of porous-coated CoCr implants plasma-sprayed with tricalcium phosphate, *J. Biomed. Mater. Res.*, 26, 93, 1992.

88. Tisdel, C.L., Goldberg, V.M., Parr, J.A., et al., The influence of hydroxyapatite and tricalcium-phosphate coating on bone growth in titanium fiber-metal implants, *J. Bone Joint Surg.*, 76A, 159, 1994.

89. Berlemann, U., Cripton, P., Nolte, L.P., et al., New means in spinal pedicle hook fixation. A bio-mechanical evaluation, *Eur. Spine J.*, 4, 114, 1995.

90. Berlemann, U., Cripton, P.A., Rincon, L., et al., Pullout strength of pedicle hooks with fixation screws: influence of screw length and angulation, *Eur. Spine J.*, 5, 71, 1996.

91. Lim, T.H., An, H.S., Evanic, C., et al., Strength of anterior vertebral screw fixation in relation to bone mineral density, *J. Spinal Disord.*, 7, 121, 1995.

92. Kwok, A.W., Finkelstein, J.A., Woodside, T., et al., Insertional torque and pullout strengths of conical and cylindrical pedicle screws in cadaveric bone, *Spine*, 21, 2429, 1996.

93. Kido, H., Schulz, E.E., Kumar, A., et al., Implant diameter and bone density: effect on initial stability and pullout resistance, *J. Oral Implantol.*, 23, 163, 1997.

94. Ohrnell, L.O., Brånemark, R., Nyman, J., et al., Effects of irradiation on the biomechanics of osseoin-tegration. An experimental *in vivo* study in rats, *Scand. J. Plast. Reconstr. Surg. Hand Surg.*, 31, 281, 1997.

95. Brånemark, R., Öhrnell, L.O., Skalak, R., et al., Biomechanical characterization of osseointegration: an experimental *in vivo* investigation in the beagle dog, *J. Orthop. Res.*, 16, 61, 1998.

96. Jinno, T., Goldberg, V.M., Davy, D., and Stevenson, S., Osseointegration of surface-blasted implants made of titanium alloy and cobalt-chromium alloy in a rabbit intramedullary model, *J. Biomed. Mater. Res.*, 42, 20, 1998.

97. Okada, Y., Suka, T., Sim, F.H., et al., Comparison of replacement prostheses for segmental defects of bone: different porous coatings for extracortical fixation, *J. Bone Joint Surg.*, 70A, 160, 1988.

98. Chin, H.C., Frassica, F.J., Markel, M.D., et al., The effects of therapeutic doses of irradiation on experimental bone graft incorporation over a porous-coated segmental defect endoprosthesis, *Clin. Orthop.*, 289, 254, 1993.

99. Roy, R.G., Markel, M.D., Lipowitz, A.J., et al., Effect of homologous fibrin adhesive on callus formation and extracortical bone bridging around a porous-coated segmental endoprosthesis in dogs, *Am. J. Vet. Med.*, 54, 1188, 1993.

100. Cook, S.D., Baffes, G.C., Palafox, A.J., et al., Torsional stability of HA-coated and grit-blasted titanium dental implants, *J. Oral Implantol.*, 18, 354, 1992.

101. Gotfredsen, K., Wennerberg, A., Johansson, C., et al., Anchorage of TiO_2-blasted, HA-coated, and machined implants: an experimental study with rabbits, *J. Biomed. Mater. Res.*, 29, 1223, 1995.

102. Pebé, P., Barbot, R., Trinidad, J., et al., Countertorque testing and histomorphometric analysis of various implant surfaces in canines: a pilot study, *Implant Dent.*, 6, 259, 1997.

30 The Validity of a Single Pushout Test

Wouter J.A. Dhert and John A. Jansen

CONTENTS

I. INTRODUCTION

The long-term clinical success of hard-tissue implants is based on the presence and maintenance of a proper bone response.[1] Basically, two types of bone response to implant materials can be distinguished. The first type involves the formation of a collagenous connective tissue capsule around the implant.[2] The second type of bone response is characterized by a direct bone–implant contact, without an intervening connective tissue layer, or even by direct bone bonding.[3-5] Generally, this second type of bony fixation is considered to be the preferable situation for implant fixation.

Various histological and histomorphometrical techniques can be used to analyze and quantify the bone response to implanted biomaterials. However, a thorough histological description cannot be used as the only criterion for implant–bone biocompatibility. For example, histological procedures do not provide information about the bone–implant interfacial strength and perhaps the development of chemical bonding between implant and surrounding bone. Since a major purpose in implant-related research in orthopaedic surgery is to achieve a proper fixation of the implant in the surrounding bone (as a result of bone bonding or bone ingrowth), a mechanical test that actually measures this implant fixation is desired. Various test methods are now available for the mechanical evaluation of retrieved implants. Two tests that have been developed to provide the investigator with absolute numbers for the mechanical fixation of an implant in the surrounding bone are the pushout test and the tensile test. Both tests measure the force that is necessary to move an implant in the surrounding tissue (usually cortical or trabecular bone), and allow the calculation of a so-called pushout or tensile strength. Pushout and tensile tests are simple tests which can easily be performed with limited biomechanical knowledge and low-cost instruments. On the other hand, the ease of use of these tests in experiments on implant fixation does not mean that tests performed by various investigators in various experiments are comparable. When pushout data from various studies are compared (see Table 30.1), a large scatter in data is seen,

TABLE 30.1
Example Overview of Various Studies on Press-Fit-Inserted Implants in Which Pushout Strengths Were Measured

Substrate	Surface Treatment	Surface Texture	Follow-up	Animal	Bone Type	Shear Strength	Ref.
Polyurethane	HA coated	—	4	Rabbit	Cortical	5.9	9
		—	12			8.2	
c.p. Ti	Noncoated	Porous coated	3	Dog	Cortical	7.7	10
			6			12.6	
			12			18.1	
	HA coated		3	Dog	Cortical	7.5	
			6			14.2	
			12			17.9	
c.p. Ti	Noncoated	Bead/grit blasted	3	Dog	Cortical	1.5	11
			6			1.5	
			10			1.0	
			32			1.2	
			3			4.0	
			6			7.0	
			10			7.3	
			32			6.0	
Ti6Al4V	Noncoated	Bead/grit blasted	12	Goat	Cortical	7.4/6.7	12
			26			9.6/7.5	
	HA coated		12	Goat	Cortical	13.3/11.1	
			26			17.3/13.3	
Ti6Al4V	Noncoated	Bead/grit blasted	6	Dog	Cortical		13
			12			49.1	
	HA coated		6	Dog	Cortical	54.8	
			12				
Ti6Al4V	Noncoated	Porous coated	4	Dog	Trabecular	7.0	14
	HA coated		4	Dog	Trabecular	6.7	
c.p.Ti	Noncoated	Macrotexture	3	Dog	Cortical	4.4	15
			5			4.8	
			10			10.5	
	HA coated		3	Dog	Cortical	6.0	
			5			9.6	
			10			14.1	
c.p. Ti	Noncoated	Bead/grit blasted	12	Goat	Cortical	2.9	16
	Ti coated		12	Goat	Cortical	6.9	

The variation in pushout data can most likely not only be explained by differences between implant materials and/or surfaces.

even for identical implant materials. The problem of comparability and reproducibility of a pushout test has been subject to various discussions in the past,[6,7] and in 1989, Black stated that when a pushout test is used, the test conditions need to be described thoroughly.[8]

It is now obvious that pushout and tensile tests are valuable instruments for the study of implant fixation in bone. However, past experience indicates that comparison of results from different investigators is difficult, and that variations in results can most likely not only be attributed to differences in bone bonding ability between implants but also to variations in methods of testing. The present chapter discusses various biomechanical and biological aspects that determine the validity of pushout and tensile testing.

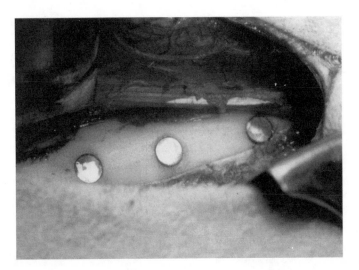

FIGURE 30.1 Photograph of surgical procedure where various cylindrical implants were placed in the diaphyseal femoral cortex of a goat. After a defined healing period, the mechanical fixation of the implants in the cortical bone is measured in a "pushout test."

II. PRACTICAL ASPECTS OF PUSHOUT AND TENSILE TESTING

The design of a pushout test is based upon a cylindrical implant that is placed in cortical or trabecular bone (Figure 30.1). The implant is prepared of the specific material to be tested, and has a certain diameter (usually 2 to 5 mm), length (usually 3 to 7 mm), and surface characteristics (coating and surface topography).

For an extensive description of the practical aspects of the pushout test, see Chapter 29, "Implant Pushout and Pullout Tests." Briefly, the following procedure is used for pushout testing. After surgical placement of the implant in the bone, the wound is closed, with or without suturing the periosteum over the implant top. The implant is then allowed to heal, and after a certain follow-up period, the animal is sacrificed and the bone with the implant(s) *in situ* is excised. By using a diamond saw, specimens are removed from the retrieved bones, taking care not to damage the interface and ensuring adequate bone remains next to the implant. Some authors use only part of an implant–bone specimen by making a cross section,[14,17] but in most studies the entire implant is used in a pushout test. Figure 30.2 shows a schematic drawing of a pushout setup. To prevent disturbance of the test by periosteal or endosteal bone that has grown over the implant top/bottom surface, this tissue should be removed by polishing or grinding. This will also allow for an accurate alignment of the specimen (loaded surface perpendicular to bone–implant interface). The specimen is positioned on a support jig above a hole which is larger than the implant diameter, and pushed out of the surrounding bone by a force that is applied from the opposite side of the implant. The pushout load is applied by a test bench with a constant displacement speed of 0.5 to 1.0 mm/min. The resulting forces are registered by a load cell, and a load–displacement curve is recorded (Figure 30.3). The peak force on the load–displacement curve is considered as the pushout force and is usually the force at which the implant starts to move in the surrounding bone. A pushout test measures the force that is necessary to move the implant in the surrounding bone (ultimate load), and since from a theoretical standpoint this is a shear force, subsequently an interface shear strength is calculated:

$$\sigma = F/A \tag{30.1}$$

where σ is the interface shear strength (Pa), F is the ultimate load (N), and A is the implant surface (mm^2).

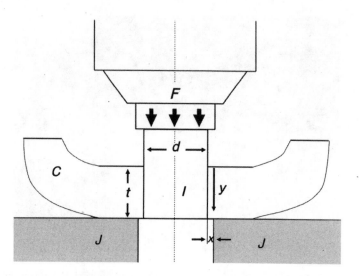

FIGURE 30.2 Schematical drawing of the pushout test. F = force applied on implant; C = cortical bone; J = support jig; y = position along interface; t = cortical thickness; d = implant diameter; x = clearance of hole in support jig.

It is clear from the formula that besides the ultimate load *F* that was measured, the implant surface *A* will determine the pushout strength. Although most scientific reports only mention the pushout strength, it is important to explain how the surface area was measured. The surface area *A* should represent the actual interface area, i.e., only that part of the implant that was fixed in the bone. From a macroscopic point of view, *A* is the part of the implant that is surrounded by bone, but from a microscopic point of view, *A* can also be considered as that part of the implant that is actually in contact with the implant surface. The latter is the percentage of bone–implant contact, and can only be determined by histomorphometry. When transcortical implants are tested, upgrowth of woven or trabecular bone at the endosteal side of the implant has most likely occurred, which will have an unknown influence on the ultimate load (Figure 30.4). It will be technically difficult to remove this endosteal bone without damaging the interface in the cortical zone. Therefore, although this can be subject to dispute, the authors recommend neglecting this endosteal bone and calculate *A* as follows

$$A = \pi d\bar{h}$$

(30.2)

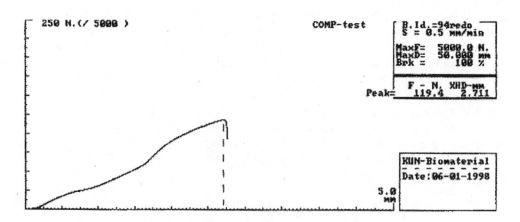

FIGURE 30.3 Example of a load–displacement curve, as registered during a pushout test.

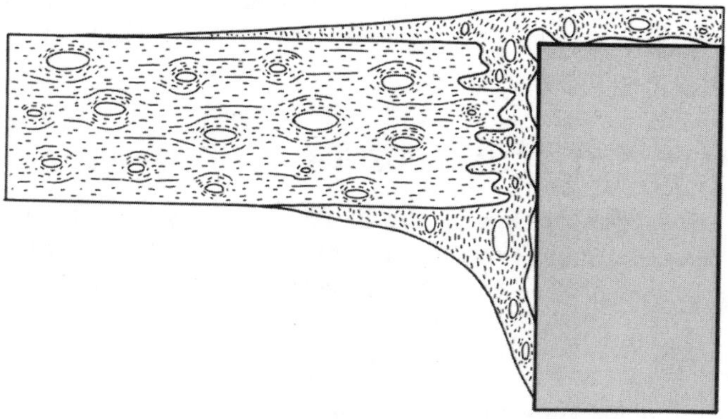

FIGURE 30.4 Graphical representation of a cross section of an implant in cortical bone, after a healing period. At the periosteal side, bone has grown over the implant, and at the endosteal side, upgrowth of woven bone along the implant surface is present. Prior to pushout testing, the periosteal bone should be removed by polishing or grinding.

where d is the implant diameter (mm) and $\bar{h}$ is the average thickness of the cortex (mm), taken from several measurements at distance of the implant, so upgrown bone at the endosteal side is excluded (Figure 30.5).

To measure (predominantly) shear strengths with pushout tests, it was suggested by Steinemann[18] to use a model for tensile testing. A hole is reamed in, but not through, the cortical bone of a test animal, and one end of a cylinder-shaped implant is placed in the hole. The implant can be kept in position by either a spring with screws next to the implant, or by a cerclage wire. A silastic spacer is placed around the implant to prevent upgrowth of bone. Hypothetically, this test has the advantage of measuring only tensile strength, being more reproducible, and allowing for a better alignment during the test. Nevertheless, calculations show that for cylindrical implants the distribution of the tensile stresses along the interface is still not uniform, unless the implant is shaped according to very specific standards.[19,20] Further, previous *in vivo* results have shown that data from this tensile test model do differ with respect to data from a pushout model. It takes, for

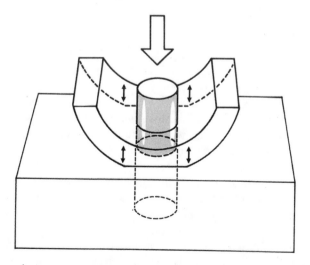

FIGURE 30.5 Schematic drawing of a piece of semicircular cortical bone prior to pushout testing. Arrows indicate the four positions at which the cortical thickness can be measured to calculate the pushout strength.

instance, a considerable follow-up period (>6 weeks in goats) to get a measurable tensile strength.[19,20] Nevertheless, the authors think that the model is very promising for tensile testing of implant fixation.

III. FACTORS AFFECTING PUSHOUT AND TENSILE TESTING

Despite the use of standardized and appropriate pushout and pullout models, the investigator needs to be aware that there are a lot of experimental variables, which can affect the finally measured bone–implant fixation strength. These influences can be test, implant, or biologically dependent.

A. EXPERIMENTAL SETUP

As explained by the formulae in the previous paragraph, pushout strength is calculated as shear force per unit area. From a biomechanical point of view, the use of this formula is justified when actual forces are measured that represent the bone–implant interface, and when these forces are shear forces. By dividing the pushout force by the contact area, local stresses along the interface are "averaged" and no longer recognized. Only for situations where there is an equal distribution of stresses along the interface does the calculated pushout strength also represent local stresses. From a theoretical standpoint, local peak stresses along the interface could initiate interface debonding/local implant loosening, after which the peak stresses move to another point that is still bonded/fixed, and the same process of following local areas of peak stresses is repeated until the implant is entirely loosened. Since these peak stresses are not recognized in a single pushout test, a pushout test setup should pursue an equal distribution of stresses along the interface. To gain insight in these interface stress distributions, several studies calculated interface stress distributions using finite-element models. In a study by Dhert et al.,[21] it was demonstrated that the implant diameter and the cortical thickness did not have much influence, but that the Young's modulus of the implant (see next paragraph) and the clearance of the hole in the support block (Figure 30.6) were of major impact for the interface stress distribution. This clearance is nothing more than the oversize of the hole in the support block as compared with the implant diameter. Several investigators mistakenly believe that the better the fit of the implant in the hole, the more accurate the test will be. Shirazi-Adl[22,23] reported that to get a uniform stress distribution along the interface, the bone surrounding the implant should be supported instead of using a support block under the implant. This will, however, introduce practical difficulties in the execution of the test.

B. IMPLANT PROPERTIES

Implant fixation can be considered as the (im)possibility of motion of an implant in the surrounding bone, and is basically a result of three parameters: friction, mechanical interlock, and chemical bonding. When two surfaces that are completely smooth and flat are tested in shear, the main parameter that will prevent movement is friction. However, when these surfaces are not smooth or have a certain macrotexture, mechanical interlock will be another factor that determines shear movement. In view of this, distinction has to be made between macro- and microtexture. Macrotexture, for example, is provided by screw threads and porous bead-shaped coatings. Microtexture is related to surface dimensions in the order of magnitude of 1 to 40 μm, like that created by grit-blasting procedures. Although macrotextured implants have been subjected to pushout testing,[15] it must be emphasized that pushout tests are not suited to measure the mechanical bone interfacial strength of such implants. Bone ingrowth in the recesses of the macrotexture will prevent a reliable interfacial disruption at the bone–implant interface.

Besides the surface condition of the implant material, specific bulk mechanical properties can affect the pushout or pullout test. As regards material-related mechanical aspects, various classes of implant materials have to be distinguished, e.g., metals, ceramics, and polymers. The modulus

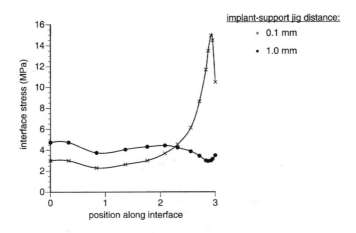

FIGURE 30.6 Interface stress distributions, as calculated with a finite-element analysis, for implant-support jig distances of 0.1 and 1.0 mm (Ti6Al4V implant; implant diameter of 5.0 mm; cortical thickness of 3.0 mm). *Y*-axis represents position along the interface from 0 mm (endosteal side) to 3 mm (periosteal side). The graph demonstrates that a closer fit of the support jig results in high stress peaks at the periosteal side of the implant.

of elasticity of metallic implant materials is in general above that of bone, while the modulus of elasticity of polymers is usually below that of bone. This will result in different patterns of load transfer through the implant, and in differences in implant deformation. Clearly, this can hamper pushout testing. Finite-element studies demonstrated that interface stress distributions are influenced by the Young's modulus of the implants.[21] At lower Young's moduli (e.g., for polymer implants), interface stress distributions become less uniform, and the higher stresses are located at the side from which the load is applied to the implant (Figure 30.7). Ceramics such as hydroxyapatite can give a favorable bone response and these materials are used frequently in mechanical interface tests. However, ceramics have intrinsic mechanical shortcomings,[24] such as a low tensile and bending strength. This low tensile strength limits the use of a tensile test for ceramic materials. Pushout tests are also limited as implant failure during the test can hamper the procedure.

C. BIOLOGICAL PARAMETERS

In addition to mechanical testing, bone contact measurements are used to evaluate how bone tissue responds to an implant surface. They are also supposed to give an indication of implant fixation since it seems logical that implants with a high percentage of bone contact will be firmly fixed into the bone. To investigate a possible relationship with the most common test for implant fixation, the pushout test, the authors plotted corresponding pushout and bone contact data from former studies[12,25] against each other, and this is presented in Figure 30.8. The correlation coefficient for these data was 0.38. Thus the expected high correlation between bone contact and pushout strength was not present in these data. This is very remarkable. Two explanations for this discrepancy can be given: first, the unequal distribution of stresses along the interface during a pushout test[21] already indicates that there cannot be a linear relationship between bone contact and pushout strength. Second, the biomechanical characteristics of the bone tissue in contact with the implant might also vary (e.g., in mineralization, collagen content, etc.), which is confirmed by Corten et al.[26] Bone mineral density measurements using dual X-ray absorptiometry (DEXA) around implants inserted into the lateral and medial femoral condyles of goats revealed that the bone of the medial condyle showed a higher density than the lateral condyle. Bone contact measurements showed that the implants in the medial condyle demonstrated more bone contact compared with similar implants in the lateral condyle. Evidently, this is due to the X-shaped anatomy of the limbs of goats. Moreover, it can be supposed that this higher density will affect the biomechanical evaluation of the bone

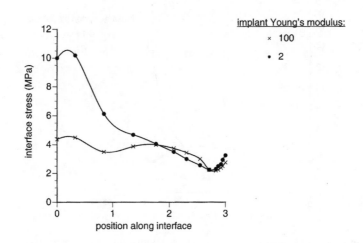

FIGURE 30.7 Interface stress distributions, as calculated with a finite-element analysis, for implants with a Young's modulus comparable to Ti6Al4V ($E = 100$ GPa) and for implants with a low ($E = 2$ GPa) Young's modulus (clearance of hole in support jig of 0.7 mm; implant diameter of 5.0 mm; cortical thickness of 3.0 mm). Y-axis represents position along the interface from 0 mm (endosteal side) to 3 mm (periosteal side). The stress distribution is less uniform for implants with a low Young's modulus, resulting in high local interface stresses at the side of the implant from which the load is applied. This could result in a stepwise implant loosening during the test at relative low loading.

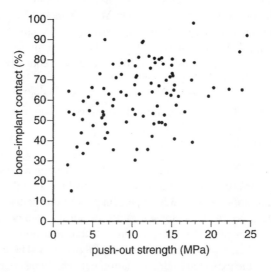

FIGURE 30.8 Scatter plot of pushout strengths as a function of corresponding bone contact measurements of the same implants. Data represent a total of 96 transcortical implants in the femur and humerus of goats, 12 and 25 weeks after implantation. Although there is clearly a trend visible, the actual correlation is only moderate.

response. These findings also prove that care has to be taken of an influence of the biomechanical properties and loading forces of the bone at the implantation site.

A second relevant biological consideration is the "freshness" of the specimens, as used for pushout or pullout studies. Considering the transportation and maintenance of the retrieved samples, an uniform method of preservation has to be recommended. Concerning this storage, the best method is to cool the specimens on ice (0°C) until measurement. However, the samples should never be frozen,[27] nor fixed in formalin[21] prior to testing. With regard to freshness, "fresh" is defined as tested within 4 h after explantation.[6]

IV. FAILURE MODE ANALYSIS

At present, no standard pushout and tensile test methods are available to evaluate the mechanical behavior of the implant–tissue interface. Therefore, it is essential that in publications as much detail as possible is provided about the test conditions.[8,21] With regard to this, besides mechanical testing, data also have to be provided about the mode of failure. Otherwise, a correct interpretation of the measured shear or tensile forces is impossible. The actual mode of failure evaluation can be most simply done by scanning electron microscopy (SEM). Following the mechanical testing, the samples are fixed, dehydrated, and embedded in methylmethacrylate. After polymerization, the specimens are hemisectioned longitudinally through the implant. After polishing the specimens, the failure site resulting from the mechanical testing can be examined with an SEM.

The relevance of a failure mode analysis can be demonstrated with two recent examples. First, Vercaigne et al.[16] inserted three types of titanium plasma-spray-coated implants with a roughness value (Ra) of 16, 21, and 38 μm, respectively, in the tibial cortical bone of goats. Mechanical pushout evaluation was performed 3 months after implantation. As expected, the pushout values showed an increase with increasing surface roughness. On the other hand, failure mode analysis revealed that the fracture line around the roughest implants was located in the bone and not at the bone–implant interface. This phenomenon is explained by the previously mentioned parameter of mechanical interlocking. In the Vercaigne study, the roughest surface provided the strongest mechanical interlock, and thus resulted in the highest pushout value. As shown in Figure 30.9, the pushout test did not measure the actual strength of the bone–implant interface, but the mechanical properties of the bone were the major determining factors. So the measured failure load can be considered only as some kind of general measure of the amount of fixation of the implant in the bone. The second example is dealing with plasma-sprayed hydroxyapatite (HA) coatings. These coatings are applied on titanium implants to improve the poor fatigue properties of HA ceramic with maintenance of the biological advantage.[28] Installation of plasma-sprayed HA-coated implants in the tibial cortex of goats resulted, after 3 months of implantation, in mean pushout strengths of about 15 MPa.[12] However, fracture analysis demonstrated that the fracture site was in some situations located at the coating–titanium interface and not at the coating–bone interface (Figure 30.10). Consequently, the measured data not only represent the bone–implant interface, but also the strength of the substrate–coating fixation.

The two above-mentioned examples clearly demonstrate that under comparable test conditions two completely different mechanical structures were measured (i.e., the mechanical properties of bone itself, and the strength of the coating–titanium interface), and that none of these structures measured the actual bone–implant interface. Of course, this raises doubts about the reliability of a pushout test to measure the strength of bone–implant interface, which concerns the clinical relevance. Therefore, a pushout test should be used to obtain data on implant fixation in a more general context. Subsequent failure analysis should give the user additional information on the actual mode of fixation of the implant. This will put the interpretation of single pushout data and comparison with other studies in perspective.

V. PRACTICAL RECOMMENDATIONS AND CONCLUSIONS

Pushout and tensile testing can be effective in demonstrating differences in the interfacial bonding strength for various types of bone implants. Unfortunately, the simplicity of these methods is associated with an easy inclusion of errors, which affect the accuracy of the finally obtained data. Therefore, it has to be recommended that researchers use a strictly designed protocol for their mechanical tests and mention as much detail as possible.[8,21] It has to be recognized that most pushout tests do not measure the shear strength of the bone–implant interface, but report

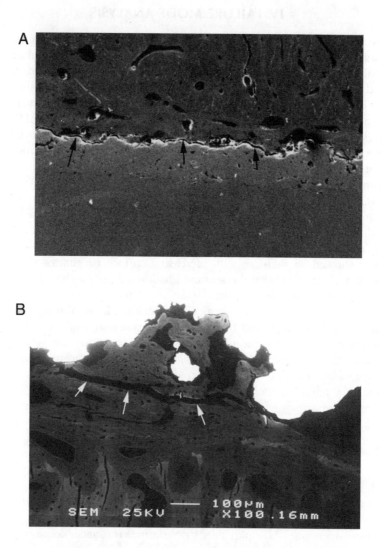

FIGURE 30.9   Example of failure mode analysis after a pushout test for two characteristic implant surfaces: (A) nonmacrotextured surface showing interface failure (arrows) at the bone–coating interface; (B) macro-textured surface showing failure of the bone (arrows) next to the interface.

a value that, although called "pushout strength," is a combination of various fixation principles (friction, mechanical interlock, and chemical bonding). From a clinical perspective, such pushout data still are valuable, since these will provide an indication of how strongly an implant is anchored in the implant bed. However, since so many parameters are of significant influence on the pushout test, extrapolation to other studies is complex and can result in misinterpretation, unless experiments were performed under identical conditions (which will hardly ever happen in practice). Therefore, the authors strongly recommend that investigators design pushout experiments such that comparisons within a single study are possible. A thorough and detailed description of the pushout test should be provided. Still, investigators should recognize that even within one experiment, implant properties, biological parameters, and test conditions may vary and prevent a proper comparison of pushout data. In view of this, to obtain the best possible impression about implant fixation, the authors recommend always combining a mechanical test with histomorphometrical measurements.

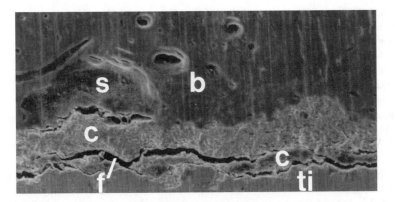

FIGURE 30.10 Example of failure mode analysis after a pushout test of a plasma-sprayed calcium phosphate–coated Ti6Al4V implant. The fracture is visible at the coating–titanium interface. c = coating; b = bone; s = soft tissue; ti = titanium alloy implant; f = fracture as a result of the pushout test.

REFERENCES

1. Zoldos, J. and Kent, J.N., Healing of endosseous implants, in *Endosseous Implants for Maxillofacial Reconstruction*, Block, M.S. and Kent, J.N., Eds., W.B. Saunders, Philadelphia, 1995, 40.
2. Weiss, C.M., Tissue integration of dental endosseous implants: description and comparative analysis of the fibro-osseous integration and osseous integration systems, *J. Oral Implantol.*, 12, 169, 1986.
3. Linder, L., Osseointegration of metallic implants. I. Light microscopy in the rabbit, *Acta Orthop. Scand.*, 60, 129, 1989.
4. Brånemark, P.I., Introduction to osseointegration, in *Tissue Integrated Prostheses, Osseointegration in Clinical Dentistry*, Brånemark, P.I., Zarb, G.A., and T.A., Eds., Quintessence, Chicago, 1985, 11.
5. Cook, S.D., Thomas, K.A., Dalton, J.E., et al., Hydroxylapatite coating of porous implants improves bone ingrowth and interface attachment strength, *J. Biomed. Mater. Res.*, 26, 989, 1992.
6. Groot de, K., Letter to the editor, *J. Biomed. Mater. Res.*, 23, 1367, 1989.
7. Thomas, K. A., Letter to the editor, *J. Biomed. Mater. Res.*, 23, 1367, 1989.
8. Black, J., Pushout tests, *J. Biomed. Mater. Res.*, 23, 1243, 1989.
9. Boone, P.S., Zimmerman, M.C., Gutteling, E., et al., Bone attachment to hydroxyapatite coated polymers, *J. Biomed. Mater. Res.*, 23, 183, 1989.
10. Cook, S.D., Thomas, K.A., Kay, J.F., and Jarcho, M., Hydroxyapatite-coated porous titanium for use as an orthopedic biologic attachment system, *Clin. Orthop.*, 303, 1988.
11. Cook, S.D., Thomas, K.A., Kay, J.F., and Jarcho, M., Hydroxyapatite-coated titanium for orthopedic implant applications, *Clin. Orthop.*, 225, 1988.
12. Dhert, W.J., Klein, C.P., Wolke, J.G., et al., A mechanical investigation of fluorapatite, magnesium-whitlockite, and hydroxylapatite plasma-sprayed coatings in goats, *J. Biomed. Mater. Res.*, 25, 1183, 1991.
13. Geesink, R.G., de Groot, K., and Klein, C.P., Chemical implant fixation using hydroxyl-apatite coatings. The development of a human total hip prosthesis for chemical fixation to bone using hydroxyl-apatite coatings on titanium substrates, *Clin. Orthop.*, 147, 1987.
14. Soballe, K., Hansen, E.S., Brockstedt-Rasmussen, H., et al., Hydroxyapatite coating enhances fixation of porous coated implants. A comparison in dogs between press fit and noninterference fit, *Acta Orthop. Scand.*, 61, 299, 1990.
15. Thomas, K.A., Kay, J.F., Cook, S.D., and Jarcho, M., The effect of surface macrotexture and hydroxylapatite coating on the mechanical strengths and histologic profiles of titanium implant materials, *J. Biomed. Mater. Res.*, 21, 1395, 1987.
16. Vercaigne, S., Wolke, J.G., Naert, I., and Jansen, J.A., Histomorphometrical and mechanical evaluation of titanium plasma-spray-coated implants placed in the cortical bone of goats, *J. Biomed. Mater. Res.*, 41, 41, 1998.

17. Soballe, K., Hansen, E.S., Brockstedt-Rasmussen, H., et al., Bone graft incorporation around titanium-alloy- and hydroxyapatite-coated implants in dogs, *Clin. Orthop.*, 282, 1992.

18. Steinemann, S.G., Eulenberger, J., Maeusli, P.A., and Schroeder, A., Adhesion of bone to titanium, in *Biological and Biomechanical Performance of Biomaterials. Advances in Biomaterials*, Christel, P., Meunier, A., and Lee, A.J., Eds., Elsevier Science Publishers, Amsterdam, 1986,

19. Brunski, J.B., Elias, J., Edwards, J.T., et al., Tensile bonding at bone–biomaterial interfaces. An *in vivo* test and related finite stress analysis, *Trans. Soc. Biomater.*, 17, 15, 1991.

20. Kangasniemi, I., Development of Calcium Phosphate Ceramic Containing Bioactive Glass Composites, Thesis — Biomaterials, University of Leiden, the Netherlands, 1993.

21. Dhert, W.J., Verheyen, C.C., Braak, L.H., et al., A finite element analysis of the pushout test: influence of test conditions, *J. Biomed. Mater. Res.*, 26, 119, 1992.

22. Shirazi-Adl, A., Finite element stress analysis of a pushout test. Part 1: Fixed interface using stress compatible elements, *J. Biomech. Eng.*, 114, 111, 1992.

23. Shirazi-Adl, A. and Forcione, A., Finite element stress analysis of a pushout test. Part II: Free interface with nonlinear friction properties, *J. Biomech. Eng.*, 114, 155, 1992.

24. Aoki, H., *Science and Medical Applications of Hydroxyapatite*, Takajima Press System Center Co., Tokyo, 1991,

25. Dhert, W.J., Klein, C.P., Jansen, J.A., et al., A histological and histomorphometrical investigation of fluorapatite, magnesiumwhitlockite, and hydroxylapatite plasma-sprayed coatings in goats, *J. Biomed. Mater. Res.*, 27, 127, 1993.

26. Corten, F.G., Caulier, H., van der Waerden, J.P., et al., Assessment of bone surrounding implants in goats: *ex vivo* measurements by dual X-ray absorptiometry, *Biomaterials*, 18, 495, 1997.

27. Thomas, K.A., Cook, S.D., Dalton, J.E., and Baffes, G.C., Effects of storage upon interface attachment characteristics: testing of fresh vs. frozen samples, *Trans. Soc. Biomater.*, 16, 251, 1990.

28. Groot de, K., Geesink, R., Klein, C.P., and Serekian, P., Plasma sprayed coatings of hydroxylapatite, *J. Biomed. Mater. Res.*, 21, 1375, 1987.

31 Tensile Testing of Bone–Implant Interface

Takashi Nakamura and Shigeru Nishiguchi

CONTENTS

I. INTRODUCTION

Tests of interfacial bonding strength have been pursued using a variety of test methods, implant geometries, and surface configurations. One type of test is a torque test, frequently involving screw-shaped implants in the rabbit tibia or femur.[1] Another type of interfacial test is a pushout or shear test. In the typical form of this test, cylindrical implants are placed through the cortex of a long bone, such as the femur of a dog, and then pushed out following animal sacrifice.[2]

Besides torque and pushout tests, another method for investigating interfacial strength is the tensile test, in which loads are applied in a direction normal to the tissue–biomaterial interface. It is considered that in the tensile test, the strength of a direct biochemical bonding between the bone and the biomaterial can be measured, thereby eliminating the resistive force due to surface roughness of the biomaterial.[3] However, among various tensile testing methods, there is no standard method in widespread use at the present time.

This chapter describes in detail the tensile testing method the authors have developed,[3] discussing its advantages and one disadvantage. The methods are compared to the tensile test methods used by other research groups.

II. TENSILE TEST METHOD (NAKAMURA'S METHOD)

A. IMPLANTATION

The biomaterial to be tested is shaped into a rectangular plate, of size $15 \times 10 \times 2$ mm. A rabbit is anesthetized by intravenous injection of sodium pentobarbital (50 mg/kg). The operation is performed under standard aseptic conditions with local administration of 0.25% xylocaine. For

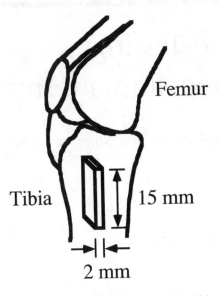

FIGURE 31.1 Implantation method: implant is inserted into rabbit tibia from medial side through both medial and lateral cortices parallel to the frontal plane of the tibia. The plate protrudes from both cortices.

implantation of the implant into the proximal tibial condyle, a 3-cm skin incision is made on the anteromedial aspect of the tibial metaphysis of the rabbit, and the skin, muscle, and periosteum are retracted. By using a dental burr and saline coolant, a hole (15 × 2 mm) is made parallel to the longitudinal axis of the tibial metaphysis with the proximal end located 5 mm distal to the joint. The medial cortex is drilled as slowly as possible so that the heat generated does not damage the remaining bone. At this stage, care is taken to ensure that the hole for the implant is kept parallel to the frontal plane of the tibia. After making the hole, a test insertion of the implant into the hole is attempted. If the implant cannot be inserted, the hole is enlarged little by little.

When the preparation of the hole in the medial cortex is complete, the hole in the tibial metaphysis for implantation is extended from the medial cortex to the lateral cortex. After the medial cortex has been penetrated, the dental burr immediately reaches the inner side of the lateral cortex because of the scant amount of cancellous bone in the proximal tibial metaphysis. Since the lateral cortex cannot be visualized directly due to constant bleeding from the medullary cavity of the tibia, careful cutting is required at this stage. Once again, care is taken to ensure that the hole in the lateral cortex is kept parallel to the frontal plane of the tibia. The lateral hole is enlarged step by step and it is confirmed whether the implant can be inserted into the tibia through both medial and lateral cortices. The hole is irrigated with saline before the plate is implanted in the frontal plane, perforating the tibia and protruding from both tibial cortices (Figure 31.1). The muscle and skin are closed in layers.

B. Sample Preparation

The rabbit is killed at a given postimplantation time. A segment of the tibia containing the implant is excised (Figure 31.2a) and the bone is sectioned transversely with a disk cutter by parallel cuts 2 mm above and below each end of the plate (Figure 31.2b). The bony tissues located on the lateral sides of the plate are removed with a dental burr. Cuts of the same width as those of the implants are made with a dental burr, extending from both ends of the bone tissue to the ends of the implant (Figure 31.2c). After such sectioning, the bony segments on either side of the implant are not directly connected but are now joined only through the intervening implant. Extreme care is taken to remove the bone completely from the sides of the implant and to keep the bones and implant moist throughout the dissection and subsequent testing.

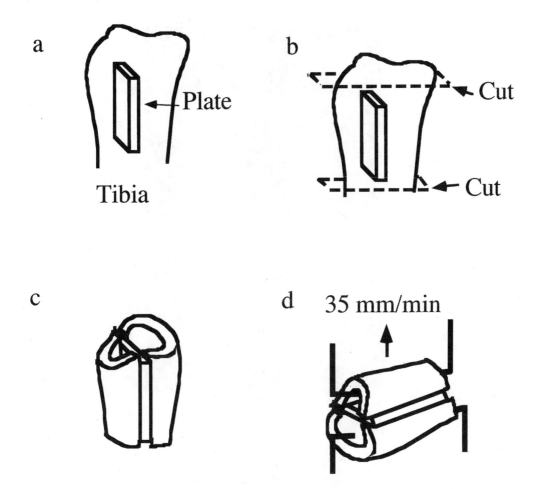

FIGURE 31.2 Schematic drawing of preparation of tensile specimen. (a) Retrieve the proximal tibia containing the implant. (b) Cut the tibia at 2 mm proximal and distal at the end of the plate. (c) Remove bone connecting anterior and posterior cortices. (d) Apply tensile load through hooks holding anterior and posterior cortices until the bone is detached from the plate.

C. Measurement of Tensile Failure Load

Each segment is held by a hook that is connected to an Instron-type testing machine (either Autograph Model S-500, Shimadzu Seisakujo Ltd., Kyoto, Japan, or Model 1011, Aikoh Engineering Co. Ltd., Nagoya, Japan; Figures 31.2d and 31.3). The plate is placed horizontally and pulled in opposite directions at a crosshead speed of 3.5 cm/min. The load at which an implant is detached from the bone or at which the bone is broken is designated as "failure load." In the authors' study, the pressure or tensile stress cannot be calculated because the true contact area cannot be measured adequately by X-ray or light microscopic techniques. Thus, the results of this method are shown by a unit of force, such as kgf or N, not by a unit of stress, such as MPa.

D. Advantages and Disadvantages

This method possesses four advantages. First, the detachment test is simple and easy to perform and quite reproducible. On account of the relatively low invasive nature of the surgical procedure, this test method can be performed on both tibias. Second, since the shape of the biomaterial to be tested is rectangular ($15 \times 10 \times 2$ mm), it is relatively easy to prepare the material for implantation

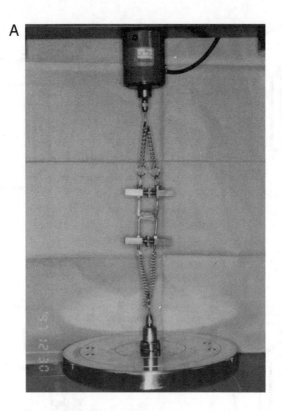

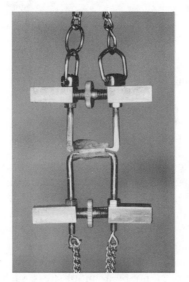

FIGURE 31.3 Photographs of detaching test. (A) Overall configuration. (B) Close-up of the hooks and the bone.

and testing. Third, the implant has two bone–implant interfaces, only one of which is broken after a single tensile test. Thus, on the remaining bone–implant interface, one can either perform a second tensile test or carry out a histological examination. Finally, this tensile test has been performed since 1985, mainly at the authors' institute, in order to evaluate the bone-bonding abilities of many different kinds of biomaterials. The accumulated results are quite useful for comparing the bone-bonding

TABLE 31.1
Bone-Bonding Strength of Biomaterials Using the Nakamura's Tensile Test Method (mean value)

	4 weeks, kgf	8 weeks, kgf	10 weeks, N	16 weeks, kgf	25 weeks
AW-glass ceramic (AW-GC)[3]		7.43			8.15 kgf
Dense hydroxyapatite[3]		6.28			7.90 kgf
45S5 Bioglass[3]		2.75			
Alumina[3]		0.13			
β-Calcium phosphate[5]			31.65		47.04 N
β-Tricalcium phosphate (TCP)[5]			72.81		71.34 N
Tetracalcium phosphate[5]			43.22		62.03 N
Ti6Al4V[7]	0.0014	0.029		0.334	2.852 kgf
Bioglass-coated Ti6Al4V[7]		1.04		2.72	
AW-coated Ti6Al4V[7]		2.03		2.39	
TCP-coated Ti6Al4V[7]		3.91		4.23	
Alkali- and heat-treated Ti[6]		2.71		4.13	
Pure titanium[6]		0.02		0.33	
Demineralized bone powder + AW-GC[4]	7.21	9.00			11.91 kgf
PMMA cement[8]			0.29		0.2 N
Bioactive bone cement					
(bis-GMA) + (MgO-CaO-SiO$_2$-P$_2$O$_5$-CaF$_2$) glass powder[8]			29.52		33.42 N
(bis-GMA) + (MgO-CaO-SiO$_2$-P$_2$O$_5$-CaF$_2$) glass ceramic powder[8]			41.48		41.27 N
(bis-GMA) + (MgO free CaO-SiO$_2$-P$_2$O$_5$-CaF$_2$) glass powder[8]			28.22		33.64 N

strengths of different biomaterials. One can better estimate the bone-bonding ability of a new material by comparing its performance with the results obtained from preexisting biomaterials.

On the other hand, this tensile test method has one disadvantage; the force intensity or tensile stress cannot be calculated because the true contact area cannot be measured easily.

E. Previous Results Using the Detachment Test

As mentioned previously, since 1985, when Nakamura et al. developed this testing method, several different researchers at Kyoto University have carried out this test in order to evaluate the bone-bonding strength of different biomaterials, such as bioactive ceramics,[3,4,5] bioinert ceramics,[3] titanium,[6,7] bioactive cements,[8] and titanium coated with bioactive materials.[7] These results are summarized in Table 31.1. Since the tensile tests in these studies are based completely upon the detachment test method of Nakamura, the results can be compared directly with each other.

F. A Second Type of Tensile Test

Yoshii et al.[9] examined the bonding strength of A-W glass ceramic to the surface of bone cortex. They used semicolumnar-shaped blocks (4 × 10 × 8 mm) with holes 2 mm in diameter at their centers (Figure 31.4), made of A-W glass ceramic and fixed with screws on the surface of the tibias of rabbits. The tensile load required to detach the implant from the surface of the bone cortex was measured at 2, 4, 8, and 25 weeks after the implantation.

Mature male rabbits each weighing 3.0 to 3.5 kg were anesthetized with sodium pentobarbital (50 mg/kg). The operations were performed under aseptic conditions. A skin incision (2 cm long) was made on the anteromedial aspect of the proximal tibial metaphysis of the rabbit. The cortex of the tibia was exposed subperiosteally about 10 × 10 mm. A hole 1.8 mm in diameter was made with a drill at the center of the exposed cortex, penetrating into the posterior cortex. The implant

a.   b.

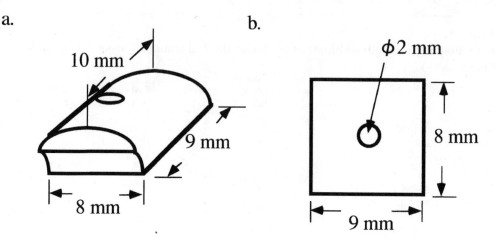

FIGURE 31.4   Implant. (a) Schema of the implant. (b) The base of the implant (approximately 70 mm²).

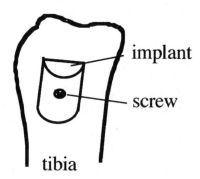

FIGURE 31.5   The method of fixation of the implant to the surface of the medial cortex of the tibia with a screw.

was placed on the flat surface of the medial cortex and fixed with a stainless steel screw 2 mm in diameter (Figure 31.5). The screw was driven securely into the drilled hole through the hole in the implant. The wound was cooled and cleaned with sterile saline solution during the operation, before being closed in layers.

At 2, 4, 8, and 25 weeks after implantation, the tibia was excised with the implant and sectioned transversely 3 mm proximal and distal to the implant. The bony tissue that had grown over the margins of the implant was removed completely in order to prepare the implant so that it was in contact with bone only at its base. The screw was removed gently.

The implant and the piece of bone were held by the use of hooks. The hooks were connected to an Instron-type tensile load tester (Autograph S-500, Shimadzu, Kyoto, Japan). The implant was pulled perpendicularly to the base of the implant contacting the bony cortex (Figure 31.6). The crosshead speed was set at 3.5 cm/min. The load required to detach the implant from the bone, or to break the bone, was measured. In this type of tensile test, the bonding area between bone and implant is the same as the area of implant surface. Thus, the tensile strength can be calculated if necessary, by dividing tensile force by implant surface area.

III. OTHER TENSILE TESTS

Lin et al.[10] carried out another type of tensile strength testing in order to evaluate bonding strength between bone and a plasma-sprayed, hydroxyapatite (HA)-coated titanium and titanium alloy. Their implant had a semicircular shape, 5.5 mm in diameter and 2.2 mm thick. Both sides of the implant

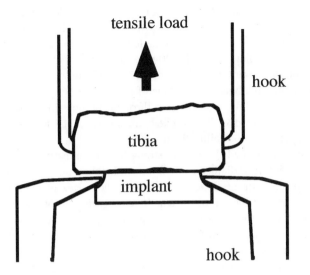

FIGURE 31.6 Tensile interface testing method. The implant and the piece of bone were held with hooks. The bone was pulled perpendicularly to the surface of the implant.

had a thin layer of plasma-sprayed HA coating. They used male Japanese white rabbits. About 2 cm below the knee, a 2.2-mm-long semicircular piece of the diaphyseal cortex was removed, using a parallel dental disk cutter and a dental burr under saline coolant. The implant was placed into this defect using light thumb pressure. After sacrifice, the left tibia was removed and sectioned into 3-cm-long segments with the implant in the middle. The extra bony tissue surrounding the implant was carefully removed using a dental burr, so that only the distal and proximal sides of the bone contacted the implant. A 1-mm hole was made in both of the bone segments, and ligatures were attached and fixed in the clamps of a Universal test machine (Autograph, DCS-5000, Shimadzu, Kyoto, Japan). A pulling force was applied to the bone–implant segment in a direction perpendicular to the bone–implant interfaces, with cross-head speed set at 2.5 mm/min. The load that broke the bone–implant interface was automatically recorded.

To calculate the bone–implant interfacial area, the bony side of the sample was measured after tensile fracture by means of image analysis. The whole bony surface that contacted the implant was used as the interfacial area. The tensile strength was determined by dividing the load obtained during testing by the interfacial area.

The advantages of the testing method used by Lin et al.[11] are that tensile testing can be performed twice with one sample and, because the bonding area between bone and implant can be determined using an image analysis system, the true tensile strength can be obtained.

The disadvantages of their tensile testing method are that a small implant of complicated shape has to be employed. In addition, the operative procedure is difficult to perform and a precise preparation of the bony recess is necessary in order to obtain an optimal fit between bone and the implant. Furthermore, this method has not been used in any other study and therefore lacks the accumulated data from the results on other biomaterials using the one method. Another concern about their method is whether the contact area between the bone and the plate can be determined exactly.

Previously, Lin et al.[11] evaluated the tensile strength of the interface between hydroxyapatite and bone using a rabbit tibia model. However, in that study, they used an implant of yet another geometry, namely, a 3-mm-long semicylindrical shape (U-shape).

Several other research groups have developed their own tensile testing methods. Steinemann et al.[12] performed tensile testing to evaluate the bond strength between bone and titanium implants of different surface roughness. They placed disk-shaped implants on the flattened surface of the monkey ulna and held the implants in place with a spring. Tensile testing was performed 3 to 7 months after implantation. The load was applied with a crosshead displacement speed of 1 mm/min.

Edwards et al.[13] also carried out a study on the tensile strength of the bone–HA interface. They used HA disks (5.25 mm in diameter and 2.30 mm thick) and fixed these disks on the flattened surface of the cortex of the rabbit femur. An additional small bony plate was used to stabilize each test specimen in position on the bone. At the time of testing, the bony plate was removed. A tensile load was applied through a stainless steel cable through the hole in the top of the Ti6Al4V part that had been bonded to the HA disk. The stroke control was set at 1 mm/min and the greatest load during the test was reported as the failure load.

Kangasniemi et al.[14] examined the tensile strength of fluorapatite and coatings sprayed with HA-plasma. A cylinder 5 mm in diameter and 3 mm in height was coated with bioactive material. The cylinder was implanted on the flattened surface of the cortex of the femur of goats and was fixed with wire bound around the femur. In tensile testing, the pulloff wires were attached to the implant, and the whole system was placed in the support jig with wires downward so that the bone could be left resting freely during testing. A crosshead speed of 0.1 mm/min was used in the Hounsfield testing apparatus.

As reviewed above, all these tensile testing methods are characterized by differences in experimental animals, implantation sites, surgical techniques, implant-fixation methods, testing machines, and crosshead speeds. Furthermore, most testing methods were used in one study only, and the results cannot be compared easily with other studies.

IV. CONCLUSION

In recent years, several tensile testing methods have been developed to evaluate the bonding strength between bone and biomaterials. However, a standardized method, with respect to choice of animal, implantation site, surgical technique, method of implant fixation, testing device, and crosshead speed has not yet been established. In order to evaluate the bonding abilities of biomaterials and to compare the bonding strengths of biomaterials with each other, it is desirable to establish a standard method of tensile testing as soon as possible. The testing method described is simple to perform. The method has the additional advantage that it has already been used to accumulate significant amounts of data on many different kinds of biomaterials. The authors believe that it is an appropriate method of choice for tensile testing of biomaterials.

REFERENCES

1. Johansson, C. and Albrektsson, T., Integration of screw implants in rabbit: a 1-year follow-up of removal torques of Ti implants, *Int. J. Oral Maxillofac. Implants*, 2, 69, 1987.
2. Cook, S.D., Thomas, K.A., Kay, J.F., and Jarcho, M., Hydroxyapatite-coated titanium for orthopedic implant application., *Clin. Orthop.*, 232, 225, 1988.
3. Nakamura, T., Yamarumo, T., Higashi, S., et al., A new glass-ceramic for bone replacements: evaluation of its bonding ability to bone tissue, *J. Biomed. Mater. Res.*, 23, 631, 1985.
4. Kotani, S., Yamamuro, T., Nakamura, T., et al., Enhancement of bone bonding to bioactive ceramics by demineralized bone powder, *Clin. Orthop.*, 278, 1311, 1992.
5. Kitsugi, T., Nakamura, T., Oka, M., et al., Bone-bonding behavior of plasma-sprayed coatings of Bioglass, AW-glass ceramic, and tricalcium phosphate on titanium alloy, *J. Biomed. Mater. Res.*, 30, 261, 1996.
6. Nishiguchi, S., Nakamura, T., Kobayashi, M., et al., Effect of heat treatment on bone bonding ability of heat-treated titanium, *Biomaterials*, 29, 491, 1999.
7. Takatsuka, K., Yamamuro, T., Nakamura, T., and Kokubo, T., Bone-bonding behavior of titanium alloy evaluated mechanically with detaching failure load, *J. Biomed. Mater. Res.*, 29, 157, 1995.

8. Tamura, J., Kitsugi,T., Iida, H., et al., Bone bonding ability of bioactive bone cements, *Clin. Orthop.*, 343, 183, 1997.

9. Yoshii, S., Kakutani,Y., Yamamuro, T., et al., Strength of bonding between A-W glass-ceramic and the surface of bone cortex, *J. Biomed. Mater. Res.*, 22(3 Suppl.), 327, 1988.

10. Lin, H., Xu, H., and de Groot, K., Tensile strength of the interface between hydroxyapatite and bone, *J. Biomed. Mater. Res.*, 26, 7, 1992.

11. Lin,H., Xu, H., Zhang, X., and de Groot, K., Tensile tests of interface between bone and plasma-sprayed HA coating-titanium implant, *J. Biomed. Mater. Res.*, 43, 113, 1998.

12. Steinemann, S.G., Eulenberger, J., Maeusli, P.A., and Schroeder, A., Adhesion of bone to titanium, in *Biological and Biomechanical Performance of Biomaterials*, Christel, P., Meunier, A., and Lee, A.J., Eds., Elsevier Science, Amsterdam, 1986.

13. Edwards, J.T., Brunski, J.B., and Higuchi, H.W., Mechanical and morphologic investigation of the tensile strength of a bone-hydroxyapatite interface, *J. Biomed. Mater. Res.*, 36, 454, 1997.

14. Kangasniemi, I.M., Verheyen, C.C., Velde, E.A., and de Groot, K., *In vivo* tensile testing of fluorapatite and hydroxyapatite plasma-sprayed coatings, *J. Biomed. Mater. Res.*, 28, 563, 1994.

32 Fracture Toughness Tests of the Bone–Implant Interface

Xiaodu Wang, Kyriacos A. Athanasiou, and C. Mauli Agrawal

CONTENTS

I. INTRODUCTION

Interfacial strength between bone and implants is critical to the success of both orthopaedic and dental implant systems. To evaluate an implant system, it is imperative for researchers to assess the intrinsic interfacial strength between bone and implant. Currently, there are no standardized test techniques. However, some interfacial fracture toughness tests have been developed and are used in orthopaedic and dental research. This chapter presents three relatively well-defined interfacial fracture toughness test specimens: compact sandwich specimen, mixed mode specimen, and short-bar or short-rod specimen.

Interfacial debonding between tissue and implant surfaces is a major reason for failure of both orthopaedic and dental implant systems. The mechanical strength of bone–implant interfaces not only has a direct impact on short-term success, but also influences long-term stability of the prosthesis.[9,15] There are many variables that influence the mechanical integrity of the interface such

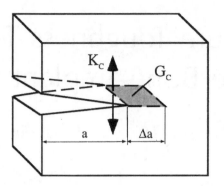

FIGURE 32.1 A conceptual diagram showing definitions of the fracture toughness parameters. K_C is the critical stress intensity factor, and G_C is the critical strain energy release rate.

as interfacial bonding, the intrinsic properties of implanted materials and surrounding tissues, and structural characteristics and external loading modes. For instance, porous surfaces and bioactive materials have been proved to be beneficial for the stability of implant systems due to enhanced interfacial bonding between implant and bone tissue. On the other hand, wear debris from the articulating surfaces of total joint prostheses can induce bone loss (osteolysis) around the implant and consequently lead to loosening of the prosthesis. Furthermore, high-cycle, low-magnitude loading may cause a combination of fatigue failures at the interface, in the implant, and in the surrounding bone tissues. To understand fully the implications of all these variables on the intrinsic fracture properties of the interface, it is imperative that a suitably reliable and accurate mechanical test be developed.

Over the years, the "pushout" test has been commonly used for evaluating the interface[1,5,6,15] because it is straightforward and simple. Use of simple tensile tests also has been suggested by some researchers.[9,10,16] From an engineering perspective, both pushout and tensile tests are akin to structural tests, which yield the nominal strength of interfaces, but not the intrinsic interfacial strength. In recent years, fracture mechanics approaches have drawn an interest in testing interfacial bonding of biological systems. Because fracture mechanics estimates the interfacial strength in terms of the energy or stress intensity required to propagate an interfacial crack along the interface,[6,7,13] this critical energy or stress intensity may be a fundamental and meaningful measure of the intrinsic fracture properties of the interface. There are two major parameters commonly used to assess the fracture toughness: critical stress intensity factor, K_C, and critical energy release rate (driving force), G_C. Figure 32.1 shows a schematic representation of these parameters. K_C defines the magnitude of stress at the crack tip from where the crack starts to propagate, while G_C gives a measure of energy which is needed to create new fracture surfaces concomitant with an initial crack extension (Δa). As illustrated in Figure 32.2, there are three modes of loading that a crack can experience. In Mode I loading, the principal load is applied normal to the crack plane; since the crack tends to open under such loading, this type of loading is also known as the opening mode. Mode II is characterized by the sliding of one crack face against the other in the direction of crack propagation, and so it is regarded as the shearing mode. Mode III refers to a twisting mode because the shear load is applied in a direction normal to the crack propagation direction. In reality, an interfacial crack can be loaded in any of these modes, or a combination of two or three of them. In general, a crack tends to propagate along the path of least resistance, which is not necessarily confined to its initial plane. However, in the case of interfacial fractures of bone–implant interfaces, crack propagation commonly occurs at the interfaces.

There are no standard interfacial fracture toughness tests for biological systems. Among the techniques that have been developed thus far, "sandwich" (Figure 32.3) and the short-rod or short-bar (Figure 32.4) specimens are relatively well defined. The short-rod or short-bar specimen has been widely used in dental biomaterials research,[6,8,12] while the sandwich specimen was developed

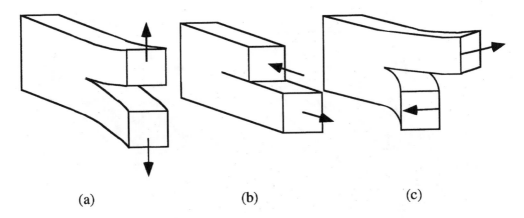

FIGURE 32.2   Three loading modes that a crack can experience: (a) opening mode (tension); (b) shear mode; and (c) tear mode.

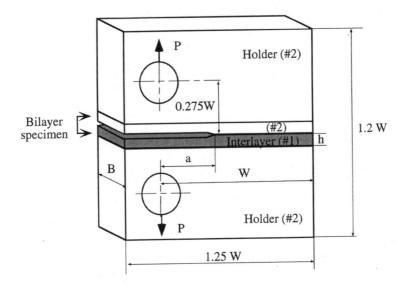

FIGURE 32.3   A schematic representation of the compact sandwich specimen. This specimen shares a similar overall configuration with the standard compact tension specimen, but has a bilayer specimen sandwiched between two holders. The holder material must be the same, or similar to one of the layers of the bilayer specimen.

for biological systems in general.[18,19] The distinguishing feature of these specimens is that a layer of one material is sandwiched between two layers of another material with a precrack lying at one of the two interfaces. In fact, these specimens were originally developed for testing adhesive joints and interfacial bonding strength of composite laminates. These techniques have been adapted to testing the interfacial bonding strength between bone and implant.

It should be borne in mind that these fracture toughness tests have their own limitations, because they are developed mainly based on linear elastic fracture mechanics. First of all, these tests are not suitable for testing material systems with large plastic deformation, although some corrections can be made to take into account small-scale plastic deformation at the vicinity of the crack tip. Second, these tests cannot be used to assess time-dependent fracture behavior. If viscoelastic materials are involved in the material system, a slow and constant loading speed is recommended for these tests. Third, these tests can be used only for those interfaces that are formed between

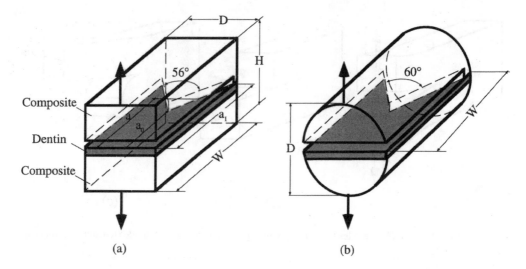

FIGURE 32.4 Schematic diagrams of the short bar (a) and short rod (b) specimens used for testing dentin–dental composite interfaces. A chevron notch is made at the interface between dentin and the biomaterial tested.

relatively smooth surfaces; otherwise, most assumptions on which the techniques are derived become invalid. Finally, these tests require relatively rigorous specimen preparation procedures, such that well-developed skills and hands-on experience are needed to ensure the accuracy of these tests.

II. COMPACT SANDWICH FRACTURE TOUGHNESS TEST

The compact sandwich specimen is designed to measure interfacial fracture toughness under an opening mode (Mode I, tension). Except for the interlayer (see Figure 32.3), this specimen is similar to a homogeneous compact tension specimen described in ASTM standard E399-90.[2]

A. Specimen Preparation

A compact sandwich specimen consists of two components: a bilayer specimen and two holders (see Figure 32.3). The bilayer component comprises the interface between bone and a biomaterial of interest. As far as the overall geometry is concerned, the proportions and tolerances of the specimen follow those recommended by the ASTM standard for compact tension specimens.[2] This technique requires that the holder material be the same as or similar to either the bone or the biomaterial in the bilayer component. As shown in Figure 32.3, the layer in the bilayer which has material properties different from the holders is defined as the interlayer.

The interface can be formed either *in vivo* or *in vitro* depending on the purpose of one's study. Figure 32.5 shows an example of preparing *in vivo* formed bilayer specimens.[1] A coupon made of the test biomaterial had dimensions of $20 \times 3.5 \times 2$ mm. This specimen was implanted with one surface fixed flush against a defect made on the proximal tibia of a rabbit. Briefly, the rabbit was anesthetized and the incision region was shaved and sterilized. In order to ensure a consistent surgical outcome, a custom-designed fixture was utilized to create the defect. The leg was then secured to the fixture, draped, and a longitudinal incision was made just below the tibial tuberosity to expose the subperiosteal surface of the medial aspect of the proximal tibia (Figure 32.5). Then, a shallow, trough-shaped groove (about 0.2 mm deep) was created on the subperiosteal surface of the tibia using a 4-mm carbide router. Finally, the implant was secured in the groove using sutures with the surface of interest against the defect in the bone. The incision was closed in a routine fashion. In order to facilitate initiation of the precrack at the bone–implant interface, one third of

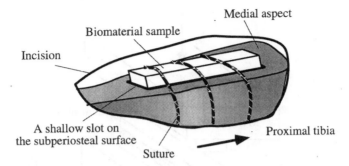

FIGURE 32.5   An example showing the preparation of an *in vivo* formed bilayer specimen. An implant was placed against a shallow slot previously made on the medial subperiosteal surface of the proximal tibia in a rabbit. Sutures were used to secure the implant in position.

the surface of these implants were covered with a thin layer of bone wax (Ethicon Inc., Somerville, NJ) so as to prevent bone ingrowth from occurring. At sacrifice, the implant was excised with the bone tissue attached. All extra tissue was carefully removed using a diamond circular saw and a bench-top milling machine to form a rectangular bilayer specimen. Extra precautions were taken during the specimen preparation to avoid damage to the bone–implant interface. The bilayer specimen was cemented between the two holders using a cyanoacrylate adhesive to form the compact sandwich specimen.[19] The overall dimensions of the specimen were $20 \times 19 \times 3.5$ mm. The holder was made of bovine femur to ensure that no significant differences in elastic properties would occur between the holders and the bony layer of bilayer specimens; such differences would violate the assumptions on which this technique is based and consequently affect accuracy of the test. In this case, the interlayer was the biomaterial to be tested.

The next example considers a bilayer specimen consisting of an *in vitro*–formed bone-to-bone cement interface (Figure 32.6).[19] In this test, the interfacial strength of bone-to-bone cement was tested. Bone coupons were obtained from a bovine femur and machined to final dimensions of $21.9 \times 3.5 \times 2.0$ mm. To prepare the bone cement, liquid monomer and polymer powder were mixed at room temperature ($23°C$) following the manufacturer's instruction. The cement was then poured on the top of the bone coupon which was placed in the base of a mold (see Figure 32.6). Pressure was applied uniformly through the mold cap for approximately 20 min. Because it is difficult to obtain very accurate specimen dimensions from the molding process, the bilayer specimens were initially made larger than the required size and machined to the final desired dimensions. The bilayer was carefully cemented between two PMMA (polymethylmethacrylate) holders using a cyanoacrylate adhesive (Quicktite™, Loctite Corp.). Any extra adhesive on either side of the specimen was polished off using fine sandpaper. A starter notch was cut at the interface using a circular saw with a 0.5-mm-thick blade, then a precrack was introduced at the tip of the notch using a sharp razor blade. In this case, the interlayer material was bone.

Several precautions need to be taken to ensure testing success. First, the elastic properties (i.e., elastic modulus and Poisson's ratio) of the holder must be the same as or similar to the bone specimens or biomaterial to be tested, as the governing equations are derived based on this assumption. Second, the accuracy of specimen shape and size is critical to the results obtained using the compact sandwich specimen because the results are very sensitive to these parameters. Finally, extreme care has to be taken during specimen preparation to avoid damaging the interface of interest.

B. TEST PROCEDURE

Precaution needs to be taken while mounting the compact sandwich specimen in a material testing machine not to prestress the interface. The specimen is loaded until failure of the interface. Clevises (U-shaped fixtures) are needed to facilitate loading of the compact sandwich specimens. The design

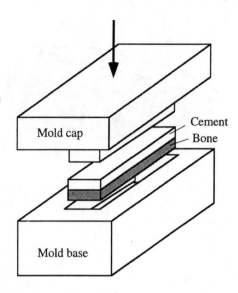

FIGURE 32.6 An example of preparing bone-to-bone cement bilayer specimen. Bone cement was press molded onto a bone coupon to form a bilayer specimen in a mold.

of the clevises is outlined in ASTM standard E399-90.[2] A water-soluble dye can be used at the crack tip to facilitate the measurement of the crack length (a) under an optical microscope. The specimen width (W) and thickness (B) can be determined using a digital caliper micrometer. To avoid time-dependent effects (viscoelasticity), the loading rate at the crack tip, defined as the increment of stress intensity factor in unit time ($\Delta K/s$), should be kept low and constant (e.g., 0.15 to 0.30 MPa$\sqrt{m}$ /s) by adjusting the crosshead speed of the test machine. The curve of force vs. displacement is recorded, and the peak load is determined as the critical load, P_C.

C. DATA INTERPRETATION

The sandwich technique was originally developed to test engineering material systems.[11,16] Based on the same concept, this technique was successfully adapted to measuring tissue–biomaterial interfacial bonding strength.[18,19] The interfacial fracture toughness or critical stress intensity factor (K_C) can be calculated using the following equation developed in a previous study:[19]

$$K_C = \frac{\lambda^{\psi} P_C Y}{B\sqrt{W}}$$

(32.1)

where K_C is the interfacial fracture toughness, P_C is the critical load, λ is a scale factor determined by elastic properties of bone and the biomaterial bilayer materials, ψ is a correction factor which is a function of the normalized interlayer thickness h/W,[19] B is the thickness of specimen, W is the specimen width, and the remaining parameter Y is a constant determined by W and initial crack length a. Parameter λ can be determined using

$$\lambda = \sqrt{\frac{1-\alpha}{1-\beta^2}}$$

(32.2)

where α and β are Dundurs' parameters, which estimate the elastic mismatch across an interface of two dissimilar materials [4] and are given by

$$\alpha = \frac{E_1(1-v_2^2)-E_2(1-v_1^2)}{E_1(1-v_2^2)+E_2(1-v_1^2)} \tag{32.3}$$

$$\beta = \frac{E_1(1-v_2-2v_2^2)-E_2(1-v_1-2v_1^2)}{2E_1(1-v_2^2)+2E_2(1-v_1^2)} \tag{32.4}$$

where E_1, E_2, and v_1, v_2 are elastic moduli and Poisson's ratios of the interlayer and the other material of the bilayer specimen, respectively. Additionally, in Equation 32.1, ψ is the correction factor for the finite interlayer thickness h, and is expressed as a polynomial function of h/W (in the range of $0.0 < h/W < 0.12$) as

$$\psi = 1.00 - 14.07\left(\frac{h}{W}\right) + 136.0\left(\frac{h}{W}\right)^2 - 538.8\left(\frac{h}{W}\right)^3 \tag{32.5}$$

Here, h is the thickness of the interlayer.

Finally, Y can be directly calculated using the standard equation for compact tension specimens recommended in ASTM standard E 399-90,[2]

$$Y = \left(2+\frac{a}{W}\right)\frac{\left(0.886+4.64\frac{a}{W}-13.32\left(\frac{a}{W}\right)^2+14.72\left(\frac{a}{W}\right)^3-5.6\left(\frac{a}{W}\right)^4\right)}{\left(1-\frac{a}{W}\right)^{3/2}} \tag{32.6}$$

From K_C, the critical strain energy release rate can be calculated as follows:

$$G_C = \frac{E_1(1-v_2^2)+E_2(1-v_1^2)}{2E_1E_2\cosh^2(\pi\varepsilon)}|K_C|^2 \tag{32.7}$$

where ε is a parameter determined by one of the Dundurs' parameters of material mismatch, β:

$$\varepsilon = \frac{1}{2\pi}\ln\left(\frac{1-\beta}{1+\beta}\right) \tag{32.8}$$

An extremely important aspect of compact sandwich specimens is the existence of complex loading modes at the crack tip. Unlike homogeneous test specimens, the interfacial crack of compact sandwich specimens is actually loaded under both tension and shear loads because of the material mismatch across the interface.[9] However, the interfacial fracture toughness cannot be simply separated into conventional Mode I (tension) and Mode II (shear).[9] To address this issue, a nominal-phase angle, ξ, can be used to assess the ratio of the shear component with respect to the tensile component of the interfacial fracture toughness.

$$\xi = \tan^{-1}\left(\frac{\text{Shear component of } K_C}{\text{Tensile component of } K_C}\right) \tag{32.9}$$

TABLE 32.1

Values of ω as a Function of α and β

					α				
β	-0.8	-0.6	-0.4	-0.2	0.0	0.2	0.4	0.6	0.8
-0.4	2.2	3.5							
-0.3	3.0	4.0	3.3	1.4					
-0.2	3.6	4.1	3.4	2.0	-0.3	-3.3			
-0.1	4.0	4.1	3.3	2.0	0.1	-2.3	-5.5	-10.8	
0.0	4.4	3.8	2.9	1.6	0.0	-2.1	-4.7	-8.4	-14.3
0.1			2.3	1.1	-0.5	-2.3	-4.5	-7.4	-11.6
0.2					-1.3	-3.0	-4.9	-7.3	-10.5
0.3							-5.8	-7.8	-10.4
0.4									-11.1

This table was reproduced based on the work by Suo and Hutchinson.[11]

TABLE 32.2

Values of α, b, ε, λ, and ω for Some Bone–Biomaterial Systems

Holder/Interlayer	E (GPa)	ν	α	β	ε	λ	ω (°)
Human bone/CoCr	11.8/234	0.25/0.30	-0.907	-0.304	0.10	1.450	2
PMMA/bovine bone	2.8/20	0.35/0.25	-0.764	-0.164	0.051	1.336	3.5
Bovine/human bone	20/11.8	0.25/0.25	0.258	0.086	-0.027	0.865	-2.7
Ti alloy/bovine bone	110/20	0.30/0.25	0.70	0.24	-0.078	0.564	-9.1
CoCr/human bone	234/11.8	0.30/0.25	0.907	0.304	-0.10	0.320	-12

PMMA: polymethylmethacrylate; CoCr: cobalt–chrome alloy; Ti: titanium.

ξ can be determined using the following procedure:[19] First, a material system having very small ε (< 0.01) is selected arbitrarily as control, and then the relative discrepancy in phase angle, $\Delta\xi$, between the test specimen and the control is calculated using the following equation:

$$\Delta\xi = \omega - \omega_0 - \ln\left(h^\varepsilon / h_0^{\varepsilon_0}\right) \tag{32.10}$$

where ω is an auxiliary parameter determined by α and β (Table 32.1), ε is the parameter outlined in Equation 32.8, and h is the interlayer thickness for the test specimen. ω_0, h_0, and ε_0 are the values for the control. Then, ξ can be obtained as

$$\xi = \xi_0 + \Delta\xi \tag{32.11}$$

where ξ_0 ($= \omega_0 + \varepsilon_0 \ln r/h_0$) is the phase angle of the control as outlined in a previous study.[19] Although r is an arbitrary number in this case,[9] for simplicity r is fixed at $1/10$ of h_0. Table 32.2 shows the values of ω, ε, λ, α, and β for the material systems often seen in orthopaedic applications. In fact, the loading modes at the crack tip are primarily determined by the material mismatch, and interlayer thickness, h, of the compact sandwich specimen.

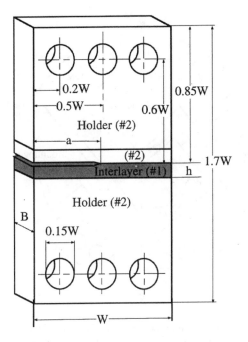

FIGURE 32.7 A schematic diagram of the mixed-mode sandwich specimen. A bilayer specimen is sand-wiched between two holders. The specimen is mounted onto a loading fixture through the holes in the holders.

D. LIMITATIONS

The compact sandwich test is not valid for measuring the fracture toughness of very rough or irregular interfaces. Currently, there are no accurate means to assess the fracture toughness of such interfaces. In addition, linear elasticity and isotropy are assumed for this test. However, the elastic-plastic behavior at the crack tip may play an important role in determining interfacial fracture toughness. Liechti and Liang[5] have shown that the plastic zone at the interfacial crack tip might be extremely large if a shear component is present, and it may become acute when the interlayer is much more compliant compared with the holders. Also, this test does not account for visco-elasticity, a time-dependent factor, which may also affect the measurement of interfacial fracture properties. To avoid such effects, one should use a constant loading speed for all specimens to be compared. Because specimen sizes may vary to accommodate the diverse sizes of *in vivo* samples, the overall specimen size may affect the accuracy of the test. A previous study has shown that the effect of overall specimen size can be ignored as long as the specimen dimensions are proportional.[19] In addition, elastic properties of bone and the biomaterial of the bilayer specimen are needed for determining the interfacial fracture toughness. Although in most cases these properties can be obtained from standard mechanical tests or from the literature, it is cumbersome to perform additional experiments.

III. MIXED-MODE SANDWICH FRACTURE TOUGHNESS TEST

The mixed-mode test for measuring interfacial fracture toughness is an extension of the aforementioned sandwich technique. In this test, the interfacial crack is loaded in both tension and shear simultaneously. The specimen configuration is shown in Figure 32.7. The mixed mode specimen has a different geometry compared with the compact sandwich specimen.

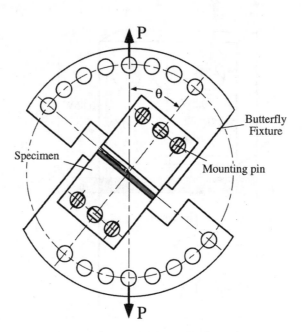

FIGURE 32.8   A custom-designed loading fixture (butterfly-loading fixture) to facilitate variation of load-ing direction (θ) with respect to the crack plane. Trough-shaped mounting pins are used to reduce the contact area between the pins and holes to avoid uneven load transfer to the test specimens. The lateral movement of the specimen is restricted by the middle holes, and axial movement of the specimen is restricted by the side holes.

A. Specimen Preparation

Similarly to the compact sandwich specimen, the mixed-mode specimen also consists of two components: a bilayer test specimen and two holders (see Figure 32.7). There are three pinholes in each holder to facilitate load transfer from the loading fixture to the specimen (Figure 32.8). The procedure for preparing the bilayer specimen is the same as described for the compact sandwich specimen. In this test, the bilayer specimen is carefully cemented between the two holders using a cyanoacrylate adhesive. The extra adhesive on both sides of the specimen is polished off using fine sandpaper. A starter notch is cut at the interface using a circular saw with a 0.5-mm-thick blade. Then, a precrack can be introduced at the tip of the notch using a sharp razor blade.

B. Test Procedure

The test specimen is mounted onto a two-piece butterfly-shaped loading fixture, which can alter the loading direction with respect to the interfacial crack plane as shown in Figure 32.8. The loading direction is changed by selecting corresponding loading holes which are evenly distributed along the perimeter of the fixture. Clevises (U-shaped fixtures) are needed to facilitate loading of the mixed-mode sandwich specimen. The design of the clevis should follow ASTM standard E399-90.[2] A water-soluble dye can be used at the crack tip to facilitate the measurement of the initial crack length (a) under an optical microscope. The specimen width (W) and thickness (B) can be deter-mined using a caliper micrometer. In order to avoid time-dependent effects (e.g., viscoelasticity), the loading rate at the crack tip, defined as the increment of stress intensity factor in a unit time ($\Delta K/s$), should be kept slow and constant (e.g., 0.15 to 0.30 MPa$\sqrt{m}$/s) by adjusting the crosshead speed of the test machine. The critical load, P_C, can be determined as the peak load from the force vs. displacement curve recorded.

C. Data Interpretation

The mixed-mode test is designed to assess the interfacial fracture toughness of a bone–biomaterial system under a mixture of different loading modes (shear and tension). Its overall effect can be assessed using a mixed-mode fracture toughness, K_C, which can be calculated using the following equation:[17]

$$K_C = \frac{\lambda^\psi P_C \sqrt{\pi a}}{WB} \sqrt{(A_I \cos \theta)^2 + (A_{II} \sin \theta)^2} \tag{32.12}$$

where P_C is the critical load, a is the initial crack length, W and B are the width and thickness of the specimen, θ is the loading angle, and A_I and A_{II} are functions of a and W:[10]

$$A_I = \frac{1}{1-\frac{a}{W}} \sqrt{\frac{0.26 + 2.65 \frac{a}{W-a}}{1 + 0.55 \frac{a}{W-a} - 0.08 \left(\frac{a}{W-a}\right)^2}} \tag{32.13}$$

$$A_{II} = \frac{1}{1-\frac{a}{W}} \sqrt{\frac{-0.23 + 1.40 \frac{a}{W-a}}{1 - 0.67 \frac{a}{W-a} + 2.08 \left(\frac{a}{W-a}\right)^2}} \tag{32.14}$$

Parameter ψ is the correction factor for finite interlayer thickness, h, and is expressed as a function of h/W and loading angle, θ.[17]

$$\psi = e^{p(h/W)^k} \tag{32.15}$$

where p and k are functions of loading angle, θ, and are given as:

$$p = 5.056 - 1.20\theta + 266\theta^2 \tag{32.16}$$

$$k = 0.777 - 0.124\theta - 0.028\theta^2 \tag{32.17}$$

Here, θ is in radians. The interfacial fracture toughness of the mixed-mode specimen cannot be simply separated into conventional Mode I (tension) and Mode II (shear).[9] As outlined for the compact sandwich specimens, the nominal phase angle, ξ, for the mixed-mode specimen can be calculated as:

$$\xi = \xi_0 + \theta - \theta_0 + \omega - \omega_0 - \ln \left(\frac{h^\varepsilon}{h_0^{\varepsilon_0}}\right) \tag{32.18}$$

where θ is the loading angle, ω is an auxiliary parameter determined by α and β, ε is determined by β as outlined in Equation 32.8, and h is the interlayer thickness for the test specimen, while ξ_0, θ_0, ω_0, ε_0, and h_0 are the values for the control. For the mixed-mode specimens, the loading modes at the crack tip are primarily affected by the material mismatch across the interface and the interlayer thickness, h.

D. LIMITATIONS

The mixed-mode specimen has the same limitations outlined for the compact sandwich specimen.

IV. SHORT-BAR AND SHORT-ROD FRACTURE TOUGHNESS TEST

The short-bar or short-rod specimen was first developed by Barker[3] to evaluate engineering materials. Because it has a small and simple shape, and no precracking procedure is needed, this technique has been successfully adapted for testing of interfacial bonding at dentin/biomaterial interfaces.[6,8,14] The short-bar or short-rod specimen consists of two halves with a bone–biomaterial interface between, as shown in Figure 32.4. Half of the specimen is made of the biomaterial, and the other half is a bone–biomaterial laminate. Thus far, two different procedures have been used;[6,8,14] one of them using the short-bar specimen to determine the critical strain energy release rate, G_C, and the other using the short-rod specimen to assess the critical stress intensity factor, K_C, of the interfaces. The following are examples of these two procedures.

A. DETERMINATION OF G_{IC} USING A SHORT-BAR SPECIMEN

1. Specimen Preparation

Lin and Douglas[6] proposed a procedure to determine the critical strain energy release rate, G_C, using a short-bar specimen. In this test, equal compliance for the two halves of the specimen was required. Specifically, the two halves of the short bar had the same load–deformation relationship. This was achieved by experimentally determining the height of each half of the short-bar specimen which would give the same compliance. Figure 32.9 shows the schematic diagram of the short-bar specimen used in their study. Two steps were involved for this procedure; first, a short-bar specimen was made by cementing a layer of dentin between two blocks of dental composite (biomaterial). A chevron notch was made in the middle of the dentin layer. This specimen was loaded at a loading rate of 0.001 mm/s until the specimen split into two halves. One half of the fractured specimen was used as the dentin–composite laminate for fabricating the interfacial fracture toughness test specimens. The fractured surface of dentin of the dentin–composite specimen was wet polished to a flat surface using 600-grit sandpaper. The load vs. mouth-opening displacement curve of the specimen was recorded and the slope of the linear part of the curve was used to calculate the compliance of the dentin–composite laminate, C_1, as

$$C_1 = \frac{\delta}{P} \tag{32.19}$$

where δ is the mouth-opening displacement of the notch and P is the load. C_1 was used to determine the height of the other half of the specimen (composite), which should have the same compliance as the dentin–composite laminate. To do so, another set of short-bar specimens of the composite were made with the same specimen length (W) and width (D) but varying specimen height (H) compared with the dentin–composite specimen described above. The compliance of these specimens was measured and the height of the specimens was adjusted until the compliance of the specimen was equal to C_1. Finally, the dental composite half with the new height was molded on the dentin–composite laminate to form the final short-bar specimen. Teflon tape was used to cover all but the V-shaped dentin-bonding surface of the dentin-composite laminate during the molding process to form a chevron notch.

    To calculate fracture toughness using the short-bar specimen, a parameter called the minimum geometry factor coefficient, Y_m, must be determined. Lin and Douglas[6] used a three-dimensional finite-element model for this purpose. This model was generated to simulate a

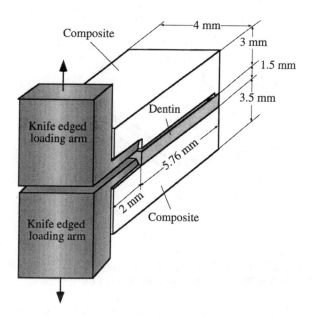

FIGURE 32.9 An example of the short-bar specimen used by Lin and Douglas.[6] The specimen was loaded through two knife-edged loading arms, which were placed between the two lips at the head of the specimen.

short-bar specimen of the dental composite with the height determined earlier. A previous study has shown that the values of the geometry factor coefficient of the specimen, Y, can be calculated using the following equation:[3]

$$Y = \left(\frac{DE}{2} \frac{\alpha_1 - \alpha_0}{\alpha - \alpha_0} \frac{dC}{d\alpha} \right)^{1/2} \tag{32.20}$$

where α is the normalized crack length (a/W), α_0 is the normalized initial crack length (a_0/W), α_1 is the normalized chevron-notch length (a_1/W), a is the crack length from loading line to crack front, a_0 is the initial crack length from loading line to the vertex of the chevron, a_1 is the maximum depth of chevron flanks from the loading line to the base of the chevron, C is the specimen compliance, D is the specimen thickness, and E is the elastic modulus of the composite. Since D, E, α_0, and α_1 are constants, Y is a function of $dC/d\alpha$ and α. By altering the crack length in the model, the compliance (C) of the specimens was calculated with respect to the normalized crack length (α). The curve of the compliance vs. the normalized crack length was then used to determine the values of $dC/d\alpha$ with respect to the normalized crack length (α). Finally, the value of Y_m was determined from the curve of Y vs. α. In the case of this example, the value of Y_m was determined as 17.3 at the normalized crack length $\alpha = 0.48$.

2. Test Procedure

The short-bar specimen is mounted onto a material-testing machine using a custom-designed fixture, in which the specimen is held in knife-edged loading arms as shown in Figure 32.9. Precautions need to be taken to ensure that the orientation of the loading line is perpendicular to the chevron-notch fracture plane of the specimen. The test is run at a constant loading rate of 0.001 mm/s by adjusting the crosshead speed of the test machine. Several loading–unloading cycles are performed during the test until the maximum failure load is reached. The cycle which includes the maximum load is defined as the effective cycle. Load and displacement values are recorded to plot the curve of load vs. mouth-

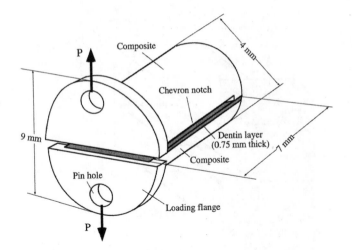

FIGURE 32.10 An example of the short-bar specimen developed in previous studies.[12] The specimen was loaded through the holes in the two loading flanges at the head of the specimen.

opening displacement. From the curve, the average load of the effective cycle was determined as the critical load, P_C. Details for obtaining the critical load can be found elsewhere.[3]

3. Data Interpretation

The critical strain energy release rate, G_{IC}, for a short-bar specimen can be calculated using the following equation:[6]

$$G_{IC} = \frac{P_C^2 Y_m^2}{ED^2 W}$$

(32.21)

where P_C is the critical load measured at time of fracture, D is the specimen thickness for the short-bar specimen, E is the elastic modulus of the composite, W is the specimen length, and Y_m is the minimum geometric factor coefficient.

B. DETERMINATION OF K_{IC} USING A SHORT ROD SPECIMEN

1. Specimen Preparation

Tam and Pilliar[12,14] have used short-rod specimens (Figure 32.10) to assess the interfacial bonding of dentin and dental biomaterials. In their studies, slices were sectioned from animal teeth and cut with a high speed burr, under constant water irrigation, to a rectangular coupon ($7 \times 4 \times 1.5$ mm). The slice was inserted into a stainless steel mold, and the dental composite was packed into the mold to form a half specimen. The dentin surface of the half specimen was wet polished with 600-grit sandpaper, rinsed, and dried. The dried dentin surface was then pre-treated, dried with compressed air, and coated with primer. Thereafter, the half specimen was placed in another mold and a spacer made of highly polished stainless steel was placed on top of it to form a chevron-shaped notch after molding. The adhesive agent was brushed onto the dentin surface and light-cured without prior air thinning. The dental composite was then packed into the remainder of the mold. After complete polymerization was ensured, the specimen was separated from the mold. The minimum geometry factor coefficient, Y_m, was required for the short-rod specimen in order to calculate fracture toughness values. In this test, Y_m was determined experimentally with the compliance calibration curves of the specimens using a similar procedure outlined earlier.

2. Test Procedure

The short-rod specimen is mounted on a mechanical testing machine using clevises. Precaution is taken to avoid prestressing the interface during the process. A load is applied to the specimen at a loading rate of 0.5 mm/min until failure of the interface. The peak load, P_C, is recorded at the time of failure. The initial crack length (a_0), specimen length (W), and specimen diameter (D) were determined by the dimensions of the mold.

3. Data Interpretation

The critical stress intensity factor, K_{IC}, can be obtained from this test using the following equation:[12,15]

$$K_{IC} = \frac{P_C Y_m}{D\sqrt{W}} \tag{32.22}$$

where P_C is the peak load measured at time of fracture, D is the diameter of the short-rod specimen, W is the specimen length, and Y_m is the minimum stress intensity factor coefficient.

C. Limitations

A drawback of the short-bar or short-rod specimen is that for each configuration and material combination preliminary experiments are needed to determine the specimen geometry, to ascertain the geometry factor coefficient, and to ensure equal compliance for the two halves of the specimen. Thus, investigators must be quite experienced in specimen preparation. They also must be quite knowledgeable in the nuances of fracture mechanics. The short-bar and short-rod specimens, which are similar to sandwich specimens, are developed based on the assumption of linear elasticity. Thus, this approach is not valid for a specimen with large plastic deformation. Additionally, Liechti and Liang[5] have shown that the plastic zone at the interfacial crack tip might be extremely large if there is a shear component present, and it may become acute when the material mismatch is significant across the interface. Moreover, this test is valid only for measuring the fracture toughness of smooth interfaces because it has been developed based on this assumption. Also, this approach does not account for viscoelasticity. To avoid such effects, one should use a constant loading speed for all specimens to be compared.

REFERENCES

1. Agrawal, C.M., Wang, X., and Mabrey, J., Bone ingrowth into porous coated implants impregnated with PLA-PGA and TGF-β, unpublished.
2. ASTM, E399-90 Standard test method for plane strain fracture toughness of metallic materials, in *1993 Annual Book of ASTM Standards*, ASTM, West Conshohocken, PA, 1993.
3. Barker, L.M., Theory for determining K_{IC} from small, non-LEFM specimens, supported by experiments on aluminum, *Int. J. Fract.*, 15, 515, 1979.
4. Dundurs, J., Edge-bonded dissimilar orthogonal elastic wedges under normal and shear loading, *J. Appl. Mech.*, 36, 650, 1969.
5. Liechti, K.M. and Liang, Y.-M., The interfacial fracture characteristics of biomaterial and sandwich strip blister specimens, *Int. J. Fract.*, 55, 95, 1992.
6. Lin, C.P. and Douglas, W.H., Failure mechanism at the human dentin-resin interface: a fracture mechanics approach, *J. Biomech.*, 27, 1037, 1994.
7. Pilliar, R.M., Davies, J.E. and Smith, D.C., The bone–biomaterial interface for load-bearing implants, *MRS Bull.*, 155, 55, 1991.

8. Pilliar, R.M., Smith, D.C., and Maric, B., Fracture toughness of dental composites determined using the short-rod fracture toughness test, *J. Dent. Res.*, 65, 1308, 1986.

9. Rice, J.R., Elastic fracture mechanics concept for interfacial cracks, *J. Appl. Mech.*, 55, 98, 1988.

10. Richard, H.A., Examination of brittle fracture criteria for overlapping mode I and mode II loading applied to cracks, in *Proceedings of the International Conference on Application of Fracture Mechanics to Materials and Structures*, Freiburg, F.R.G., 1983, 309.

11. Suo, Z. and Hutchinson, J.W., Sandwich test specimen for measuring interface crack toughness, *Mater. Sci. Eng.*, A107, 135, 1989.

12. Tam, L.E. and Pilliar, R.M., Fracture toughness of dentin/resin-composite adhesive interfaces, *J. Dent. Res.*, 72, 953, 1993.

13. Tam, L.E. and Pilliar, R.M., Effects of dentin surface treatments on the fracture toughness and tensile bond strength of a dentin–composite adhesive interface, *J. Dent. Res.*, 73, 1530, 1994.

14. Tam, L.E. and Pilliar, R.M., Fracture surface characterization of dentin-bonded interfacial fracture toughness specimens, *J. Dent. Res.*, 73, 607, 1994.

15. Wang, C.T. and Pilliar, R.M., Short-rod elastic-plastic fracture toughness test using miniature specimens, *J. Mater. Sci.*, 24, 2391, 1989.

16. Wang, J.S. and Suo, Z., Experimental determination of interfacial toughness curves using Brazil-nut sandwiches, *Acta Metall. Mater.*, 38, 1279, 1990.

17. Wang, X. and Agrawal, C.M., Mixed mode fracture toughness of bone–biomaterial interfaces, *Trans. Orthop. Res. Soc.*, 22, 46, 1997.

18. Wang, X., Subramanian, A., Dhanda, R., and Agrawal, C., Testing of bone–biomaterial interfacial bonding strength: a comparison of different techniques, *J. Biomed. Mater. Res.*, 33, 133, 1996.

19. Wang, X.D. and Agrawal, C.M., Interfacial fracture toughness of tissue–biomaterial systems, *J. Biomed. Mater. Res.*, 38, 1, 1997.

33 *In Vitro* Measurements of Implant Stability

Aivars Berzins and Dale R. Sumner

CONTENTS

I. INTRODUCTION

The purpose of this chapter is to review some of the basic principles involved in performing *in vitro* tests of implant stability. After introducing the topic, the motions analyzed in the different setups are first considered. Then, the various approaches to applying loads to implant and host bone are discussed. In general, citations are restricted to papers that have appeared in peer-reviewed journals.

From the early days of joint replacement surgery, there has been interest in determining how prosthetic design and surgical technique influenced fixation of the implant to the host bone.[1] This has been investigated by measuring the relative motion between the bone and the implant. Since the variety of prosthetic designs has increased and concepts of biological fixation have evolved, *in vitro* measurements are commonly used to test the initial stability of orthopaedic devices implanted in cadaver bones or synthetic bones. Technically similar tests have also been applied to *postmortem* retrieved specimens to evaluate the long-term stability *ex vivo*.

Femoral or acetabular components of hip replacement systems and femoral or tibial components of knee replacement systems are the most frequently tested implants, mainly due to concerns about loosening. A number of studies have used *in vitro* stability tests not only to address fixation design features but also to test new surgical techniques, particularly those used in revision surgery in the presence of insufficient bone stock. In addition to tests on human cadaver bones, numerous investigators have used animal models to study implant stability, predominantly with hip and knee replacement systems.

It is worth mentioning at this point that implant stability has also been investigated *in vivo* in patients, most commonly with a technique called roentgen stereophotogrammetric or radiostereometric analysis (RSA).[2] In general, this technique has a detection limit of 0.2 to 0.3 mm and is far superior to conventional radiographic assessment, but is one to two orders of magnitude less sensitive than many of the *in vitro* techniques described below. RSA and the techniques described below can measure both the inducible or recoverable motion and the nonrecoverable motion (often referred to as migration). The recoverable motion is the difference in position of the implant from the unloaded to the loaded state. After a few load cycles this value usually becomes constant, but

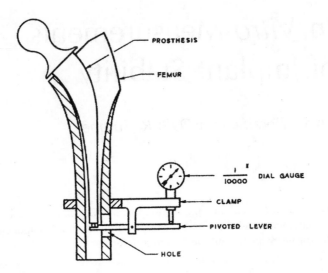

FIGURE 33.1 Test setup used by Charnley and Kettlewell in a paper published in 1965.[1] In this case the authors were interested in axial motion at the distal aspect of the femoral component in cemented hip replacement. (From Charnley, J. and Kettlewell, J., *J. Bone Joint Surg.*, 47B, 56, 1965. With permission.)

typically is below the detection limit of RSA. The nonrecoverable motion is the difference in position of the implant from the first to the last load cycle.

In vivo, it is easier to measure migration than the recoverable motion because of the limited sensitivity of RSA and because measurement of recoverable motion requires the subject or investigator to load and unload the joint repeatedly, and it is difficult to do this reproducibly in the living subject. In contrast, *in vitro* one can measure either quantity, although it is often simpler to measure the recoverable motion because only a limited number of load cycles are required (often as few as ten).

II. STABILITY MEASUREMENTS AND THE NUMBER OF MEASURED MOTION COMPONENTS

In vitro implant stability testing setups can first be characterized by the number of separate motion components (degrees of freedom) which the motion monitoring system is capable of sensing and recording. Table 33.1 summarizes an immense amount of information and is arranged from relatively simple setups (e.g., one translation or one rotation) to the most complete description of motion (three translations and three rotations) for femoral stems, tibial trays, and acetabular components. With the simplest systems, a motion at a specific location is measured by determining the displacement at that location (Figure 33.1). In this situation, no assumptions are needed, although it should be recognized that the investigator has had to decide *a priori* the most important motion component and its location.

To measure all six components of motion, one typically uses an array of dial gauges, extensometers, linear variable differential transformers, or eddy current transducers (Figure 33.2). These are grounded to the surrounding bone in order to sense the displacement of a target device rigidly attached to the implant. From these motions, the motion at a given point on the implant with respect to the bone is then calculated. In this type of system, the assumption is made that the bone and implant behave as two rigid bodies (i.e., neither deform while being loaded). While this is obviously not always true globally (e.g., along the length of the femoral stem in hip replacement), it has been shown that the assumption allows for accurate local estimates of motion.[3,4] If one is interested in motion at different parts of the bone–implant interface (e.g., the proximal and distal aspects of the femoral stem) and it is known that significant deformation of the bone and/or implant occurs between these sites, then the array of transducers must be set up at each local site.[3] In this situation,

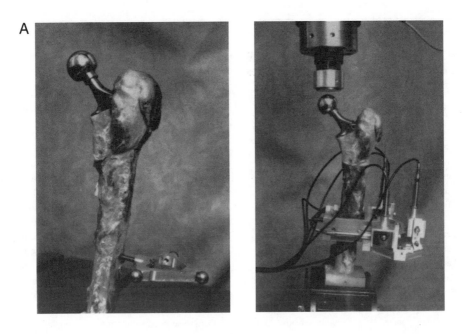

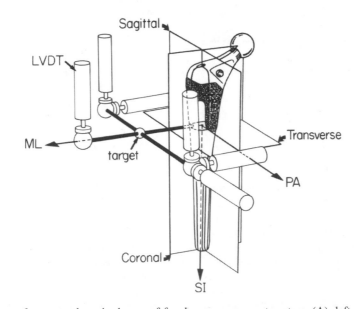

FIGURE 33.2 Setup for a complete six-degree-of-freedom measurement system. (A), left, shows a femur with an implant *in situ* and the target device attached to the distal aspect of the implant through a hole in the cortex. (A), right, shows that the six linear variable displacement transducers were attached to the bone via a rigid collar that did not interfere with the motion of the implant or target device. In the (B) schematic, the attachment of the six linear variable displacement transducers to the femoral cortex is not shown. Note that the target was rigidly attached to the implant and that the transducers measured motion of this target. Based on these measurements, three translations (PA = posterior-anterior, ML = medial-lateral, and SI = superior-inferior) and three rotations (in the sagittal, transverse, and coronal planes) of the point and axes, respectively, defined by the intersection of the three planes were calculated. (From Berzins, A., et al., *J. Orthrop. Res.,* 11, 758, 1993. With permission. The published matrix used in the calculations contained a typographic error and an erratum was published in the *J. Orthop. Res.,* 13, 151, 1995).

TABLE 33.1

Summary of Implants Tested, Sensors Used, Number of Motion Components Determined and the Location of the Measurement Sites

Ref.	Implants Tested	Sensors Used	Number of Motion Components Determined	Location of Measurement Sites
1	Femoral stem	Dial gauge	Axial translation	Distal tip of the stem
46	Femoral stem	Extensometer	Axial translation	Proximal and distal stem
14	Femoral stem	LVDT	Axial translation	At the crosshead
38	Canine femoral stem	LVDT	One translation (medial-lateral)	Proximal stem
47	Tibial component	Two LVDTs	Axial translation	Medial and lateral plateau
48	Femoral stem	LVDT	Transverse rotation[a]	Prosthetic neck
49	Femoral stem	LVDT	Transverse rotation[a]	Prosthetic neck
50	Femoral stem	LVDT	Transverse rotation[a]	Prosthetic neck
24	Femoral stem	LVDT	Transverse rotation[a]	At the crosshead
51	Femoral stem	LVDT	Transverse rotation[a]	Prosthetic neck
52	Femoral stem	LVDT	Transverse rotation[a]	Prosthetic neck
16	Tibial component	Pressure-sensitive film	Transverse interface motion	Implant–bone interface
53	Tibial component	LVDT	Load–displacement curve	At the crosshead
21	Femoral stem	Video digitizing system	Axial translation; transverse rotation[a]	Proximal stem
54	Femoral stem	LVDT and rotational transducer[b]	Axial translation; transverse rotation[a]	At the crosshead
41	Canine femoral stem	Two extensometers	Two translations (axial and medial-lateral)	Proximal stem (anterior and posterior)
55	Canine femoral stem	Two eddy current transducers	Two translations (axial and medial-lateral)	Proximal stem
35	Femoral stem	Extensometer	Two translations (axial and medial-lateral)	Proximal stem (anterior and posterior)
56	Femoral stems	Extensometer	Two translations (axial and medial-lateral)	Proximal stem (anterior and posterior)
39	Femoral implant (stemless)	Four LVDTs	Two translations (anterior-posterior and medial-lateral)	Prosthetic neck
34	Femoral stem	Three strain gauge displacement transducers	Two translations (axial and medial-lateral); transverse rotation[a]	Proximal stem
57	Femoral stems	Dial gauge, extensometer	Two translations (axial and medial-lateral); transverse rotation[a]	Proximal stem
36	Femoral stem	Extensometers	Three translations; transverse rotation	Proximal and distal stem
58	Femoral stem	Six LVDTs	Three translations (axial-proximal, anterior-posterior and medial-lateral distal); transverse rotation (proximal)	Proximal and distal stem
59	Femoral stem	Five dial gauges	Three translations proximal; two translations distal (no axial)	Prosthetic head; proximal and distal stem

TABLE 33.1 (continued)
Summary of Implants Tested, Sensors Used, Number of Motion Components Determined
and the Location of the Measurement Sites

Ref.	Implants Tested	Sensors Used	Number of Motion Components Determined	Location of Measurement Sites
42	Femoral stems	Six eddy current transducers	Three translations and two rotations (transverse and frontal)	Proximal stem
60	Femoral stem	Seven LVDTs	Three translations distal; two translations proximal (no axial); transverse rotation	Proximal and distal stem
61	Femoral stem	Six LVDTs	Three translations proximal; two translations distal; transverse rotation[b]	Proximal and distal stem; prosthetic neck
9	Femoral stems	Two linear resistive transducers, LVDT; rotary potentiometer; four strain gauge-based interface transducers	Three translations and transverse rotation of the distal femur; interface motion in two planes (sagittal and frontal)	Distal femur; proximal and distal stem (interface motion)
40	Femoral stems	Six LVDTs	Three translations and three rotations	Distal stem
3	Femoral stems	Six LVDTs	Three translations and three rotations	Proximal and distal stem
33	Femoral stem	Seven LVDTs	Three translations and three rotations	Proximal and distal
17	Femoral stem (goat model)	RSA	Three translations; three rotations	Femoral stem
62	Tibial component	Three LVDTs	Axial translation	Anterior, medial, and posterior aspects
63	Tibial component	Four liquid metal strain gauges	Axial translation	Anterolateral, anteromedial, posterolateral, and posteromedial aspects
64	Simulated tibial component	Four strain gauge transducers	Axial translation	Anterolateral, anteromedial, posterolateral, and posteromedial aspects
65	Tibial component	Four LVDTs	Axial translation	Anterior, posterior, medial, and lateral rims
20	Tibial component	Video camera via a stereomicroscope	Interface motion	Implant–bone interface
66	Tibial component	Three LVDTs	Two translations (axial in two locations and medial-lateral)	Lateral plateau, medial rim
23	Tibial component	LVDTs	Axial translation; posterior-anterior translation (separate tests)	Anterolateral and posteromedial plateau, medial and lateral rims
45	Tibial component	LVDTs	Axial translation; posterior-anterior translation; transverse rotation[a] (separate tests)	Lateral plateau, medial and lateral rims

TABLE 33.1 (continued)
Summary of Implants Tested, Sensors Used, Number of Motion Components Determined
and the Location of the Measurement Sites

Ref.	Implants Tested	Sensors Used	Number of Motion Components Determined	Location of Measurement Sites
22	Tibial component	Two dial gauges; four LVDTs	Posterior-anterior translation; axial translation	Medial and lateral rims, anterior, lateral, posterior, posteromedial points
4	Canine tibial component	Six LVDTs	Three translations, three rotations	Central aspect of the component
10	Tibial component	Seven LVDTs	Three translations, three rotations	Medial and lateral rims
44	Acetabular component	Load cell	Force required to loosen the component	
11	Acetabular component	Preset angular velocity in a displacement- controlled test	Twist angle to loosen the component	Actuator (estimated)
13	Acetabular component	Rotational transducer[b]	Polar rotation (displacement controlled loading)	Actuator
67	Acetabular component	Two extensometers	Interface motion at two locations	Dome of the cup, posterior wall
68	Acetabular component	Strain gauge displacement transducer	Translation within the equatorial plane (superior-lateral)	Superior-lateral edge of the cup
69	Acetabular component	Three LVDTs	Interface motion within equatorial plane	Adjacent to implant–bone interface
70	Acetabular component	Three eddy current transducers	Axial translation	At the cup edge
71	Acetabular component	Six LVDTs	Three translations (resultant translation reported)	Anteromedial and posterolateral rim
19	Acetabular component (goat model)	RSA	Three translations; three rotations	Acetabular component

Note: The table is organized from simple systems (e.g., determination of one motion component) to complex (determination of all six motion components).

[a] Indicates that rotations were reported as projected linear displacements in μm within arbitrary distance from the axis of rotation.

[b] Indicates that the transducer is a part of the materials testing machine and senses the displacement of the actuator or the crosshead.

LVDT = linear variable displacement transducer; RSA = roentgen stereophotogrammetric analysis.

---

if it were important to have a map of the motions everywhere at the interface, then a finite-element model would be needed,[5,6] with the actual *in vitro* measurements serving as a validation of the model. If one is interested in micromotion at only a few relevant locations of the bone–implant interface, it is possible to use custom-built sensors specifically designed to measure three-dimensional micromotion at the point of their location.[7-9]

In the presence of a full six-degree-of-freedom motion data set and a model of the geometry of both the implant and bone, it is possible to calculate the exact amount of displacement for any specific point of the bone–implant interface (keeping in mind the limitation of the rigid-body assumption, discussed above).[3,4,10] Thus, maps of each of the components of motion or of various combinations can be displayed to help interpret how the component moves with respect to the bone (see, e.g., Reference 4). In addition, the number of motion descriptors can be reduced to a single measure of interface motion (e.g., the resultant translation) that can then be used for interpretation.

Between the one-motion and complete six-degree-of-freedom systems, there are a variety of motion-sensing setups that provide a subset of motions (see Table 33.1). Most of these include at least an axial displacement and/or rotational motion around the longitudinal axis for hip femoral components and subsidence and lift-off for knee tibial components.

In addition to motions determined from static testing (e.g., the application of one or a very limited number of load cycles), recoverable and nonrecoverable motion can be characterized from cyclic tests. The nonrecoverable motion should be analogous to migration measured *in vivo* by RSA. Thus, some authors report both the recoverable (inducible) motion and the nonrecoverable (migratory) motion.

While most studies use the implant–bone displacement to describe implant stability, there are a few studies where the ultimate force required to loosen the implant has been used to characterize implant stability.[11-15] In addition, imprints on a precalibrated pressure-sensitive film have been used to describe a stability of tibial components of total knee replacements,[16] RSA has been used to evaluate acetabular component and femoral stem stability *ex vivo* in a goat model[17-19] and direct visualization by a video camera was used to document bone–implant interface movement in a canine tibial hemiarthroplasty model[20] and in femoral stems implanted in cadaveric human bones.[21]

III. STABILITY MEASURING SYSTEMS AND THE LOADING SETUPS

The value of results from *in vitro* stability tests depends on the representativeness of the loading protocol with respect to the known magnitude and direction of joint reaction forces measured *in vivo*. It is generally agreed that using simplified loading protocols with high forces acting in a nonphysiological direction can result in misleading test results. As an example, testing prosthetic components by application of an isolated load in the transverse direction without a normal axial component of load will almost certainly lead to the failure of implant fixation[22-24] in a fashion which is not comparable to loosening mechanisms observed *in vivo*.

Ideally, resultant joint reaction forces are preferred to isolated components of load. On the one hand, the reports on force measurements obtained from telemetrized hip prostheses provide an excellent database for hip loading conditions in humans,[25-31] canines,[26,32] and sheep.[26] On the other hand, attempts to replicate the exact *in vivo* loading conditions *in vitro* can lead to the introduction of nonphysiological constraints and excessive stresses imposed by the test setup. Because the loads affecting the hip joint are fairly well understood and have received the most attention of those investigating implant stability, the trade-offs involved, using the hip as an example, will be illustrated. This discussion is followed by much briefer descriptions of loading of the acetabular components and the tibial component.

In a simple setup for testing the stability of the femoral stem in hip replacement, the distal femur typically is rigidly fixed to maintain the shaft angle against the test loads simulating the stance phase of level walking or stair climbing.[3,17,18,21,33,34] By using this type of loading setup, despite the perfect projection of the resultant force against the proximal joint surface of the implant, the whole femoral shaft is subjected to bending and torsion due to its distal constraint.

So, even though the loads applied to the head of the implant may be physiological, the moments created by the joint forces are always balanced by the activity of the muscles crossing the hip and knee joints *in vivo* and not by rigid fixation of the distal femur as is often the case *in vitro*. Therefore, if such a loading protocol is used to test the implant–bone displacement one has to recognize the

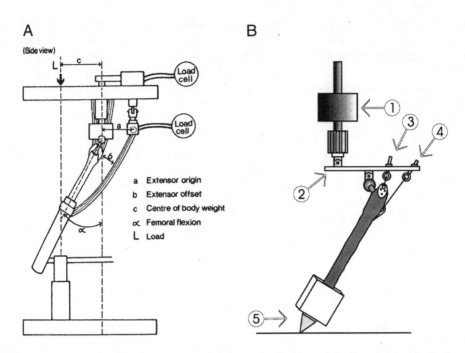

FIGURE 33.3   Schematic of loading setups to simulate stair climbing originally published by Burke et al.[35] (A) and Berzins et al.[40] (B). Note for (B), 1 = load cell, 2 = loading plate, 3 = gluteus medius cable, 4 = gluteus maximus cable, and 5 = the distal support (which allowed rotation). ((A) from Burke, D.W. et al., *J. Bone Joint Surg.,* 73B, 33, 1991. With permission. (B) from Berzins, A., et al., *J. Arthroplasty,* 11, 500, 1996. With permission.)

potential bias due to excess deformation of the proximal femur. With these setups, it is not uncommon for the specimen to fail (i.e., the femur to break) as a result of stress concentration at the distal fixity.

More accurate reproductions of hip loading conditions can be achieved by simulation of the abductors and adding one degree of rotational freedom (hinge) to the distal femur for level walking.[35-38] Hip loading conditions for fast walking have been replicated using two actuators and a system of cables simulating the action of three muscles.[39] Stair climbing can be represented by a combination simultaneous axial and torsion load[36] or by simulation of the abductors and extensors in stair climbing[35,40] (Figure 33.3). Similar setups with added support to the proximal femur can be used to reach realistic peak joint reaction forces without the risk of losing the specimen due to femoral fracture in bending. Three muscle groups have been used to simulate femoral component loading conditions in the canine.[41] However, these more sophisticated loading regimes have drawbacks — simulating muscle forces through the application of nylon straps[36,42] or steel cables[40] attached to the proximal femur may lead to nonphysiological local strain concentrations in the bone.

The next logical step toward more accurate loading simulation would be a complete release of the distal femur (except for the projected ground reaction force) in the presence of perfectly balanced simulation of all major muscle groups. This type of setup has been used to investigate the biomechanical effects of relocation of the hip center,[43] but has not been used in conjunction with implant stability experiments. Technically, it would be difficult to have the complex instrumentation needed for both.

Acetabular components of hip replacement are typically subject to either oblique axial loads or to torque tests.[44] Since the axial load is estimated to be the predominant component of the resultant force within the knee joint, most tibial components are tested by eccentric application of an axial load, with only a few studies adding torsion or a transverse load component.[45]

There certainly is no single perfect loading apparatus for a given joint. After all, an implant tested in a cadaver bone is just a model. So, it is up to the researcher to understand the inherent limitations and to design the experiment and the experimental set up to permit specific questions to be addressed.

Another issue that merits consideration is the number of load cycles, frequency, and rate of load application. In the studies concerned with recoverable motions of the implant against the bone, it is important to apply a sufficient number of cycles to accomplish the initial settling and to record the motion after it has become repeatable.[4] If the study is more concerned with migration (non-recoverable motion) between the implant and bone, a larger number of load cycles should be used to simulate the shift in implant position after hundreds or even thousands of *in vivo* load cycles. Loading frequency should always be representative of physiological loading rates. In studies where a large number of loading cycles are applied and time constraints call for an accelerated test protocol, the higher test speeds involving dynamic loading conditions (inertial forces, etc.) should be avoided.

IV. CONCLUSION

The authors would like to emphasize that *in vitro* experiments of implant stability fall at the crossroads of two complex issues — deciding how to make the stability measurements and deciding how to apply the loads to the system. In terms of implant motion, one can measure from one to six components of motion. In terms of loading, one can apply a simple unidirectional load or attempt more physiological loading. The complexity of the experimental setup increases significantly, as the experiment becomes more "realistic." It is always important to keep in mind that the research question being asked determines how complex the experimental setup needs to be.

ACKNOWLEDGMENTS

Research was supported by NIH Grants AR16485 and AR42862.

REFERENCES

1. Charnley, J. and Kettlewell, J., The elimination of slip between prosthesis and femur, *J. Bone Joint Surg.*, 47B, 56, 1965.
2. Nilsson, K.G. and Karrholm, J., RSA in the assessment of aseptic loosening, *J. Bone Joint Surg.*, 78B, 1, 1997.
3. Berzins, A., Sumner, D.R., Andriacchi, T.P., and Galante, J.O., Stem curvature and load angle influence the initial relative bone–implant motion of cementless femoral stems, *J. Orthop. Res.*, 11, 758, 1993.
4. Sumner, D.R., Berzins, A., Turner, T.M., et al., Initial *in vitro* stability of the tibial component in a canine model of cementless total knee replacement, *J. Biomech.*, 27, 929, 1994.
5. Keaveny, T.M. and Bartel, D.L., Effects of porous coating, with and without collar support, on early relative motion for a cementless hip prosthesis, *J. Biomech.*, 26, 1355, 1993.
6. Weinans, H., Huiskes, R., and Grootenboer, H.J., Quantitative analysis of bone reactions to relative motions at implant–bone interfaces, *J. Biomech.*, 26, 1271, 1993.
7. Buhler, D.W., Oxland, T.R., and Nolte, L.P., Design and evaluation of a device for measuring three-dimensional micromotions of press-fit femoral stem prostheses, *Med. Eng. Phys.*, 19, 187, 1997.
8. Schneider, E., Schonenberger, U., Giraud, P., and Burgi, M., [Initial stability and pelvic deformation in cemented and non-cemented acetabular components], *Orthopade,* 21, 57, 1992 [in German].
9. Schneider, E., Eulenberger, J., Steiner, W., et al., Experimental method for the *in vitro* testing of the initial stability of cementless hip prostheses, *J. Biomech.*, 22, 735, 1989.
10. Stern, S. H., Wills, R. D., and Gilbert, J. L., The effect of tibial stem design on component micromotion in knee arthroplasty, *Clin. Orthop.*, 345, 44, 1997.
11. Ohlin, A. and Balkfors, B., Stability of cemented sockets after 3–14 years, *J. Arthroplasty,* 7, 87, 1992.

12. Jansson, V., Zimmer, M., Kuhne, J.H., and Sailer, F.P. [Initial stability of an implanted cement-canal prosthesis. Results in experimental studies on human cadaver femurs], *Z. Orthop.*, 131, 377, 1993 [in German].

13. Curtis, M.J., Jinnah, R.H., Wilson, V.D., and Hungerford, D.S., The initial stability of uncemented acetabular components, *J. Bone Joint Surg.*, 74B, 372, 1992.

14. Whiteside, L.A., Amador, D., and Russell, K., The effects of the collar on total hip femoral component subsidence, *Clin. Orthop.*, 231, 120, 1988.

15. Kendrick, J.B., Noble, P.C., and Tullos, H.S., Distal stem design and the torsional stability of cementless femoral stems, *J. Arthroplasty*, 10, 463, 1995.

16. Walker, P.S., Hsu, H.P., and Zimmerman, R.A., A comparative study of uncemented tibial components, *J. Arthroplasty*, 5, 245, 1990.

17. Schreurs, B.W., Huiskes, R., Buma, P., and Sloof, T. J., Biomechanical and histological evaluation of a hydroxyapatite-coated titanium femoral stem fixed with an intramedullary morselized bone grafting technique: an animal experiment on goats, *Biomaterials*, 17, 1177, 1996.

18. Schreurs, B.W., Buma, P., Huiskes, R., et al., Morselized allografts for fixation of the hip prosthesis femoral component, *Acta Orthop. Scand.*, 65, 267, 1994.

19. Schimmel, J.W., Buma, P., Versleyen, D., et al., Acetabular reconstruction with impacted morselized cancellous allografts in cemented hip arthroplasty, *J. Arthroplasty*, 13, 438, 1998.

20. Stulberg, B.N., Watson, J.T., Stulberg, S.D., et al., A new model to assess tibial fixation. II. Concurrent histologic and biomechanical observations, *Clin. Orthop.*, 263, 303, 1991.

21. Lee, T.Q., Lewis, D.A., Barnett, S.L., et al., Structural integrity of implanted WMT infinity hip and osteonics omnifit hip in fresh cadaveric femurs, *J. Biomed. Mater. Res.*, 39, 516, 1998.

22. Miura, H., Whiteside, L.A., Easley, J.C., and Amador, D.D., Effects of screws and a sleeve on initial fixation in uncemented total knee tibial components, *Clin. Orthop.*, 259, 160, 1990.

23. Yoshii, I., Whiteside, L.A., Milliano, M.T., and White, S.E., The effect of central stem and stem length on micromovement of the tibial tray, *J. Arthroplasty*, 7, 433, 1992.

24. Phillips, T.W., Nguyen, L.T., and Munro, S.D., Loosening of cementless femoral stems: a biomechanical analysis of immediate fixation with loading vertical, femur horizontal, *J. Biomech.*, 24, 37, 1991.

25. Bergmann, G., Graichen, F., Rohlmann, A., and Linke, H., Hip joint forces during load carrying, *Clin. Orthop.*, 335, 190, 1997.

26. Bergmann, G., Siraky, J., Rohlmann, A., and Koelbel, R., A comparison of hip joint forces in sheep, dog and man, *J. Biomech.*, 17, 907, 1984.

27. Bergmann, G., Graichen, F., and Rohlmann, A., Hip joint loading during walking and running, measured in two patients, *J. Biomech.*, 26, 969, 1993.

28. Bergmann, G., Graichen, F. and Rohlmann, A., Is staircase walking a risk for the fixation of hip implants? *J. Biomech.*, 28, 535, 1995.

29. Davy, D.T., Kotzar, G.M., Brown, R.H., et al., Telemetric force measurements across the hip after total arthroplasty, *J. Bone Joint Surg.*, 70A, 45, 1988.

30. Kotzar, G.M., Davy, D.T., Berilla, J., and Goldberg, V.M., Torsional loads in the early postoperative period following total hip replacement, *J. Orthop. Res.*, 13, 945, 1995.

31. Kotzar, G.M., Davy, D.T., Goldberg, V.M., et al., Telemeterized *in vivo* hip joint force data: a report on two patients after total hip surgery, *J. Orthop. Res.*, 9, 621, 1991.

32. Page, A.E., Allan, C., Jasty, M., et al., Determination of loading parameters in the canine hip *in vivo*, *J. Biomech.*, 26, 571, 1993.

33. Gilbert, J.L., Bloomfeld, R.S., Lautenschlager, E.P., and Wixson, R. L., A computer-based biomechanical analysis of the three-dimensional motion of cementless hip prostheses, *J. Biomech.*, 25, 329, 1992.

34. McKellop, H., Ebramzadeh, E., Niederer, P.G., and Sarmiento, A., Comparison of the stability of press-fit hip prosthesis femoral stems using a synthetic model femur, *J. Orthop. Res.*, 9, 297, 1991.

35. Burke, D.W., O'Connor, D.O., Zalenski, E.B., et al., Micromotion of cemented and uncemented femoral components, *J. Bone Joint Surg.*, 73B, 33, 1991.

36. Callaghan, J.J., Fulghum, C.S., Glisson, R.R., and Stranne, S.K., The effect of femoral stem geometry on interface motion in uncemented porous-coated total hip prostheses: comparison of straight-stem and curved-stem designs, *J. Bone Joint Surg.*, 74-A, 839, 1992.

37. Maloney, W.J., Jasty, M., Burke, D.W., et al., Biomechanical and histologic investigation of cemented total hip arthroplasties, *Clin. Orthop.*, 249, 129, 1989.

38. Finkelstein, J.A., Anderson, G.I., Waddell, J.P., et al., A study of micromotion and appositional bone growth to a canine madreporic-surfaced femoral component, *J. Arthroplasty*, 9, 317, 1994.

39. Munting, E. and Verhelpen, M., Fixation and effect on bone strain pattern of a stemless hip prosthesis, *J. Biomech.*, 28, 949, 1995.

40. Berzins, A., Sumner, D.R., Wasielewski, R.C., and Galante, J.O., Impacted particulate allograft for femoral revision total hip arthroplasty: *in vitro* mechanical stability and effects of cement pressurization, *J. Arthroplasty*, 11, 500, 1996.

41. Jasty, M., Krushell, R.J., Zalenski, E., et al., The contribution of the nonporous distal stem to the stability of proximally porous-coated canine femoral components, *J. Arthroplasty*, 8, 33, 1993.

42. Walker, P.S., Schneeweis, D., Murphy, S., and Nelson, P., Strains and micromotion of press-fit femoral stem prostheses, *J. Biomech.*, 20, 693, 1987.

43. Doehring, T.C., Rubash, H.E., Shelley, F.J., et al., Effect of superior and superolateral relocations of the hip center on hip joint forces. An experimental and analytical analysis, *J. Arthroplasty*, 11, 693, 1996.

44. Volz, R.G. and Wilson, R.J., Factors affecting the mechanical stability of the cemented acetabular component in total hip replacement, *J. Bone Joint Surg.*, 59, 501, 1977.

45. Kraemer, W.J., Harrington, I.J., and Hearn, T.C., Micromotion secondary to axial, torsional, and shear loads in two models of cementless tibial components, *J. Arthroplasty*, 10, 227, 1995.

46. Markolf, K.L., Amstutz, H.C., and Hirschowitz, D.L., The effect of calcar contact on femoral component micromovement, *J. Bone Joint Surg.*, 62A, 1315, 1980.

47. Lee, R.W., Volz, R.G., and Sheridan, D.C., The role of fixation and bone quality on the mechanical stability of tibial knee components, *Clin. Orthop.*, 273, 177, 1991.

48. Sugiyama, H., Whiteside, L.A., Engh, C.A., and Otani, T., Late mechanical stability of the proximal coated AML prosthesis, *Orthopedics*, 17, 583, 1994.

49. Sugiyama, H., Whiteside, L.A., and Kaiser, A.D., Examination of rotational fixation of the femoral component in total hip arthroplasty. A mechanical study of micromovement and acoustic emission, *Clin. Orthop.*, 249, 122, 1989.

50. Sugiyama, H., Whiteside, L.A., and Engh, C.A., Torsional fixation of the femoral component in total hip arthroplasty, *Clin. Orthop.*, 275, 187, 1992.

51. Ohl, M.D., Whiteside, L.A., McCarthy, D.S., and White, S.E., Torsional fixation of a modular femoral hip component, *Clin. Orthop.*, 287, 135, 1993.

52. Otani, T., Whiteside, L.A., White, S.E., and McCarthy, D.S., Reaming technique of the femoral diaphysis in cementless total hip arthroplasty, *Clin. Orthop.*, 311, 210, 1995.

53. Channer, M.A., Glisson, R.R., Seaber, A.V., and Vail, T.P., Use of bone compaction in total knee arthroplasty, *J. Arthroplasty*, 11, 743, 1996.

54. Mahomed, N., Schatzker, J., and Hearn, T., Biomechanical analysis of a distally interlocked press-fit femoral total hip prosthesis, *J. Arthroplasty*, 8, 129, 1993.

55. Manley, P.A., Vanderby, R., Kohles, S., et al., Alterations in femoral strain, micromotion, cortical geometry, cortical porosity, and bony ingrowth in uncemented collared and collarless prostheses in the dog, *J. Arthroplasty*, 10, 63, 1995.

56. Fischer, K.J., Carter, D.R., and Maloney, W.J., In *vitro* study of initial stability of a conical collared femoral component, *J. Arthroplasty*, 7 (Suppl.), 389, 1992.

57. Maloney, W.J., Jasty, M., Burke, D.W., et al., Biomechanical and histologic investigation of cemented total hip arthroplasties. A study of autopsy-retrieved femurs after *in vivo* cycling, *Clin. Orthop.*, 249, 129, 1989.

58. Hua, J. and Walker, P.S., Relative motion of hip stems under load. An *in vitro* study of symmetrical, asymmetrical, and custom asymmetrical designs, *J. Bone Joint Surg.*, 76A, 95, 1994.

59. Whiteside, L.A. and Easley, J.C., The effect of collar and distal stem fixation on micromotion of the femoral stem in uncemented total hip arthroplasty, *Clin. Orthop.*, 145, 1989.

60. Otani, T., Whiteside, L.A., White, S.E., and McCarthy, D.S., Effects of femoral component material properties on cementless fixation in total hip arthroplasty, *J. Arthroplasty*, 8, 67, 1993.

61. Whiteside, L.A., White, S.E., Engh, C.A., and Head, W., Mechanical evaluation of cadaver retrieval specimens of cementless bone-ingrown total hip arthroplasty femoral components, *J. Arthroplasty*, 8, 147, 1993.

62. Kaiser, A.D. and Whiteside, L.A., The effect of screws and pegs on the initial fixation stability of an uncemented unicondylar knee replacement, *Clin. Orthop.*, 259, 169, 1990.

63. Branson, P.J., Steege, J.W., Wixson, R.L., et al., Rigidity of initial fixation with uncemented tibial knee implants, *J. Arthroplasty*, 4, 21, 1989.

64. Wyatt, R.W., Alpert, J.P., Daniels, A.U., et al., The effect of screw fixation on initial rigidity of tibial knee components, *J. Appl. Biomater.*, 2, 109, 1991.

65. Shimagaki, H., Bechtold, J.E., Sherman, R.E., and Gustilo, R.B., Stability of initial fixation of the tibial component in cementless total knee arthroplasty, *J. Orthop. Res.*, 8, 64, 1990.

66. Volz, R.G., Nisbet, J.K., Russel, W.L., and McMurtry, M.G., The mechanical stability of various noncemented tibial components, *Clin. Orthop.*, 226, 38, 1988.

67. Kwong, L.M., O'Connor, D.O., Sedlacek, R.C., et al., A quantitative *in vitro* assessment of fit and screw fixation on the stability of a cementless hemispherical acetabular component, *J. Arthroplasty*, 9, 163, 1994.

68. Lachiewicz, P.F., Suh, P.B., and Gilbert, J.A., *In vitro* initial fixation of porous-coated acetabular total hip components. A biomechanical comparative study, *J. Arthroplasty*, 4, 201, 1989.

69. Won, C.H., Hearn, T.C., and Tile, M., Micromotion of cementless hemispherical acetabular components. Does press-fit need adjunctive screw fixation? *J. Bone Joint Surg.*, 77B, 484, 1995.

70. Perona, P.G., Lawrence, J., Paprosky, W.G., et al., Acetabular micromotion as a measure of initial implant stability in primary hip arthroplasty, *J. Arthroplasty*, 7, 537, 1992.

71. Stiehl, J.B., MacMillan, E., and Skrade, D.A., Mechanical stability of porous-coated acetabular components in total hip arthroplasty, *J. Arthroplasty*, 6, 295, 1991.

34   *In Vitro* Testing of the Stability of Acetabular Components

James R. Davis, Robert A. Lofthouse, and Riyaz H. Jinnah

CONTENTS

I. INTRODUCTION

Measurement of acetabular stability is difficult to perform *in vivo*. Every day in the clinical situation, surgeons make a judgment on whether or not an acetabular component is stable. If there is doubt, a number of dome screws may be used in conjunction with the cup. The decision when to insert screws is arbitrary. If asked closely about screw insertion and the rationale behind it, many surgeons will answer that if it feels stable on insertion they will not use screws, but if the position of the cup has to be changed due to initial malpositioning, then screws will be inserted. Many will always use screws and others will select a prosthesis with fins, pegs, spikes, or altered geometries in an attempt to gain increased initial stability. The use of screws in the revision setting is more prevalent, especially when using modified implants such as the oblong or bilobed cups.[1]

The use of cups with dome screw holes has been of concern. Polyethylene will creep through these holes when repetitively loaded and generate wear debris which may induce pelvic osteolysis and lead to premature failure.[2] If correctly placed, the use of screws will increase the initial stability, but they may loosen causing extensive cavitary acetabular defects which can result in a more difficult revision procedure. Screw placement is also not without immediate hazards; in the literature, there are reported cases of vital vessel or organ damage.[3,4] Concerns also arise with respect to screw fretting at the prosthetic interface as this may cause debris generation and promote a histological response resulting in component loosening.[5]

Initial acetabular prosthetic stability is important for optimal biological fixation.[6,7] Figures for the level of micromotion at the cup–bone interface preventing osseointegration and predisposing to fibrous fixation vary between 40 μm and 1 mm.[8-10] Gaps between the prosthesis and bone are theoretically not so problematic; in a canine model with a stable implant–bone environment, gaps of 1.5 mm have been bridged by new bone.[11] The correlation between the canine model and humans is, however, questionable with respect to predicting the osseous response to implants.[12]

Stability from bony ingrowth occurs by the apposition and generation of new bone, which incorporates into pores or surface defects on the acetabular cup surface. The most important factor for providing optimum conditions for this to occur is stability at the bone–prosthesis interface.[7,10,13] This, in conjunction with pore sizes of 200 to 400 μm, availability of cancellous bone, and close proximity of the implant to bone provide the most likely environment for successful integration.[7,13-15] Retrieval studies of porous-surfaced implants have confirmed this.[15-19] Prosthetic designs that pre-load the bone in compression and eliminate tensile and shear loading at the interface are likely to provide the best initial fixation and the correct conditions for bony ingrowth.[20] In animal studies, weight-bearing stresses are important for the stimulation of bony ingrowth into acetabular implants. There is an optimal configuration for these force vectors and, if imbalance exists, they can lead to abnormal micromotion and disruption of early trabecular ingrowth.[21] Other factors influencing the process of ingrowth include porous surface geometry, hydroxyapatite coating, accuracy of press-fit, and implant design.[13,22-24]

The difference in the modulus of elasticity of the acetabular prosthesis and bone at the bone–prosthetic interface will lead to differential strains across the area of the cup. Most uncemented acetabular prostheses are significantly stiffer than the surrounding bone. It has been shown that on axial loading of a press-fit acetabular component without augmentation, more motion is consistently detected at the ilium than the pubis or ischium, respectively. This suggests that the ilium is the least supportive structure contributing to initial stability. Furthermore, the ilium bears the greatest load across the hip joint and gains the majority of its load-bearing capabilities from an intact subchondral bone plate.[25] This reinforces the importance of retaining the subchondral plate when implanting an acetabular component.

Direct measurement of the true motion at the interface is difficult. Most studies rely on detecting movement in a rigid cup–jig construct and assume this reflects the movement at the interface.[9,21,26,27] To measure the motion between cup and subchondral bone the strain gauge would need to be applied directly at the interface. This is not possible, so the closest is to measure the motion between the cup and the bone just behind the subchondral plate. Many authors thus incorporate in their results the deformation at three sites: compression or torque in the prosthesis itself, deformation in cancellous bone, and the true movement at the bone–prosthesis interface. Consideration needs to be given in respect to the changing Young's modulus of cancellous bone; as it is crushed, the lattice structure becomes more compact and therefore stiffer. This deformation may be plastic and not recoverable. If more than one load is applied to the cancellous bone, the subsequent results will include less displacement at this level.[28]

There are reported differences between embalmed and fresh acetabula and their behavior under load. Embalmed specimens display changes in mechanical properties; commonly, the modulus of elasticity of cortical bone is increased and its compressive strength diminished.[21,29] The bone mineral density becomes an important factor when comparisons between pelvises are made. This requires standardization as the extrapolation of stability in pelvises with different densities may not be linear. There are also inherent variations between cadaveric pelvises. To some extent this has been addressed by comparing different implants in the two acetabula of one pelvis (matched pairs). However, this does not address the effect of macroscopic or microscopic individual local acetabular defects.[30]

To overcome the variables in cadaveric bones, comparisons between prostheses can be made by standardizing the material into which the prosthesis is implanted. Many studies have used foam blocks into which the acetabular prosthesis is seated. Comparisons can be made by either varying the implant diameters with the same acetabular prosthesis or maintaining constant cup diameters and comparing different cup designs.[31]

One important comparative parameter that requires consistency is the external diameter of the acetabular components. As the radius becomes greater, the surface area and the linear rim length in contact with bone increase, and this may influence the initial stability, particularly in torsion.[30] To compare a cohort of the same prosthesis, the cup size requires standardization. Problems can arise with preparation of the acetabulum. It is known that acetabula reamed to cancellous bone offer less support to the uncemented press-fit cup than those where the subchondral bone is left intact.[32] Choice of acetabula to test becomes critical, the demographics of normal acetabular size show a large variance and a certain number of pelvises will be unsuitable because the acetabular preparation to accept the same diameter of cup across the experimental cohort will be different. Additionally, those with similar diameters may show disparities in the amount and thickness of the subchondral bone plate remaining after preparation.

Implantation technique is important; the method requires consistency and repeatability and preferably should be performed by the same surgeon.[32,33] The acetabula require reaming accurately to remove remaining hyaline cartilage but to leave the subchondral bone plate, particularly in the acetabular dome, relatively undisturbed. The dome in conjunction with the posterior column offers extremely important means of acetabular stability. The acetabulum acts as a dynamic structure in obtaining stability, which differs from that of a fixed-ring construct. Under load, the dome is compressed while the columns are pushed apart by tensile stresses.[34] Implantation of the cup is critical as bone has inherent viscoelasticity, meaning that the stiffness of bone varies depending on the rate of loading. The faster the load rate, the stiffer and thus more brittle the bone. If a cup is inserted with a heavy blow, macro- or microfractures may be created, weakening the cup bone construct. Conversely, if the cup is not seated properly, the interface may not be optimized.

Testing of the implant–bone construct requires isolating the acetabulum and holding it in such a way that the inherent elasticity of the pelvis is minimized and that the deformation detected will be at the bone-prosthesis interface. This requires mounting, usually in resin, gypsum, or low-melting-point metal. The orientation for each specimen needs to be consistent to eliminate errors. The implant must be tested under the same conditions in a standard manner and determination of the parameters measured must be established prior to the test to prevent cup–bone interface disturbance and, thus, inaccurate data acquisition.

Guidelines for the amount of torque force experienced at the cup–bone interface vary depending on bearing surface, femoral head size, cup radius, and individual patient characteristics.[9] Torsional moments of 6.8 N·m are not uncommon for metal-on-metal bearing surfaces, with polyethylene–metal forces about half of that value. These forces are thought to be the most damaging to the bone–implant interface; their values increase as the static load across the acetabulum increases.[35,36] Compressive forces between prosthetic femoral head and cup have been found to be as high as 4.3 times body weight in the middle-aged man.[36] The strains imparted on the prosthesis bone interface can be presumed to be significantly higher in the young adult.[9] When using an instrumented total hip arthroplasty the forces experienced during passive movements of physical therapy were as high as 50% of body weight, and during protected weight bearing with two crutches forces between 85 and 200% of body weight were observed.[9] The frictional moments experienced by the acetabular prosthesis have been reported to be between 0.4 to 10.8 N·m; these are the baselines on which many trials are founded.[1,37] The importance of initial protected weight bearing is confirmed by studies showing that by increasing the applied static load from 110 to 840 N the frictional torque forces increase by 2.5 to 3.5 times.[38] Increasing the femoral head diameter has a limited effect on the frictional torque forces, progression from 22.5 to 50 mm elevates them by 1.5 times. These forces are magnified when there is no lubrication, which is seen in prolonged weight bearing without movement.[36]

II. VARIOUS METHODS AND PARAMETERS IN THE LITERATURE

A. TORSIONAL STABILITY

A number of studies have measured this variable which was felt to be a reproducible means of assessing acetabular component fixation *in vitro*.[32,33,39] In one study 52-mm porous-coated cups with two pegs were implanted in fresh frozen cadaveric acetabula which had been underreamed by 1, 2, 3, and 4 mm. The cups were implanted at 45° of abduction and 10° of anteversion. Seating of the cup was measured through the dome holes in the cup with a modified depth gauge. No screws were used to augment the initial stability. The acetabula were mounted in resin and tested on a material testing machine (MTS). A ten-sided foil, shaped to fit the metal shells, was machined. To determine the initial stability a compressive load of 686 N was applied perpendicular to the cup rim to simulate loading comparable to a 70-kg human. A torque of 6.8 N·m (within physiological limits) was applied to the cup as a triangular wave over 3 s for five cycles. The angular deformation was then measured. Second, a 100-N·m force was applied over a 0.5-s ramp and the moments required to produce 1°, 2°, and 20° of rotation of the prosthesis in the bone were recorded.[26] Measurement of the displacement was achieved through the actuator attached to the MTS. This assumes that the acetabulum–pelvis-resin mount does not move in relation to the cup and that the deformation is occurring only at the bone–prosthesis interface.

A second study compared the porous-coated two-pegged cup to a porous-coated cup with screw holes. The cups were implanted using the manufacturer's guidelines into one pelvis. This was repeated five times in five fresh-frozen cadaver pelvises. The authors used meticulous care to spare the subchondral bone. A prosthesis of the same final diameter as the final reamer used was implanted. Three screws were used to fix the second cup. The same surgeon implanted all prostheses. The hemipelvises were then embedded into epoxy resin blocks known to have negligible torsional instability. A four-pronged removable jig was constructed from two orthogonally placed stainless steel pins locked into a hemispherically surfaced aluminum block. The pins were placed in predrilled slots on the implanted acetabular prostheses after mounting on the MTS (Figure 34.1).

The loading cycle consisted of an axial 686-N force directed medially with a 6.8-N·m moment applied in both directions over 1.5 s for five cycles. The resultant angular deformation was then measured. The construct was then tested to failure over a 0.5-s period with 100 N·m moment.

Failure was defined as 20° of rotation of the prosthesis within the pelvis.[31] This was determined to be an excessive level and a failure limit of 2° was adopted which approximates to 1-mm linear displacement.[9]

Again the degree of movement that is taken to cause failure of optimum fixation is too great, as the displacement is being measured indirectly by assuming that the acetabulum remains stationary

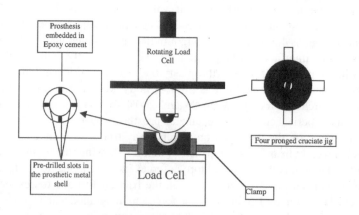

FIGURE 34.1   Testing configuration for measurement of torsional stability.

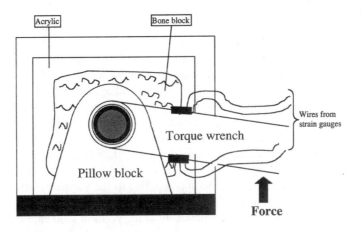

FIGURE 34.2 Testing in torque. A strain gauge instrumented torque wrench is mounted to the acetabular prosthesis. A 1.25-cm bolt was passed through the pillow block after attachment to the strain gauge. Load was delivered to the torque wrench by the MTS.

while the cup rotates within it. This is not measuring the motion at the interface but is giving a relative value. If the specimens are mounted in the same way and the pelvises are all matched, then the errors are limited. The study was performed with matched pairs standardizing the variables to some degree. Direct medial axial compression does not simulate the direction of physiological load bearing *in vivo*. There is no mention of the torsional stiffness of the jig used to impart the moment to the cup or its fit within the machined slots; these could be sources of error.

The third study of torsional stability investigated the stability of three component designs, one with dome screws, one with three-spike fixation, and the third with two-peg fixation. Six of each were implanted into 8 fresh-frozen and 12 embalmed cadaveric acetabula. All prostheses were implanted in accordance with the manufacturer's guidelines by one surgeon. An anteroposterial (AP) radiograph of each pelvis was then taken and the acetabula removed from the pelvis, potted in acrylic resin and placed on the testing frame. Each liner was drilled and two screws were used to secure the polyethylene to the outer shell. The liner was then drilled and tapped to accept a torque wrench. The torque wrench was instrumented with four strain gauges and secured to the liner with four screws. A 1.25-cm steel rod was screwed to the torque wrench at its center of rotation and passed through a pillow block, which was bolted to the test frame. Load was delivered at 4.06 cm/min over a 25° arc with a moment arm of 25 cm. The load curve had reached a plateau by the end of each arc[28] (Figure 34.2).

One must not forget the stability issues of cemented prostheses whose problem is not so much the initial but the long-term stability. However, comparative studies of torsion have been done between autopsy retrieval specimens and cups cemented into cadaveric pelvises. In one such study Charnley cups were cemented into 11 cadaveric acetabula. The acetabula were prepared with a hemispherical reamer preserving the subchondral bone plate. Ten holes were then drilled with a diameter of 4 and 10 mm deep and the cups were implanted after cement pressurization. Eight holes were drilled in the periphery of the cup to accept a holder through which torque could be imparted to the specimen. The acetabula were mounted in a cubiform mount. A torque force was applied to the cup by means of an AC motor revolving at an angular velocity of 2.12°/s. The forces were recorded a load cell. Instability was defined as the point at which the torque–displacement curve reached a plateau.[40]

B. OFFSET CUP LOADING

This form of loading is thought to be a more stringent test of initial fixation than axial load or torsion.[7] This mechanism tests the resistance of the interface to shear loads. In one study, metal-backed acetabular cups were implanted into a dense, homogeneous, isotropic closed-cell polyethylene foam. The compressive modulus and Poisson's ratio of this were within the range for cancellous bone.[29,41-45] A 54-mm hemispherical socket was reamed and debris removed with compressed air. A custom jig and centering hole were employed to assure consistency of implantation. Five different cup designs were tested, three with external threads, one with four external fins, and a press-fit design. The finned cup was tested in two ways, loading over one fin, then loading between fins. The press-fit cup was loaded in three ways; with no screws, with three dome screws, and finally with three peripheral screws. For each trial a new polyethylene block was used.

The threaded cups were inserted using the rotary capabilities of the MTS with minimal axial compression. The cups were inserted to a final torque of 125 N·m. Press-fit cups were slowly lowered until fully seated.

The cups were then tested with an axial load applied to the periphery of the cup until shear failure. A load of 0 to 2000 N applied over a 3-min period producing a torsional moment of 54 N·m was used. Displacement was measured continuously at the point of load application by the MTS. Each cup was tested in seven freshly prepared polyethylene blocks with a minimum of five repetitions of the loading cycle to each specimen.[31]

In a second study six different 56-mm cups were seated in artificial bone blocks according to the manufacturer's guidelines. A radiograph was then obtained to confirm seating of each component and an offset load applied to the rim of the cup until failure.[46]

Studies in prosthetic bones can only at best give relative values of stability. Screw placement not only depends on the position within the cup but the quality of the surrounding bone. One can standardize for position in this model but it is not applicable to the clinical situation. Displacement measured at the point of load application will give very rough values of the actual interface displacement as it is purely a two-dimensional measure. The prosthetic bone will, however, have the same characteristics between samples. One concern is that the cups have different geometries and will occupy a different volume in the same-sized block of prosthetic material, thus compromising the standard behavior of the material. Important information can be gained by testing in the prosthetic bone model; however, as already discussed, bone is a heterogeneous, anisotropic material and behaves differently from homogeneous substitutes.

C. Axial Loading in a Superioposteriomedial Direction 30° to the Plane of Cup Rim, Adduction Torsion

In this experiment, 12 fresh-frozen cadaver pelvises were obtained; each hemipelvis was mounted in low-melting-point metal with the acetabula parallel to the horizontal plane. The acetabula were then reamed to subchondral bone level, a trial implant was then implanted to assess fit, and if the fit was not uniform the cavity was re-reamed. A component with a 2-mm peripheral flare was implanted. The size of the flare was 2 mm greater than the last reamer used. Three titanium screws were inserted in a triangular configuration either centrally or at the rim of the prosthesis. The rim screws were cortical and the dome screws cancellous. The screws were tightened and, if any stripped, a supplementary screw was repositioned and tightened with a torque wrench to 5 in.-lb. Six linear variable differential transformers (LVDT) were attached between the bone and the rim of the implant. The same individual placed each LVDT, in reference to anatomical landmarks. Each transformer was capable of resolution to 1 μm. The implants were tested in axial load to 500 N and then 1000 N in a superioposteriomedial direction at 30° to the plane of the rim of the implant. The axial load was applied through a 28-mm femoral head. The implant was then tested in adduction torsion from 1.1 to − 1.1 N·m and 22.2 to −22.2 Nm. One of two different acetabular defects was then created; either 50% of the acetabular rim (peripheral) or 50% of the dome of the acetabulum (central), using an osteotome and oscillating saw. The size of the defect was recorded by lining the acetabulum with pressure-sensitive film both before and after the defect had been created. Cups were then implanted into the defective acetabula; the cups implanted into the acetabula with peripheral defects were secured with central screws and those with central defects with peripheral screws. The acetabula were all rotated by 30° to allow the screws to gain purchase in fresh bone. The specimens were then tested as before.

Each acetabulum was used for these experiments: rim and center screws in intact acetabulum, either rim or central screws with a created defect. The order of screw placement, either central or peripheral, was reversed in each specimen.

The effect of larger acetabular cups were then assessed by reaming the acetabulum to 66, 72, and 78 mm. Bone apposition was determined with pressure-sensitive film.

The bone mineral density was determined in all specimens.

In order to simplify data collection the data from the LVDT showing the greatest displacement were analyzed. For comparison of torsion the most distal transducer was used and for axial load the most proximal. The torque or axial load that produced 50 μm of motion and the maximal implant motion were used for comparison. The screw torques for each specimen were added together.[30]

The preparation of test specimens in this study appears to be meticulous. The number of tests performed on a single specimen is excessive. The axial load is smaller than that expected in clinical practice. Torsion studies were performed after axial loading; it is unlikely that the values gained in the torsional experiment would be similar if this part had been performed first. It is difficult then to create a defect in the acetabula that is consistent within the test group. Retesting the acetabula with defects by rotating the cup through 30° to achieve screw purchase in fresh bone is difficult. There is no way of knowing that the screw is not crossing a previous tract and thus will offer less support than in fresh bone. Prior testing has also already compromised the remaining acetabular surface and the values for stability are likely to be lower than those in a fresh specimen. This method of testing, however, gives a more realistic picture of what a surgeon might face in the clinical environment.

D. AXIAL LOAD ORIENTATED AT 12° OF FLEXION AND 21° OF ADDUCTION

Eight fresh frozen and 12 embalmed cadaver pelvises were randomly distributed into three test groups. Three acetabular prosthesis were tested; one with dome screws, one with three-spike fixation, and the third with two-peg fixation. Six of each type of prosthesis were implanted according to the manufacturer's guidelines. The acetabula were removed and potted in acrylic resin. The construct was then placed in the MTS and oriented so that the resultant force would act at 12° of flexion and 21° of adduction of the femur. This is the orientation achieved during postoperative partial weight bearing with ambulatory supports.[47] Load was applied to the construct via the appropriately sized femoral head at a rate of 2.44 mm/min until a resultant load of 100 kg was reached. Motion was sensed by a strain gauge transducer mounted between two 1.5-mm threaded rods 13 mm apart and implanted either side of the prosthetis–bone interface. The transducer consisted of a 0.25-mm-thick and 5.5-mm-wide strip of brass bent into a rectangle. A gap of 4 mm was present at the free end of the rectangle. Four foil-type strain gauges were mounted to the transducer and connected in a Wheatstone bridge configuration. The transducer was calibrated by attaching two similar rods to the MTS and advancing the actuator at 0.001 in. and the resolution of the system determined at 10 μm (Figure 34.3).[28]

There is no information given on the diameters of prosthesis implanted and these may vary both within and between the study cohorts. The selected load of 100 kg represents about 1.4 times body weight and the predicted partial weight-bearing values are between 0.5 to two times body weight.[36,43] The values obtained for motion again are not pure interface values and reflect both compression of the prosthesis but also that of subchondral cancellous bone. The measurement was only recorded in one direction and may be misleading. Theoretically, six degrees of freedom with rotation about three perpendicular axes and translation along these could be present. No mention is made of whether the acetabula were matched pairs and it is difficult to compare embalmed with fresh-frozen pelvises because of their mechanical differences.

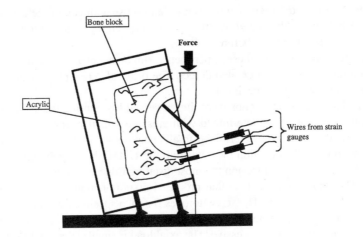

FIGURE 34.3   Testing under physiological load.

E. Axial Load Orientated at 10° of Flexion and 15° of Adduction

Three fresh cadaver pelvises were harvested. High-contrast radiographs were taken in five projections: AP, iliac oblique, obturator oblique, pelvic inlet, and outlet. This ruled out any underlying skeletal disease. The AP projection was used as a template for the correct acetabular component size. The hemipelvises were then mounted by the iliac crests in polymethylmethacrylate. Each acetabulum was under-reamed by 2 mm, preserving 50% of the subchondral bone plate and the cups were implanted at 45° of abduction and 20° of anteversion. An acetabular impactor and mallet were used to seat the prostheses. Prior to implantation the cups were modified slightly; the polar screw hole at the apex of the dome and one peripheral screw hole were bored and threaded. Threaded metal pins were then screwed into place and passed through overdrilled holes in the pelvis. The dome pin passed through the medial wall and the peripheral screw through the posterior wall of the acetabulum. Cylindrical brass platforms were then placed around each motion pin and attached to the bone with epoxy-cement; these platforms served as a reference point against which movement of the pins could be measured. Extensometers were used to assess the relative movement between pin and platform (Figure 34.4). Motion of the implant was measured in three planes under simulated stance loads: anteroposterior tilt, representing move-

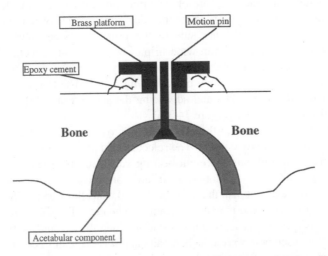

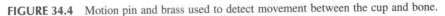

FIGURE 34.4   Motion pin and brass used to detect movement between the cup and bone.

ment in anteversion and retroversion; lateral tilt, representing movement in abduction-adduction plane; and axial motion, representing movement parallel to the motion of the axis of the micromotion pin. Assessment of seating of the component was carried out in two ways: (1) visualization of the contact through the screw holes and (2) 5-mm disks of pressure-sensitive film were placed at multiple sites in the acetabulum prior to implantation. Five standard radiographic projections were taken. The specimens were then mounted in the loading jig oriented in the position of single-legged stance with 15° of abduction and 10° of forward flexion relative to the vertically directed load. A load of 200 lb resulting in a joint reaction force of approximately 250 lb was applied with an appropriately sized femoral head. The relative motion of the prosthesis in relation to the bone was assessed. The cups were then secured with four 6.5-mm cancellous screws, two in the vertical position, one in the resultant position, and one in an anteriosuperior direction. All screws were tightened to a torque of 12 in.-lb. A second set of radiographic projections was taken to assess cup position. When measurements with four screws had been made, the screws were successively removed to give values for three, two, and one screw. After testing was complete, the acetabular component was removed and reamed to give a 1-mm press-fit and then 0 mm of discrepancy. The experimental procedure was repeated.[49]

Errors are inherent in the results obtained with this testing regime. Implantation of pressure-sensitive film will to some degree compromise the fixation, particularly in the press-fit cups. Some problems are encountered when performing multiple experiments on one specimen, as not only will the screw holes alter the performance of the acetabular prosthetic interface but re-reaming the same acetabulum will give results that are likely to be different from those achieved in a fresh specimen. Initially, 50% of the subchondral bone plate was preserved. After reaming to leave no discrepancy between cup and acetabulum it is likely that very little would be left, altering the mechanical properties significantly. One may assume from the methodology that as the AP radiograph was used as a template for the correct size of prosthesis that the component size may not be the same between the pelvises. The measurement apparatus is ingenious but again is not measuring the deformation purely at the bone–prosthesis interface but also the deformation of the prosthesis and subchondral cancellous bone.

F. Axial Load with the Pelvis Orientated in the Anatomical Position

In this experiment, 11 fresh-frozen cadaver pelvises were selected and the acetabula evaluated to remove those with fractures or lesions. The posterior aspect of each pelvis was mounted in gypsum dental stone to minimize rigid-body motion during loading. The acetabula were then reamed to the medial pelvic wall with size-matched reamers and debris cleared with pressurized water. Three types of acetabular prosthesis were implanted: (1) a porous-coated titanium press-fit hemispherical cup; (2) a porous-coated titanium cup with dome screws; and (3) a porous-coated titanium cup with three spikes. For comparison a cemented metal-backed prosthesis was also tested. The cups were implanted in accordance with the manufacturer's guidelines. To gain consistency with positioning a preangled rod was used to place the cups in 40° abduction and 15° anteversion. Seating was obtained with a soft mallet. The specimens were then mounted on the MTS and a 32-mm femoral head with a 125° neck–shaft angle was seated in the acetabulum in anatomical orientation. The first four pelvises tested incorporated pressure-sensitive film at the bone–prosthesis interface to verify the position of load application. Three 1.5 × 1.5 cm aluminum blocks were secured to the periacetabular bone with small Kirschner wires and cement. Eddy current transducers were used to measure the movement of the cup rim relative to these plates. The sensitivity of these transducers was 1 μm. The first transducer was placed slightly posterior to the ilium and the remaining two staggered by 120° (Figure 34.5).

Five cycles of axial load of 0 to 2354 N at crosshead speed of 10 to 20 mm/min was selected to seat the prosthesis initially, followed by three consecutive trials from 0 to 2354 N at a crosshead speed of 0.5 mm/min increasing in 392-N increments. The prosthesis was then augmented in the

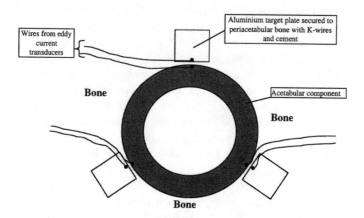

FIGURE 34.5   Transducers plates in the ilium, publis, and ischium.

same sample with one, then two 4.5-mm screws. The experimental procedure was then repeated. Each type of testing was carried out on the same acetabulum.[36]

The experiments appear to utilize the same acetabulum for each test, so here again the mechanical behavior of the bone will change once it has been loaded in the first experiment. It is difficult then to compare the results of one- and two-screw fixation accurately in the same sample. The screws were tightened until "snug"; there is a wide variation in the torque that is imparted to screws and the security in bone is reliant on this. Once the prosthesis has been tested, there is no doubt that the purchase of the screw will have changed. There is great difficulty in measuring the movement at the interface. This form of data collection has the same inherent errors as previously discussed. Implantation of pressure-sensitive film will also affect the interface performance.

G. Repetitive 100,000 Cycle Axial Loading in Full Extension, Load to Failure in Same Orientation

In this experiment, 33 embalmed cadaver hemipelvises were mounted in gypsum dye stone to a neutral frame. Five different types of porous-coated acetabular components were selected for testing, 1-mm press-fit, 1-mm press-fit with peg fixation, 1-mm press-fit with screw fixation, line-to-line press-fit with screw fixation, and 1.5-mm peripheral expansion press-fit. Each prosthesis was implanted in accordance with the manufacturer's guidelines. Micromotion and subsidence of the cup were measured three dimensionally by six LVDTs accurate to 3 μm. Two aluminum blocks were mounted to the anteriomedial and posteriolateral metal rim of each cup. Six LVDTs were attached to the cup with two cube transducer holders. The LVDTs were fixed perpendicular to the three sides of the block to determine three-dimensional movement (Figure 34.6). The construct was then placed on the MTS and loaded with the hip in full extension. The specimens were loaded with a sinusoidal profile from a preload of 10 kg to a peak of 100 kg at 5 Hz for 100,000 repetitions. At the completion of this loading cycle static load-to-failure analysis was repeated at successive loads of 150, 200, 250, and 300 kg. Five cycles at each increment were performed until gross motion was detected.[21]

This study uses a sophisticated method of three-dimensional cup movement. However, again it is not measuring the interface displacement directly, but is testing only one parameter in each sample. The peak load is slightly lower than those predicted postoperatively and the loading is performed in extension, which is an unlikely position.

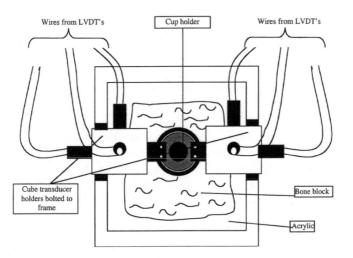

Wires from LVDT's   Cup holder   Wires from LVDT's

Cube transducer
holders bolted to
frame

Bone block

Acrylic

FIGURE 34.6   Setup for three-dimensional displacement detection.

H. FINITE-ELEMENT ANALYSIS TO CALCULATE ACETABULAR DEFORMATION

Acetabular strain distribution was studied using finite-element analysis (FEA) applied to different cup designs: 1- and 2-mm oversized hemispherical cups, an elliptical shape, a dual-radius geometry, a cup with a hemispherical dome and a wider outer cup diameter, and a cup with low-profile geometry. The magnitude and distribution of acetabular strains were assessed with an axisymmetric finite-element model. The shape of the bone section was based on the geometry described by Pedersen et al.[50] The cup was fixed by the ilium and was displaced toward the center of the dome until contact occurred at the medial wall of the acetabulum. The acetabular notch was not included. This increases the rigidity of the acetabulum; to compensate, the modulus of elasticity of cortical bone was reduced over that used in two-dimensional FEA.[34] A five-stage linear transition from the cortical rim to the subchondral bone was added. The Poisson's ratio was set at 0.3. The finite-element mesh was created with I-DEAS (version V.I, Structural Dynamics Research, Milford, OH) and solved using ABAQUS (version 5.4-1, Hibbitt, Karlsson, and Sorensen, Pawtucket, RI). The acetabular prosthesis was modeled as rigid and the coefficient of friction between bone and cup set at 0.15. Higher values for this have been previously reported.[51] Increasing the frictional coefficient led to incomplete seating of the cup in this model. Overall acetabular deformation was determined by calculating the strain energy absorbed by the finite model. Strain energy is the recoverable work due to deformation.[2]

As acetabular strains were calculated in a finite-element model the values obtained might not be those seen *in vivo*. It does, however, compare the differences in the geometries of each cup under stringent conditions. The main problem is that it cannot measure the initial stability of the bone–prosthetic interface.

I. PULLOUT FORCE

Aluminum models of the five-cup geometries in the previous section were machined. The models were coated with glass beads with no porous coating in order to assess the effect of the geometric differences. Each prosthesis was implanted into foam bones after reaming on a drill press which produced consistent hemispherical shapes. A rod was threaded into the center of each cup and mounted on the MTS. A gradually increasing tensile force was then applied to the rod until failure.[2] The results obtained cannot be directly translated to the clinical situation but it isolates the cup geometries as the only variable. The method of failure is not physiological unless a constrained acetabular liner were to be implanted.

III. CONCLUSION

There is no fault-free method of testing the stability of the acetabular cup. None of the published methods can measure the micromotion at the prosthesis–bone interface directly. All rely on indirect methods. It is noticeable in the literature that authors have become aware of this and are employing many varieties of strain gauges and configurations to record values for micromovement. Methodology does require elimination of variables by using consistent techniques of both implantation and testing. It is tempting to test more than one parameter on one acetabulum. It is imperative that testing conditions and design are standardized, as by doing this comparisons between centers and thus different prostheses can be made, which at the moment is difficult because of the wide variety of parameters measured. If a single test method were adopted, results could become more consistent and thus accurate. The authors feel that torsional stability is the most important parameter and therefore test this at their institution.

REFERENCES

1. Cameron, H.U., Modified cups, *Orthop. Clin. North Am.*, 29, 277, 1998.
2. Ries, M.D., Harbaugh, M., Shea, J., and Lambert, R., Effect of cementless acetabular cup on strain distribution and press fit stability, *J. Arthroplasty*, 12, 207, 1997.
3. Keating, E.M., Ritter, M.A., and Faris, P.M., Structures at risk from medially placed acetabular screws, *J. Bone Joint Surg.*, 72A, 509, 1990.
4. Zalenski, E., Jasty, M., Page, A., et al., Micromotion of porous-surfaced, cementless prosthesis following 6 months of *in vivo* bone growth in a canine model, presented at *The 35th Annual Meeting of the Orthopaedic Research Society,* Las Vegas, NV, February 6–9, 1989.
5. Letournel, E., Failures of biologically fixed devices: causes and treatment, in *The Hip, Proceedings of the 14th Open Scientific Meeting of the Hip Society,* Mosby, St. Louis, MO, 1987, 318.
6. Gallante, J.O., Overview of current attempts to eliminate methyl methacrylate, in *The Hip, Proceedings of the 11th Open Scientific Meeting of the Hip Society,* Mosby, St. Louis, MO, 1984, 181.
7. Pilliar, R.M., Bony ingrowth into porous metal coated implants, *Orthop. Rev.*, 9, 85, 1980.
8. Burke, D.W., Bragdon, C.R., O'Connor, D.O., et al., Dynamic measurement of interface mechanics *in vivo* and the effect of micromotion on bone ingrowth into a porous surface device under controlled loads *in vivo*, *Orthop. Res. Soc. Trans.*, 16, 103, 1991.
9. Clarke, H.J., Jinnah, R.H., Warden, K.E., et al., Evaluation of acetabular stability in uncemented prostheses, *J. Arthroplasty*, 6, 335, 1991.
10. Pilliar, R.M., Lee, J.M., and Maniatopoulos, C., Observations on the effect of movement on bone growth into porous-surfaced implants, *Clin. Orthop.*, 208, 108, 1986.
11. Haddad, R.J., Cook, S.D., and Thomas, K.A., Biological fixation of porous-coated implants: current concepts review, *J. Bone Joint Surg.*, 69A, 1459, 1987.
12. Phillips, T.W., Johnston, G., and Wood, P., Selection of an animal model for resurfacing hip arthroplasty, *J. Arthroplasty*, 2, 111, 1987.
13. Cameron, H.U., Pilliar, R.M., and McNab, I., The effect of movement on the bonding of porous metal to bone, *J. Biomed. Mater. Res.*, 7, 301, 1973.
14. Bobyn, J.D., Pilliar, R.M., Cameron, H.U., and Weatherly, G.C., The optimum pore size for the fixation of porous surfaced metal implants by ingrowth of bone, *Clin. Orthop.*, 150, 263, 1980.
15. Pilliar, R.M., Powder metal-made orthopaedic implants with porous surface for fixation by tissue ingrowth, *Clin. Orthop.*, 176, 42, 1983.
16. Bobyn, J.D., Pilliar, R.M., Cameron, H.U., and Weatherly, G.C., Osteogenic phenomena across endosteal bone implant spaces with porous surfaced intramedullary implants, *Acta Orthop. Scand.*, 52, 145, 1981.
17. Cook, S.D., Barrack, R.L., Thomas, K.A., and Haddad, R.J., Quantitative analysis of tissue growth into human porous total hip components, *J. Arthroplasty*, 3, 249, 1988.
18. Cook, S.D., Renz, E.A., Barrack, R.L., et al., Clinical and metallurgical analysis of retrieved internal fixation devices, *Clin. Orthop.*, 194, 236, 1985.

19. Cook, S.D., Thomas, K.A., and Haddad, R.J., Jr., Histologic analysis of retrieved human porous-coated total joint components, *Clin. Orthop.*, 234, 90, 1988.
20. Bobyn, J.D., Pilliar, R.M., Cameron, H.U., et al., The effects of porous surface configuration on the tensile strength of fixation of implants by bony ingrowth, *Clin. Orthop.*, 149, 291, 1980.
21. Stiehl, J.B., MacMillan, E., and Skrade, D.A., Mechanical stability of porous-coated acetabular components in total hip arthroplasty, *J. Arthroplasty*, 6, 295, 1991.
22. Hedly, A.K., Kabo, N., Kim, W., et al., Bone ingrowth fixation of a newly designed acetabular component in a canine model, *Clin. Orthop.*, 176, 12, 1983.
23. Jasty, M. and Harris W.H., Observation on factors controlling bony ingrowth into weight-bearing porous canine total hip replacement, in *Non-Cemented Total Hip Arthroplasty*, Fitzgerald, R., Ed., Raven Press, New York, 1988.
24. Pilliar, R.M., Cameron, H.U., Welsh, R.P., and Binnington, A.G., Radiographic and morphologic studies of load-bearing porous surface structural implants, *Clin. Orthop.*, 156, 249, 1981.
25. Bourne, R.B., Finlay, J.B., Rorabeck, C.H., and Landsberg, R.P., The effect of endoprosthetic mismatch and metal or non-metal-backed acetabular components on *in vitro* pelvic stresses, in *The Hip, Proceedings of the 13th Open Scientific Meeting of the Hip Society*, Mosby, St. Louis, 1985, 114.
26. Curtis, M.J., Jinnah, R.H., Wilson, V.D., and Hungerford, D.S., The initial stability of uncemented acetabular components, *J. Bone Joint Surg.*, 74B, 372, 1992.
27. Perona, P.G., Lawrence, J., Paprosky, W.G., et al., Acetabular micromotion as a measure of initial implant stability in primary hip arthroplasty, *J. Arthroplasty*, 7, 537, 1992.
28. Lachiewicz, P.F., Suh, P.B., and Gilbert, J.A., in *vitro* initial fixation of porous-coated acetabular total hip components a biomechanical comparative study, *J. Arthroplasty*, 4, 201, 1989.
29. Evans, F.G., *Mechanical Properties of Bone*, Charles C Thomas, Springfield, IL, 1972.
30. Hadjari, M.H., Hollis, J.M., Hoffman, O.E., et al., Initial stability of porous coated acetabular implants, *Clin. Orthop.*, 307, 117, 1994.
31. Litsky, A.S. and Pophal, S.G., Initial mechanical stability of acetabular prostheses, *Orthopedics*, 17, 53, 1994.
32. Andersson, G.B., Freeman, M.A., and Swanson, S.A., Loosening of the cemented acetabular cup in total hip replacement, *J. Bone Joint Surg.*, 54B, 590, 1972.
33. Oh, I., A comprehensive analysis of the factors affecting acetabular cup fixation and design in total hip replacement arthroplasty: a series of experimental and clinical studies, in *The Hip, Proceedings of the 11th Open Scientific Meeting of the Hip Society*, Mosby, St. Louis, MO, 1984, 129.
34. Vasu, R., Carter, D.R., and Harris, W.H., Stress distribution in the acetabular region: I. Before and after total joint replacement, *J. Biomech.*, 15, 155, 1982.
35. Rydell, N.P., Forces acting on the femoral head-prosthesis: a study on strain gauge supplied prosthesis in living persons, *Acta Orthop. Scand.*, 37(Suppl.) 88, 1966.
36. Simon, S.R., Paul, I.L., Rose, R.M., and Radin, E.L., "Stiction friction" of total hip prostheses and its relationship to loosening, *J. Bone Joint Surg.*, 57A, 226, 1975.
37. Wilson, J.N. and Scales, J.T., Loosening of total hip replacements with cement fixation, *Clin. Orthop.*, 72, 145, 1970.
38. Ma, S.M., Kabo, J.M., and Amstutz, H.C., Frictional torque in surface and conventional hip replacement, *J. Bone Joint Surg.*, 65A, 366, 1985.
39. Volz, R.G. and Wilson, R.J., Factors affecting the mechanical stability of the cemented acetabular component in total hip replacement, *J. Bone Joint Surg.*, 59A, 501, 1977.
40. Ohlin, A. and Balkfors, B., Stability of cemented sockets after 3–14 years, *J. Arthroplasty*, 7, 87, 1992.
41. Brown, T.D. and Ferguson, A.B., Jr., Mechanical property distributions in the cancellous bone of the human proximal femur, *Acta Orthop. Scand.*, 51, 429, 1980.
42. Carter, D.R. and Hayes, W.C., The compressive behavior of bone as a two phase porous structure, *J. Bone Joint Surg.*, 59, 954, 1977.
43. Lindahl, O., Mechanical properties of dried defatted spongy bone, *Acta Orthop. Scand.*, 47, 11, 1976.
44. McElhaney, J.H. and Byars, E.F., Dynamic response of biologic materials, American Society of Mechanical Engineers, Publ. 65-WA/HUF 9, 1, 1965.
45. Van Audekercke, R. and Martens, M., Mechanical properties of cancellous bone, in *Natural and Living Biomaterials*, Hastings, G.W. and Ducheyne, P., Eds., CRC Press, Boca Raton, FL, 1984, 89.

46. Bear, B., Bostrom, M., and Sculco, T., Press fit acetabular cups, an evaluation of initial torsional stability, *AAOS Scientific Exhibit,* San Francisco, CA, 1997.

47. Engh, C.A., Bobyn, J.D., and Matthews, J.G., III, Biologic fixation of a modified Moore prosthesis, in *The Hip, Proceedings of the 11th Open Meeting of the Hip Society,* Mosby, St. Louis, MO, 1984, 95.

48. Bergmann, G., Rohlmann, A., and Graichen, F., Hip joint forces during physical therapy after joint replacement, *Orthop. Trans.,* 14, 303, 1990.

49. Kwong, L.W., O'Connor, D.O., Sedlacek, R.C., et al., A quantitative *in vitro* assessment of fit and screw fixation on the stability of a cementless hemispherical acetabular component, *J. Arthroplasty,* 9, 163, 1994.

50. Pedersen, D.R., Crowninsheild, R.D., Brand, R.A., and Johnston, R.C., An axisymmetric model of acetabular components in total hip arthroplasty, *J. Biomech.,* 15, 305, 1982.

51. Shirazi-Adl, A., Dammak M., and Paiement G., Experimental determination of friction characteristics at the trabecular bone/porous-coated metal interface in cementless implants, *J. Biomed. Mater. Res.,* 27, 167, 1993.

35 *In Vitro* Testing of the Stability of Femoral Components

Sanjiv H. Naidu, Fadi M. Khoury, and John M. Cuckler

CONTENTS

I. INTRODUCTION

The success of a cementless femoral component during *in vivo* service is a direct function of osseointegration. Initial stability of cementless femoral devices is paramount for biological ingrowth leading to mechanical fixation.[1] A universal conclusion of clinical experiences with cementless fixation is that immediate stable fixation is fundamental to a successful hip arthroplasty.[2,3]

Primary fixation of a femoral stem is accomplished by surgical preparation of the bone cavity to optimally fit the implant. Impaction of the femoral stem during implantation leads to a press-fit between the implant and the bone interface; the intention is to create an interface with minimal relative motion, a condition crucial to the permanent fixation of the implant stem with the bone. If such a primary condition of minimal relative motion is met, secondary fixation with bone ingrowth will follow, ensuring a successful outcome. Burke and associates[4] showed that rotational moments caused by out-of-plane forces sustained in activities such as stair climbing cause interface slippage of an order of magnitude greater than coronal, in-plane loading. Cook[5] concluded that lack of proximal fit and poor bone quality significantly increased the magnitude of stem micromotion when torsional moment was applied.

It has long been recognized that relative motions of human joints involve six degrees of freedom.[6] The following setup provides for rigorous measurement of micromotion in three dimensions: translations measured along and rotations are measured about the three axes, accounting for all six degrees of freedom of the femoral stem motion relative to the femur. A modular femoral stem with metaphyseal augmentation pads and distal cylindrical sleeves was used to vary the proximal and distal canal fill in composite femurs. The modular system allows one to vary the proximal and distal fit/fill values reliably; by further adding consistency in bony anatomy and material properties, the following experimental setup with composite bones clearly delineates the role of canal fit and fill on the initial stability of femoral stems.

0-8493-0266-9/00/$0.00+$.50

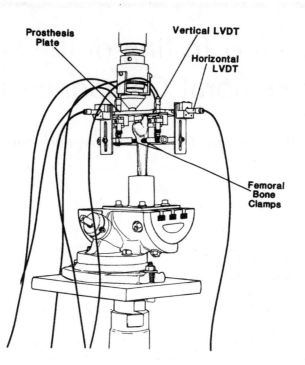

FIGURE 35.1 Experimental apparatus for evaluating the initial stability of a cementless femoral stem in anatomically consistent composite bones. The prosthesis plate is fixed to the prosthetic head. The femoral bone clamps affix the bottom plate to the femur. LVDTs attached to the two plates measure the relative motion between the prosthesis and bone. (From Naidu, S.H. et al., *Am. J. Orthop.,* 25, 829, 1996. With permission).

II. METHODS

A. MATERIALS AND METHODS

Test fixtures that will attach to the femur and prosthesis were designed to permit the measurement of the micromotion of the prosthesis relative to the femur. The test fixtures consist of several parts that, when fastened to the femur and the prosthetic femoral head, enable the calculation of the motion of the prosthesis relative to the femur at a critical location, namely, the prosthetic center and the bone interface. Six linear variable displacement transducers (LVDTs) were positioned as shown in Figure 35.1 (RDP Electronics, Phoenixville, PA). The following will describe the manner in which the test fixtures are assembled together for data acquisition.

The plate that attaches to the femoral head is formed by fastening, with two screws, the two "half plates" illustrated in Figure 35.2A. Both half plates were designed and machined such that the cavity that forms when both plates are fastened together has the exact geometric conformation of the femoral head. This will allow a very rigid connection of the top plate around the prosthetic head.

The bottom plate shown in Figure 35.2B fastens to the femur via long screws that all meet at the midpoint of the plate. This midpoint coincides with both the axis of the implanted prosthesis and the midpoint of the top plate. Gauges 5 and 6, of the six LVDTs, are fastened vertically at the top plate such that the gauges are in contact with the upper surface of the bottom plate. The top and bottom plates are aligned by two long screws to ensure that the plates are parallel in assembly.

The plate in Figure 35.2C fastens vertically to the medial edge of the bottom plate such that the midpoint between gauges 1 and 2 is aligned with the horizontal plane bisecting the top plate. The plate in Figure 35.2D mounts vertically onto the medial edge of the top plate. Gauges 1 and 2 are fastened to the plate in Figure 35.2C such that they are inferior and superior to the horizontal bisecting plane of the top plate.

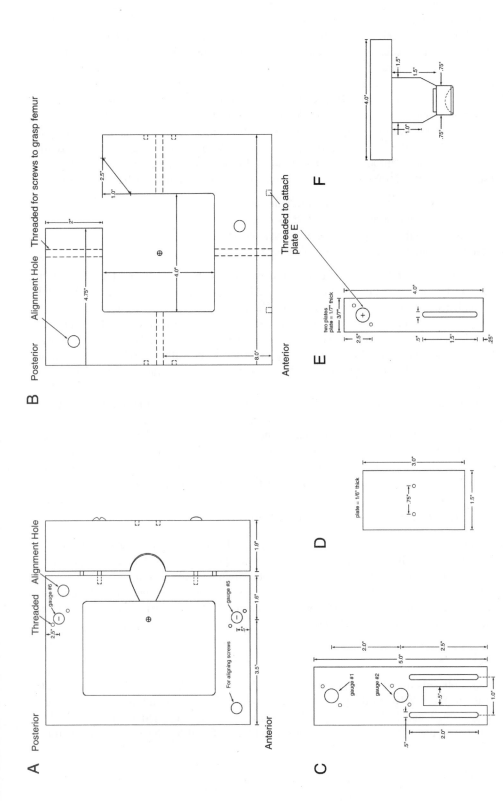

FIGURE 35.2 Plate fixtures to hold the femoral component: (A) The femoral head or the top plate where LVDTs 5, and 6 are fastened; (B) the bottom plate with screw clamps for holding the femur; (C) plate to hold LVDTs 1 and 2; (D) this plate mounts vertically onto the medial edge of the top plate; (E) two of these plates are mounted medial and lateral to the femur to hold LVDTs 3 and 4, respectively; (F) plate to transfer load from the Instron crosshead to the femoral head. (From Naidu, S.H., *Am. J. Orthop.*, 25, 829, 1996. With permission.)

The two plates shown in Figure 35.2E are fastened vertically to the anterior edge of the bottom plate, anterior to the coronal plane of the femur, such that gauges 3 and 4 align with the top plate. Gauges 3 and 4 are placed such that they are medial and lateral, respectively, to the sagittal plane of the femur. The load transfer from the Instron 1331 to the femoral head is facilitated by the component illustrated in Figure 35.2F.

Modular femoral stems (Smith and Nephew, Memphis, TN) were implanted in composite bones (Pacific Research Labs, Vashon Island, WA) with a section modulus equal to that of human femora.[7] They were used for consistency in anatomy and in mechanical properties. In all, 20 bones were randomly prepared to receive one of four prosthesis configurations. A size 14 large femoral stem was modified by either adding a 6-mm proximal anterior pad or a 17-mm distal sleeve, by adding both, or by using only a 0-mm anterior pad without a distal sleeve. Therefore, five femurs, and thus five tests for each of the following configurations, were prepared and mechanically tested:

0/–S = 0-mm proximal anterior pad, no distal sleeve;
6/–S = 6-mm proximal anterior pad, no distal sleeve;
0/+S = 0-mm proximal anterior pad, 17-mm distal sleeve;
6/+S = 6-mm proximal anterior pad, 17-mm distal sleeve.

The 20 bones were randomly prepared to receive five stems of each of the above four configurations. Osteotomy was made 1.5 cm above the lesser trochanter, and serial reaming with appropriate rigid reamers and broaching was done. The reconstructed femora were aligned in an aluminum pot and cemented in place with polyester resin. They were then cyclically loaded on a servohydraulic Instron 1331 (Canton, MA) between 130 and 1500 N at 1 H; the assembly was positioned in 7° of adduction and loaded in neutral to mimic level walking and at 20° of flexion to mimic stair climbing. Before mechanical testing, prosthetic seating was confirmed by radiograph as shown in Figure 35.3.

After mechanical testing, one 6/+S, and one 0/–S were sectioned on the accutome without embedding. The sections were radiographed and analyzed on the Macintosh image analysis system to determine fit/fill values. Fit was determined as the percentage of prosthetic surface in close apposition with the endosteum (<1 mm); fill was calculated as the percentage of the endosteal canal that the prosthesis occupied. Data from four proximal sections and four distal sections were averaged to obtain the fit/fill values for each of the four prosthetic configurations.

B. DERIVATION OF DISPLACEMENT AND ROTATION EQUATIONS

In these equations, the prosthesis and the bone are considered to be rigid bodies. The design of the test assembly necessitated the LVDTs to be centered about a point in the center of the upper plate. In order to give a better estimate of the relative motion at the real interfaces, motions were calculated using the point in the center of the lower plate of the test assembly as a reference. In each direction, the translation at this point is the translation in the center of the top plate plus an additional displacement due to the rotation of the prosthesis.

C. ROTATION

Rotation in each plane is found from the arctangent of the difference between the two appropriate LVDTs and the distance between them. Transverse plane rotations are found using LVDTs 3 and 4 (θ_T); coronal from 1 and 2 (θ_c); and sagittal from 5 and 6 (θ_S). The calculation is identical in each plane. For example, if S_{56} is the distance between LVDTs 5 and 6, the rotation in the coronal plane (θ_c) is

$$\theta_c = \arctan (\#6 - \#5)/S_{56} \qquad (35.1)$$

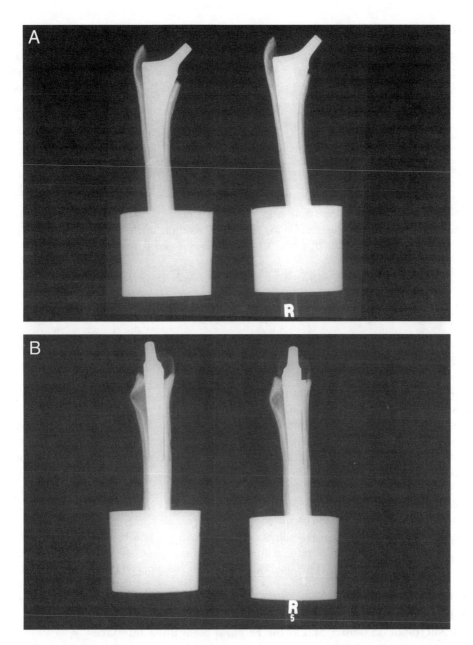

FIGURE 35.3   Anteroposterior (A) and lateral (B) radiographs of the prosthesis with 6-mm anterior proximal pad without the distal sleeve, confirming prosthetic seating in the composite bones. (From Naidu, S.H. et al., *Am. J. Orthop.*, 25, 829, 1996. With permission).

D. VERTICAL (SUPERIOR-INFERIOR) TRANSLATION

This is the easiest case, since there is no contribution from a rotation. That is, the vertical displacement of the prosthesis is the same for all the points along the axis of the prosthesis. Since LVDTs 5 and 6 were centered about this axis, the vertical displacement is given by

$$\delta_{SI} = (\#5 + \#6)/2 \qquad\qquad (35.2)$$

E. Medial-Lateral Displacement

This displacement is found by adding the mediolateral displacement in the top plate to a translation resulting from rotation in the coronal plane. If h is the distance between the top plate and the bottom plate, and S_{12} is the distance between LVDTs 1 and 2, then the translation along the mediolateral plane is

$$\delta_{ML} = (\#1 + \#2)/2 + h \tan\theta_c = (\#1 + \#2)/2 + h\,(\#2 - \#1)/S_{12} \qquad (35.3)$$

F. Anterior-Posterior Displacement

Anteroposterior displacement is calculated in the same manner using LVDTs 3 and 4 for the translational component and the rotation in the sagittal plane (LVDTs 5 and 6). The rotational component is subtracted in this case since a positive rotation in the coronal plane results in a posterior translation. If S_{56} is the distance between LVDTs 5 and 6, then

$$\delta_{AP} = (\#3 + \#4)/2 - h \tan\theta_S = (\#3 + \#4)/2 - h\,(\#6 - \#5)/S_{56} \qquad (35.4)$$

III. RESULTS

From Table 35.1 it is clear that none of the four groups showed significant differences in translational interfacial micromotion when tested with neutral loading and flexion loading. However, it is evident that prostheses in all four groups showed increased translational micromotion when tested in flexion, compared with neutral loading. While the mean anteroposterior displacements in flexion ranged from 56.4 to 72.4 μm, it ranged from 8.7 to 12.2 μm in neutral loading.

Similarly, Table 35.2 shows that rotation of the prosthesis is consistently increased in all three planes when tested in flexion for all four configurations. This increase is significant along both the prosthesis vertical and anteroposterior axes ($p < 0.05$). The mean rotation ($° \times 10^{-3}$) in flexion along the vertical axis ranged from 43.5 to 74.5; whereas in neutral loading, mean vertical rotation ($° \times 10^{-3}$) ranged from 6.3 to 13.4. The anteroposterior rotation in flexion also showed a six- to sevenfold increase when compared with neutral loading.

Although the rotation in flexion consistently increased for all four configurations in comparison with neutral loading, there are some notable differences in rotation between the four groups in flexion. Prosthesis with the larger proximal pad, without the distal sleeve, 6/-S, showed a mean rotation ($° \times 10^{-3}$) of 43.5, whereas the one with the smaller proximal pad, without the distal sleeve,

TABLE 35.1
Relative Micromotion (mm ± SD) at the Femoral Stem Bone Interface

Group	Vertical (Z Axis)		Mediolateral (X Axis)		Anteroposterior (Y Axis)	
	Neutral $n = 5$	Flexon $n = 5$	Neutral $n = 5$	Flexion $n = 5$	Neutral $n = 5$	Flexion $n = 5$
0/–S	13.9 ± 0.4	19.8 ± 1.0	44.9 ± 1.4	47.4 ± 2.3	8.7 ± 1.4	56.4 ± 8.9[a]
6/–S	13.6 ± 0.7	19.0 ± 0.5	45.9 ± 2.4	47.5 ± 1.2	10.1 ± 0.9	72.4 ± 6.1[a]
0/+S	17.1 ± 0.5	22.3 ± 1.4	46.7 ± 1.2	45.7 ± 1.8	10.8 ± 1.4	69.4 ± 4.7[a]
6/+S	16.5 ± 1.0	21.7 ± 2.9	49.9 ± 1.9	51.2 ± 3.5	12.2 ± 1.9	67.0 ± 10.3[a]

Note: For group descriptions, see text in methods section.

[a] Significantly higher than displacements along Y axis in neutral loading (one-way ANOVA $p < 0.05$).

Source: Naidu, S.H., *Am. J. Orthop.*, 25, 829, 1986. With permission.

TABLE 35.2
Relative Rotation at the Bone Stem Interface (degrees × 10⁻³ ± SD)

Group	Vertical (Z Axis)		Mediolateral (X Axis)		Anteroposterior (Y Axis)	
	Neutral $n = 5$	Flexon $n = 5$	Neutral $n = 5$	Flexion $n = 5$	Neutral $n = 5$	Flexion $n = 5$
0/–S	8.4 ± 2.0	56.4 ± 8.9[a]	60.2 ± 2.6	75.6 ± 5.6	7.0 ± 0.3	49.0 ± 2.9[a]
6/–S	6.3 ± 1.0	43.5 ± 3.6[a,b]	62.3 ± 3.8	72.2 ± 2.9	6.4 ± 1.0	47.8 ± 3.2[a]
0/+S	12.1 ± 1.8	74.5 ± 5.9[a]	65.8 ± 2.5	79.3 ± 6.5	7.7 ± 0.9	53.9 ± 2.3[a]
6/+S	13.2 ± 2.4	73.1 ± 12.6[a,b]	69.9 ± 4.2	84.8 ± 11.4	8.4 ± 1.0	57.0 ± 5.0[a]

[a] Significantly higher than its neutral rotation along the same axis (one-way ANOVA $p < = 0.05$).
[b] Significant intergroup difference (one-way ANOVA $p < = 0.05$).

Source: Naidu, S.H., *Am. J. Orthop.*, 25, 829, 1996. With permission.

0/–S, showed an average rotation of 56.4 along the vertical axis. Although this difference is not statistically significant, all five tests in the 6/–S group consistently showed less rotation than did those of the 0/–S group.

When the 17-mm distal sleeve was added to the smaller, 0-mm proximal pad stem, the 0/+S group showed a mean rotation ($° × 10^{-3}$) of 74.5 along the vertical axis; this is a definite increase over its sleeveless counterpart, 0/–S, which showed a mean rotation of 56.4 ($° × 10^{-3}$). When the distal sleeve was added to the larger 6-mm proximal pad augmented stem, the 6/+S stem showed a significant increase in mean rotation along its vertical axis at $73.1 × 10^{-3}°$, compared with its sleeveless counterpart, which displayed vertical rotation of $43.5 × 10^{-3}°$.

From Table 35.3, it is apparent that proximal fill is essentially unchanged at 63% for all the configurations. Addition of the 17-mm distal sleeve increased the distal canal fill from 71 to 96%. Although proximal fill was unchanged by the 6-mm proximal pad, proximal fit was markedly improved from 6 to 37%. Distal fit was increased from 16 to 57% by adding the distal sleeve.

IV. DISCUSSION

The increase in anteroposterior displacements in flexion may be explained by the increase in the posteriorly directed component of the loading force when the potted femur is flexed. Although no other axis shows such a dramatic increase in translational micromotion, rotational instability is evident along both the anteroposterior and vertical axes. The six- to sevenfold increase in both anteroposterior and vertical rotation when compared with neutral loading suggests that the pros-

TABLE 35.3
Intramedullary Canal Fit and Fill Percentages

Configuration	Proximal Fill	Distal Fill	Proximal Fit	Distal Fit
0/–S	63% $n = 3$	71% $n = 4$	6% $n = 3$	16% $n = 4$
6/–S	63% $n = 4$	71% $n = 4$	37% $n = 4$	16% $n = 4$
0/+S	63% $n = 3$	96% $n = 4$	6% $n = 3$	57% $n = 4$
6/+S	63% $n = 4$	96% $n = 4$	37% $n = 4$	57% $n = 4$

Note: Configurations are the same as the group descriptions in the methods section.

Source: Naidu, S. H., *Am. J. Orthop.*, 25, 829, 1996. With permission.

thesis is unstable in more than one dimension when out-of-plane forces are applied. Burke and colleagues, in a cadaver femora study, reported that torsional interface slippage increased by a factor of ten in uncemented devices, when the implant bone assembly was loaded on the materials testing system assembly in 30° of flexion.

Crowninshield and colleagues[8] estimated the greatest loads on the hip to be during stair climbing, when the resultant was predicted to be more than seven times the body weight, with the component of force acting on the pelvis in the anteroposterior direction being up to five times the body weight. They commented that this force affects the torque that is transmitted to the bone–prosthesis interface and may be related to implant loosening. Our observation of increased rotation in flexion loading in more than one axis is consistent with their findings.

Although most *in vitro* studies on implant stability use cadaver femora, the validity of our model is confirmed by Walker and Robertson's[9] experiments. They tested the so-called exact fit stem in cadaver femora, both in vertical loading and with an added out-of-plane force. In vertical loading, similar to coronal neutral stance loading, the anteroposterior displacement ranged from 8.8 to 26.3 μm; however, when they added a 100 N anterior force to the 1000 N vertical load, the anteroposterior displacements increased to a range of 42.2 to 51.0 μm. The vertical rotational angles increased from 19×10^{-3} to 73×10^{-3}° by adding the anterior force. Since the measured translational micromotion and rotational angles are of the same magnitude under similar loading regimens, the use of composite bones for initial stability study is justified.

Gilbert and colleagues,[10] in a cadaver femora study, compared a porous-coated anatomical stem and a custom prosthesis with higher proximal fill; the authors demonstrated no significant difference between the porous-coated anatomical stem and the custom prosthesis in both migration and micromotion. The authors hypothesized that stability appears to be provided by the relatively small areas of cortical contact between the stem and the bone. The authors' data appear consistent with their observations. The 0-mm proximal pad gave a proximal fit value of 6%; adding a 6-mm proximal pad increased the fit to 37%. This improved fit decreased the prosthesis rotation along its vertical axis, as shown in Table 35.3.

Huiskes,[11] in his study of cementless stems using finite-element analysis, hypothesized that press-fit devices require elastic subsidence to develop interface compression to balance the axial joint compressive forces. Since the proximal femoral mediolateral stem curvature dictates the amount of mediolateral compressive forces generated, it follows that the anteroposterior taper angle will influence the amount of anteroposterior compressive forces generated to stabilize the prosthesis. Since there is no ingrowth, initial stability provided by the larger anterior pad depends solely on prosthetic elastic subsidence and the shear stress generated by the porous proximal coating (Figure 35.4). With the larger anterior pad, the anteroposterior taper angle increases, thereby allowing more anteroposterior compressive forces to be generated. These larger anteroposterior compressive forces reduce the prosthesis rotation about the vertical axis.

The addition of the distal sleeve increased the average distal fill to 96%, and the average distal fit to 57%. From Table 35.3 it is evident that the addition of the distal sleeve significantly increased the rotation of the 6/+S group compared with the 6/–S group along the prosthesis vertical axis. The distal canal was rigidly reamed to 17 mm, and, therefore, distal fixation is unlikely to be the reason for the increase in rotation. The increase in distal fit probably diminishes the elastic subsidence of the stem. Because of decreased stem subsidence, the effect of proximal pad wedging is effectively negated. Since the composite bone was reamed anteriorly to accommodate the proximal pad, the observed rotational instability of the 6/+S configuration is not surprising.

In the above *in vitro* study, the authors demonstrate that the modular uncemented femoral stem investigated is more unstable when subject to flexion loading than in neutral loading. This study also suggests that it is probably the proximal fit, and not the fill, that contributes to initial stability of an uncemented system where stabilization by bony ingrowth has yet to occur.

FIGURE 4: LOAD TRANSFER AT WEDGE CYLINDER
INTERFACE IN UNCEMENTED STEMS

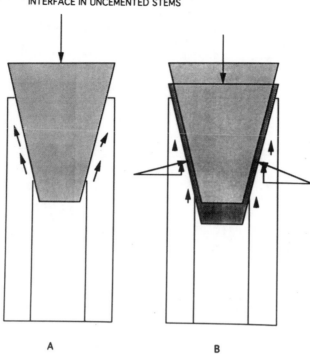

A   B

FIGURE 35.4   Load transfer at the wedge cylinder interface in uncemented stems. (A) With a porous coat, shear stress (the force tangent to the wedge surface, divided by the area on which the force acts; shown by the angled arrows) is developed to equilibrate the compressive force which is the weight applied. (B) Since there is no bony ingrowth, initial equilibrium relies on the magnitude of the vertical component (N) of the normal force (N, the force perpendicular to the surface of the wedge) of the compressive interface stress. The wedge must subside to develop the required compressive stress values. (From Naidu, S.H. et al., *Am. J. Orthop.*, 25, 829, 1996. With permission.)

REFERENCES

1. Pilliar, R.M., Lee, J.M., and Maniatopoulos, C., Observations on the effect of movement on bone ingrowth into porous surfaced implants, *Clin. Orthop.*, 208, 108, 1986.
2. Engh, C.A. and Bobyn, J.D., The influence of stem size and the extent of porous coating on femoral bone resorption after primary cementless hip arthroplasty, *Clin. Orthop.*, 1988; 231, 1988.
3. Engh, C.A., Bobyn, J.D., and Glassman, A.H., Porous coated hip replacement: the factors governing bone ingrowth, stress shielding, and clinical results, *J. Bone Joint Surg.*, 69B, 45, 1987.
4. Burke, D.W., O'Connor, D.O., Zalenski, E.B., and Harris, W.H., Biomechanics of the femoral total hip components in simulated stair climbing, *Trans. Orthop. Res. Soc.*, 13, 345, 1988.
5. Cook, S.D., Walsh, K.A., Haddad, R.J., Jr., Interface mechanics and bone growth into porous Co-Cr-Mo alloy implants, *Clin. Orthop.*, 193, 271, 1985.
6. Noyes, F.R., Grood, E.S., and Torizilli, P.A., Current concepts review. The definition of terms for motion and position of the knee and injuries of the ligaments, *J. Bone Joint Surg.*, 71B, 465, 1989.
7. Miller, D., Saw Bones 1994, Pacific Research Labs, Washington, 1994, 22.
8. Crowninshield, R.D., Johnston, R.C., Andrews, J.G., and Brand, R.A., Biomechanical investigation of the human hip, *J. Biomech.*, 11, 75, 1978.
9. Walker, P.S. and Robertson, D.D., Design and fabrication of cementless hip stems, *Clin. Orthop.*, 235, 25, 1988.

10. Gilbert, J.L., Bloomfield, R.S., Lautenschlager, E.P., et al., An *in vitro* investigation of the migration and micromotion of custom and off-the-shelf cementless prostheses, *Trans. Orthop. Res. Soc.*, 16, 543, 1991.

11. Huiskes, R., The various patterns of press fit, ingrown, and cemented femoral stems, *Clin. Orthop.*, 261, 27, 1990.

36 Screw Pullout Testing

Lisa A. Ferrara and Timothy C. Ryken

CONTENTS

I. INTRODUCTION

The bone–screw interface is a critical component of spinal stabilization. In general, bone has a smaller modulus of elasticity than the screw and is therefore weaker than the various metals used in screw constructs. Screw loosening as a result of bony failure can significantly compromise the stabilizing effect of the implant.[1,2] Differences between the elastic moduli of bone and metal can have detrimental effects regarding stability. Placement of a significantly stiffer penetrating implant into bone disperses the forces nonuniformly, and regions of increased stress result within the screw and within the bone. Eventually, the bone will fail due to microfracturing of the trabeculae or fracturing within the cortical bone, or the screw will break at the region of peak stress. Therefore, the quality of the bone and the biomechanics of screw fixation must be respected when using instrumentation to stabilize an injury. This symbiotic relationship must exist between the bone and the screw for a successful fusion or stabilization to occur.

To enhance screw purchase to the bone and increase resistance to pullout, certain design features of the screw have been implemented. Screw diameter, in particular the major diameter, screw design, insertion techniques, and bone integrity all affect the strength of the screw fixation.[3-7] The clinical objective is, theoretically, to increase the volume of bone the screw can hold between the threads. This relationship of bone volume to screw thread contributes to the degree of purchase the screw has to the bone.

Many types of screws are used in bone fixation. The standard machine screw design is used for hard materials that are less compressible, such as metals and cortical bone. Cortical screws are used in hard, compact, dense bone and possess the machine screw design with shallow threads that have approximately a 60° thread angle.[2] Tapping the insertion hole for cortical screw placement is optimal to avoid microfracturing within the bone and increased insertional torques which could result in screw breakage.[1,2,6,8] The self-tapping machine screw is used for minimizing the steps during cortical bone screw insertion while optimizing the cutting capabilities. Self-tapping screws have a tapered outside diameter to eliminate additional steps of bone preparation to receive the screw. These screws tap during insertion and have leading-edge flutes to guide the debris and maintain it within the confine of the screw–bone interface region. The self-tapping machine screw is conventionally used in cortical bone and provides similar stabilizing properties as screws that are placed after tapping.[1,9]

The standard wood screw design is used for softer compressible materials such as cancellous bone. Its deep thread design and tapering permits easy insertion into the material. This design forms threads within the material by compressing the surrounding material during the insertion process.[6] Tapping is not recommended in cancellous bone because it can weaken the bone–implant interface and decrease the pullout strength of the screw.[9,10]

Screw insertion into cancellous bone and resistance to pullout requires that an optimal amount of bone be captured between the screw threads. The structural characteristics of the screw and the integrity of the cancellous bone can significantly alter the performance of the screw. Enhancement of the screw performance within the bone can be achieved by altering the thread depth, shape, and interthread distance of the screw. This enables a larger volume of bone to surround the screw, thereby increasing the resistance to backout.

II. SCREW ANATOMY

Screws function as fixation devices that stabilize bony abnormalities and injuries.[3,6,11,12] Understanding the biomechanical principles of screw fixation and its stabilizing features, such as compression generation, can help reduce failure rates. The function of the screw is to change rotational motion into translational motion while providing mechanical stability to the injured site.[6,8,13] In order to achieve correction of the deformity in bone, there are some basic design features of the screw that contribute to maintaining the mechanical stability within bone. The main components of the screw consist of the head, the core, and the threads (Figure 36.1).[1,2,6] Each component plays a crucial role in the performance of the screw.[6]

The head (Figure 36.1) of the screw serves to transmit the insertion torque to the core and threads. It also functions as a stop when it comes into contact with the surface of the bone, hence ceasing the translational motion of the screw. Once the translational motion has stopped, the screw generates a compressive force. Continued rotation of the screw can result in failure of the screw or the material into which it is inserted.[6]

The core (see Figure 36.1) is the main shaft of the screw around which the threads wrap. Geometrically, the screw has a major and minor diameter. The major diameter, or outside diameter, is the largest diameter of the screw and is measured from the outside tip of one side of the thread to the outside tip of the other side. The minor diameter, or inner diameter, is the smallest diameter of the screw measured across the base of the threads. It is the minor diameter that is referred to as the core of the screw.

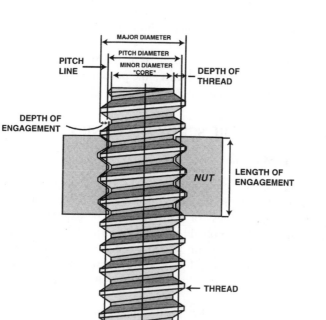

FIGURE 36.1 Anatomy of the screw. The three main components of the screw are the head, core (minor diameter), and thread. The major diameter is the outer diameter of the screw measured at the crest of the threads. Length of the engagement of the screw is measured by the number of threads seated in the material.

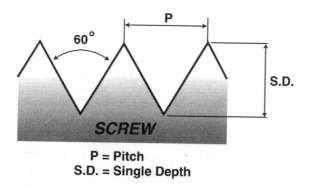

FIGURE 36.2 The pitch is the distance between the threads of the screw and can be calculated from the inverse of the number of threads per inch. The single depth of the thread is calculated from the root to the crest of the thread.

The thread (see Figure 36.1) is defined as the ridge in the form of a helix on the external or internal surface of a cylinder that does the work of an inclined plane.[1,2]

Pitch (Figures 36.1 and 36.2) is the distance between the threads on the screw, provided the measurements are taken consistently from the base or apex of one thread to the exact point on the adjacent thread. Pitch can also be defined as the inverse of the number of threads per inch (T.P.I.):

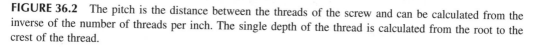

$$\text{Pitch} = 1/\text{T.P.I.} \qquad (36.1)$$

The lead is the distance a screw advances with one turn.[1,2] This is equal to the pitch (distance between threads).

Thread depth is the distance from the apex of the thread to the base of the thread (see Figure 36.1). The depth of the thread influences the purchase of the screw into the bone and can significantly influence pullout resistance.[1,2,8,13-15]

III. SCREW MECHANICS

A. THE MECHANICS OF MATERIALS

The bone–implant interface in screw fixation is the site of greatest load transfer. The load is transferred from the head of the screw along the core and into the material in which the screw is placed. The elasticity or stiffness of a material can be expressed as the amount of elastic deformation that results from an applied force. This is termed the elastic modulus of the material and describes the stress (force per unit of cross-sectional area) per unit of strain (the linear deformation per unit of original length).[2] There are three types of elastic moduli that exist: Young's modulus, bulk modulus, and shear modulus. All are dependent on the type of loading the material endures.

A high modulus of elasticity implies a stiffer material. A low modulus of elasticity suggests that the material is less rigid. Given this information, bone screws are commonly constructed from various grades of titanium or 316L stainless steel with high moduli of elasticity ranging from 100 to 200 GPa.[2] Steel and titanium are roughly eight times stiffer than bone, whose modulus of elasticity is approximately 20 GPa. A material whose modulus of elasticity is similar to that of a screw will transfer the force to the screw core. As the core is deformed from the loading, a force is generated between the screw head and the material, creating a region of high stress localized at the head of the screw. When a material with a lower modulus of elasticity is used with screw insertion, the material is deformed, transferring the force between the head of the screw and the material.[6,14] Applying this to bone suggests that any loosening that occurs at the bone–screw interface will result in loss of compression, leading to loss of fixation.

B. SCREW STRENGTH

Complex forces act upon a screw once it is inserted into bone (Figure 36.3). Therefore, it is essential that the screw be of sufficient strength to accommodate these forces. The bending strength of a screw can be expressed in terms of the section modulus (Z).[1,16]

$$Z = (\pi D^3)/32 \qquad (36.2)$$

In bending, the strength of a screw is proportional to the third power of its minor diameter.[1,2] Thus, the core diameter of a screw significantly affects the bending strength of the screw. A small increase in the diameter can yield a large increase in the bending strength of the screw.

C. HOLDING STRENGTH OF A SCREW

The holding power of a screw in bone is associated with the mechanical properties of the screw itself and the shear strength of the bone.[17] The main constituents of screw pullout resistance with respect to screw design are thread depth and the major diameter.[18] Other variables, however, contribute to the pullout behavior of the screw, such as the extent of cortical purchase, depth of screw penetration, thread angulation, pitch diameter, screw placement within the bone, physical changes to the screw or bone between the time of insertion and the time of withdrawal, speed at which the screw is withdrawn, the occurrence of predrilled holes, and the quality of the

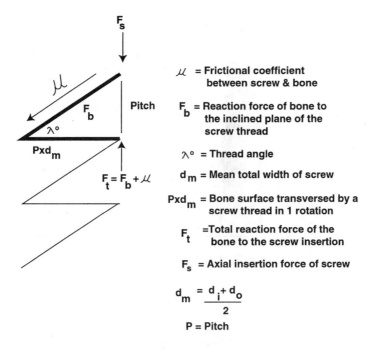

μ = Frictional coefficient between screw & bone

F_b = Reaction force of bone to the inclined plane of the screw thread

$\lambda°$ = Thread angle

d_m = Mean total width of screw

Pxd_m = Bone surface transversed by a screw thread in 1 rotation

F_t = Total reaction force of the bone to the screw insertion

F_s = Axial insertion force of screw

$$d_m = \frac{d_i + d_o}{2}$$

P = Pitch

FIGURE 36.3   The forces acting upon a screw thread. μ = the frictional coefficient between the screw and the bone, F_b = the reaction force of the bone to the inclined plane of the screw thread, λ = thread angle, d_m = mean total width of the screw, Pxd_m = bone surface transversed by the screw thread in one rotation, F_t = total reaction force of the bone to the screw insertion, F_s = axial insertion force of the screw, P = pitch.

bone.[6,8,10,14,19,20-22,24] Consideration of all of these variables will minimize screw failure and loss of bone stabilization. When a screw is inserted into a material such as bone, pullout failure of the screw implies failure of the bone as well. As the screw is loosened and begins to back out, the bone breaks and the screw toggles within the bone yielding a large void. The trabecular structure within cancellous bone forms a matrix. When the screw toggles, it breaks the individual trabeculae, disrupting the natural matrix, and enlarges the void between each trabecula. However, in soft uniform materials, the void is smaller and similar in size to the outer diameter of the screw. It is a concept best visualized by placing a screw into a soft uniform material, such as wax (Figure 36.4). When the screw is pulled out, a smooth cylinder is left inside the block of wax due to the screw threads shearing the wax from the side wall as it is pulled out.[8,16] The area of the hole is that of a cylinder; area = depth × perimeter. Therefore, the maximum holding strength a screw can have is (area of the cylinder) × (shear strength of the material).

D. INCREASING THE HOLDING STRENGTH

The repetitive cyclical loading from motion in the human body can contribute to screw loosening in bone. Many factors can affect the loss of screw fixation in bone.[1,2,10,14,20-25] Failures can be attributed to poor screw design, application of an improper screw type for the material of choice, misconception of the forces applied on the screw, shallow screw threads that do not grasp a sufficient amount of bone to prevent backout, and other limiting factors that do not respect the symbiotic relationship that must exist between the screw and the material. Fortunately, alterations in screw design and an understanding of the mechanical principles of the material used for screw fixation can provide better resistance to screw loosening and reduce the risk of stabilization failure. These issues are discussed in detail below.

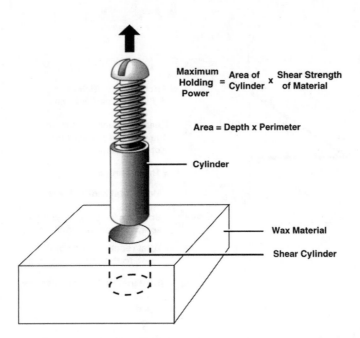

FIGURE 36.4 Screw pullout from a soft homogenous material. After screw withdrawal, a smooth cylinder is left within the wax block due to shearing of the screw threads from the side walls of the wax.

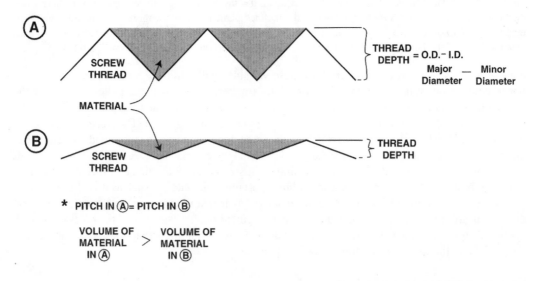

FIGURE 36.5 The difference in thread depth can significantly alter the pullout strength of a screw. Altering the thread depth while keeping the pitch constant will change the amount of bone that surrounds the threads of the screw. A greater pullout resistance exists for greater thread depth (A). Less bone surrounds the screw in (B); hence, pullout resistance is decreased.

1. Thread Depth

Screw pullout resistance can be greatly influenced by the thread design (Figure 36.5). The volume of bone the threads capture contributes to the pullout performance of the screw. The pitch can alter the amount of bone captured by changing the distance between one thread and the adjacent thread. The thread depth can alter the bone volume obtained by modifying the length of the thread. A deeper thread allows more bone to reside between each thread and increases pullout resistance.

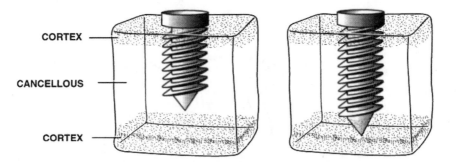

CORTEX

CANCELLOUS

CORTEX

FIGURE 36.6 Increased depth of screw penetration is achieved with longer screws. Screw pullout strength is significantly increased with longer screw penetration for both a unicortical or bicortical purchase. However, bicortical screw purchase is superior to unicortical purchase in pullout performance. The ideal situation is the use of a longer screw to obtain bicortical purchase, provided there are no neurological risks.

2. Depth of Screw Penetration

The length of the screw has a dramatic effect on the pullout strength (Figure 36.6). Deeper screw insertion has been shown to increase pullout resistance and strength in flexion and extension loading.[26] The benefits of using a longer screw must be balanced against increased operative risk. Radiographic assessment may help reduce this possibility.

3. Unicortical vs. Bicortical Purchase

Since cortical bone is denser than cancellous bone and has a significantly greater pullout strength, studies have shown bicortical screw purchase to be superior in pullout strength to unicortical screw purchase.[4,22,27] The two layers of cortex surrounding the cancellous bone provide greater stability to the screw with respect to wobbling and pullout than when only one cortical surface is purchased (Figure 36.6).[27]

4. Triangulation of the Screws

Bone is a heterogeneous material. The trabecular architecture of cancellous bone varies and tends to be denser proximal to the cortical margins.[28] Triangulation of the screws into these concentrated regions of bone will significantly increase pullout resistance.[2,3,29-31] The "toeing-in" of the screws prevents backing out along the direction of the applied axial force. It also purchases a larger wedge of bone between the two screws requiring more force to pull the screws out (Figure 36.7).[3,29,31] Triangulated constructs are biomechanically beneficial and offer stronger opposition to the forces that cause the screw to back out.

E. TORQUE INSERTION

The torsional forces during screw insertion have been shown to correlate with pullout strength. Some studies have shown that high insertional torques measured during screw insertion into material correlate very well with high pullout strengths for certain screws and uniform materials such as synthetic bone blocks and calf vertebrae.[7,14] However, pullout studies conducted in cadaver bone did not yield strong correlations between insertional torque and pullout strength.[21,32]

The peak torque that is generated during screw insertion can depend on screw type, screw diameter, screw design, and whether the screw hole was tapped prior to insertion.[12,21,24,32,33] A screw with a larger diameter in composite bone is more likely to engage the region of denser cortical bone. In contrast to this, a smaller diameter screw placed in composite bone would yield lower

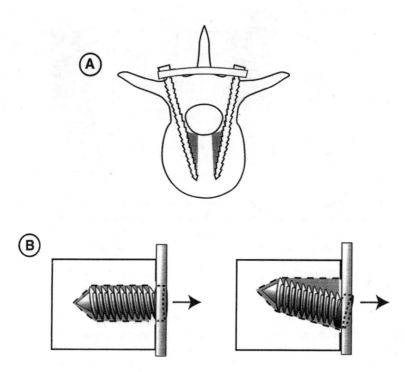

FIGURE 36.7 (A) Triangulation of the screws, or "toeing-in," provides increased screw purchase and resistance to pullout. Angulation of the screw resists backing out along the direction of the applied load. Furthermore, a large wedge of bone surrounds each of the angled screws, which increases the resistance to screw pullout. (B) If the two triangulated screws are cross-linked, there is an even greater resistance to pullout. It is far more difficult to pull out bilateral screws simultaneously. If the screws are angled toward the cortical margins while fixed to a plate, greater screw purchase will be acquired due to the increased density of the bone as it approaches the cortex. Resistance to pullout will be greater as well, due to the larger quantity of bone surrounding the angled screw.

insertional torques because it primarily engages cancellous bone.[10,21,32] Tapping of the screw hole prior to insertion also yields lower peak torques during insertion.[21,34]

F. Thread Angulation

The thread angle defines the shape of the thread (Figure 36.8). This is measured as an angle that deviates from a perpendicular line drawn to the shaft of the screw.[2] Altering this angle changes the shape of the threads and alters the amount of bone that the screw grasps directly. The larger the bone volume the screw carries within each thread, the greater the pullout resistance. However, there is a balance between optimal thread depth, shape, pitch, and thread angle. A large thread depth with few threads per inch may not provide optimal resistance to screw backout.

G. Bone Mineral Content

When a metal screw is inserted into bone, the shear strength of the screw is considerably greater than the bone. Thus, it is the bone that fails initially in pullout testing. The more dense the bone, the smaller the risk of bone failure, and the higher the pullout resistance.[3,17,31] A bending force applied to a screw in any material creates a stress concentration at the initial two or three threads of the screw. This region is often the area where screw breakage or failure (pullout) will occur.[1,2] It is the superficial two or three threads of the screw that are responsible for the transfer of the

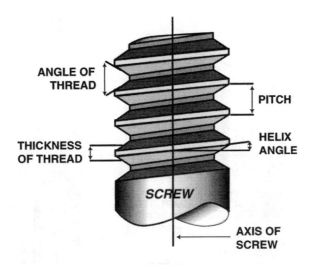

FIGURE 36.8   The thread angle defines the shape of the thread. Altering the thread angle changes the shape of the thread and the amount of bone that will be captured. In turn, this will alter the pullout strength of the screw.

load to the bone. Therefore, thread configuration and bone density correlate well with pullout resistance, especially at the bone–screw interface.

H. Screw Performance Based on Implant Material

Screw material can significantly impact performance. Currently, 316L stainless steel with a 480-MPa ultimate tensile strength is the conventional material used in biological implants.[2] Titanium has gained popularity due to its resistance to corrosion within the human body and the similarities in terms of mechanical properties to that of stainless steel.

Bioabsorbable screws have been developed in an effort to increase patient rehabilitation time postoperatively. Polylactic acid is a common component of these types of screws. *In vivo* degradation of these screws occurs over time by the process of hydration, depolymerization, loss of morphological supporting structure, absorption, and elimination.[33] Pena et al.[33] conducted a tensile pullout study on bioabsorbable screws and compared their results with metal screws. The metal screws performed favorably and had significantly higher insertional forces than the bioabsorbable screws. They also demonstrated significantly greater failure loads than the bioabsorbable screws.

IV. EXPERIMENTAL METHODOLOGY FOR SCREW PULLOUT TESTING

The purpose of quantifying the pullout strength of screws is to measure their ability to attach and hold an object.[35] There are several ways to quantify screw performance and the holding strength of the screw implant. Quantification of the tensile forces required to pull a screw out of a particular material determines the pullout strength of that screw. Measurement of the axial forces necessary for insertion of the screw as it is tightened into a material will also describe biomechanical characteristics of the screw.

A. Testing Apparatus

Any testing apparatus is suitable to perform a screw pullout study, provided it has a testing platform that can move at a constant rate and has an accuracy of ±1% after calibration.[35] A "uniaxial materials testing system" capable of operating in tension and compression that is hydraulically or electrically controlled is the highest-quality testing apparatus.

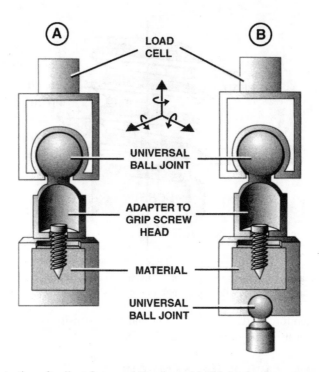

FIGURE 36.9   Illustration of pullout fixtures: (A) universal ball joint for the top grip with the bottom grip fixed to the platen of the testing apparatus, allowing the top grip to toggle during the application of tensile forces, and (B) universal ball joint for the top and bottom grip allowing both to toggle during the application of tensile forces. Use of these devices eliminates residual stresses that occur within the pulling fixtures during tension.

B.   GRIPPING FIXTURES

The fixtures that are used to grip the screw and the material into which it is inserted can dramatically affect the results of a pullout study. According to the American Society for Testing and Materials standards (ASTM), a true pullout assessment of a screw would require that the grips used to grasp the screw head be shaped to fit accurately and that the grips provide a true axial load.[35] An ideal withdrawal study performed on screws should allow the grips to pivot or toggle. This would reduce any residual stresses that may occur within a rigid gripping device and diminish the transfer of these stresses to the screw during the pullout. Universal ball joints and pinned joints are commonly used as mounting devices because of their mobility, standard design, and ease of use (Figure 36.9). Compatibility of these joints to standard machinery makes them adaptable to any materials testing system with the aid of attachment fixtures. However, there are pullout studies that do not require gripping devices to toggle during tensile loading. An example of this would be a triangulated screw study using fixtures that toggle. Hence, the effect of angulation observed on the pullout strength would be reduced.

C.   SPECIMEN PREPARATIONS

1.   Synthetic Bone Specimens

Often materials of uniform density are used during screw pullout studies to provide a standardized experiment. Currently, rigid polyurethane foams are used as bone substitutes for pullout studies. The uniformity of the material and consistent mechanical properties similar to that of human bone make it a good substitute for screw strength quantification. It can be purchased in a variety of densities that represent good bone integrity, as well as osteoporotic bone models. The uniform nature eliminates

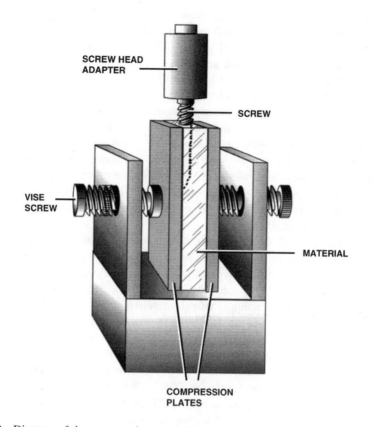

SCREW HEAD
ADAPTER

SCREW

VISE
SCREW

MATERIAL

COMPRESSION
PLATES

FIGURE 36.10   Diagram of the test sample mounted into clamping fixtures. These fixtures are positioned into the machine grips and a tensile force is applied at a uniform rate. The platens separate and the top grip pulls the screw out of the material. The load cell of the testing apparatus records the force required to separate the screw from the material. The peak force during pullout usually occurs within the first few threads that are pulled out of the material.

the variability that exists between normal bone samples and provides a standardized method for determining screw pullout resistance. Therefore, it can provide an accurate assessment of the pullout strength of the screw. Use of synthetic bone is limited in its clinical applicability because bone is an inhomogeneous substance in most regions of the body.

A general rule of thumb when determining the size of the synthetic bone sample is to maintain a constant pattern of failure within the synthetic bone by keeping the screw diameter approximately less than 5% of the circumference of the synthetic bone block.[11,19] When mounting the synthetic bone into the bottom grip on the testing apparatus, it is crucial to apply a uniform pressure across the material (Figure 36.10). This can be done by using plates that are similar in size to the synthetic bone block attached to the clamping arms of the vise. The plates distribute the forces applied by the vise screws over a larger surface area and transmit these forces uniformly across the block. The ideal situation is to have four plates clamping four sides of the block for a uniform application of pressure. This eliminates discrepancies in the screw pullout data due to regions of high stresses within the synthetic bone blocks caused by nonuniform clamping.

2. Bone Specimens

In order to assess the clinically relevant nature of screw fixation, pullout experiments are commonly conducted in various types of bone. Bovine, porcine, and unembalmed cadaver bone are common bone sample types. However, bone is not homogeneous in composition. In the vertebral bodies, the bone density is significantly higher at the cortical margins and lowest in the center of the body.[28] Human cortical bone, such as that found in the long bones of the appendages, is extremely dense and can generate screw pullout strengths approximately four times greater than that of cancellous bone.[7,17,18,20,36-39]

It is essential to prepare each of the bone samples meticulously, especially when using cadaver bone samples.[38] All soft tissue should be cleanly dissected off the bone in order to provide a better gripping surface. The oils secreted from the musculature can cause the bone sample to slip out of the grips during the tensile pull. Although Kaab et al.[40] found no significant changes in pullout strength with cadaver bone that was allowed to undergo structural degradation caused by time-dependent autolytic processes, Simonian et al.[5] found that the process of freeze-drying the bone significantly weakened the pullout resistances of the screw. Therefore, it is best to conduct pullout studies with bone specimens that have been subjected to minimal thawing and freezing cycles and have not undergone any processing treatments.

A significant factor in the holding strength of bone instrumentation is the quality of the bone itself. There are many techniques currently used to assess the integrity of the bone samples.[4,36] Dual X-ray absorptiometry (DEXA), quantitative computed tomography (QCT), and magnetic resonance imaging (MRI) are used clinically to study the bone mineral density for studies on osteoporosis.[4,19,20,22,28] DEXA is a common scanning method for determining bone quality because of its ease of use, speed, and accurate assessment. However, it provides an overall average bone mineral density (BMD) for the regions of bone measured. QCT is another common method used for determining BMD. When bone specimens are scanned with this technique, it is suggested that a phantom be used with each scan taken. The advantage of this technique is the ability to measure distinct regions of bone for the quantification of BMD. This can yield a more localized BMD for the region where the screw will be placed. Proper CT algorithms should be used for cancellous and cortical bone and the regions measured within the bone can be calibrated against the phantom for each scan. MRI is the most accurate method for BMD quantification and can be used to characterize trabecular architecture.[36] The inhomogeneity of tissue induces signal intensity differences in response to the magnetic stimulation; thus differences in the trabeculae can be visualized and quantified for specific regions of interest.

The manner in which the specimens are secured into the bottom fixture that sits in the grip of the testing apparatus can affect the pullout resistances of the screw.[38] The fixture is responsible for holding the specimen in place and resisting the tensile forces placed on the screw. In contrast, the grip is attached to the testing apparatus and holds onto the fixture housing the testing specimen. Typically, the specimens are secured in a vise and may initially be embedded in a polyester resin (see Figure 36.10). The resin provides additional support to the bone specimen and can prevent rotation of the specimen when clamped within the vise. It also serves to distribute the axial forces evenly across the surface between the specimen and fixture by allowing a greater surface area. The extensive porosity of bone can prompt intrusion of the resin into it. Pfeiffer et al.[38] demonstrated this occurrence by examining the trabecular architecture after failure, and characterizing the biomechanical behavior of screw pullout in bone that had been invaded with resin. Their data demonstrated significantly greater pullout resistances with bone that had been intruded by the resin than those without resin intrusion. Therefore, if an embedding material is to be used, the bone specimens should be wrapped in a substance that will not allow the material, such as latex or plastic wrapping, to seep into the bone.

D. Screw Insertion Technique

To initiate screw insertion, the screw holes can be drilled with bits that are approximately 10% larger than the minor diameter of the screw without compromising pullout strength.[11,19] If the bone is cortical bone or has a cortical shell, it is suggested that the cortex be drilled and tapped to avoid microfracturing at this layer. Since the cortical shell is usually at the bone–screw interface and may surround the initial few threads of the screw, microfractures could reduce the pullout strength. Guides must be used to ensure the proper orientation of the screw within the bone. If the screws are to be placed at an angle, special guides must be constructed to ensure the screw will follow the correct insertion angle. Radiographs can document the screw orientation and screw depth within the test sample. After insertion, the peak insertional torque should be quantified by using a finely graded torque wrench.

E. Testing Protocol

The test specimen should be placed onto the loading platform of the testing machine into a top and bottom grip that is in perfect alignment. This avoids bending moments and additional stresses transferred to the screw as a result of misalignment. Depending on the type of testing apparatus, the protocol for screw pullout should be withdrawal of the screw using an axial force in tension moving at a constant rate. This causes the platens on which the grips are secured to separate at a uniform speed. For material testing systems such as an MTS model (MTS Systems, Inc., Minneapolis, MN), the test should be performed under stroke control (actuator displacement). According to ASTM standards,[35] the basic speed of withdrawal should be the application of the tensile force throughout the test at a uniform rate of platen separation of 0.10 in./min ± 25% (2.54 mm/min).[35] Some common pull rates range from 0.1 to 5 mm/s depending on the type of screw and the material into which it is inserted.[4,19,34,38] It is recommended that a screw be used only once within a pullout study. Repetition of pullout on a screw can weaken and dull the threads.[35] Placement of this used screw into another piece of bone will reduce its purchase capability and may decrease its pullout resistance.

F. Grouping Specimens

Randomization of the test specimens, especially if bone samples are used in the study, is recommended to ensure an unbiased statistically relevant study. Differences in gender, age, bone densities, anatomical alignment, and size can all be randomized for each testing group. Test samples should be selected to cover an appropriate range of densities and properties that would be clinically pertinent. The number of tests conducted should be extensive enough to provide reliable results. ASTM standards suggest that the coefficient of variation from screw testing ranges from 15 to 30%.[35] An optimal sample size of pullout testing for each group of screws is to conduct at least ten replications. Often, a power analysis can be conducted to validate the sample size.

G. Data Analysis

Statistical comparisons between testing groups and the pullout results commonly use a Student's t-test analysis and/or a multivariate analysis of variance to detect differences between the testing groups and the corresponding results. To define the relationship among bone mineral density, insertional torque, and pullout force, a regression analysis or multivariate regression analysis should be conducted. The regression analysis is defined here on the amount of linearity that the pullout force has when compared with one of the other variables, such as bone mineral density. It will determine if there is a strong statistical association between bone mineral density and screw pullout strength. An r value closer to 1 characterizes a strong relationship between the two variables, whereas an r value of 0 indicates no correlation. A multivariate regression analysis will evaluate the relative contribution of both dependent variables, bone mineral density and insertion torque, on the variability observed with the independent variable, pullout force.

REFERENCES

1. Bennett, G.J., Materials and materials testing, in *Spinal Instrumentation*, Benzel, E.C., Ed., American Association of Neurological Surgeons, Chicago, 1994, 31.
2. Benzel, E.C., Implant–bone interfaces, in *Biomechanics of Spine Stabilization: Principles and Clinical Practice*, Benzel, E.C., Ed., McGraw-Hill, New York, 1995, 127.
3. Ruland, C.M., McAfee, P.C., Warden, K.E., and Cunningham, B.W., Triangulation of pedicular instrumentation. A biomechanical analysis, *Spine*, 16, S270, 1991.
4. Ryken, T.C., Clausen, J.D., Traynelis, V.C., and Goel, V.K., Biomechanical analysis of bone mineral density, insertion technique, screw torque, and holding strength of anterior cervical plate screws, *J. Neurosurg.*, 83, 325, 1995.
5. Simonian, P.T., Conrad, E.U., Chapman, J.R., et al., Effect of sterilization and storage treatments on screw pullout strength in human allograft bone, *Clin. Orthop.*, 302, 290, 1994.
6. Uhl, R.L., The biomechanics of screws, *Orthop. Rev.*, 18, 1302, 1989.
7. Zdeblick, T.A., Kunz, D.N., Cooke, M.E, and McCabe, R., Pedicle screw pullout strength. Correlation with insertional torque, *Spine*, 18, 1673, 1993.
8. Asnis, S.E., Ernberg, J.J., Bostrom, M.P., et al., Cancellous bone screw thread design and holding power, *J. Orthop. Trauma*, 10, 462, 1996.
9. Boyle, J.M., Frost, D.E., Foley, W.L., and Grady, J.J., Torque and pullout analysis of six currently available self-tapping and emergency screws, *J. Oral Maxillofac. Surg.*, 51, 45, 1993.
10. Phillips, J.H. and Rahn, B.A., Comparison of compression and torque measurements of self-tapping and pretapped screws, *Plast. Reconstr. Surg.*, 83, 447, 1989.
11. Pratt, W.B. and Yazdani, S., Laboratory testing of bolts and screws in cancellous bone, *Orthop. Rev.*, 18, 1073, 1989.
12. Wittenberg, R.H., Lee, K.S., Shea, M., et al., Effect of screw diameter, insertion technique, and bone cement augmentation of pedicular screw fixation strength, *Clin. Orthop.*, 296, 278, 1993.
13. Chapman, J.R., Harrington, R.M., Lee, K.M., et al., Factors affecting the pullout strength of cancellous bone screws, *J. Biomech. Eng.*, 118, 391, 1996.
14. Daftari, T.K., Horton, W.C., and Hutton, W.C., Correlations between screw hole preparation, torque of insertion, and pullout strength for spinal screws, *J. Spinal Disord.*, 7, 139, 1994.
15. Horton, W.C., Blackstock, S.F., Norman, J.T., et al., Strength of fixation of anterior vertebral body screws, *Spine*, 21, 439, 1996.
16. Brod, J.J., The concepts and terms of mechanics, *Clin. Orthop.*, 146, 9, 1980.
17. Stromsoe, K., Kok, W.L., Hoiseth, A., and Alho, A., Holding power of the 4.5 mm AO/ASIF cortex screw in cortical bone in relation to bone mineral, *Injury*, 24, 656, 1993.
18. Skinner, R., Maybee, J., Transfeldt, E., et al., Experimental pullout testing and comparison of variables in transpedicular screw fixation. A biomechanical study, *Spine*, 15, 195, 1990.
19. DeCoster, T.A., Heetderks, D.B., Downey, D.J., et al., Optimizing bone screw pullout force, *J. Orthop. Trauma*, 4, 169, 1990.
20. Halvorson, T.L., Kelley, L.A., Thomas, K.A., et al., Effects of bone mineral density on pedicle screw fixation, *Spine*, 19, 2415, 1994.
21. Kohn, D. and Rose, C., Primary stability of interference screw fixation. Influence of screw diameter and insertion torque, *Am. J. Sports Med.*, 22, 334, 1994.
22. Maiman, D.J., Pintar, F.A, Yoganandan, N., et al., Pullout strength of Caspar cervical screws, *Neurosurgery*, 31, 1097, 1992.
23. Ellis, J.A. and Laskin, D.M., Analysis of seating and fracturing torque of bicortical screws, *J. Oral Maxillofac. Surg.*, 52, 483, 1994.
24. Schwimmer, A., Greenberg, A.M., Kummer, F., and Kaynar, A., The effect of screw size and insertion technique on the stability of the mandibular sagittal split osteotomy, *J. Oral Maxillofac. Surg.*, 52, 45, 1994.
25. Soshi, S., Shiba, R., Kondo, H., and Murota, K., An experimental study on transpedicular screw fixation in relation to osteoporosis of the lumbar spine, *Spine*, 16, 1335, 1991.
26. Krag, M.H., Beynnon, B.D., Pope, M.H., and DeCoster, T.A., Depth of insertion of transpedicular vertebral screws into human vertebrae: effect upon screw–vertebra interface strength, *J. Spinal Disord.*, 1, 287, 1988.

27. Ryken, T.C., Goel, V.K., Clausen, J.D., and Traynelis, V.C., Assessment of unicortical and bicortical fixation in a quasistatic cadaveric model. Role of bone mineral density and screw torque, *Spine*, 20, 1861, 1995.
28. Keaveny, T.M. and Hayes, W.C., A 20-year perspective on the mechanical properties of trabecular bone, *J. Biomech. Eng.*, 115, 534, 1993.
29. Baldwin, N.G. and Benzel, E.C., Sacral fixation using iliac instrumentation and a variable-angle screw device. Technical note, *J. Neurosurg.*, 81, 313, 1994.
30. Benzel, E.C. and Baldwin N.G., Crossed-screw fixation of the unstable thoracic and lumbar spine, *J. Neurosurg.*, 82, 11, 1995.
31. Hadjipavlou, A.G., Nicodemus, C.L., Al-Hamdan, F.A., et al., Correlation of bone equivalent mineral density to pullout resistance of triangulated pedicle screw construct, *J. Spinal Disord.*, 10, 12, 1997.
32. Kwok, A.W., Finkelstein, J.A., Woodside, T., et al., Insertional torque and pullout strengths of conical and cylindrical pedicle screws in cadaveric bone, *Spine*, 21, 2429, 1996.
33. Pena, F., Grontvedt, T., Brown, G.A., et al., Comparison of failure strength between metallic and absorbable interference screws. Influence of insertion torque, tunnel-bone block gap, bone mineral density, and interference, *Am. J. Sports Med.*, 24, 329, 1996.
34. Hearn, T.C., Schatzker, J., and Wolfson, N., Extraction strength of cannulated cancellous bone screws, *J. Orthop. Trauma*, 7, 138, 1993.
35. Standard Test Methods for Mechanical Fasteners in Wood. *Annual Book of ASTM Standards*, Vol. 4, ASTM, Philadelphia, 1999, 268.
36. Eysel, P., Schwitalle, M., Oberstein, A., et al., Preoperative estimation of screw fixation strength in vertebral bodies, *Spine*, 23, 174, 1998.
37. Lieberman, I.H., Khazim, R., and Woodside. T., Anterior vertebral body screw pullout testing. A comparison of Zeilke, Kaneda, Universal Spine System, and Universal Spine System with pullout-resistant nut, *Spine*, 23, 908, 1998.
38. Pfeiffer, M., Gilbertson, L.G., Goel, V.K., et al., Effect of specimen fixation method on pullout tests of pedicle screws, *Spine*, 21, 1037, 1996.
39. Sell, P., Collins, M., and Dove, J., Pedicle screws: axial pullout strength in the lumbar spine, *Spine*, 13, 1075, 1988.
40. Kaab, M.J., Putz, R., Gebauer, D., and Plitz, W., Changes in cadaveric cancellous vertebral bone strength in relation to time. A biomechanical investigation, *Spine*, 23, 1215, 1998.

37 Finite Element Analysis for Evaluating Mechanical Properties of the Bone–Implant Interface

Keith R. Williams

CONTENTS

I. INTRODUCTION

An example of a mechanical interaction between the implant and bone occurs following the loading of titanium dental pins surgically implanted in the mandible. Titanium pins are now used routinely for fixed and removable bridge and single implant restorations in edentulous and partially dentate patients. The clinical implantation technique has remained as established by Brånemark[1] and colleagues some 20 years ago, although the actual pin design has undergone various modifications by subsequent workers. The ability of titanium to osseointegrate[2,3] into bone has resulted in very high success rates for this type of clinical restoration. For these reasons this chapter will concentrate mainly on assessing the mechanical stability of titanium dental implants in bone, although a static analysis of a knee ligament prosthesis in cancellous bone is also investigated.

Osseointegration is defined as a direct contact between an implant and adjacent hard tissue.[1-3] The chemical and biological processes that take place at the interface between a solid implant and biological tissue depend on various factors. These include the implant biocompatibility, the presence of infection, the interval between the operation and the distribution of load to the pin, and the clinical procedure followed. Variations in these factors can lead to different rates of osseointegration and degrees of stability of the pin in the surrounding tissue, ranging from complete bone fixation to fibrous encapsulation. It is therefore important that an assessment be made of the state of pin stability before fixed or removable metal work or other attachments are made to titanium implants. Indeed, a non-invasive technique whereby an assessment of the fixity of the implant in tissue with time would appear an ideal clinical situation. It is believed that the natural frequency of vibration of the implant in the surrounding tissue offers the best method of estimating this interaction. However, natural frequency analysis alone provides no indication of the type and quality of bone supporting the implant. X-ray radiography does not offer a high enough resolution to be able to indicate the bone quality at the interface; hence, the current adoption of the finite-element approach to the problem.

Certain noninvasive methods for the evaluation of fracture healing of long bones have been developed over the past 10 years [4-7] relying on vibrational methods [8-10] for the assessment of bone healing with time. Essentially, two techniques have been devised; in the first, the resonances are measured by the impedance probe technique, while the second relies on impulse excitation by hammer impact. Both techniques give good reproducibility when the experimental conditions are idealized in the laboratory on cadaver material.[5]

A similar approach has been attempted within the broad area of dental treatment. The equipment developed again makes use of an impulse excitation in order to assess the state of periodontal health. The test relies on measurement of the deceleration of an impacting probe on the surface of the tooth and provides a subjective measure of the viability of the periodontium. This test method may be useful in assessing the preliminary stages of osseointegration since it is probable that the material properties of the initial amorphous zone surrounding the implant may be similar to those of the periodontium [11] resulting in similar displacements and decelerations. However, when an implant is supported by bone with significantly higher elastic moduli and density, the probe method becomes unreliable. This unreliability may be due to the low frequency of probe excitation (4 Hz). Thus, vibrational methods are being developed [12] relying on higher excitation frequencies in order to measure implant fixity in bone. Indeed, natural frequency analysis of the implant in tissue offers a more sensitive means of measuring the implant movement following the application of physiologically acceptable excitation loads.

These vibrational techniques have been simulated using finite-element methodologies.[13,14] Results from these computer models suggest the natural frequencies of vibration of the implant are extremely sensitive to the fixity conditions at the implant–bone interface or the degree of osseointegration. These simulation studies provide a reasonable understanding of the range and importance of the variables that require measuring experimentally and clinically in order to allow an assessment of bone healing and eventual osseointegration following surgery. The finite-element method has also been used to study the behavior of endosseous implants in tissue and related problems,[15-22] as well as the biomechanics of the osseointegration process.[23-26]

In this work, the natural frequencies and mode shapes of vibration of a single titanium implant fixed in various media and the mandible have been calculated using a cantilever bar attached to the dental pin and excited using an attached piezoelectric plate.[27] Additionally, due to the clinical complexities in attaching such a cantilever *in situ,* a simpler impulse technique has also been examined in which the dental pin was excited directly by hammer impact and the resulting dynamic response observed. In this way, the natural frequencies of vibration may be identified with healing time and hence the exact level of integration existing around the implant. It is possible using modern numerical analysis techniques to discretize the various tissues and their anatomy existing around the implant and assign various mechanical properties to these volumes in order to evaluate the degree of osseointegration or pin fixity with time. Since the discretized volumes may be of the order of size of trabecular processes, a correlation may be established between the pin frequency and its fixity in the bone. Furthermore, the numerical procedures allow a variety of bone properties to be input to the model ranging from isotropic to more realistic anisotropic nonlinear behavior. In this work, both homogeneous and recently measured orthotropic properties [28] have been used. A reasonably simple discretization of trabecular bone based on a plate model in contact with a titanium implant has also been examined and the resultant interfacial stresses and strains compared with recently acquired experimental data.

Accordingly, a variety of possible implant support conditions, bone types and properties, and bone adaptation parameters have been set up and interfacial stresses, displacements, and natural frequencies calculated. The sensitivity of the natural frequencies to these variable conditions have been analyzed over a time interval sufficient to be able to offer data that lead to a clinical interpretation of the osseointegration condition.

II. MODELING AND METHODS

The experimental methodology for the measurement of the natural frequencies of vibration of implants in supporting media has been the subject of a recent study.[27] Essentially, the setup consists of a small cantilever between 15 and 22 mm long and 2 by 2.6 mm in cross section, to which are attached piezoelectric plates and which is then screwed onto the implant. The external frequency excitation is then increased until the first natural frequency of vibration of the pin is reached and then recorded. Various cantilever designs have been produced, but in this work an axial and right-angled cantilever attachment to the dental implant has been modeled.

A. AXIAL CANTILEVER

The finite-element discretization initially modeled the dental implant as an axially symmetric arrangement using axisymmetric triangular and quadrilateral elements (Figure 37.1). Pin support was initially provided by assigning various levels of spring fixity to the threaded portion of the implant over a range 1 to 10^6 N/mm (10^{-3} to 10^3 N/m). Subsequently, in order to increase the sensitivity of the model to the support provided by the surrounding tissue a full three-dimensional (3D) discretization was established using six- and eight-noded continuum elements incorporating both axial and right-angled cantilevers (Figure 37.1 shows the axial model). The refinement of this mesh allowed the tissue properties to be changed between that of collagenous fiber to cortical bone at the implant–bone interface and also allowed the incorporation of crestal and basal bone elements adjacent to the implant in order to simulate a more realistic *in vivo* model. The volume of bone was gradually extended radially from the implant to a maximum of 22 mm in order to simulate increasing support and the possibility of bone growth around the dental pin during healing.

B. DENTAL IMPLANTS IN THE MANDIBLE

A 3D discretization of a section of the human mandible is shown in Figure 37.2 with both a single implant and an implant with right-angled cantilever attachment.

The basic geometric model reported in the present work derives from the anatomical measurement of several mandibles by tomographic scanning. The mandible is assumed to be symmetric, and accordingly only one half is discretized with the inclusion of two osseointegrated but unconnected dental pins as shown in Figure 37.2. This figure illustrates the conditions for the cantilever setup on the dental pin. The local z direction is along the axis of the dental pins while the x direction is parallel to the crestal ridge and the y direction is orthoradial at the symmetry interface. The material properties assumed for pin, cortical, and cancellous bone are taken from those indicated earlier.[28] Fixity of the model discretization is assumed at the symmetry interface and all nodes surrounding the condyle head.

Initially, a simple eigenvalue extraction of the discretized model was carried out in order to provide the first few natural frequencies as calculated for the axial model (see Figure 37.2). However, this numerical approach is not sufficiently sensitive to the local pin–bone interface condition in the current model and yields only bending modes for the complete mandible. Accordingly, a dynamic analysis procedure was implemented.

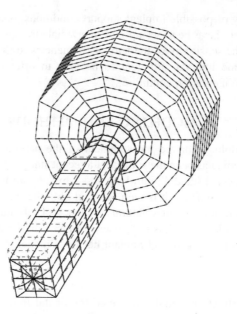

FIGURE 37.1 Axial cantilever attached to a dental implant. Axisymmetric and 3D discretization (mode 1 resonance dotted).

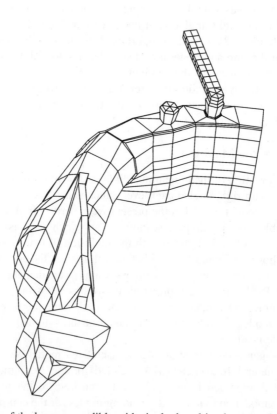

FIGURE 37.2 Section of the human mandible with single dental implants, one with attached cantilever.

In order to examine the natural frequency of vibration of the cantilever model, an impulse excitation was applied at the end of the cantilever (node 8499) in the z direction rather than the use of piezoelectric plates described earlier. The impulse length, t_o, was varied between 5×10^{-4} and 5×10^{-6} sec in order to assess the effect of impulse strength on frequency. With the cantilever removed as indicated in Figure 37.2 impulse loads of 100 N were applied in two different directions, the first in an orthoradial direction (local y direction) and the second series in a direction along the cortical crestal ridge (essentially local x direction). Under these conditions the impulse length was varied between 10^{-4} and 2×10^{-6} s. In all these initial loading conditions the pin is assumed fixed to the surrounding bone; i.e., osseointegration is assumed to have taken place. Subsequently, partial osseointegration of the implant was modeled by incorporating spring elements at the pin–bone interface.

Prior to implementing the dynamic approach, a forced harmonic response analysis was completed which provided vibration data over the whole of the discretized volume allowing the movement of each node to be identified. This approach provides valuable information on the displacement at the pin–bone interface at the first few natural frequencies for the pin–cantilever model unlike the initial natural frequency extraction procedure of the whole discretized volume.

The equation of motion of a system with one degree of freedom and an excitation $F(t)$ is

$$m\ddot{x} + c\dot{x} + kx = F(t) \tag{37.1}$$

where m is the mass matrix, c is the damping matrix, k is the stiffness matrix, x is the displacement, $\dot{x}$ is the velocity, and $\ddot{x}$ is the acceleration.

The system response due to a unit impulse input with zero initial conditions is called its impulse response. A unit impulse is impossible to realize in applications but an excitation can be considered an impulse if its duration is very short compared with the natural period $(1/f_n)$ of the system.[29]

If a shock $F(t)$ is applied to a mass m, the equation of motion is that given by Equation 37.1 and the response $x(t)$ is

$$x(t) = \int_0^t F(t)h(t)dt \tag{37.2}$$

where

$$h(t) = \frac{1}{\omega m} e^{\zeta \omega t} \sin \omega t \tag{37.3}$$

For a shock of time length t_o and for $t > t_o$ the maximum value of $x(t)$ can be expressed as

$$\frac{x_{max}}{F_o/k} = \frac{2r}{r^2 - 1} \cos \frac{\pi}{2r} \tag{37.4}$$

which gives the residual shock spectrum since it occurs after the shock has terminated,

where

$$r = \frac{\omega_i}{\omega_n}, \quad \omega_n^2 = \frac{k}{m}, \quad \omega_n t_o = \frac{\pi}{r}, \quad \text{and} \quad \omega_n = 2\pi f_n$$

or more simply

$$\frac{d_{max}}{d_i} = 2\sin\pi\frac{t_o}{T}$$
(37.5)

for

$$\frac{t_o}{T} \leq \frac{1}{2}$$

where d_{max} is the maximum displacement, d_i is the initial displacement, T is the initial period of vibration $= 2\pi/\omega_n$, and d_{max}/d_i is the magnification factor, R.

C. KNEE LIGAMENT CONNECTOR IN CANCELLOUS BONE

The value of this type of study is quantification of the holding of a screw in cancellous bone with different bone trabeculae directions. The finite-element analysis should help in allowing modifications to the screw design as well as providing an indication of the fixation in tissue. It is also of value to be able to quantify stresses at the microstructural level in order to gain knowledge of possible mechanically induced bone remodeling or excessive loading leading to local bone fracture

Previously, effective stiffness and microstructural stresses have been approximated using a representative volume element (RVE) approach.[30] This involves modeling and analyzing small volumes of the composite material under a set of arbitrary boundary conditions. Other investigators of the mechanical properties of trabecular bone have idealized the bone geometry as intersecting plates[31] or as spherical voids within a cube.[32] Each of these approaches can only supply upper or lower bounds on the effective stiffness because boundary conditions are unknown.

The current methodology again relies on a RVE approach using plates, but here the boundary conditions should be better defined from a knowledge of the experimentally available pullout test results. The finite-element discretizations are based on radiographic and histological observations of the trabeculae directions and dimensions. The intersecting trabecula plates were arranged to be at 0°, 45°, and 90° to the direction of loading of the bone. The model employed quadrilateral brick and pentahedral continuum elements. Elastic properties of the trabeculae were varied between 10 and 20 GPa and the intratrabecular property as 1 GPa. These two values provided global trabecular bone elastic behavior of

$$E = 12.3 \text{ GPa} \quad \nu = 0.26$$

and

$$E = 7.9 \text{ GPa} \quad \nu = 0.24$$

The failure loads obtained from the pullout tests[33] were used in the model as applied loads for each trabecula direction, thereby allowing location and magnitude of stresses at the screw–bone interface. An elastic modulus and Poisson's ratio of $E = 7.9$ GPa and $\nu = 0.24$ were judged to be most representative of bovine bone properties and were used subsequently in the stress and displacement calculations. The bone–screw assembly was axisymmetric, allowing computation to be reduced by modeling a 60° section of the whole. The finite-element discretization for the 0° and 90° calculations used a model containing 2982 elements while it was necessary to use 5964 pentahedral elements to model the 45° trabeculae. Concentrated loads of 3.6, 2.8, and 2.4 N were applied to each of the 39 nodes at the screw surface providing total loads over the modeled screws of 840, 655, and 560 N for the 0°, 45°, and 90° trabecula directions, respectively. The total loads were obtained from the screw pullout tests. The nodes at the base of the trabecular bone block were fixed in the x, y, and z global directions.

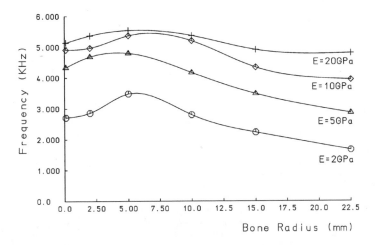

FIGURE 37.3 Variatiozn in natural frequency of vibration of a dental implant with bone modulus and bone support.

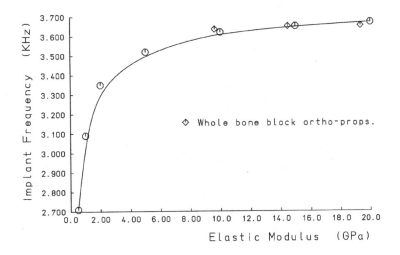

FIGURE 37.4 First natural frequency of the implant in a cylindrical bone block (Figure 37.1) for changing homogeneous and orthotropic bone properties.

III. RESULTS

A. Axial Model

Figure 37.3 shows the change of the first natural frequency with bone density/modulus and the position of bone support around the implant for the axisymmetric case. Following a shallow maximum at a position 5 mm from the pin, the frequencies gradually fall away as the volume of bone surrounding the implant increases. The frequencies are also seen to increase with bone modulus in the range 2×10^9 to 20×10^9 Pa. The effect of changing the bone properties from homogeneous to orthotropic were investigated using a right-angled cantilever arrangement similar to that shown in Figure 37.1. The results are shown in Figure 37.4 which indicates a rapid rise in frequency as the modulus of the supporting tissues changes from that near fibrous material to cortical bone. Superimposed on this graph is the frequency when the whole-bone block assumes orthotropic properties (diamonds).

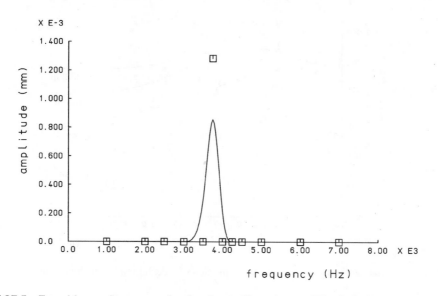

FIGURE 37.5 Forced harmonic response for the pin–cantilever in mandible discretization with excitation at the cantilever extremity indicating the first natural frequency.

TABLE 37.1
Impulse Response Values for Pin and Cantilever

$t_0 \times 10^{-6}$ (s)	T (s)	d_i (mm)	d_{max} (mm)	$R = \dfrac{d_{max}}{d_i}$	f_n (kHz)	$\dfrac{t_o}{T} = \dfrac{\omega_n}{\omega_i}$	$\dfrac{\omega_i}{\omega_n}$
			100 N Load				
5	3.5×10^{-4}	0.55×10^{-4}	0.75×10^{-4}	1.36	2.86	0.014	71.4
10	3.5×10^{-4}	1.0×10^{-4}	1.53×10^{-4}	1.53	2.86	0.028	35.0
50	3.8×10^{-4}	3.5×10^{-4}	6.7×10^{-4}	1.91	2.63	0.130	7.69
100	4.4×10^{-4}	8.5×10^{-4}	11.2×10^{-4}	1.31	2.27	0.230	4.34
200	5.8×10^{-4}	14.2×10^{-4}	14.6×10^{-4}	1.03	1.72	0.345	2.9
500	11.0×10^{-4}	17.5×10^{-4}	16.0×10^{-4}	0.91	0.91	0.450	2.22
			10 N Load				
100	4.4×10^{-4}	0.85×10^{-4}	112×10^{-4}	132	2.27	0.230	4.34

B. Mandible Model

The forced harmonic response spectrum is shown in Figure 37.5 and indicates a first natural frequency of the pin of about 3.6 kHz.

Table 37.1 shows the results of the dynamic analysis of the pin/cantilever model over the impulse duration periods from 5×10^{-4} to 5×10^{-6} s. These data are plotted in Figure 37.6 where the change in frequencies with impulse duration are indicated. The corresponding results for this dynamic analysis of pin only are shown in Table 37.2 for excitation in the local x and y directions. The variation in frequency with pulse length ratio for the pin with the cantilever removed is shown in Figure 37.6.

Partial integration of the implant was modeled using spring elements at the bone–implant interface. The change in frequency for different spring support conditions for an impulse strength of $t = 5.0 \times 10^{-5}$ is shown in Figure 37.7.

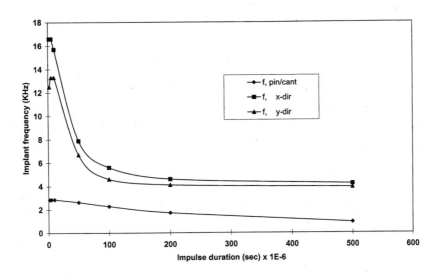

FIGURE 37.6   Change in implant frequency with impulse strength for the pin–cantilever and pin-only model (full integration).

TABLE 37.2
Impulse Response Values for the Pin-Only Discretization (100 N load)

$t_0 \times 10^{-6}$ (s)	T (s^{-1})	d_i (mm)	d_{max} (mm)	$R = \dfrac{d_{max}}{d_i}$	f_n (kHz)	$\dfrac{t_o}{T} = \dfrac{\omega_n}{\omega_i}$
		Impulse Local x Direction				
2	6×10^{-5}	1.4×10^{-6}	3.5×10^{-6}	2.5	16.6	0.033
5	6.0×10^{-5}	3.5×10^{-6}	8.5×10^{-6}	2.4	16.6	0.09
10	6.3×10^{-5}	8.7×10^{-6}	13.7×10^{-6}	1.57	15.8	0.16
50	1.25×10^{-4}	24×10^{-6}	30×10^{-6}	1.25	7.9	0.40
100	1.8×10^{-4}	34×10^{-6}	25×10^{-6}	0.73	5.56	0.54
		Impulse Local y Direction				
2	8×10^{-5}	1.25×10^{-6}	3.7×10^{-6}	2.84	12.5	0.03
5	7.5×10^{-5}	3.0×10^{-6}	8.3×10^{-6}	2.76	13.3	0.07
10	7.5×10^{-5}	7.5×10^{-6}	14.5×10^{-6}	1.93	13.3	0.13
50	15.0×10^{-5}	40.0×10^{-6}	22×10^{-6}	0.55	6.7	0.33
100	2.2×10^{-4}	50×10^{-6}	28×10^{-6}	0.56	4.55	0.45

C. KNEE LIGAMENT CONNECTOR

The experimental results of the screw pullout tests indicate a stress of 54.9 MPa obtained when the trabeculae are orientated in the same direction as the implant axis. This direction is the normal load-bearing direction of the bone. At 90° to this direction, a stress of 37.1 MPa was obtained and an intermediate value of 42.8 MPa at a 45° direction. The finite-element model was employed to explain these failures at a microscopic level.

Following an examination of the types of stress present at the screw–bone interface, it was concluded that an effective shear stress best explained failure. An example of this stress distribution at the bone–screw interface for the 0° trabeculae direction is shown in Figure 37.8. Relative stress values are shown as contours and the bone plates of the model can be observed. The highest stresses in the bone occur at the minor diameter of the screw threads and fall away rapidly along the interface

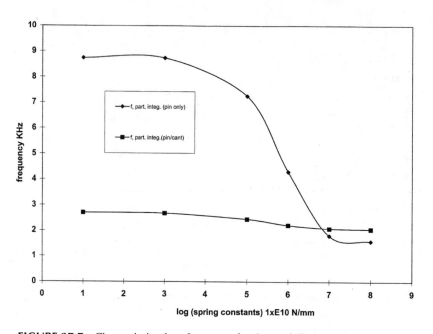

FIGURE 37.7   Change in implant frequency for the partially integrated condition.

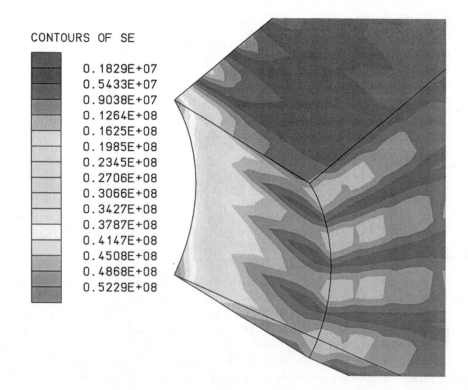

FIGURE 37.8   Effective stress contours at the implant trabecular bone interface. Screw pullout calculation for a simple plate discretization of trabecular bone.

away from the nodal support positions. The maximum effective stress predicted by the finite-element analysis model was for the 0° trabecula direction. The value of 54 MPa is in good agreement with experimentally measured values. For the 90° trabecula direction an effective stress of 37 MPa was calculated and 43 MPa for the intermediate 45° direction.

IV. DISCUSSION

The natural frequencies of vibration of cantilever sections can be associated normally with three distinct modes of propagation, namely, transverse, torsional, and longitudinal. The lowest natural frequencies in a solid beam are due to resonant transverse modes, followed by torsional and longitudinal modes. In this work, the initial dental pin/axial cantilever finite-element discretization was modeled using axisymmetric solid elements. The transverse and torsional vibration modes are therefore excluded and only the higher-frequency longitudinal mode allowed.

The frequencies calculated for the axisymmetric pin–bone block shown in Figure 37.1 are longitudinal modes and have been reduced by a value of 17.5 in Figure 37.3[13] for comparison with the nonaxisymmetric cases plotted subsequently.

Nevertheless, the natural frequencies of vibration of the implant plotted in this figure suggest a marked sensitivity to the type and quality of supporting bone. Thus, when the bone–tissue modulus or density surrounding the pin increases by a factor of ten, the first natural frequency increases by 1000 Hz. Additionally, the natural frequencies are dependent on the volume and quality of bone supporting the pin. If, as suggested clinically, cortical bone gradually builds around the implant during the healing process, then it would appear about 5 mm thickness is sufficient for optimum support (see Figure 37.3).

The calculated natural frequencies with changing homogeneous bone modulus for the full 3D discretization of pin, cantilever, and supporting bone are shown in Figure 37.4. In this analysis, the bone was fully fixed at the periphery of the bone block. Figure 37.4 also shows the effects of changing to orthotropic bone properties. These new frequency values are superimposed on the homogeneous data already indicated. The frequencies shown are somewhat different in magnitude compared with the axial cantilever model shown in Figure 37.1, due to the different geometric conditions imposed in the analysis. From these data, it is possible to calculate rates of pin integration using frequency plots such as Figure 37.4, since it is to be expected that increasing implant support is a result of increasing bone density and modulus. Thus, if a period of time P is required to obtain a final bone density/modulus during the healing period, then Figure 37.4 (i.e., frequency vs. modulus) may be converted into a plot indicating the change in frequency with time. Implant osseointegration plots similar to Figure 37.4 suggest substantial pin support is obtained early in the healing process and little change occurs after approximately 40% of the elapsed healing time.

In the earlier section of this chapter, the natural frequencies of vibration of a single dental implant with attached cantilever in a cylindrical block of bone were calculated. For a completely osseointegrated pin with approximately 5 mm of surrounding bone, a first natural frequency of about 3.3 kHz was obtained. A forced harmonic response analysis for a similar implant–cantilever setup in the human mandible shown in Figure 37.2 yields a first natural frequency of about 3.6 kHz (see Figure 37.5) which compares favorably with the earlier simplified model. The result suggests that a bone model discretization local to the implant may be adequate for dynamic analysis.

From a clinical perspective, the attachment of devices to a dental implant can prove problematical as well as involving patient stress. Thus, in the dynamic analysis approach, the cantilever has been removed and an impulse excitation applied directly to the top of the dental implant. This work follows on from an earlier analysis[34] where this methodology was attempted purely as a means of examining the type of implant response to be expected in a clinical situation. However, in this earlier work,[34] an arbitrary impulse excitation was applied at the top of the pin and while still providing valuable displacement information may not necessarily yield the correct natural frequencies required for comparison with a parallel clinical study.

In the present work, this problem has been addressed by examining a range of impulse durations/ strengths for both the cantilever model and pin-only model shown in Figure 37.2. A listing of all the frequency information obtained from a range of impulse values is shown in Table 37.1 for the cantilever configuration. Figure 37.6 shows the change in frequency with impulse strength when the cantilever is excited at the extremity. Clearly, true dynamic frequency values are only obtained at short impulse durations ($\sim 5 \times 10^{-6}$ s) and small displacements. As the impulse duration increases, the first natural frequency falls to unrealistic values near 1 kHz. The frequency obtained at an impulse of 5×10^{-6} s ($\sim$3.0 kHz) is in close agreement with that obtained from the forced harmonic analysis (see Figure 37.5) and the calculated value from the pin–cantilever–bone block model. The effect of changing the impulse load from 100 to 10 N has no effect on the frequency values, only on pin displacement.

The frequency data for the pin-only configuration (Figure 37.2) are shown in Table 37.2. These data were obtained from impulse loads applied in the local x and y directions. Due to the varying stiffness values of bone in the different directions,[34] it would be expected that different frequency values emerge from this analysis. This appears to be the case with the frequency peaking at 16.6 kHz in the x direction where more bone support for the pin is to be expected compared with the orthoradial direction (y) with a maximum frequency of 13.3 kHz

The frequencies are plotted against pulse length in Figure 37.6 for both loading directions. The displacement and frequency values are sensitive to pulse duration, and as for the cantilever model, small impulse durations are required to establish the correct frequency values, in this case near 2×10^{-6} s.

The frequency data calculated above was based on full integration of the implant with bone. Any changes in frequency calculated with time thus demonstrate a change in the type and quality of bone supporting the implant. In order to explore the condition of less than full integration, spring elements were included at the implant–bone interface. By varying the value of the spring constants, a range of partial integration conditions were simulated. Figure 37.7 demonstrates the changing implant frequency with changing spring support for an intermediate impulse loading of $t_o = 5 \times 10^{-5}$ s. In these partial integration calculations, the supporting bone properties were maintained constant. The calculations indicate the extreme sensitivity of the natural frequency of vibration of the implant to the support offered by the tissue at the implant–bone interface.

The mechanical data values used for the axial cantilever and mandible models outlined above use essentially homogeneous and orthotropic bone properties for estimating the implant fixity. This is an idealized situation since it is known that bone properties are markedly directional.

A relatively simple perpendicular plate model for cancellous bone has yielded excellent agreement with experiment (Figure 37.8). The model was effective in explaining the quantitative differences observed in screw pullout tests and also explained the radiographic features observed.[33] The calculated stiffness values were somewhat higher than those measured experimentally, which was attributed to the rigid boundary conditions imposed in the model discretization. However, the calculations confirm the directionality of properties of cancellous bone and demonstrate a significant difference in screw-holding ability depending upon the direction of the cancellous bone spicules.

V. CONCLUSION

The dynamic analysis by impulse excitation of a dental pin osseointegrated in bone has indicated a sensitivity of the implant response to both impulse duration and direction. The analysis provides response data from the implant for a range of impulse strengths. These data may be used with clinically measured experimental data for a correct interpretation of implant osseointegration, rate of bone healing, or the onset of infection or pin integration failure. Refinements to these models should include discretization of bone volumes closer to the implant which will allow more-detailed stress evaluation, a more exact representation of the bone structure, and relaxation of the rigid boundary conditions which produce high stiffness values. It is the intention in future work to develop and refine further the mesh by the introduction of material and geometric nonlinearities in order to simulate the early stages of bone healing. These new procedures will allow full validation of the numerical technique and extend its use to a noninvasive clinical assessment of osseointegration.

REFERENCES

1. Brånemark, P.-I., Osseointegration and its experimental background, *J. Prosthet. Dent.,* 50, 399, 1983.
2. Albrektsson, T., Hansson, H.A., and Ivarsson, B., Interface analysis of titanium and zirconium bone implants, *Biomaterials*, 6, 97, 1985.
3. Brånemark, P.-I., Hansson, B.O., and Adell, R., Osseointegrated implants in the treatment of the edentulous jaw. Experience from a 10 year period, *Scand. J. Plast. Reconstr. Surg.*, 16 (Suppl.), 1977.
4. Collier, R.J., Nadan, O., and Thomas, T.G., The mechanical resonances of a human tibia: Part I — *in vitro*, *J. Biomech.*, 15, 545, 1882.
5. Christensen, A.B., Ammintzboll, F., Dyrnbye, C., et al., Assessment of tibial stiffness by vibration testing *in situ*. I. Identification of mode shapes in different supporting conditions, *J. Biomech.*, 19, 53, 1986.
6. Collier, R.J. and Donarski, R.J., Non-invasive method of measuring resonant frequency of a human tibia *in vivo*. Parts I and II, *J. Biomed. Eng.*, 9, 321, 1987.
7. Bull, D.R., Nokes, L.D.M., and Frampton, R., Detection of internal fixation plate loosening by means of an analysis of vibratory response, *J. Biomed. Eng.*, 13, 321, 1991.
8. Doherty, W.M., Dynamic Response of Human Tibia, Ph.D. dissertation, University of California, Berkeley, 1971.
9. Jurist, J.M. and Kianion, K., Three models of the vibrating ulna, *J. Biomech.*, 6, 331, 1973.
10. Lewis, J.L., A dynamic model of a healing fractured long bone, *J. Biomech.*, 9, 17, 1975.
11. Albrektsson, T. and Hansson, H.A., An ultrastructural characterisation of the interface between bone and sputtered titanium or stainless steel surfaces, *Biomaterials*, 7, 201, 1986.
12. Meredith, N., Alleyne, D., and Cowley P., Quantitative determination of the stability of the implant–tissue interface using resonance frequency analysis, *Clin. Oral Implants Res.*, 7, 1, 1996.
13. Williams, K.R. and Natali, A.N., Simulation of the stability of dental implants in bone by natural frequency analysis, in *2nd Symposium on Computer Methods in Biomechanics and Biomedical Engineering*, Middleton, J.M., Pande, G.R., and Jones, M., Eds., Edward Arnold, London, 1995, 415.
14. Williams, K.R. and Williams, A.D.C., Impulse response of a dental implant in bone by numerical analysis, *Biomaterials*, 715, 18, 1997.
15. Awadalla, H.A., Azarbal, M., Ismail, Y.H., and el-Ibiari, W., Three-dimensional finite element stress analysis of a cantilever fixed partial denture, *J. Prosthet. Dent.*, 68, 243, 1992.
16. Chen, J., Lu, X., Paydar, N., et al., Mechanical simulation of the mandible with and without an endosseous implant, *Med. Eng. Phys.*, 16, 53, 1994.
17. Hart, R.T., Hennebel, V.V., Thongpreda, N., et al., Modeling the biomechanics of the mandible: a three-dimensional finite element study, *J. Biomech.*, 25, 261, 1992.
18. Holmes, R.T., Grigsby, W.R., Goel, V.K., and Keller, J.C., Comparison of stress transmission in the IMZ implant system with polyoxymethylene or titanium intramobile element: a finite element stress analysis, *Int. J. Oral Maxillofac. Implants*, 7, 450, 1992.
19. Ko, C.C., Kohn, D.H., and Hollister, S.J., Micromechanics of implant/tissue interfaces, *J. Oral Implantol.*, 18, 220, 1992.
20. Meijer, H.J., Starmans, F.J., Bosman, F., and Steen, W.H.A., A comparison of three finite-element models of an edentulous mandible provided with implants, *J. Oral Rehabil.*, 20, 147, 1993.
21. Meijer, H.J., Starmans, F.J., Bosman, F., and Steen, W.H.A., A three dimensional finite element analysis of bone around dental implants in an edentulous mandible, *Arch. Oral Biol.*, 38, 491, 1993.
22. Rieger, M.R., Adams, W.K., and Kinzel, G.L., A finite element survey of eleven endosseous implants, *J. Prosthet. Dent.*, 63, 457, 1990.
23. Richter, E.J., Basic biomechanics of dental implants in prosthetic dentistry, *J. Prosthet. Dent.*, 61, 602, 1989.
24. Hart, R.T., Davy, D.T., and Heiple, K.G., A computational method for stress analysis of adaptive elastic materials with a view toward applications in strain-induced bone remodeling, *J. Biomech. Eng.*, 106, 342, 1984.
25. Natali, A.N., Nonlinear interaction phenomena between pin and bone, *Clin. Mater.*, 9, 109, 1992.
26. Natali A.N., and Meroi, E., Pin–bone interface: a geometric and material nonlinear analysis, *Proc. Interfaces 90*, Elsevier Science, London, 1991, 104.
27. Meredith, N., Cawley, P., and Alleyne, D., The application of modal vibration analysis to study bone healing *in vivo*, *J. Dent. Res.*, 73, 793, 1994.

28. Natali, A.N. and Meroi, E., A review of the mechanical properties of bone as a material, *J. Biomed. Eng.*, 11, 266, 1989.
29. Crede, C.E., *Shock and Vibration Concepts in Engineering Design*, McGraw-Hill, New York, 1965, 138.
30. Hashin, Z., Analysis of composite materials — a survey, *J. Appl. Mech.*, 50, 481, 1983.
31. Pugh, J.W., Rose, R.M., and Rodin, E.L., A structural model for the mechanical behavior of trabecular bone, *J. Biomech.*, 6, 657, 1973.
32. Beaupre, G.S. and Hayes, W.C., Finite element analysis of a three-dimensional open-celled model for trabecular bone, *J. Biomech. Eng.*, 107, 249, 1985.
33. Young, F.A., private communication.
34. Natali, A.N., Meroi, E., Williams, K.R., and Calabrese, L., Investigation of the integration process of dental implants by means of a numerical analysis of dynamic response, *Dent. Mater.*, 13, 325, 1997.

38 Fatigue Testing of Bioabsorbable Screws in a Synthetic Bone Substrate

William S. Pietrzak, David R. Sarver, and David H. Kohn

CONTENTS

I. INTRODUCTION

The use of rigid internal fixation (RIF) to maintain the apposition and stability of skeletal fractures and osteotomies during osseous union is one of the primary techniques employed by orthopaedic and craniomaxillofacial surgeons. Historically, such fixation devices, consisting of plates, screws, and pins, were made of medical-grade metals such as stainless steel, titanium and its alloys, and cobalt–chromium alloys. Despite the success of this mode of fixation, there has been increasing concern over certain consequences that may originate from the use of these implants. The high stiffness of these materials, relative to bone, may cause stress shielding in the vicinity of the implant, thereby weakening the bone; implant migration and growth restriction, particularly in pediatric patients, can be an issue; long-term tissue reactions to the presence of metal implants have been documented; palpability can be problematic; key radiographic information can be obscured by their presence; and they can interfere with therapeutic applications of irradiation.[1-7] All of the above can result in the need for a secondary surgical procedure to remove the implant with its attendant risks and costs. In an attempt to address this wide spectrum of issues, a new class of RIF devices has evolved over the past 30 years, and has achieved status as a viable alternative to metallic internal fixation over the past 10 years.[8-12] These devices, fabricated from bioabsorbable polymers, gradually degrade commensurate with tissue healing and are eliminated by the body. In this fashion, a temporary implant serves a temporary fixation need without the requirement of further surgical intervention to remove the implant.

There is increasing interest in the use of absorbable fixation of mandibular fractures and osteotomies, including absorbable screw fixation of sagittal split mandibular osteotomies for the correction of occlusal deficiencies.[13-17] Not only is this a significant load-bearing application, but the dynamic, cyclic nature of the applied loads mandate that not only must this fixation be capable of withstanding the magnitude of the expected loads, but also the fatigue characteristics of such fixation must be demonstrated to be capable of withstanding the expected number of cycles until osseous union occurs. Absorbable implants present special considerations with respect to characterization of their fatigue properties, and, to date, few studies have investigated the subject.[18] Presented here is a basic background of absorbable technology and the unique methods employed to determine the fatigue characteristics of such implants in a synthetic bone substrate. Clinical relevance to the case of sagittal split mandibular fixation is discussed, although the concepts presented are broad and have general applicability.

II. BACKGROUND

A. BIOABSORBABLE POLYMER TECHNOLOGY

Ideally, an absorbable polymer fixation implant should provide adequate fixation for approximately 6 to 8 weeks to permit primary healing to occur.[19] During this period, a decrease in fixation strength due to implant degradation should be matched by a corresponding increase in strength from the healing biological union. The degrading implant should not cause any deleterious physiological reaction necessitating surgical intervention. The implant should fully absorb and be totally eliminated. Once gone, the body should "forget" that the implant was ever there.[20]

In general, absorbable polymers degrade, *in vivo*, in a two-phase process.[5,20] In the first phase, water molecules infiltrate the polymer and hydrolyze the polymer chains, thereby reducing the molecular weight and causing a reduction in mechanical strength of the implant. As the polymer degrades and fragments, a cellular macrophage response ensues, with the macrophages phagocytizing the polymer debris, metabolically converting them to water and carbon dioxide which is eliminated via the kidneys and the lungs.

These degradation phases result in a timed sequence of molecular weight reduction, strength loss, and mass loss, often with a significant difference in the times between strength loss and mass loss.[20] Consequently, the implant will generally lose all mechanical strength before significant mass is lost. Many factors influence the rate of polymer degradation, including the chemical identity and microstructure of the polymer, the molecular weight, the size and shape of the implant, the vascularity of the implant site, the tissue environment (bone or soft tissue), and the state of stress application to the implant.[20-23]

The strength-loss profiles of absorbable implants are often tested under controlled laboratory conditions that simulate the *in vivo* environment, i.e., pH 7.4 phosphate-buffered saline (PBS) at 37°C.[24] The implants, submersed in the buffer either alone or attached to a substrate, are periodically removed from the bath for mechanical testing. While such testing probably provides a good approximation to the expected initial *in vivo* strength-loss profiles, it cannot mimic the *in vivo* mass-loss profiles due to the lack of a metabolizing, cellular response.

The most commonly used absorbable polymers are from the class of constituents known as alpha-hydroxy acids.[25] Such compounds include lactic acid (both D and L), glycolic acid, and *p*-dioxanone, with polymers of L-lactic acid, glycolic acid, and copolymers thereof the most prevalent. Historically, homopolymers of glycolic acid (PGA) and L-lactic acid (PLLA) have dominated clinical use. Late inflammatory reactions in response to these degrading polymers have been documented in several clinical series.[23,26-31] As the homopolymers tend to possess a high degree of crystallinity, crystalline release is thought to play a role in this reaction.[23,26-29] Additionally, PGA, which degrades very quickly, may overwhelm the local ability of the body to clear the acidic

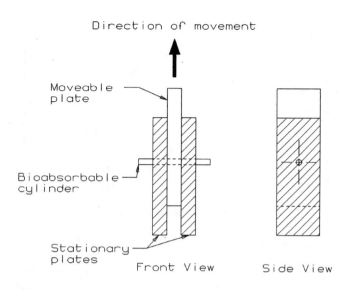

FIGURE 38.1 Schematic showing the measurement of shear strength of the bioabsorbable LactoSorb®
cylinders.

degradation products, and may be a factor in these reactions. There is a trend toward the increasing
use of amorphous copolymers which appear to have little or no incidence of these late reactions.
One such copolymer, LactoSorb® (Biomet, Inc., Warsaw, IN), is composed of 82% L-lactic acid
and 18% glycolic acid and has been used in over 10,000 clinical cases for internal fixation. This
material retains significant strength for 6 to 8 weeks,[24] requires approximately 12 months to
completely absorb,[19,32,33] and results in no late inflammatory response as demonstrated in both
animal testing[19,32] and human clinical series.[33] Coupled with appropriate implant design, LactoSorb®
appears to be suitable for many internal fixation needs. The absorbable screw implants discussed
below are made from LactoSorb® copolymer.

B. LACTOSORB® COPOLYMER *IN VITRO* STRENGTH-LOSS PROFILE

The modes by which screws can experience load *in situ* include axial pullout or extraction forces,
bending or flexural forces, and shear forces. For sagittal split mandibular osteotomies, it is the
resistance to shear that is the primary material property of interest.[13] To determine the *in vitro* shear
strength-loss profile of LactoSorb® copolymer, a model system was tested. This model consisted
of small-diameter (1.5-mm) cylindrical rods of LactoSorb® copolymer that provided a uniform
cross-sectional area for the tests. The cylinders were submersed in pH 7.4 PBS at 37°C for
predetermined periods up to 12 weeks, then removed from the bath and mechanically tested at the
various intervals.

Shear strength testing consisted of placing the cylinders through a continuous hole drilled through
a sequence of three steel plates, placed directly alongside each other, as shown in Figure 38.1. The
clearance between the plate holes and the cylinders was sufficiently tight to just permit introduction
of the cylinders without notable excess clearance. The two outer plates were fixed to the base of the
mechanical test system (Sintech 1/S, Sintech, Inc., Research Triangle Park, NC) while the central
plate was attached to the movable crosshead of the apparatus. With the crosshead engaged to move
upward at the rate of 5.0 mm/min, force–displacement curves were recorded. Shear strength was
defined as the peak shear stress at failure (severance of the cylinder) as calculated by the Testworks
software (Sintech, Inc. Research Triangle Park, NC). Five specimens were tested in this fashion at
each *in vitro* time point. The statistical significance of differences between means was determined
by ANOVA and subsequent Student–Newman–Keuls test at $p < 0.05$.

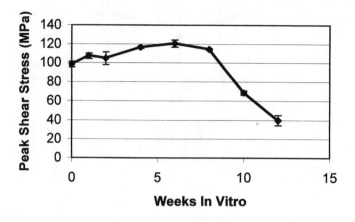

FIGURE 38.2　Peak shear stress of LactoSorb® cylinders *in vitro*. Error bars represent ±1 SD.

Figure 38.2 shows the *in vitro* shear strength-loss profile. In this model, the shear strength increased significantly over the first 8 weeks and did not significantly diminish, relative to initial values, until after 10 weeks of hydrolysis in PBS. Although not fully understood, this phenomenon of initial strength increase has also been observed by the authors when performing similar tests on LactoSorb® copolymer screws (unpublished data). This may be due to the occurrence of two competing reactions, with hydrolytic strength loss dominating after several weeks.

C. Mathematical Model of Screw Fixation of a Mandibular Osteotomy

During orthognathic mandibular surgery to correct occlusal deficiencies, the mandibular ramus is bilaterally sagittally split. The distal fragment, or the body of the mandible, is then advanced or set back. The fragments are typically internally fixed with three screws on each side. Generally, the patient is placed in maxillomandibular fixation (MMF) and on a soft diet for a period of time, followed by MMF removal and a program of progressively more demanding rehabilitation.[34]

The analysis of the state of stress in the screws used to fix sagittal split mandibular osteotomies is complex, as has been derived by Kohn et al.[13] In its simplest form, the distal bone fragment can be treated as a cantilever beam bolted onto a rigid plate. A measure of the stability of such fixation can be defined as the deflection of the tip of the beam under the influence of the loading pattern, with greater stability associated with less deflection. A mathematical model was derived for such a loading pattern that related the deflection of the tip of the distal bone fragment to the applied load, considering such factors as bone geometry, modulus, load lever arm, screw size, shear strength, and screw pattern. Typically, there is a "critical" screw in the fixation pattern that sustains the greatest shear stress and governs the stability of the fixation. The position of the critical screw varies with the screw pattern employed. Consequently, the equation relating the load on the distal fragment to the deflection of the tip of the distal fragment is dependent upon the fixation screw configuration. For a linear pattern, the relationship may be expressed as

$$\delta^{\text{total}} = L \tan \left\{ \cos^{-1}[1 - (R^2/4 + RS + S^2)D^2/2l^2G^2] \right\} + PL^3/3E \tag{38.1}$$

$$R = PL/Al \tag{38.2}$$

$$S = P/3A \tag{38.3}$$

where δ^{total} is the total deflection of the tip of the distal fragment; P is the load on the distal fragment; L is the distance between the point of load application and the centroid of the fixation screw pattern, i.e., the lever arm; D is the screw diameter; G is the shear modulus of the screws; l is the interscrew distance; A is the screw cross-sectional area; E is the elastic modulus; and I is the cross-sectional moment of inertia of the distal bone fragment.[13]

The model was validated by empirically testing both LactoSorb® copolymer and titanium screws in various substrates, including cadaver mandibles and synthetic mandibles. It was found that the dominant effect causing deflection was rotation of the distal fragment about the centroid of the screw pattern, in response to the shear deformation of the screws. Bending of the distal bone fragment under the action of the applied load had an effect that was three orders of magnitude less. Consequently, in this type of model, the quality of the substrate was not important, and, in fact, comparing predicted deflections with both synthetic and natural substrates yielded no significant differences.[13]

D. Fatigue Testing of Absorbable Materials

In general, a material specimen, exposed to fluctuating loads and deformations above a certain threshold, will eventually fail suddenly and catastrophically after a period of time. This process is known as fatigue.[35] The loads and deformations that cause fatigue failure are typically far below those that cause static failure, or failure after the application of a single stress cycle. The mechanism behind this process is the initiation and propagation of cracks to an unstable size. Once this critical size of defect is reached, the next cycle of applied stress causes catastrophic failure. Fatigue behavior is highly statistical in nature since the nucleation sites for crack initiation include material defects which, themselves, are statistically distributed. Many engineered parts, including implants, undergo cyclic loads in actual use conditions, making an understanding of their fatigue behavior an essential part of the design process.

The formal theory and practice of fatigue analysis is complex and beyond the scope of this chapter.[35] In general, the number of applied load cycles to failure (*fatigue life*) will increase with decreasing load, or stress, applied per cycle. Some materials may approach a *fatigue limit,* which is defined as the stress cycle at which the specimen can survive an infinite number of cycles, i.e., does not exhibit fatigue. Specimens can be loaded in a variety of configurations (tension, compression, shear, torsion, bending, etc.). The load cycles can be tailored by adjusting the minimum and maximum load values, the frequency, the amplitude profile, etc. A given specimen will typically be cycled until failure. Alternatively, a "run-out" can be established in which the test on a given specimen is terminated if it survives a predetermined number of load cycles, N.

Testing the fatigue characteristics of absorbable polymers presents special challenges due to the deteriorating physical properties of the polymer in a hydrolytic environment. Thus, a fatigue test performed on an absorbable polymer in dry air, where the changes in the material properties are attributed only to the applied cyclic load, will be considerably different than a test performed while the specimens are submersed in aqueous buffer, because of the combination of degradation due to cyclic loading and hydrolysis. Both of these effects may be synergistic; that is, the formation of microcracks during cyclic loading may create pathways to facilitate the penetration of water into the interior of the specimen, thereby increasing the rate of hydrolysis. Conversely, during hydrolysis, absorbable polymers typically embrittle, which would be expected to reduce fatigue performance. Consequently, the concept of a fatigue limit would not be expected since pronounced degradation would ultimately lead to failure regardless of the magnitude of the applied cyclic load.

A novel approach to the determination of the fatigue properties of absorbable polymer specimens is to preincubate the specimens, *in vitro,* in a load-free manner to create a given amount of hydrolytic degradation. Then, the specimens are cyclically loaded over a period of time that is relatively small compared with the unloaded incubation time in an effort to obtain fatigue "snapshots" of the material as hydrolysis is occurring. Thus, a composite curve can be constructed that can indicate the point of hydrolysis at which the number of cycles to failure is adversely affected.

If an absorbable polymer implant is to be used as an osteosynthesis fracture fixation device, then the implant should be inserted into an appropriate substrate, with the implant(s) and substrate

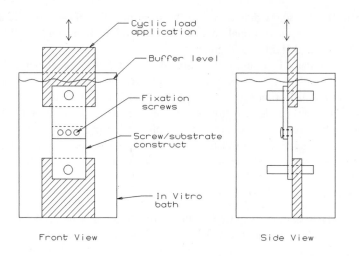

FIGURE 38.3   Schematic of synthetic substrate–absorbable screw constructs.

tested as a complex. For an osteosynthesis device, one choice of substrate is bone. However, there are many problems with the use of this substrate (see below) that make desirable the use of a synthetic substrate. Following are the details of a unique procedure to determine the fatigue characteristics of absorbable screws in synthetic bone substrate.

III. FATIGUE TESTING OF BIOABSORBABLE SCREW–SYNTHETIC BONE

A. METHODS AND MATERIALS

The absorbable osteosynthesis implants used were 2.5-mm-diameter by 11-mm-long fully threaded screws fabricated from LactoSorb® absorbable copolymer (supplied by Lorenz Surgical, Jacksonville, FL). The substrate was solid, polyurethane synthetic cortex (Pacific Research, Vashon Island, WA) with an elastic modulus of approximately 15 GPa. The synthetic cortical substrate was 3.2 mm in thickness and cut into rectangles of dimensions 26 mm wide by 37.5 mm long. Two of the cortical specimens were overlapped by 13 mm and fixed together using three of the screws in a linear pattern, directed perpendicular to the long axis of the cortical specimens, as shown in Figure 38.3. Screws were administered by drilling 2.2-mm-diameter pilot holes through the overlapping segments and tapping the holes to a threadform identical to that of the screws. The screw heads had a twist-off drive mechanism that sheared off once the screws were fully seated. Thus, all screws experienced the same final insertion torque. Screws were used positionally without lagging with an interscrew distance of approximately 7 mm. At the end of each of the two cortical specimens (opposite the center of the construct), a 6.5-mm-diameter hole was drilled to permit attachment of each end to the mechanical test apparatus with pins.

The constructs were first submersed in a circulating, temperature-controlled bath of PBS (pH 7.4, 37°C), without load, from 0 to 8 weeks prior to fatigue testing. Fatigue testing was then performed with the constructs submersed in a similar bath with the two ends of the constructs attached to the stationary base and movable crosshead of the servohydraulic custom-testing machine (Endura-Tec, Eden Prairie, MN), respectively.

During the fatigue test, a sinusoidal tensile load was applied to the construct with magnitudes from 4.5 to 45.5 kg_f (corresponding to 11.6 to 116 MPa of shear stress based on a screw minor diameter of 2.2 mm) at the rate of 1 Hz. The test apparatus was under closed-loop load control; i.e., the apparatus generated whatever displacement was required to maintain this load cycle. The bodies of the screws at the interface between the blocks were in shear. Due to the finite thickness

TABLE 38.1
Summary of Fatigue Test Results

Nonload PBS Incubation Time (weeks)	Average No. Cycles	S.E.M.	N	Log (no. cycles)
0	2.60×10^5	0	5	5.41
1	1.75×10^5	5.25×10^4	3	5.24
2	2.58×10	2.06×10^3	5	5.41
3	1.72×10^5	3.30×10^4	4	5.24
4	1.36×10^5	1.73×10^4	4	5.13
8	8.64×10^2	7.2×10^1	3	2.94

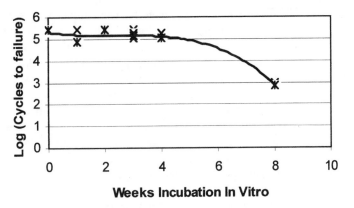

FIGURE 38.4 Plot of the log of the number of cycles to run-out (2.5×10^5) or failure as a function of weeks of initial unloaded incubation in PBS (pH 7.4, 37°C).

of each synthetic cortex, there was a distance of 3.2 mm between their centers. The high stiffness and minimal relative motion of the cortical blocks ensured that the screws did not bend during cyclic loading.

Three to five repetitions were performed for each period of "pre-soaking" the unloaded specimens. Individual runs were terminated when the screws failed by shear (a displacement greater than 2 mm detected) or a maximum of 260,000 cycles (run-out) was attained. Statistical significance of the differences between means was determined by ANOVA and subsequent application of the Student–Newman–Keuls test at $p < 0.05$.

B. RESULTS

Table 38.1 summarizes the data while Figure 38.4 shows a plot of the log of the number of cycles corresponding to run-out (2.6×10^5 cycles) or failure as a function of unloaded incubation time. The specimens attained 5.1 to 5.4 log units of cycles up to at least 4 weeks of unloaded incubation in PBS. After 8 weeks of unloaded incubation in buffer the number of cycles to failure was significantly less than those of all of the preceding time points. The trendline shows a "knee" in the curve at a time equivalent to about 6 weeks of exposure to PBS, meaning that the corresponding degree of hydrolysis is sufficient to affect the fatigue characteristics of the LactoSorb® specimens under the conditions tested. Failure of the substrate was not observed at any of the time periods.

C. Discussion

Synthetic substrates provide a number of advantages over cadaver bone for the testing of fixation implants. First, the quality of cadaver bone varies widely, requiring a large number of specimens to be tested per configuration to establish significant differences. Second, fixation implants are often used in relatively young patients whose bone quality can be poorly represented by the often fragile, osteoporotic bone characteristic of the elderly donors from whom most cadaver bone is derived. Third, cadaver bone is typically obtained "fresh-frozen," hence has not been sterilized, creating stringent handling requirements for the prevention of disease transmission. Fourth, for a long-term *in vitro* study to be performed, deterioration of the properties of the cadaver bone over time must be considered.

The use of synthetic substrates in the testing of internal fixation screws is an established method.[36-40] Such substrates, typically polymeric, have been used as models for many skeletal sites, including the mandible, the pedicles of the spine, the femur, and the metatarsals.[38,39,41,42] In one study, the interfemur mechanical variability for the synthetic models was 20 to 200 times less than that of cadaver femurs.[42] The polyurethane synthetic cortex used in the current study had a similar modulus to that of cortical bone, i.e., about 15 GPa for the synthetic vs. about 12 to 17 GPa for natural bone.[43] It has been stated that plastic models may simulate the mechanical properties of natural bone in tests in which only elastic deformation of the substrate is achieved.[41] During the fatigue testing, the substrate did not undergo noticeable plastic deformation since no alteration of the screw hole geometry was seen. Consequently, for the purpose of generating preliminary fatigue data on absorbable polymer screws used for the fixation of sagittal split mandibular osteotomies, the synthetic substrate model served as a reasonable approximation to natural healthy bone.

Maximum mean unilateral molar bite forces measured in skeletally normal adults have been reported as ranging from approximately 30 to 86 kg.[44-46] Patients requiring orthognathic surgery typically exhibit lower bite forces than normal controls.[47] For patients requiring mandibular setback surgery, mean maximal molar bite forces were measured at 13.7 kg before surgery, 7.6 kg at MMF removal, and 14.2, 19.7, and 26.1 kg at 3, 6, and 12 months postsurgery, respectively.[48] In normal chewing, the forces exerted on the occlusal surface seldom exceed 5 to 7 kg.[49] As such, the load range of 4.5 to 45 kg used in the current study may be considered to be the worst case since patients undergoing postoperative rehabilitation following mandibular surgery are unlikely to exceed normal chewing activities. It has been reported that a typical bite cycle in a normal patient is about one per second.[50] Assuming that a patient eats three meals per day and is chewing an average of 10 min per meal, then this corresponds to about 2000 masticatory cycles per day. Over the course of 8 weeks, this represents 112,000 cycles. Thus, the 1 Hz load frequency and the run-out limit of 260,000 cycles chosen for the fatigue test were also clinically relevant.

At the rate of 1 Hz, approximately 3 days are required to accumulate 260,000 cycles. From Figure 38.2, it is apparent that little hydrolysis occurs over this short an interval. Consequently, Figure 38.4 may be interpreted as a true composite curve whereby each data point represents the fatigue characteristics of the LactoSorb® copolymer screw–synthetic bone constructs for a given level of hydrolysis.

Under the conditions of the fatigue test employed, it is apparent that the fatigue properties of the LactoSorb® copolymer screws diminish greatly after the equivalent of about 6 weeks of hydrolysis in simulated *in vivo* conditions. Tested statically, the LactoSorb® copolymer cylinders did not begin to lose strength until after 8 weeks. This may be evidence of a synergistic effect of hydrolysis and cyclic loading.

The major goal of this study was to develop a novel method of characterizing the fatigue characteristics of an absorbable screw–synthetic bone substrate system. The composite curve that was created, showing fatigue "snapshots" corresponding to various degrees of screw hydrolysis, demonstrated the interrelated dynamics of hydrolysis and cyclic loading. It was demonstrated that fixation of synthetic bone substrate with three 2.5-mm-diameter LactoSorb® copolymer screws could withstand cyclic loads nearly one order of magnitude greater than typical loads developed during chewing. Additionally, even after considerable hydrolysis, the screws withstood the number of chewing cycles expected from a patient during healing. This provides strong evidence of the utility of this method of fixation for sagittal split mandibular osteotomies. This method provides a unique analytical tool upon which future studies can be based.

There were, however, several limitations in the current study that can be addressed with more sophisticated methods. First, as was discussed above, the mathematical analysis of the stability of screw fixation of sagittally split mandibular osteotomies is complex, requiring that a series of vector equations be solved to characterize the shear stress pattern in the critical screw in response to the moment placed on the distal fragment. In the current study, a simple model was chosen for the preliminary study of the fatigue properties of an absorbable screw–synthetic bone complex. The substrate segments were loaded in tension without an applied moment. As such, the stresses resisted by each of the three screws were equivalent to each other, unlike the clinical situation in the mandible. The testing, as it was performed, may have more correlation with the stress pattern in screws used to fix fractures of the extremities and other regions. Second, soaking the implants, unloaded, in buffer prior to accelerated fatigue testing does not replicate the short periods of cyclic loading during eating followed by long periods of non-load-bearing between meals characteristic of the clinical pattern. The interplay between hydrolysis and fatigue would be expected to differ between the two cases. Third, only one set of loading parameters was used in the study. A different loading cycle may have produced a different composite curve than the one shown in Figure 38.4. Although the applied loads were extreme and can be considered to be worst case, future studies should include the generation of a family of composite curves in which each individual curve corresponds to a different cyclic load cycle. In this manner, the variables of hydrolysis, loading pattern, and number of cycles to failure could be combined.

An important concept governing the use of absorbable fixation devices is that of *variable load sharing*. When an osteotomy or fracture is united with absorbable fixation, initially the absorbable fixation provides 100% of the support. After healing occurs and the absorbable devices are eliminated, all of the support is provided by the osseous union. At intermediate times, the load will be partially shared between the healing union and the residual strength of the absorbable implants. This important load-sharing concept cannot be mimicked by any *in vitro* study with cadaver or synthetic bone substrates.

IV. CONCLUSIONS

The fatigue testing of bioabsorbable fixation devices presents significant challenge due to the time-varying properties of the materials under the influence of hydrolysis. To avoid the limitations of a cadaver bone substrate, a synthetic bone substrate that resembled the modulus of natural cortical bone was used in conjunction with absorbable copolymer screws. Under the test conditions employed, it appeared that the fatigue characteristics of the absorbable screws did not begin to diminish greatly until about 6 weeks of hydrolysis had occurred. The results indicate that these absorbable screws may be useful to fix sagittal split mandibular osteotomies based on documented loading patterns in the mandible.

REFERENCES

1. Viljanen, J., Kinnunen, J., Bondestam, S., et al., Bone changes after experimental osteotomies fixed with absorbable self-reinforced poly-L-lactide screws or metallic screws studied by plain radiographs, quantitative computed tomography and magnetic resonance imaging, *Biomaterials*, 16, 1353, 1995.
2. Velkes, S., Nerubay, J., and Lokiec, F., Stress fracture of the proximal femur after screw removal, *Arch. Orthop. Trauma Surg.*, 115, 61, 1996.

3. Ebraheim, X.R., Nadaud, M.C., and Phillips, E.R., Local tissue of the lumbar spine response to titanium plate–screw system. Case reports, *Spine,* 21, 871, 1996.
4. Thomas, K.A., Cook, S.D., Harding, A.F., and Haddad, R.J., Jr., Tissue reaction to implant corrosion in 38 internal fixation devices, *Orthopedics*, 11, 441, 1988.
5. Pietrzak, W.S., Sarver, D.R., and Verstynen, M.L., Bioabsorbable polymer science for the practicing surgeon, *J. Craniofac. Surg.*, 8, 87, 1997.
6. Jorgenson, D.S., Mayer, M.H., and Ellenbogen, R.G., et al., Detection of titanium in human tissues after craniofacial surgery, *Plast. Reconstr. Surg.*, 99, 976, 1997.
7. Rubin, J.P. and Yaremchuk, M.J., Complications and toxicities of implantable biomaterials used in facial reconstructive and aesthetic surgery: a comprehensive review of the literature, *Plast. Reconstr. Surg.*, 100, 1336, 1997.
8. Cutright, D.E., Hunsuck, E.E., and Beasley, J.B., Fracture reduction using a biodegradable material, polylactic acid, *J. Oral Surg.*, 28, 393, 1971.
9. Viljanen, V.V. and Lindholm, T.S., Background of the early development of absorbable fixation devices, *Tech. Orthop.*, 13, 117, 1998.
10. Pietrzak, W.S., Verstynen, M.L., and Sarver, D.S., Bioabsorbable fixation devices: status for the craniomaxillofacial surgeon, *J. Craniofac. Surg.*, 8, 92, 1997.
11. Middleton, J.C. and Tipton, A.J., Synthetic biodegradable polymers as medical devices, *Med. Plast. Biomater.*, Mar/Apr, 30, 1998.
12. Barber, F.A., Resorbable fixation devices: a product guide, *Orthopedics, Spec. Ed.,* 4, 11, 1998.
13. Kohn, D.H., Richmond, E.M., Dootz, E.R., et al., *In vitro* comparison of parameters affecting the fixation strength of sagittal split osteotomies, *J. Oral Maxillofac. Surg.*, 53, 1374, 1995.
14. Bos, R.R., Rozema, F.R., Boering, G., et al., Bio-absorbable plates and screws for internal fixation of mandibular fractures. A study in six dogs, *Int. J. Oral Maxillofac. Surg.*, 18, 365, 1989.
15. Suuronen, R., Comparison of absorbable self-reinforced poly-L-lactide screws and metallic screws in the fixation of mandibular condyle osteotomies: an experimental study in sheep, *J. Oral Maxillofac. Surg.*, 49, 989, 1991.
16. Suuronen, R., Pohjonen, T., Vasenius, J., and Vainionpää, S., Comparison of absorbable self-reinforced multilayer poly-l-lactide and metallic plates for the fixation of mandibular body osteotomies: an experimental study in sheep, *J. Oral Maxillofac. Surg.*, 50, 255, 1992.
17. McManners, J., Moos, K.F., and El-Attar, A., The use of biodegradable fixation in sagittal split and vertical subsigmoid osteotomy of the mandible: a preliminary report, *Br. J. Oral Maxillofac. Surg.*, 35, 401, 1997.
18. Gerlach, K.L. and Derichs, D., Comparative studies on the fatigue strength of absorbable polymers used in oral and maxillofacial surgery, *Dtsch. Zahnarztl. Z.,* 43, 376, 1988 [in German].
19. An, Y.H, Friedman, R.J., Powers, D.L., et al., Fixation of osteotomies using bioabsorbable screws in the canine femur, *Clin. Orthop.*, 355, 300, 1998.
20. Pietrzak, W.S., Sarver, D., and Verstynen, M., Bioresorbable implants: practical considerations, *Bone,* 19(Suppl. 2), 109S, 1996.
21. Athanasiou, K.A., Agrawal, C.M., Barber, F.A., and Burkhart, S.S., Orthopaedic applications for PLA-PGA biodegradable polymers, *Arthroscopy*, 14, 726, 1998.
22. Hutmacher, D., Hurzeler, M.M., and Schliephake, H., A review of material properties of biodegradable and bioresorbable polymers and devices for GTR and GBR applications, *Int. J. Oral Maxillofac. Implants*, 11, 667, 1996.
23. Bucholz, R.W., Henry, S., and Henley, M.B., Fixation with bioabsorbable screws for the treatment of fractures of the ankle, *J. Bone Joint Surg.*, 76A, 319, 1994.
24. Pietrzak, W.S., Sarver, D.R., Bianchini, S.D., and D'Alessio, K., Effect of simulated intraoperative heating and shaping on mechanical properties of a bioabsorbable fracture plate material, *Appl. Biomater.*, 38, 17, 1997.
25. Simon, J.A., Ricci, J.L., and DiCesare, P.E., Bioresorbable fracture fixation in orthopedics: a comprehensive review. Part I. Basic science and preclinical studies, *Am. J. Orthop.*, 26, 665, 1997.
26. Böstman, O.M., Pihlajamaki, H.K., Partio, E.K., and Rokkanen, P.U., Clinical biocompatibility and degradation of polylevolactide screws in the ankle, *Clin. Orthop.*, 320, 101, 1995.

27. Eitenmuller, J., David, J., Pommer, A., and Muhr, G., Die Versorgung von Sprunggelenksfrakturen unter Verwendung von Platten und Schrauben aus resorbierbarem Polymermaterial, in Abstracts of 53 *Jahrestagung der Deutschen Gesellschaft für Unfallheilkunde*, No. 64, Springer, Berlin, 1990.

28. Simon, J.A., Ricci, J.L., and DiCesare, P.E., Bioresorbable fracture fixation in orthopaedics: A comprehensive review Part II. Clinical studies, *Am. J. Orthop.*, 26, 754, 1997.

29. Bergsma, J.E., de Bruijn, W.C., Rozema, F.R., et al., Late degradation tissue response to poly (L-lactide) bone plates and screws, *Biomaterials*, 16, 25, 1995.

30. Böstman, O., Hirvensalo, E., Makinen, J., and Rokkanen, P., Foreign body reactions to fracture fixation implants of biodegradable synthetic polymers, *J. Bone Joint Surg.*, 74B, 592, 1990.

31. Casteleyn, P., Handelberg, F., and Haentjens, P., Biodegradable rods vs. Kirschner wire fixation of wrist fractures, *J. Bone Joint Surg.*, 76A, 319, 1994.

32. Eppley, B.L. and Reilly, M., Degradation characteristics of PLLA-PGA bone fixation devices, *J. Craniofac. Surg.*, 8, 116, 1997.

33. Eppley, B.L., Prevel, C.D., and Sadove, A.M., Resorbable bone fixation: does it have a role in craniomaxillofacial trauma? *J. Craniomaxillofac. Trauma*, 2, 56, 1996.

34. Salyer, K.E., *Aesthetic Craniofacial Surgery*, J.B. Lippincott, Philadelphia, 1989, chap. 7.

35. Collins, J.A., *Failure of Materials in Mechanical Design — Analysis, Prediction, Prevention*, John Wiley & Sons, New York, 1981, chaps. 7 and 11.

36. DeCoster, T.A., Heetderks, D.B., and Downey, D.J., et al., Optimizing bone screw pullout force, *J. Orthop. Trauma*, 4, 169, 1990.

37. Hearn, T.C., Schatzker, J., and Wolfson, N., Extraction strength of cannulated cancellous bone screws, *J. Orthop. Trauma*, 7, 138, 1993.

38. McKinley, T.O., McLain, R.F., Yerby, S.A., et al., The effect of pedicle morphometry on pedical screw loading. A synthetic model, *Spine*, 22, 246, 1997.

39. Ziccardi, V.B., Scheider, R.E., and Kummer, F.J., Wurzburg lag screw plate vs. four-hole miniplate for the treatment of condylar process fractures, *J. Oral Maxillofac. Surg.*, 55, 602, 1997.

40. Thompson, J.D., Benjamin, J.B., and Szivek, J.A., Pullout strengths of cannulated and noncannulated bone screws, *Clin. Orthop.*, 341, 241, 1997.

41. Landsman, A.S. and Chang, T.J., Can synthetic bone models approximate the mechanical properties of cadaveric first metatarsal bone? *J. Foot Ankle Surg.*, 37, 122, 1998.

42. Cristofolini, L., Vicconti, M., Cappello, A., and Toni, A., Mechanical validation of whole bone composite femur models, *J. Biomech.*, 29, 525, 1996.

43. Hayes, W.C. and Bouxsein, M.L., Biomechanics of cortical and trabecular bone: implications for assessment of fracture risk, in *Basic Orthopaedic Biomechanics*, 2nd ed., Mow, V.C. and Hayes, W.C., Eds., Lippincott-Raven, Philadelphia, 1997, 85.

44. Hellsing, E. and Hagberg, C., Changes in maximum bite force related to extension of the head, *Eur. J. Orthodontol.*, 12, 148, 1990.

45. Floystrand, F., Kleven, E., and Oilo, G., A novel miniature bite force recorder and its clinical application, *Acta Odontol. Scand.*, 40, 209, 1982.

46. Waltimo, A. and Kononen, M., A novel bite force recorder and maximal isometric bite force values for health young adults, *Scand. J. Dent. Res.*, 101, 171, 1993.

47. Iwase, M., Sugimori, M., Kurachi, Y., and Nagumo, M., Changes in bite force and occlusal contacts in pateints treated for mandibular prognathism by orthognathic surgery, *J. Oral Maxillofac. Surg.*, 56, 850, 1998.

48. Kim, Y.G. and Oh, S.H., Effect of mandibular setback surgery on occlusal force, *J. Oral Maxillofac. Surg.*, 55, 126, 1997.

49. De Boever, J.A., McCall, W.D., Jr., Holden, S., and Ash, M.M., Jr., Functional occlusal forces: an investigation by telemetry, *J. Prosthet. Dent.*, 40, 326, 1978.

50. Youssef, R.E., Throckmorton, G.S., Ellis, E., and Sinn, D.P., Comparison of habitual masticatory cycles and muscle activity before and after orthognathic surgery, *J. Oral Maxillofac. Surg.*, 55, 699, 1997.

39 Testing Intervertebral Stability after Spinal Fixation

Kenneth S. James and A. U. Daniels

CONTENTS

I. INTRODUCTION

Implant components used to stabilize the spine are generally referred to as "spinal instrumentation," and the affected portion of the spine with instrumentation in place is described as a "spine construct." Too much intervertebral motion occurring in a spine construct is deleterious to achieving spine fusion that the surgeon initiates to maintain long-term correction of spinal injury or deformity. By measuring the amount of motion present within a spinal construct in the laboratory, it is possible to assess the contribution that instrumentation design and specific construct components make to the intervertebral stability the instrumentation provides.

Spinal instrumentation load-to-failure experiments,[1-3] individual component testing,[4,5] and construct fatigue tests[6-8] are excellent mechanisms for initial screening of new instrumentation designs. Less strong, less durable, less secure designs are weeded out early by these testing protocols. Subsequent spinal construct intervertebral stability testing is an essential additional step in pursuing a meticulous, clinically relevant spinal instrumentation analysis. Intervertebral stability can be defined as the amount of intervertebral displacement that occurs when a construct is subjected to a load–displacement regimen believed to be clinically relevant.

Ashman et al.,[9] Smith,[10] Wilke et al.,[11] and Panjabi[12] have reviewed a number of *in vitro* methods for applying and measuring spinal loads and intervertebral displacements in instrumented spines. Limitations and pitfalls of such systems have similarly been discussed.[13,14] Many investigators have adapted standard material testing devices to load and move spines. Others have developed an apparatus specifically for testing spines. This chapter describes the authors' methodology for providing an accurate means to control gross spine movements while concurrently measuring intervertebral micromotion and the sacral load profile. The spine motion control system developed here is capable of moving uninstrumented and instrumented cadaver spines through physiological ranges of flexion, extension, lateral bending, and torsion. Parameters such as cycling frequency and motion excursion amplitude are controlled through a custom software interface. Intervertebral micromotion is recorded in three dimensions with a custom-built optoelectronic laser/charge-coupled device (CCD) system. Motion and load data are computed and recorded concurrently in real time by an Intel microprocessor-based personal computer. Differences in spinal instrumentation and stability are assessed by comparing intervertebral motion and load data.

II. SPINE TESTING METHODS

A. INTERVERTEBRAL MOTION MEASUREMENT DEVICES

Displacement transducers can be divided into linked and nonlinked types. Linked types generally are electromechanical and introduce the possibility of altering normal spinal motion through their linkages from one vertebra to another. A popular linked motion transducer is the LVDT (linear variable differential transducer). Panjabi et al.[15] produced a displacement transducer system based on LVDTs. Another popular linked motion transducer is the electrogoniometer. This mechanism is capable of measuring relative vertebral movement in all six degrees of freedom by using linkages connected to the vertebral bodies and potentiometers oriented in each plane of motion.[16]

Nonlinked motion measurement methods do not affect the intervertebral motion and are potentially superior to linked methods. Systems have been devised using optoelectronic and stereophotogrammetry techniques.[17,18] Stereophotogrammetry has the disadvantage that the accuracy is inversely related to the viewing volume.[19] Historically, optoelectronic systems had proved too bulky for measuring intervertebral micromotion. This changed with the development of the laser-CCD device–based motion measurement system.[17,20] This device made very accurate, noncontacting three-dimensional measurement of multilevel intervertebral micromotion possible. Advantages of this system include miniaturization of the components, the elimination of the need for mechanical linkages between the bodies, and a high degree of accuracy which is not dependent on viewing volume.[19,21]

B. SPINE TESTING — LOAD- AND DISPLACEMENT-CONTROL METHODS

The spine is one of the most complex mechanical structures of the body and is able to produce and undergo complicated three-dimensional movements. *In vitro* spine testing protocols attempt to replicate the *in vivo* situation. However, simulating active paraspinous musculature, intraabdominal pressure, intercostal muscles, and the dynamic fluid exchange through the disk and vertebra, for example, is currently not practical in the laboratory. Only the mechanical contributions of the passive bony and cartilaginous components of the spine to strength or stability can generally be tested.

One spine testing method available to the researcher is to control the load applied to the spine, e.g., 10 N·m flexion moment, and measure the resulting vertebral displacements — a load-controlled

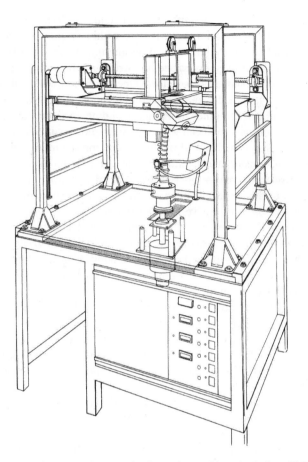

FIGURE 39.1 The spine motion control system is shown here with a single laser/CCD unit attached to the mounted spine. See text for details. (From James, K.S., Ph.D. thesis, University of Utah, Salt Lake City, 1995.)

experiment. This is a popular testing method, partly arising from the relative ease with which load-controlled experiments can be performed.[9,12,15,22] However, the alternative testing approach, controlling gross spine displacement and measuring the resulting loads and intervertebral motion — a displacement-control protocol — offers the benefits of better simulating *in vivo* motions, has the best supporting data for most biomechanical situations and, consequently, offers the opportunity for obtaining data of greater clinical relevance.[23, 24]

For the present displacement control studies to mimic, *in vitro*, the natural movements of the spine, a motion control system was built to guide the spine through defined physiological ranges of flexion, extension, lateral bending, and torsion. The system duplicates *in vitro* the direction and amount of vertebral motions seen *in vivo* on radiographs by applying the loading needed to achieve natural spine movement. What is more, controlling gross spine motion and measuring the resultant loading and intervertebral motion grounds the resulting intervertebral stability data in the clinical realm of actual patient spine bending or torsional movements.

III. SPINE MOTION CONTROL AND ANALYSIS SYSTEM

A. SPINE MOTION CONTROL SYSTEM

Located at the center of the spine motion load frame (Figure 39.1) are two 4-in. steel specimen mounting cups. The inferior cup is fixed to a stepper motor (25,000 motor steps per 360° of axial rotation; Compumotor PC23, Parker Hannifan Corp, Petaluma, CA); (hereafter referred to as the torsional stepper motor), and the superior cup is housed within a rigid, movable crosshead structure. Each end of the crosshead is rigidly mounted to an aluminum carriage (Thomson System 2DA, Port Washington, NY) with four close-tolerance, low-friction, linear bearings. Each carriage slides on a vertically mounted dual-shaft rail assembly. One of these horizontally sliding carriages is mounted to a drive screw, which is driven by a second identical stepper motor (25,000 motor steps per 2.54 cm of linear motion). The other horizontally sliding carriage travels freely upon its rail. The result is a horizontally driven crosshead which is free to move passively in the vertical direction. A gimbal system within the crosshead allows the superior mounting cup to pivot about two orthogonal axes (flexion/extension and lateral bending) while remaining fixed about the torsional axis. The horizontal crosshead, free to move in the vertical direction, is initially counterbalanced to apply zero axial load to the spine specimen. Static weights may be applied to the crosshead to provide vertical distractive or compressive loads, if required.

To take advantage of the accuracy of the actuators and achieve reproducible mechanical performance, a rigid loading frame supports the aforementioned horizontally mounted dual shaft rail assemblies. The height of the mounted rails can be adjusted to accommodate spine specimens of any length normally seen in humans, e.g., the entire thoracolumbar spine.

To produce flexion or extension, the spine specimen is placed in the mounting cups such that the anterior-posterior (AP) plane of the spine corresponds with the plane of primary crosshead movement. Under microcomputer control, the linear motion stepper motor is actuated, moving the crosshead and therefore the cephalad-most vertebral body at a software-controllable frequency, number of cycles, and range of motion. The inferior cup is held fixed by the locked torsional stepper motor, thereby immobilizing the sacral region of the spine specimen, much the same way the pelvis does in the intact human.

Lateral bending of the spine specimen is made possible by rotating the spine 90° such that the AP plane of the spine is perpendicular to the primary crosshead movement. In addition, the most caudal vertebral body can be subjected to cyclic torsion about the spine axis by the torsional motion stepper motor, either while the spine is held in place or during bending motion, thereby simulating trunk rotation. The motors are controlled by a custom-designed software interface and can resolve the position of the horizontal crosshead to within ±0.005 mm, and the position of the torsional motor to ±5 arc-min.

B. Relative Intervertebral Micromotion Measurement

Three-dimensional intervertebral micromotion is measured with an optical transducer system consisting of a mutually orthogonal cluster of three miniature AlGaAS laser diodes (LDs) (ML4102A, Mitsubishi Electronic America, Inc., Sunnyvale, CA) which is mounted to one vertebral body with bone screws and is directed at a corresponding array of three mutually orthogonal plane CCDs (CCD222, Fairchild Weston Systems, Inc., Sunnyvale, CA) mounted to an adjacent body (Figure 39.2, 39.3). The CCDs are light-sensitive video screens with over 185,000 (380 × 488) sensing elements in a rectangle of 8.8 × 11.4 mm, a density high enough to detect the motion of a collimated laser beam at a resolution of 30 μm. The collimated laser beams effectively originate from the same point in space. Both the CCDs and LDs are packaged in custom-made brackets occupying the volume of a 4-cm cube, and weigh approximately 80 g. As one vertebra moves relative to another, the three points illuminated by the lasers on the CCDs change accordingly, and uniquely determine the spatial orientation of the laser array with respect to the CCD array. The maximum translation measurable in any one direction is 8.8 mm. If the axis of rotation is located at the laser origin, the system is capable of measuring angulation up to 20°. In practice, however, the axis of rotation is located within the vertebral bodies, permitting angulation up to 10° to be measured. With proper mounting, the entire typical range of intervertebral motion of the lumbar or thoracic spinal motion segments can be measured.[25]

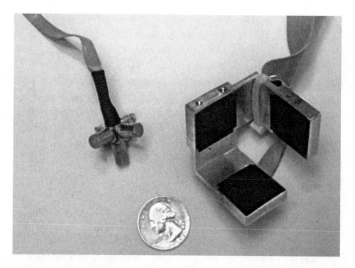

FIGURE 39.2 The laser/CCD motion measurement arrays used to measure relative intervertebral motion. (From James, K.S., Ph.D. thesis, University of Utah, Salt Lake City, 1995.)

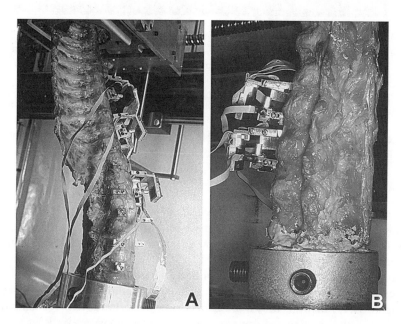

FIGURE 39.3 The laser/CCD motion measurement system mounted on prepared human cadaver spines, to measure relative intervertebral motion as the spine specimens are moved through physiological motion excursions.

The static orientations of the LD and CCD, with respect to an anatomically based coordinate system of the vertebral body to which they are mounted, are determined prior to dynamic testing of the spine utilizing a three-dimensional digitizer (see below). The relative three-dimensional motion of a vertebral pair itself is derived through a series of coordinate transformations which relate the motion sensed by the laser/CCD arrays to the actual relative motion of the vertebral bodies. The mathematical basis of this system is thoroughly described by Dean et al.[17] The system is calibrated with a six-degree-of-freedom micrometer (Edmund Scientific, Barrington, NJ). Tests with this micrometer have established the accuracy of the system to be 50 µm in translation and 0.1° in rotation.[17] Newer, higher-resolution CCDs (over a million pixels) now available offer the

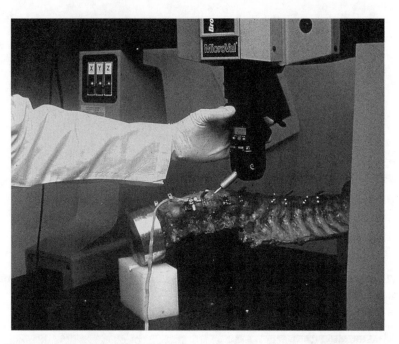

FIGURE 39.4   The three-dimensional, relative position relationships between the vertebral bodies and the corresponding mounted laser and CCD arrays are established with a highly accurate three-dimensional digitizer. The geometry of the vertebral bodies is digitized to approximate the vertebral body centers. Other anatomical points are digitized to establish the orientation of the local coordinate system for each vertebral body. Similarly, when relative motion between two specific points is of interest, e.g., the facet joint, additional points are digitized on the adjacent vertebrae.

promise of even greater accuracy. It is possible to use multiple LD/CCD systems to measure intervertebral motion at several levels simultaneously.

C. ANATOMICAL CHARACTERIZATION

To be of value, motion data recorded by the measurement system must be related to the anatomy of the vertebral bodies and their initial relative positions. Many researchers reference motions and positions to the center of the vertebral body, and a vertical axis which passes through it identifies the orientation of the body in space.[9,22]

A method for repeatably determining a coordinate system for the vertebral bodies is based on measuring external geometries with a highly accurate three-dimensional coordinate measuring machine (Figure 39.4, Microval, Brown & Sharpe, North Kingstown, RI). The anterior surface of each vertebral end plate is digitized down to the bases of the transverse processes. A centroid is calculated based upon each semiellipse, and a line through the two centroids represents the vertical coordinate axis, with the midpoint as the local origin. The tip of the spinous process is digitized to provide a posterior planar direction and subsequently to establish the anterior axis. The third axis, in the left lateral direction, is easily resolved from the previously determined axes.

Once the CCDs and lasers are mounted anterolaterally to their respective vertebral bodies, their positions are digitized relative to the spine anatomy. The final relationship appears as rotation matrices and translation vectors[17] which are used in online calculations to resolve dynamically relative vertebral body position in real time.

If the vertebral bodies are treated as rigid bodies, the relative translation between any two anatomical points can be calculated so long as the relative positions of these points, e.g., points on the facet joint, have likewise been digitized (Figure 39.5).

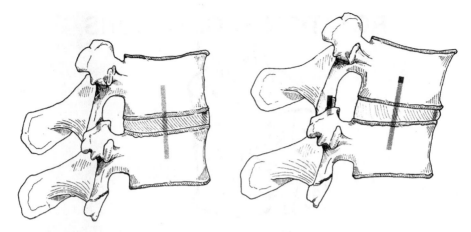

FIGURE 39.5 Relative vertebral motion is commonly referenced to the vertebral body centers. However, because the vertebrae are treated as rigid bodies, the motion between other sites, e.g., the facet or midsagittal anterior disk, can also be calculated so long as the positional relationships have been established during the digitization step. For instance, calculating the translations at additional sites is helpful in analyzing the motion present at the fusion site.

D. LOAD MEASUREMENT SYSTEM

A load cell (AMTI, Newton, MA) is mounted between the inferior mounting cup and the torsional motion stepper motor. It is capable of measuring three orthogonal forces and three orthogonal moments, thereby providing a complete load profile at the sacrum. The resolution of these forces and moments are 0.075 N and 0.015 N·m, respectively, and are recorded through a multichannel analog-to-digital board (Keithley Instruments, Cleveland, OH) mounted in the computer.

E. DATA ACQUISITION

For spine specimens subjected to dynamic motion, rates of computerized data acquisition per motion cycle depend on microprocessor speed, the number of vertebral levels under evaluation, and the number of other parameters measured (e.g., resultant loads and gross spine position). One can routinely sample and compute motion data from three spinal levels plus sacral load data concurrently at 15 Hz with an Intel microprocessor-based personal computer.

F. DATA ANALYSIS AND REDUCTION

In quantifying three-dimensional vertebral motion, every researcher is faced with the difficult problem of interpreting the results in a manner which is clinically relevant and facilitates specimen-to-specimen comparisons. The coordinate system which best relates the spatial representations of the vertebral bodies will be one whose separate planes correspond to the common clinical anatomical planes, namely, the midsagittal, transverse, and frontal. The authors have oriented their coordinate system with the x-axis aligned anteriorly, the y-axis laterally, and the z-axis pointed in the superior direction (Figure 39.6). The separate components of the translation vector therefore correspond to motion parameters familiar to the clinician, while the magnitude of the resultant vector can serve to quantify the complete amount of translation.

The rotational matrix can be somewhat more challenging to interpret due to the complex nature of three-dimensional rotation and the noncommunitivity of sequential rotation.[12,15,22] While other researchers have referenced the rotational matrix as axial rotations, the authors have chosen a projection method similar to Pearcy[26] which provides a unique solution to the interpretation of the matrix in parameters familiar to the clinician in viewing radiographic films, which are also projec-

ROTATION PROJECTIONS

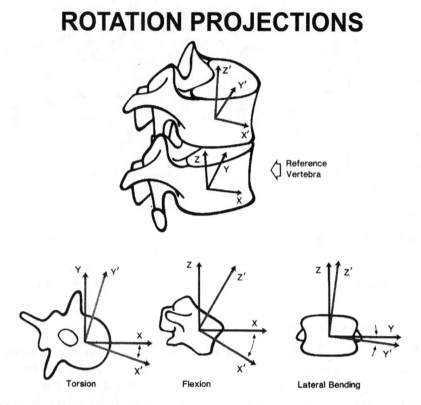

FIGURE 39.6   To aid in interpreting the three-dimensional rotation matrix, rotations of the coordinate system of the superior vertebra are projected onto the planes of the inferior coordinate system, defined as the midsagittal plane, transverse plane, and frontal plane.

tions.[17] Rotations of the coordinate system of the superior vertebra are projected onto the planes of the inferior coordinate system, defined as the midsagittal plan, transverse plane, and frontal plane.

By using this projection method, each axis of one vertebral body provides a different rotation parameter when projected onto the appropriate plane of the adjacent body (see Figure 39.5). To measure flexion/extension, for example, a line parallel to the vertical axis of the body is transformed into the x–z plane of the adjacent body, which approximates the midsagittal plane. The angles between the lines comparing the neutral position with the flexed and extended spine define the relative angular motion of flexion and extension, respectively. Similarly, the anterior axis projected onto the transverse (x–y) plane quantifies torsion of the spinal column, and the lateral axis projected onto the frontal (y–z) plane quantifies lateral bending.

IV. AN EXAMPLE — SCOLIOSIS INSTRUMENTATION TESTING

A. OVERVIEW

The evolution of scoliosis instrumentation has been marked recently by the introduction of bulkier, increasingly stiff implants. Presumably, these stiffer constructs are intended to allow less intervertebral motion within the instrumented area which, in turn, provides a more favorable environment conducive to the formation of the bony fusion mass needed to maintain correction of the deformity. The question presents itself — During patient movement, is there a significant difference in the amount of intervertebral motion present within scoliosis instrumentation systems of varying complexities, sizes, and stiffnesses?

In this example, the authors investigated how a spectrum of scoliosis instrumentation systems differs in their respective stiffnesses and their abilities to restrict intervertebral motion. This study assessed the initial effect that Harrington (the historic standard), Cotrel Dubousset (CD), and Luque instrumentation have on both intervertebral micromotion and spine stiffness when these instrumentation systems span the spinal levels commonly instrumented in scoliosis correction. In addition, a protocol was employed to examine how removal of selected components in the CD constructs decreased stiffness and whether this correlated with a measured increase in intervertebral motion. This "tear-down" protocol helps in determining specific component contribution to the stability of the scoliosis construct.

The change in relative intervertebral motion immediately caudal to the instrumentation was also investigated. In an instrumented patient, intervertebral motion in the lumbar spine increases to accommodate the flexibility lost in the fused segments. Clinically, the additional demand placed on the unfused motion segments has been implicated in accelerated adjacent disk degeneration and higher incidences of low back pain.[27, 28]

B. SPECIMEN PREPARATION

Six human cadaver spines (one female, age 57 and five males, ages 19, 36, 37, 39, and 47) were harvested and frozen within 24 h after death at $-20°$ in evacuated, heat-sealed polyethylene bags. Prolonged storage under these conditions and subsequent thawing has little effect on a spine's biomechanical properties.[29] Gross dissection involved removal of the cervical spine and the distal sacrum and pelvis from the specimen. The ribs were resected such that 5 cm remained in order to preserve the costotransverse joint and the associated ligament. All remaining associated musculature (except for the intercostal muscle associated with the remaining ribs) was removed. All ligamentous structures were left intact, and AP and lateral radiographs were taken to assess any degeneration or bony abnormalities. The specimens present a limitation for scoliosis studies in that they are normal rather than scoliotic. However, spine biomechanics researchers generally agree that this does not seem likely to change the relative ability of the instrumentation to control intervertebral motion.

The most cephalic (T1) and caudal (S1 and S2) vertebral bodies of a given spine were potted in 10-cm-diameter aluminum cups with a low-melting-point lead alloy. The specimens were potted such that the axial rotation axis of the spine is perpendicular to the L3/L4 disk. Metal pins and screws inserted through the distal and proximal end structures assured a stable fixation throughout the duration of the test.

While thawed, specimens are kept moist with saline. Loosely wrapping the specimen in household plastic film helps to prevent the specimen from drying.

C. TEST MODES

The spine was fixed with commercially available Harrington distraction/compression, CD and Luque instrumentation from T4 to L2 in a configuration typical for a right thoracic idiopathic scoliosis curve. The instrumentation test sequence performed on each spine was as follows: Harrington distraction/compression system, full CD construct, CD construct without devices for transverse traction (DTTs), a single left CD rod, and a full Luque construct. The instrumentation testing protocol had to be ordered in this manner and not randomized in order to minimize the tissue damage caused by one instrumentation system that would interfere with the fixation of another system tested.

Three laser/CCD units were used to make intervertebral motion measurements at two levels within each construct, T7–T8 and T10–T11, and at a level immediately outside the applied instrumentation, L2-L3 (see Figure 39.3A). The spines were cycled at 0.1 Hz to gross bending angles of $15°$ flexion, $10°$ extension, $15°$ right and left bending, and $15°$ right and left torsion. Clinical radiographic studies have shown that normal patients can voluntarily achieve these angles. Each specimen was precycled 20 times for each of the instrumentation configurations and gross motion imposed with intervertebral motion recorded on the subsequent cycle. A steep acceleration ramp was used to ensure that induced movements were at a constant velocity throughout the majority of a motion cycle. The neutral position used to differentiate between flexion and extension, right and left torsion, and right and left bending was defined as the position where no moments or lateral forces were measured at the base of the spine. During testing, sacral load data were recorded concurrently with intervertebral motion data. Data was recorded at 15 Hz. This yielded 150 load and position readings per spine level per motion cycle.

D. DATA ANALYSIS AND REDUCTION

The resultant relative motion between adjacent vertebra is quite small. Maximum primary projection angles are typically less than 3°, and the translation vector less than 3 mm. This confirms the need for a sensitive, accurate motion transducer system.

Primary angular micromotion was consistent with the induced gross motion. In other words, when the spine was placed in flexion and extension, the majority of the angular motion was seen in the midsagittal projection plane. Likewise, for lateral bending the primary angular motion was seen in the frontal plane, and induced torsion resulted in primary angulation in the transverse plane. Subsequent analyses focused on the changes measured in primary angulation. Similarly, although the load acquisition system provides a complete description of sacral loading, the primary moment measured is deemed sufficient for comparing construct stiffness.

Motion and stiffness data were normalized to the uninstrumented spine data. Intervertebral micromotion seen at the spinal levels monitored are present for selected gross spine motions: torsion and lateral bending at T7/T8 and T10/T11 and flexion, extension, lateral bending, and torsion at L2/L3. Flexion and extension data are not presented for the thoracic segments because the facet orientation inherently limited the motion in these planes to an extent below the measurement capabilities of the system.

E. CONSTRUCT STIFFNESS

In general, the application of the instrumentation systems increased average spine stiffness by 70% (Figure 39.7) over the uninstrumented spines. The elegantly simple Harrington rods which are attached to the spine only at the rod ends matched the stiffness of Luque instrumentation which, in contrast, is attached to the spinal column at every level within the construct. The greatest disparity in spine stiffness was in torsion, where spines instrumented with CD instrumentation were over twice as stiff as the average Harrington and Luque constructs.

Removal of the DTTs and subsequently the right rod of the CD construct resulted in stiffness decreases of approximately 15 and 55%, respectively, for all motion excursions. Notably, the one-rod CD construct approached the stiffness of the two-rod Harrington and Luque constructs. This testing method found that the CD instrumentation design, utilizing a combination of pedicle and laminar hooks (5 hooks per rod) and the largest diameter rods (6.8 mm compared with 6.4 mm diameter rods) offered the most resistance to an imposed displacement. In fact, that data suggest it may be overdesigned and could be streamlined.

F. MOTION OUTSIDE THE CONSTRUCT

Intervertebral motion (angulation and translation) at L2/L3, the segment immediately caudal to the construct, typically increased 30% upon application of the spinal instrumentation systems (Figure 39.8) except for torsion, where motion increased upward of 65% as compared with the uninstrumented spines. Torsional motion is greatly increased because most of the thoracic spine that normally accommodates torsion had been instrumented. This measured increase in motion was not a function of the instrumentation configuration used since each of the instrumentation systems were grossly comparable in fixing the intervertebral motion within the construct. Each construct, therefore, displaced similar amounts of motion caudal to the instrumentation.

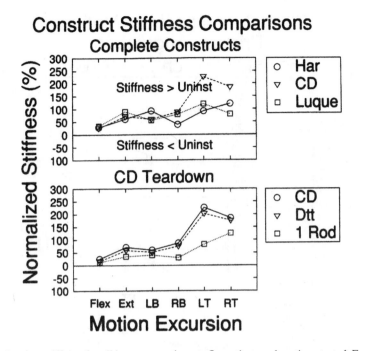

FIGURE 39.7   Average stiffness for all instrumentation configurations and motions tested. For full constructs, a 70% increase in overall spine stiffness is typically measured. Removal of instrumentation components was accompanied by a decrease in construct stiffness, with a one-rod construct being about half as stiff as the two-rod construct. (From James, K.S., Ph.D. thesis, University of Utah, Salt Lake City, 1995.)

By using such a displacement control protocol it is possible *in vitro* to measure magnitudes of displaced motion systematically as a function of the number of levels fused and other instrumentation designs. Clinically, only fusions extending below L2 have been implicated in increased back pain. Consequently, it should be possible to establish motion baselines beyond which accelerated degeneration and low back pain may result.

G. MOTION WITHIN THE CONSTRUCT

Intervertebral micromotion measurements made within the constructs at T7/T8 and T10/T11 revealed no significant difference between the Harrington, CD, and Luque instrumentation systems (Figures 39.8 and 39.9). Typically, primary angulation was reduced 40 to 50% and translation of the vertebral body centers 10 to 18%. The contribution of the DTTs and the second rod to the CD construct to restricting micromotion was unremarkable. The one-rod CD construct was, on average, equivalent to the two-rod Harrington construct in managing intervertebral motion within the instrumentation.

It is helpful to analyze motion at sites other than the vertebral body centers, e.g., the fusion site, in order to appreciate movements not immediately apparent in the data.[30] For example, in an extreme case, it is possible for a vertebra to rotate about its body center. In this case no relative translation, only rotation, would be measured. This can be misleading because at the facet, for example, where fusion is to occur, there is significant translation (see Figure 39.5). Studying the motion at different landmarks across the intervertebral joints can provide more clinically useful information regarding spinal motion than simply studying the translations of one point, especially the vertebral body centers. The authors find that referencing intervertebral micromotion to more than one landmark helps in comprehending the complex three-dimensional translations and angulations measured. Referencing motion to the area where the fusion mass forms is of special importance.

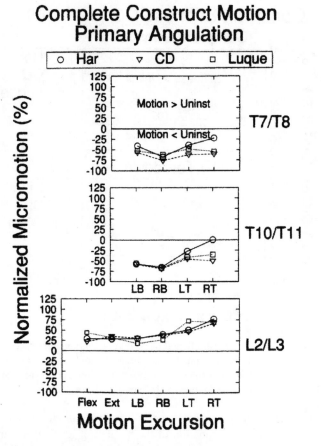

FIGURE 39.8　Normalized angulation measured inside and outside the constructs tested. Each construct provided comparable intervertebral stability within the construct. Similarly, motion increases caudal to the constructs were comparable for each type of instrumentation. (From James, K.S., Ph.D. thesis, University of Utah, Salt Lake City, 1995.)

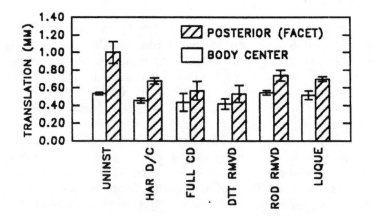

FIGURE 39.9　Through coordinate transformations, it is possible to measure the translations between any two digitized or calculated points on adjacent vertebrae. Here, the relative translation between the vertebral body centers (T7/T8) and facet are compared for right bending. Differences between instrumentation types are accentuated when the translation at the facet is calculated and analyzed. This is important because translation at the fusion site can be of greater clinical significance.

To measure motion at the facet, the relative location of the right side facet to the vertebral body centers was digitized in three dimensions. The maximum translation at the facet joint and the vertebral body center was measured as the spine was moved from the neutral position to the gross motion extremes. Figure 39.9 shows the translation between the vertebral body centers and the facet at T7/T8 for the case of right bending. Clearly, the translation is markedly different depending on the reference site. There are differences in translation at the facet site that are not readily appreciated when simply considering motion at the vertebral body centers. Translation at the facet was reduced 25 to 40% by the instrumentation systems compared with 10 to 18% when the relative motion between the vertebral body centers was considered. In general, there are greater translations at the facet than at the body center because the axis of rotation of the vertebral bodies is closer to the body center than the facet. More importantly, these motions reflect the translation of the facet joint to be fused. At the facet, the CD system appears somewhat better in inhibiting motion when compared with the Harrington and Luque systems.

Similar to the stiffness results, the one-rod CD construct proved comparable with the two rod Harrington and Luque systems in intervertebral fixation at T7/T8 and T10/T11. This again suggests the possibility of streamlining the CD design. Such data, if borne out in additional testing, raise fundamental questions regarding the significance of the added implants that are present when one uses traditional, two-rod constructs with cross-linking. At the clinical extreme, one might achieve the same fusion rate with a single rod as with a double rod while at the same time minimizing hooks and increasing the surface area available for fusion. These data are germane, however, only to the restriction of intervertebral micromotion and the respective stiffness of the constructs. The questions of yield strength, fatigue life, and loosening of a single-rod construct have to be considered in further studies.

V. SUMMARY

This approach to evaluating the stability provided by spinal constructs employs instrumented human cadaver spines which are moved through physiological ranges of motion under displacement control. Loading and intervertebral motion are measured concurrently. Systematically analyzing a variety of instrumentation systems and the contribution of individual components to the overall stability of the construct provides a means of characterizing and optimizing instrumentation design. Although the example given compared posterior scoliosis instrumentation systems, the same biomechanical testing and analysis methods are also readily adapted to anterior instrumentation, spinal fracture models, and spinal fracture instrumentation configurations.

REFERENCES

1. Gurr, K., McAfee, P., and Shih, C., Biomechanical analysis of posterior instrumentation systems after decompressive laminectomy: an unstable calf-spine model, *J. Bone Joint Surg.*, 70A, 680, 1988.
2. Jacobs, R., Nordwall, A., and Nachemson, A., Reduction, stability, and strength provided by internal fixation systems for thoracolumbar spinal injuries, *Clin. Orthop.*, 171, 300, 1982.
3. Wenger, D., Carollo, J., Wilkerson, J., and Herring, J., Laboratory testing of segmental spinal instrumentation vs. traditional Harrington instrumentation for scoliosis treatment, *Spine*, 7, 265, 1982.
4. Krag, M., Beynnon, B., Pope, M., and DeCoster, T., Depth of insertion of transpedicular vertebral screws into human vertebrae: effect upon screw–vertebra interface strength, *J. Spinal Disord.*, 1, 287, 1989.
5. Freedman, L., Houghton, G., and Evans, M., Cadaveric study comparing the stability of upper distraction hooks used in Harrington instrumentation, *Spine*, 11, 579, 1986.
6. Sutterlin, C., McAfee, P., Warden, K., et al., A biomechanical evaluation of cervical spinal stabilization methods in a bovine model: static and cyclic loading, *Spine*, 13, 795, 1988.

7. Ashman, R., Birch, J., Bone, L., et al., Mechanical testing of spinal instrumentation, *Clin. Orthop.*, 227, 113, 1988.

8. Gaines, R., Carson, W., Satterlee, C., and Groh, G., Experimental evaluation of seven different spinal fracture internal fixation devices using nonfailure stability testing: the load sharing and unstable mechanism concepts, *Spine,* 16, 903, 1991.

9. Ashman, R., Bechtold, J., Edwards, W., et al., *In vitro* spinal arthrodesis implant mechanical testing protocols, *J. Spinal Disord.*, 2, 274, 1989.

10. Smith, T., In *vitro* spinal biomechanics: experimental methods and apparatus, *Spine*, 16, 1204, 1991.

11. Wilke, H.J., Wenger, K. and Klaes, L., Testing criteria for spinal implants: recommendations for the standardization of *in vitro* stability testing of spinal implants, *Eur. Spine J.*, 7, 148, 1998.

12. Panjabi, M., Biomechanical evaluation of spinal fixation devices: I. A conceptual framework, *Spine*, 10, 1129, 1988.

13. Adams, M.A., Mechanical testing of the spine — An appraisal of methodology, results and conclusion, *Spine*, 20, 2151, 1995.

14. Kostuik, J. and Smith, T., Pitfalls of biomechanical testing, *Spine*, 16, 1233, 1991.

15. Panjabi, M.M., Krag, M.H., and Goel, V.K., A technique for measurement and description of three-dimensional six degree of freedom motion of a body joint with an application to the spine, *J. Biomech.*, 14, 447, 1981.

16. Wilke, H.J., Claes, L., Schmitt, H., and Wolf, S., A universal spine tester for *in vitro* experiments with muscle force simulation, *Eur. Spine J.*, 3, 91, 1994.

17. Dean, J.C., Wilcox, C.H., Daniels, A.U., et al., A new method for assessing relative dynamic motion of vertebral bodies during cyclic loading *in vitro*, *J. Biomech.*, 24, 1189, 1991.

18. Goel, V., Nye, T., Clark, C., et al., A technique to evalute an internal spinal device by use of the Selspot system: an application to Luque closed loop, *Spine*, 12, 150, 1987.

19. Fioretti, S., Germani, A., and Tommaso, L., Sterometry in very close-range sterophotogrammetry with non-metric cameras for human movement analysis, *J. Biomech.*, 18, 831, 1985.

20. van Wagoner, E., Method and Apparatus for Sensing and Measuring Relative Position and Motion between Two Points, *U.S. Patent* 5150169, 1992.

21. Goel, V.K., Clark, C.R., Harris, K.G., and Schulte, B.S., Kinematics of the cervical spine: effects of multiple total laminectomy and facet wiring, *J. Orthop. Res.*, 6, 611, 1988.

22. Panjabi, M.M., Brand, R.A., and White, A.A., Mechanical properties of the human thoracic spine as shown by three-dimensional load displacement curves, *J. Bone Joint Surg.*, 58A, 642, 1976.

23. Goel, V.K., Wilder, D.G., Pope, M.H., and Edwards, W., Biomechanical testing of the spine: load-controlled vs. displacement-controlled analysis, *Spine*, 20, 2354, 1995.

24. James, K.S., Scoliosis Construct and Burst Fracture Stability: *In Vitro* and Clinical Results Suggesting More Conservative Treatment Strategies for Scoliosis and Burst Fractures, Ph.D. thesis, University of Utah, Salt Lake City, 1995.

25. White, A.A. and Panjabi, M.M., The basic kinematics of the human spine. A review of past and current knowledge, *Spine*, 3, 12, 1978.

26. Pearcy, M.J., Stereo radiography of lumbar spine motion, *Acta Orthop. Scand.*, 56 (Suppl. 212), 7, 1985.

27. Fabry, G., Backpain after Harrington rod instrumentation for idiopathic scoliosis, *Spine*, 14, 620, 1989.

28. Hayes, M.A., Tompkins, S.F., Herndon, W.A., et al., Clinical and radiological evaluation of lumbo-sacral motion below fusion levels in idiopathic scoliosis, *Spine*, 13, 1161, 1988.

29. Smeathers, J.E. and Joanes, D.N., Dynamic compressive properties of human lumbar intervertebral joints: a comparison between fresh and thawed specimens, *J. Biomech.*, 21, 425, 1988.

30. Goodwin, R.R., James, K.S., Daniels, A.U., Stans, A.A., and Dunn, H.K., A new approach in analysis of intervertebral micromotion: multiple reference point evaluation of spinal instrumentation. *Trans. 39th Annual Meeting of the Orthopedic Research Society*, San Francisco, CA, February 15–18, 1993.

Appendix 1
Unit Conversions

TABLE A1.1 Force

	lb	gm	kg	N	dyne
1 lb	1	453.6	0.4536	4.448	4.448×10^5
1 gm	2.205×10^{-3}	1	10^{-3}	9.807×10^{-3}	980.7
1 kg	2.205	10^3	1	9.087	9.807×10^5
1 N	0.2248	1.020×10^2	0.1020	1	10^5
1 dyne	2.248×10^{-6}	1.020×10^{-3}	1.020×10^{-6}	10^{-5}	1

TABLE A1.2 Stress

	psi	gm/mm²	dyne/cm²	kg/cm²	Pa	MPa
1 psi	1	0.703	6.895×10^4	7.031×10^{-2}	6.895×10^3	6.895×10^{-3}
1 gm/mm²	1.422	1	9.807×10^4	0.1	9.807×10^3	9.807×10^{-3}
1 dyne/cm²	1.450×10^{-5}	1.020×10^{-5}	1	1.020×10^{-6}	0.1	10^{-5}
1 kg/cm²	14.226	10	9.807×10^5	1	9.807×10^4	9.807×10^{-2}
1 Pa 1 N/m²	1.450×10^{-4}	1.020×10^{-4}	10	1.020×10^{-5}	1	10^{-6}
1 MPa 1 MN/m² 1 N/mm²	145.05	1.020×10^2	10^7	10.20	10^6	1

TABLE A1.3 Length

	mm	cm	m	in.	ft
1 mm	1	10^{-1}	10^{-3}	3.937×10^{-2}	3.281×10^{-3}
1 cm	10	1	10^{-2}	0.397	3.281×10^{-2}
1 m	10^3	10^2	1	39.37	3.281
1 in.	25.40	2.540	2.540×10^{-2}	1	8.333×10^{-2}
1 ft	3.048×10^2	30.48	0.3048	12	1

TABLE A1.4 Area

	mm²	m²	in.²	ft²
1 mm²	1	10^{-6}	1.550×10^{-3}	1.076×10^{-5}
1 m²	10^6	1	1550	10.76
1 in.²	6.452×10^2	6.452×10^{-4}	1	6.944×10^{-3}
1 ft²	9.29×10^4	9.290×10^{-2}	144	1

Appendix 2
Useful Journals and Books
on Bone Mechanics

USEFUL JOURNALS

Acta Orthopaedica Scandinaviaca (12 issues, Scandinavian University Press)
Biomaterials (24 issues, Elsevier Science)
Bone (12 issues, Elsevier Science)
Calcified Tissue International (12 issues, Springer-Verlag, New York)
Clinical Biomechanics (10 issues, Elsevier Science)
Clinical Orthopaedics and Related Research (12 issues, Lippincott Williams & Wilkins)
Journal of Applied Biomechanics (4 issues, Human Kinetics)
Journal of Applied Physiology (12 issues, American Physiological Society)
Journal of Arthroplasty (6 issues, Churchill Livingstone)
Journal of Biomechanics (12 issues, Elsevier Science)
Journal of Biomechanical Engineering (4 issues, American Society of Mechanical Engineers)
Journal of Biomedical Materials Research (16 issues, John Wiley & Sons)
Journal of Biomedical Materials Research (Applied Biomaterials) (4 issues, John Wiley & Sons)
Journal of Bone and Joint Surgery (Am) (12 issues, Journal of Bone and Joint Surgery, Inc.)
Journal of Bone and Joint Surgery (Br) (6 issues, British Editorial Society of Bone and Joint Surgery)
Journal of Engineering in Medicine Part H (4 issues, Mechanical Engineering Publications Ltd.)
Journal of Materials Science — Materials in Medicine (4 issues, Chapman & Hall, CRC Press)
Journal of Orthopaedic Research (6 issues, Journal of Bone and Joint Surgery, Inc.)
Medical & Biological Engineering & Computing (6 issues, Peter Peregrinus Ltd.)
Medical Engineering & Physics (10 issues, Elsevier Science)

SELECTED BOOKS ON BONE BIOMECHANICS

Lucas, G.L., Cooke, F.W., and Friis, E.A., *A Primer of Biomechanics*. Springer-Verlag, New York, 1999
Cowin, S.C., *Bone Mechanics*. CRC Press, Boca Raton, 1st edition 1989, 2nd edition 2000
Bruce, M.R. and Burr, D.B., *Skeletal Tissue Mechanics*. Springer-Verlag, New York, 1998, 392 pages
Evans, F.G., *Mechanical Properties of Bone,* Charles C Thomas, Springfield, IL, 1973

Index

A

A. Ascenzi method torsion test, 283–284
Absorptiometry
 property evaluation methods, 109, 111
 techniques for measuring density, 46
Accuracy in testing, 193, 194–196
Acetabular component stability
 factors affecting *in vitro* testing
  bony ingrowth, 528
  implantation technique, 529
  modulus of elasticity differences, 528
  sample geometry, 529
  testing orientation, 529
  torque forces involved, 529
  true motion measurements, 528
  variables in test samples, 528–529
  in vivo stabilization with screws, 527
 testing methods
  adduction, 10 axial load, 534–535
  adduction, 12 axial load, 533
  adduction, 30 axial load, 532–533
  axial load from anatomical positions, 535–536
  axial loading from repetitive cycles, 536
  offset cup loading, 531–532
  pullout force, 537
  strain distribution using FEA, 537
  torsional stability, 530–531
Acoustic impedance, 371–372, 373–375
Activity levels and mechanical properties of bone, 74
Adhesives for strain gauges, 314–316
Age
 bone fragilities from, 143
 bone–implant strength and, 453–454
 bone mechanical properties and, 66–68
 bone structure and, 8, 9
Alcohol consumption and bone health, 76
Alpha-hydroxy acids in bioabsorbable polymer technology, 582
Alternate lamellae, 15, 48–49, 273
American Society for Testing and Materials (ASTM) testing designations, 177
Anelasticity, 333
Animal models in testing, 198–199
Architectural level of bone, 137–138
Areal moment of inertia for bone, 29–30, 211
Arthritis affect on bone mechanical properties, 75–76
Articular cartilage, 7
ASTM (American Society for Testing and Materials) testing designations, 177
Autoclaving, 77
Axial cantilever test of bone–implant interface, 569, 573–574

B

Backing material for strain gauges, 310
Bar wave velocity, 357
Bending tests of bone
 cantilever beam
  cancellous bone, 216
  cortical bone, 216
  single trabeculae, 296–300
  viscoelastic properties, 343–344
  whole bone, 214–216
 description of loads, 207–209
 four-point bending
  cancellous bone, 214
  cortical bone, 214
  whole bone, 161, 213–214
 loading modes, 30–31
 single osteons methods, 281–282
 three-point bending
  cancellous bone, 212
  cortical bone, 212
  whole bone, 209–212
Berkovich diamond indenter, 259–260, 263, 264
Biaxial servohydraulic testing systems, 224, 225
Bioabsorbable polymer technology fatigue testing
 materials used, 582–583
 screw fixation model, 584–585
 with synthetic bone interface, 586–589
 testing procedures, 585–586
 in vitro strength-loss profile, 583–584
 in vivo degradation process, 582
Biophosphonates and bone, 76, 451
BMC (bone mineral content)
 absorptiometric techniques for measuring, 46, 111
 defined, 45, 107
BMD (bone mineral density)
 absorptiometric techniques for measuring, 46, 111
 defined, 44–45, 107
 pQCT used to measure, 388–390, 393–395
Boiling/autoclaving, 77
Bone composition and structure
 mechanical properties affected by, 68–72
 mineral substance, 5–6
 organic matrix, 4–5
 osteons
  lamellae, 13–15
  microradiographic density, 13
  remodeling, 13
  structure, 11–13
 trabeculae, 15–16
 types of bone
  cancellous, 10
  compact, 9